Orthopaedic Knowledge Update®

OKU® 7

Foot and Ankle

Orthopaedic Knowledge Update®

OKU® 7

Foot and Ankle

EDITOR

Loretta B. Chou, MD, FAAOS
Professor and Chief of Foot and Ankle Surgery
Department of Orthopaedic Surgery
Stanford University
Stanford, California

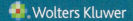

AAOS
AMERICAN ACADEMY OF
ORTHOPAEDIC SURGEONS

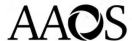

Board of Directors, 2023-2024

Kevin J. Bozic, MD, MBA, FAAOS
President

Paul Tornetta III, MD, PhD, FAAOS
First Vice President

Annunziato Amendola, MD, FAAOS
Second Vice President

Michael L. Parks, MD, FAAOS
Treasurer

Felix H. Savoie III, MD, FAAOS
Past President

Alfonso Mejia, MD, MPH, FAAOS
Chair, Board of Councilors

Joel L. Mayerson, MD, FAAOS
Chair-Elect, Board of Councilors

Michael J. Leddy III, MD, FAAOS
Secretary, Board of Councilors

Armando F. Vidal, MD, FAAOS
Chair, Board of Specialty Societies

Adolph J. Yates, Jr, MD, FAAOS
Chair-Elect, Board of Specialty Societies

Michael P. Bolognesi, MD, FAAOS
Secretary, Board of Specialty Societies

Lisa N. Masters
Lay Member

Evalina L. Burger, MD, FAAOS
Member at Large

Chad A. Krueger, MD, FAAOS
Member at Large

Toni M. McLaurin, MD, FAAOS
Member at Large

Monica M. Payares, MD, FAAOS
Member at Large

Thomas E. Arend, Jr, Esq, CAE
Chief Executive Officer (ex-officio)

Staff
American Academy of Orthopaedic Surgeons

Anna Salt Troise, MBA, *Chief Commercial Officer*

Hans Koelsch, PhD, *Director, Publishing*

Lisa Claxton Moore, *Senior Manager, Editorial*

Steven Kellert, *Senior Editor*

Wolters Kluwer Health

Brian Brown, *Director, Medical Practice*

Tulie McKay, *Senior Content Editor, Acquisitions*

Stacey Sebring, *Senior Development Editor*

Sean Hanrahan, *Lead Editorial Coordinator*

Marisa Solorzano-Taylor, *Editorial Coordinator*

Kristen Watrud, *Product Marketing Manager*

Catherine Ott, *Production Project Manager*

Stephen Druding, *Manager, Graphic Arts & Design*

Margie Orzech-Zeranko, *Manufacturing Coordinator*

TNQ Technologies, *Prepress Vendor*

The material presented in the *Orthopaedic Knowledge Update®: Foot and Ankle 7* has been made available by the American Academy of Orthopaedic Surgeons (AAOS) for educational purposes only. This material is not intended to present the only, or necessarily best, methods or procedures for the medical situations discussed, but rather it is intended to represent an approach, view, statement, or opinion of the author(s) or producer(s), which may be helpful to others who face similar situations. Medical providers should use their own, independent medical judgment, in addition to open discussion with patients, when developing patient care recommendations and treatment plans. Medical care should always be based on a medical provider's expertise that is individually tailored to a patient's circumstances, preferences and rights.

Some drugs or medical devices demonstrated in AAOS courses or described in AAOS print or electronic publications have not been cleared by the US Food and Drug Administration (FDA) or have been cleared for specific uses only. The FDA has stated that it is the responsibility of the physician to determine the FDA clearance status of each drug or device he or she wishes to use in clinical practice and to use the products with appropriate patient consent and in compliance with applicable law.

Furthermore, any statements about commercial products are solely the opinion(s) of the author(s) and do not represent an AAOS endorsement or evaluation of these products. These statements may not be used in advertising or for any commercial purpose.

All rights reserved. No part of this publication may be reproduced, stored in a retrieval system, or transmitted, in any form, or by any means, electronic, mechanical, photocopying, recording, or otherwise, without prior written permission from the publisher.

ISBN: 978-1-9752-1343-5

Library of Congress Control Number: Cataloging in Publication data available on request from publisher.

Printed in the United States of America

Published 2025 by the American Academy of Orthopaedic Surgeons
9400 West Higgins Road
Rosemont, Illinois 60018

Copyright 2025 by the American Academy of Orthopaedic Surgeons

Acknowledgments

Editorial Board, Orthopaedic Knowledge Update®: Foot and Ankle 7

Editor

Loretta B. Chou, MD, FAAOS
Professor and Chief of Foot and Ankle Surgery
Department of Orthopaedic Surgery
Stanford University
Stanford, California

Section Editors

Gregory C. Berlet, MD, FRCS(C), FAAOS, FAOA
Attending Surgeon
Department of Orthopaedics
Orthopaedic Surgery Specialist
Orthopaedic Foot and Ankle Center
Worthington, Ohio

Rebecca A. Cerrato, MD, FAAOS
Chairman, Orthopedic Surgeon
Mercy Medical Center
Institute of Foot and Ankle Reconstruction
Baltimore, Maryland

Christopher P. Chiodo, MD, FAAOS
Chairman, Department of Orthopedic Surgery
Brigham and Women's Hospital
Harvard Medical School
Boston, Massachusetts

Andrew Haskell, MD, FAAOS
Department of Molecular and Cellular Medicine
Institute for Regenerative Medicine
Texas A&M Health Science Center
Bryan, Texas

MaCalus Vinson Hogan, MD, MBA, FAAOS
Chief, Department of Orthopedic Surgery
University of Pittsburgh Medical Center
Pittsburgh, Pennsylvania

Kenneth J. Hunt, MD, FAAOS
Associate Professor
Department of Orthopaedics
University of Colorado School of Medicine
Aurora, Colorado

Sheldon S. Lin, MD, FAAOS
Associate Professor
Department of Orthopaedics
Rutgers New Jersey Medical School
Newark, New Jersey

Elizabeth A. Martin, MD, MSc, FAAOS
Attending Orthopaedic Surgeon
Department of Orthopedic Surgery
Brigham and Women's Hospital
Harvard Medical School
Boston, Massachusetts

Ariel A. Palanca, MD, FAAOS
Assistant Professor
Department of Orthopaedic Surgery
Orthopedic Surgeon
Palomar Health Medical Center
Redwood City, California

Robert D. Santrock, MD, FAAOS
Physician, Department of Foot and Ankle
Orthopaedic Foot and Ankle Center
Worthington, Ohio

Contributors

Samuel B. Adams, MD, FAAOS, FAOA
Associate Residency Program Director
Director of Foot and Ankle Research
Associate Professor
Department of Orthopaedic Surgery
Foot and Ankle Orthopaedic Surgeon
Duke University Medical Center
Morrisville, North Carolina

Amiethab Aiyer, MD, FAAOS, FAOA
Associate Professor
Department of Orthopaedics
Division Chief of Foot and Ankle Surgery
Johns Hopkins University School of Medicine
Baltimore, Maryland

Lara C. Atwater, MD, FAAOS
Assistant Professor
Department of Orthopaedic Surgery
and Rehabilitation
Orthopedist
Oregon Health and Science University
Portland, Oregon

Joseph Benevenia, MD, FAAOS
Chair, Department of Orthopaedics
Orthopaedic Surgeon
Rutgers New Jersey Medical School
Newark, New Jersey

Gregory C. Berlet, MD, FRCS(C), FAAOS, FAOA
Attending Surgeon
Department of Orthopaedics
Orthopaedic Surgery Specialist
Orthopaedic Foot and Ankle Center
Worthington, Ohio

Matthew M. Buchanan, MD, FAAOS
Orthopaedic Foot and Ankle Surgeon
Nirschl Orthopaedic Center
Arlington, Virginia

Bopha Chrea, MD
Assistant Professor
Department of Orthopaedics
and Rehabilitation
Orthopedist
Oregon Health and Science University
Portland, Oregon

David J. Ciufo, MD
Assistant Professor
Department of Orthopaedics
Orthopaedic Surgeon
University of Rochester
Rochester, New York

Justin Daigre, MD, FAAOS
Foot and Ankle Specialist
Department of Orthopaedic Surgery
Decatur Orthopaedic Clinic
Decatur, Alabama

David J. Dalstrom, MD, FAAOS
Associate Professor
Chief, Division of Foot and Ankle Surgery
Department of Orthopaedics
Orthopedic Surgeon
University of California San Diego
La Jolla, California

Richard J. de Asla, MD, FAAOS
Orthopedic Surgeon
Department of Orthopaedic Surgery
Division of Foot and Ankle Surgery
Naples Community Hospital
Naples, Florida

Malcolm R. DeBaun, MD
Assistant Professor
Department of Orthopaedic Trauma Surgery
Duke University School of Medicine
Durham, North Carolina

Benedict F. DiGiovanni, MD, FAAOS, FAOA
Professor of Orthopaedics
Department of Orthopaedics and Rehabilitation
Orthopaedic Surgeon
University of Rochester
Rochester, New York

Jesse F. Doty, MD, FAAOS
Director of Foot and Ankle Surgery
Department of Orthopaedic Surgery
Erlanger Health System
Chattanooga, Tennessee

Eric I. Ferkel, MD, FAAOS
Attending Orthopaedic Surgeon
Department of Orthopedic Surgery
Foot and Ankle Surgeon
Southern California Orthopedic Institute
Los Angeles, California

Contributors

A. Samuel Flemister Jr, MD, FAAOS
Professor, Department of Orthopaedics and Rehabilitation
Orthopedic Surgery Specialist
University of Rochester School of Medicine and Dentistry
Rochester, New York

Ian M. Foran, MD
Assistant Professor
Department of Orthopaedics
Orthopedic Surgeon
University of California San Diego
La Jolla, California

Daniel J. Fuchs, MD, FAAOS
Assistant Professor
Department of Orthopaedic Surgery
Foot and Ankle Orthopaedic Surgeon
Rothman Institute at Thomas Jefferson University
Philadelphia, Pennsylvania

Daniel J. Garcia, BS
Rutgers New Jersey Medical School
Newark, New Jersey

Michael J. Gardner, MD, FAAOS
Professor
Department of Orthopaedic Surgery
Stanford University School of Medicine
Redwood City, California

Lauren E. Geaney, MD, FAAOS
Assistant Professor, Program Director
Department of Orthopaedics
Orthopaedic Surgeon
University of Connecticut
Farmington, Connecticut

Christopher E. Gross, MD, FAAOS
Associate Professor
Director, Foot and Ankle Division
Deparment of Orthopaedics
Medical University of South Carolina
Charleston, South Carolina

Ajay N. Gurbani, MD
Assistant Professor
Department of Orthopaedic Surgery
Orthopedic Foot and Ankle Surgery Specialist
University of California, Los Angeles
Santa Monica, California

Steven L. Haddad, MD, FAAOS
Professor, Chief Clinical Officer
Department of Orthopaedic Surgery
Foot and Ankle Orthopaedic Surgeon
University of Chicago Pritzker School of Medicine
Chicago, Illinois
Extremity Medical
Parsippany, New Jersey

Nigel Hsu, MD, FAAOS
Assistant Professor
Department of Orthopaedics
Foot and Ankle Orthopaedic Surgeon
Johns Hopkins University School of Medicine
Baltimore, Maryland

Yazan Kadkoy, MS
Rutgers New Jersey Medical School
Newark, New Jersey

Meghan Kelly, MD, PhD
Assistant Professor of Foot and Ankle Surgery
Department of Orthopaedics
Mount Sinai Icahn School of Medicine
New York, New York

Trapper Lalli, MD, FAAOS
Assistant Professor
Department of Orthopaedics
University of North Carolina at Chapel Hill
Chapel Hill, North Carolina

Brian C. Lau, MD
Assistant Professor
Division of Sports Medicine
Department of Orthopaedic Surgery
Duke University School of Medicine
Durham, North Carolina

Frederick R. Lemley, MD, FAAOS
Orthopedic Foot and Ankle Surgeon
Syracuse Orthopedic Specialists
Syracuse, New York

Kshitij Manchanda, MD
Assistant Professor
Department of Orthopaedic Surgery
UT Southwestern Medical Center
Frisco, Texas

Sara Lyn Miniaci-Coxhead, MD, MEd, FAAOS
Assistant Professor
Department of Orthopaedics
Orthopaedic Surgeon
Cleveland Clinic Foundation
Cleveland, Ohio

Daniel K. Moon, MD, MS, MBA, FAAOS
Assistant Professor
Department of Orthopedic Surgery
University of Colorado School of Medicine
Aurora, Colorado

Robert F. Murphy, MD, FAAOS
Associate Professor
Department of Orthopaedics and Physical Medicine
Pediatric Orthopaedic Surgeon
Medical University of South Carolina
North Charleston, South Carolina

David E. Oji, MD, FAAOS
Clinical Assistant Professor
Foot and Ankle Surgery, Orthopedic Sports Medicine
Department of Orthopaedic Surgery
Stanford University School of Medicine
Los Gatos, California

Joseph T. O'Neil, MD
Assistant Professor of Orthopaedic Surgery
Division of Foot and Ankle Surgery
Orthopaedic Surgeon
Sidney Kimmel Medical College at Thomas Jefferson
  University
Rothman Orthopaedic Institute
Philadelphia, Pennsylvania

Ariel A. Palanca, MD, FAAOS
Assistant Professor
Department of Orthopaedic Surgery
Orthopaedic Surgeon
Palomar Health Medical Center
Redwood City, California

Chirag S. Patel, MD, FAAOS
Orthopedic Surgeon
Department of Orthopedics
OrthoCollier
Naples, Florida

Megan C. Paulus, MD, FAAOS
Assistant Clinical Professor
Department of Orthopaedic Surgery
Stony Brook University Hospital
Stony Brook Orthopaedics Associates
Stony Brook, New York

David I. Pedowitz, MD, MS, FAAOS
Professor of Orthopaedics
Department of Orthopaedic Surgery
Chief, Division of Foot and Ankle Surgery
Director, Foot and Ankle Fellowship
Sidney Kimmel Medical College
Thomas Jefferson University
Rothman Orthopaedic Institute
Philadelphia, Pennsylvania

Michael S. Pinzur, MD, FAAOS
Professor of Orthopaedic Surgery and Rehabilitation
Department of Orthopaedic Surgery
Loyola University Health System
Maywood, Illinois

Steven M. Raikin, MD, FAAOS
Professor, Department of Orthopaedic Surgery
Director of Foot and Ankle Services
Orthopaedic Surgeon
Rothman Institute and Thomas Jefferson University
Philadelphia, Pennsylvania

Christopher L. Ruland, MD, MS
Resident Physician
Department of Orthopedic Surgery
Orthopedic Sports Medicine
Stony Brook University Hospital
Stony Brook, New York

Robert D. Santrock, MD, FAAOS
Physician, Department of Foot and Ankle
Orthopaedic Foot and Ankle Center
Worthington, Ohio

Adam P. Schiff, MD, FAAOS
Assistant Professor
Department of Orthopaedic Surgery
Orthopaedist
Loyola University Medical Center
Maywood, Illinois

W. Bret Smith, DO, FAAOS
Clinical Assistant Professor
Department of Orthopedic Surgery
Orthopedic Surgery Specialist
University of South Carolina School of Medicine
Columbia, South Carolina

Niall Smyth, MD
Orthopedist, Department of Orthopaedics
Cleveland Clinic Weston
Weston, Florida

Preface

Orthopaedic Knowledge Update®: Foot and Ankle continues to be an excellent resource for the prevailing body of literature. OKU® is renowned to offer reviews and summaries of the most relevant and critical studies for the reader. Recent information can be easily accessed, and the annotated references allow for perusal. *OKU® Foot and Ankle 7* will be helpful to residents, fellows, and practicing orthopaedic surgeons.

This seventh volume contains 29 chapters contributed by more than 40 authors, all of whom are leaders in foot and ankle surgery. Like prior volumes, the chapters focus on significant discoveries, materials, methods, and studies that are new since the sixth volume was published in 2019. We are excited to include a new section titled Contemporary Surgical Techniques. This section includes chapters on surgical management of Charcot neuroarthropathy, minimally invasive surgery of the foot and ankle, and revision total ankle arthroplasty. All chapters have been updated to include the latest treatment guidelines, surgical techniques, and literature reviews, along with illustrations.

I thank the authors for completing the enormous task of reviewing and researching an immense amount of up-to-date literature. The authors have done a first-rate job of summing up these articles and adding to established knowledge. Also, I thank the section editors of *OKU® Foot and Ankle*. They are indeed leaders in the field. They, too, have expended a great deal of time and exercised their expertise to ensure the quality and comprehensiveness of the chapters. The result is chapters that are thorough and up to the rigors of OKU®.

It is a privilege to have edited the fifth and sixth volumes, and now the seventh volume, of *OKU® Foot and Ankle*. I am grateful to the American Academy of Orthopaedic Surgeons for their support and confidence in me to prepare this new volume. Special thanks to Lisa Claxton Moore, Senior Manager, Editorial, publishing team of AAOS. Her expertise and guidance were much needed and appreciated every step of the way. This acknowledgment includes Marisa Solorzano-Taylor, Editorial Coordinator, Health Learning, Research & Practice, and Stacey Sebring, Senior Development Editor, Medicine and Advanced Practice at Wolters Kluwer. I am indebted to their steady availability to answer many questions, as well as their know-how of OKU® production.

We hope this new volume of *Orthopaedic Knowledge Update®: Foot and Ankle* with up-to-date information on clinical, imaging, and surgical procedures aids the physician to evaluate, diagnose, and treat patients with disorders of the foot and ankle.

Loretta B. Chou, MD, FAAOS
Editor

Table of Contents

Section 1: General Foot and Ankle Topics

SECTION EDITOR:

Christopher P. Chiodo, MD, FAAOS

Chapter 1

Biomechanics of the Foot and Ankle . . .3

Richard J. de Asla, MD, FAAOS

Chapter 2

Shoes and Orthoses 13

Jesse F. Doty, MD, FAAOS

Chapter 3

Imaging Studies of the Foot
and Ankle 23

Daniel J. Fuchs, MD, FAAOS
Steven M. Raikin, MD, FAAOS

Chapter 4

Foot and Ankle Conditions in
Children and Adolescents. 37

Robert F. Murphy, MD, FAAOS

Section 2: Neuromuscular Disease

SECTION EDITOR:

Rebecca A. Cerrato, MD, FAAOS

Chapter 5

Cavovarus Deformity 51

Amiethab Aiyer, MD, FAAOS, FAOA
Nigel Hsu, MD, FAAOS
Niall Smyth, MD

Chapter 6

Diabetic Foot Disease 67

Bopha Chrea, MD
Lara C. Atwater, MD, FAAOS

Chapter 7

Peripheral Nerve Disorders 85

David E. Oji, MD, FAAOS

Section 3: Arthritis of the Foot and Ankle

SECTION EDITORS:

Robert D. Santrock, MD, FAAOS
Gregory C. Berlet, MD, FRCS(C), FAAOS, FAOA

Chapter 8

Ankle Arthritis: Part I. Joint
Preservation Techniques and
Arthrodesis. 109

Adam P. Schiff, MD, FAAOS
Samuel B. Adams, MD, FAAOS, FAOA

Chapter 9

Ankle Arthritis: Part II. Total Ankle
Arthroplasty. .133

Steven L. Haddad, MD, FAAOS
Justin Daigre, MD, FAAOS

Chapter 10

Midfoot and Hindfoot Arthrodesis . . .151

Kshitij Manchanda, MD
W. Bret Smith, DO, FAAOS
Trapper Lalli, MD, FAAOS

Chapter 11

Adult-Acquired Flatfoot Deformity . . .167

Matthew M. Buchanan, MD, FAAOS
Frederick R. Lemley, MD, FAAOS

Section 4: The Forefoot

SECTION EDITOR:

Elizabeth A. Martin, MD, MSc, FAAOS

Chapter 12

Disorders of the Hallux 185

Sara Lyn Miniaci-Coxhead, MD, MEd, FAAOS

Chapter 13

Lesser Toe Deformities and
Metatarsalgia 203

Lauren E. Geaney, MD, FAAOS

Section 5: Special Problems of the Foot and Ankle

SECTION EDITOR:

Sheldon S. Lin, MD, FAAOS

Chapter 14

Nondiabetic Foot Infections 225

Meghan Kelly, MD, PhD
A. Samuel Flemister Jr, MD, FAAOS

Chapter 15

Plantar Heel Pain 237

David J. Ciufo, MD
Benedict F. DiGiovanni, MD, FAAOS, FAOA

Chapter 16

Foot and Ankle Tumors 249

Yazan Kadkoy, MS
Daniel J. Garcia, BS
Joseph Benevenia, MD, FAAOS

Chapter 17

Osteonecrosis of the Talus 267

Daniel K. Moon, MD, MS, MBA, FAAOS

Section 6: Foot and Ankle Trauma

SECTION EDITOR:

Andrew Haskell, MD, FAAOS

Chapter 18

Ankle and Pilon Fractures 283

Brian C. Lau, MD
Malcolm R. DeBaun, MD
Michael J. Gardner, MD, FAAOS

Chapter 19

Talar Fractures 299

Samuel B. Adams, MD, FAAOS, FAOA

Chapter 20

Calcaneal Fractures 311

Jesse F. Doty, MD, FAAOS

Chapter 21

Midfoot and Forefoot Trauma 327

Joseph T. O'Neil, MD
David I. Pedowitz, MD, MS, FAAOS

Chapter 22

Amputations of the Foot and Ankle . . . 351

Michael S. Pinzur, MD, FAAOS

Section 7: Tendon Disorders and Sports-Related Foot and Ankle Injuries

SECTION EDITORS:

MaCalus Vinson Hogan, MD, MBA, FAAOS
Kenneth J. Hunt, MD, FAAOS

Chapter 23

Disorders of the Achilles Tendon 361

Ajay N. Gurbani, MD

Chapter 24
Sports-Related Injuries of the
Foot and Ankle....................371
Christopher E. Gross, MD, FAAOS

Chapter 25
Ankle Ligament Injuries 385
Chirag S. Patel, MD, FAAOS

Chapter 26
Arthroscopy of the Foot and Ankle and
Osteochondral Lesions of the Talus... 403
Eric I. Ferkel, MD, FAAOS
Christopher L. Ruland, MD, MS

Section 8: Contemporary Surgical Techniques

SECTION EDITOR:
Ariel A. Palanca, MD, FAAOS

Chapter 27
Surgical Management of Charcot
Neuroarthropathy................ 429
Ian M. Foran, MD
David J. Dalstrom, MD, FAAOS

Chapter 28
Minimally Invasive Surgery of the
Foot and Ankle.................... 439
Ariel A. Palanca, MD, FAAOS
Megan C. Paulus, MD, FAAOS

Chapter 29
Revision Total Ankle Arthroplasty... 449
Gregory C. Berlet, MD, FRCS(C), FAAOS, FAOA
Robert D. Santrock, MD, FAAOS

Index 461

SECTION 1

General Foot and Ankle Topics

Section Editor:

Christopher P. Chiodo, MD, FAAOS

CHAPTER 1

Biomechanics of the Foot and Ankle

RICHARD J. DE ASLA, MD, FAAOS

ABSTRACT

Understanding biomechanics and functional anatomy of the foot and ankle is mandatory if there is to be any meaningful attempt at formulating new ways of addressing pathoanatomy. It is important to provide an introduction to foot and ankle biomechanics and functional anatomy as a basis for managing disorders.

Keywords: ankle anatomy; ankle biomechanics; foot anatomy; foot biomechanics; gait cycle

INTRODUCTION

The foot is a marvelous mechanical structure. Its unique anatomy and biomechanics allow it to play several seemingly conflicting roles. During push-off, it is a rigid lever arm for efficient propulsion. In stance, it is a stable platform for balance. It is also a part-time shock absorber that adeptly navigates uneven surfaces and terrain. The average person's foot is remarkably durable, logging more than 100 million steps during an average lifetime.

With continued advancements in imaging technology, such as weight-bearing CT, knowledge of foot and ankle biomechanics continues to steadily improve.[1-5] This improved understanding of how the foot works provides better insight into disorders of the foot and ankle, which are often biomechanically based.

A thorough understanding of the biomechanics and functional anatomy of the foot and ankle is mandatory

Dr. de Asla or an immediate family member serves as a paid consultant to or is an employee of Arthrex, Inc. and has stock or stock options held in Pfizer.

to ensure successful treatment of patients and the development and advancement of new procedures.

STRUCTURAL ANATOMY

The foot is divided into three regions: the forefoot, midfoot, and hindfoot. The tarsometatarsal joints (or Lisfranc joint complex) separate the forefoot from the midfoot, and the talonavicular and calcaneocuboid joints (transverse tarsal or Chopart joint) separate the midfoot from the hindfoot.

In the forefoot, the metatarsals are unique in that they are the only long bones in the body to support weight perpendicular to their long axis. In most feet, the first metatarsal is somewhat shorter than the second, with a progressive cascade of shortening from the second to the fifth metatarsal. This metatarsal break angle encourages the foot to supinate during push-off. In the sagittal plane, all metatarsals incline to some extent; the first metatarsal has the highest inclination angle (range, 15° to 25°), and the remaining metatarsals demonstrate decreasing inclination angles from medial to lateral. Alterations and subtleties in the length and position of the metatarsals affect loading patterns that may influence alignment and contribute to the development of painful callosities, metatarsalgia, and metatarsophalangeal joint pathology.

The first, fourth, and fifth metatarsals have mobility in the sagittal plane, whereas the second and third metatarsals have relatively fixed positions. The lesser metatarsal bases are connected by a series of plantar metatarsal ligaments. No such connection exists between the base of the first and second metatarsals. The absence of an intermetatarsal ligament provides the first metatarsal a degree of mobility in the transverse plane not afforded to the lesser metatarsals. This anatomic feature may play a role in the development of hallux valgus deformities.

The forefoot is connected to the midfoot through the Lisfranc joint complex. Here, the cross-sectional wedge-shaped cuneiforms and metatarsal bases form a transverse arch across the midfoot, enhancing stability in the coronal plane (**Figure 1**). In addition, the base of the second metatarsal is recessed proximally between the medial and lateral cuneiforms, providing stability in the horizontal plane. Stability is further enhanced by a series of very strong plantar tarsometatarsal ligaments and a short, thick interosseous ligament that courses between the lateral aspect of the medial cuneiform and medial aspect of the second metatarsal base. This interosseous ligament is often referred to as the Lisfranc ligament. Disruption of the midfoot complex may result in an avulsion fracture off the base of the second metatarsal. The bony fragment, still attached to the Lisfranc ligament, can be seen between the bases of the first and second metatarsals on plain radiographs—the so-called fleck sign.

The midfoot contains the navicular, the cuboid, and three cuneiform bones. These five bones are relatively immobile with respect to one another and provide a mechanical link between the hindfoot and the more mobile forefoot. The midfoot allows for the safe passage of neurovascular structures and tendons as they course

from the leg to the foot. The disk-shaped navicular bone has a convex anterior surface and a concave posterior surface—both of which are covered with cartilage. Small vessels enter the navicular dorsally from the dorsalis pedis artery and medially from the posterior tibial artery. Blood supply to its central portion is relatively sparse, and certain foot types may accentuate shear across this portion of the bone.[6] The navicular is also the primary attachment site of the tibialis posterior tendon. These features may combine to make the navicular bone relatively susceptible to stress fracture and poor healing.

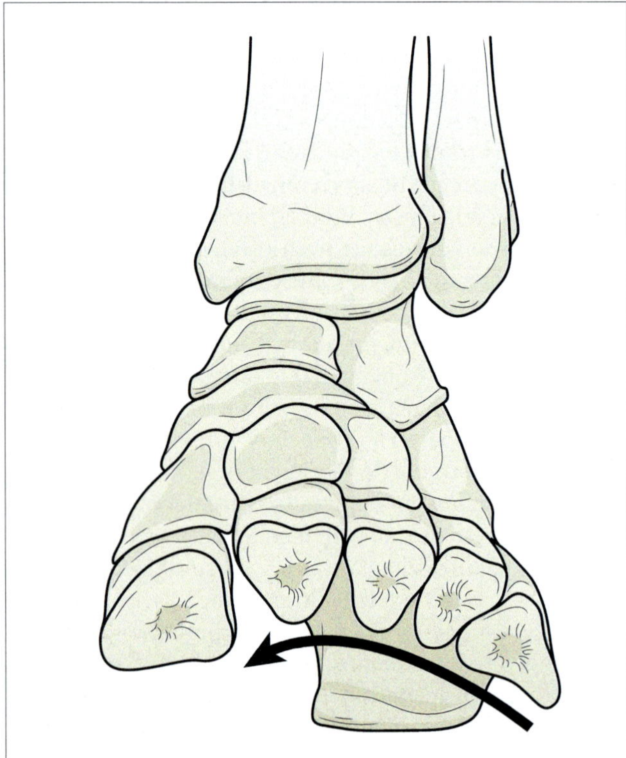

The midfoot is separated from the hindfoot by the talonavicular and calcaneal cuboid joints, known collectively as the transverse tarsal joint or Chopart joint. The talonavicular joint is a ball-and-socket–type joint. The socket that receives the talar head is deepened by the anterior and middle facets of the calcaneus, the calcaneonavicular slip of the bifurcate ligament, and the superomedial and inferior calcaneal navicular ligaments, which together comprise the spring ligament. The superomedial component of the spring ligament originates from the superomedial aspect of the sustentaculum tali and is confluent with the superficial deltoid ligament, forming a large medial ligament complex. The superomedial component of the spring ligament serves to suspend the head of the talus, functioning like an anatomic hammock. The portion in contact with the talar head is a region of fibrocartilage tissue providing a smooth surface on which to articulate. This acetabulum pedis allows for transverse, sagittal, and longitudinal planes of motion and plays a vital role in foot biomechanics (**Figure 2**). Any motion of the talonavicular joint or subtalar joint also involves motion at the calcaneocuboid joint. Maximum congruency of the calcaneocuboid joint is achieved when the hindfoot is in varus and the forefoot is supinated. This is the position the foot assumes with push-off.

The hindfoot consists of the calcaneus and the talus. Their articulation forms the subtalar joint as the talus sits sidesaddle over the superomedial aspect of the calcaneus. The subtalar joint consists of three separate articulations, or facets. More than 90% of all tarsal coalitions occur at either the anterior facet (calcaneonavicular coalition) or the middle facet (talocalcaneal coalition). For simplicity's sake, subtalar motion is often depicted as inversion and eversion around a mitered hinge. In reality, subtalar motion is quite complex, is difficult to measure, and includes rotational motions and translations in multiple planes. The subtalar joint is stabilized by the deltoid ligament, the interosseous and cervical ligaments, and a series of lateral ligaments and structures. These lateral stabilizers include the calcaneofibular ligament (CFL), the lateral talocalcaneal ligament, and the inferior extensor retinaculum. Because of its role as a subtalar joint stabilizer, the inferior extensor retinaculum is often used

Transverse arch

FIGURE 1 Illustration of the wedge-shaped bases of the second, third, and fourth metatarsals and the middle and lateral cuneiforms that create a keystone effect that stabilizes the arch in the coronal plane.

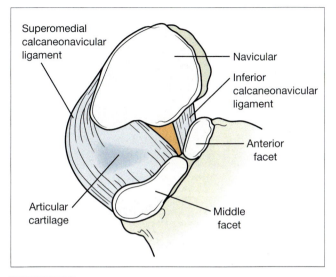

FIGURE 2 Illustration of the acetabulum pedis from a dorsal view with the head of the talus removed. (Redrawn with permission from de Asla RJ: Anatomy and biomechanics of the foot and ankle, in Thordarson DB, ed: *Orthopaedic Surgery Essentials: Foot and Ankle*, ed 2. Lippincott Williams & Wilkins, 2012.)

in Broström-type lateral ankle ligament reconstruction procedures[7-9] (**Figure 3**).

The body of the talus resides in a bony housing created by the articulation between the distal fibula and tibia. The mortise is formed by the tibial plafond and medial and lateral malleoli. Composed of the talus, distal tibia, and fibula, the ankle joint includes three articulations: tibiofibular, tibiotalar, and talofibular. The tibiofibular joint represents the inferior extent of the lower extremity syndesmosis. The syndesmosis is stabilized by four ligaments: the anterior inferior tibiofibular ligament, the posterior inferior tibiofibular ligament, the transverse tibiofibular ligament, and the interosseous tibiofibular ligament. Occasionally, a thickened accessory slip of the anterior inferior tibiofibular ligament (Bassett ligament) may insert too distally on the fibula, causing symptoms as it impinges against the anterolateral aspect of the talar dome. The transverse tibiofibular ligament originates on the posterior aspect of the fibula and extends to the posterior margin of the medial malleolus. In between, it forms the posterior labrum, which effectively deepens the tibiotalar joint. The syndesmosis allows fibula rotation and proximal migration when the wider anterior aspect of the talar body rotates into the ankle mortise during dorsiflexion. This relationship also allows the fibula to share approximately 16% of the axial load transmitted across the ankle.[10-12]

The ankle is stabilized by the inherent bony configuration of the mortise,[13] as well as the medial and lateral ligament complexes. In one study, the articular surface of the talus was compared with a truncated cone in which the medial aspect is oriented toward the apex and the lateral aspect is oriented toward the base. Therefore, this cone has a smaller medial radius and a larger lateral radius[14] (**Figure 4**). The articular surface

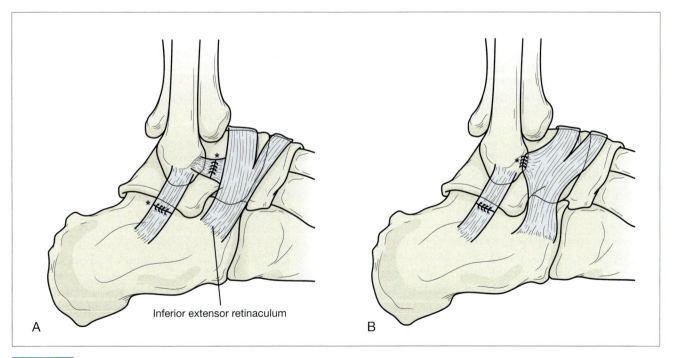

FIGURE 3 **A**, Drawing depicts a Broström procedure. **B**, Drawing depicts a modification of the Broström procedure. Note that a portion of the inferior extensor retinaculum is mobilized for incorporation into the repair.

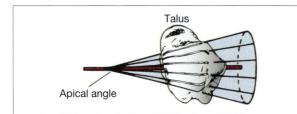

FIGURE 4 Illustration of the cone-shaped trochlear surface of the talus. The apex is oriented medially, whereas the base is oriented laterally. (Adapted with permission from Inman VT: *The Joints of the Ankle*. Williams & Wilkins, 1976 and reproduced with permission from Haskell A, Mann RA: Biomechanics of the foot and ankle, in Coughlin MJ, Saltzman CL, Anderson RB, eds: *Mann's Surgery of the Foot and Ankle*, ed 9. Saunders, 2014, pp 3-36.)

of the talus is also narrower posteriorly than anteriorly. When the ankle is dorsiflexed, the widened anterior portion of the talus fills the mortise more effectively, improving bony stability. In plantar flexion, the bony contribution to stability decreases and the surrounding ligaments assume an increased role. The deltoid ligament complex is well configured to stabilize the medial aspect of the ankle where the apex of the deltoid meets the apex of the cone. The deltoid ligament complex is divided into two anatomically distinct layers: superficial and deep. The superficial deltoid crosses both the tibiotalar and subtalar joints, whereas the deep deltoid only crosses the tibiotalar joint. The superficial layer is fan-shaped and has no discrete bands, although in the most accepted description there are four fascicles. The anatomically separate deep layer is short and thick and divided into two distinct ligaments: the anterior and posterior tibiotalar ligaments. Both layers act to resist valgus talar tilting and act as secondary restraints to anterior translation of the talus. According to a 2020 study, force probe studies performed without ligament transection found that the different fascicles of the deltoid serve differing stabilizing roles depending on the direction and rotation of the force applied[15] (**Figure 5**). The lateral ankle ligament complex is configured more broadly to accommodate a wider radius and larger arc of rotation. The lateral ankle ligament complex comprises the anterior talofibular ligament (ATFL), the CFL, and the posterior talofibular ligament. Lateral ankle stability depends on the orientation of the fibers of each of these ligaments, which changes with ankle position. The ATFL is a thickening of the anterolateral ankle joint capsule that is visible from the articular side of the capsule. Among all lateral ligaments, the ATFL has the lowest load to failure but the highest strain; it lengthens the most before failure. When the foot is plantarflexed, the fibers of the ATFL orient parallel to the leg, providing collateral restraint to inversion. The CFL is a distinct

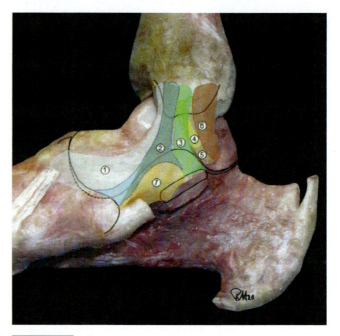

FIGURE 5 Medial view of the ankle depicting the deltoid ligament. Fascicles from the deltoid span from the medial malleolus to the navicular, talus, and calcaneus. Its fascicles are inseparable from the calcaneonavicular ligaments (spring ligament). The superficial component of the deltoid consists of the tibionavicular (1), tibiospring (2), tibiocalcaneal (3), and superficial posterior tibiotalar fascicles (4). The deep component of the deltoid ligament is composed of the anterior tibiotalar (5), posterior tibiotalar fascicles (6) and superomedial component of the spring ligament (7).

extracapsular, cordlike ligament that spans the ankle and the subtalar joints. This ligament is always perpendicular to and stabilizes the subtalar joint.

However, when the ankle is plantarflexed, this ligament assumes a relatively horizontal orientation with respect to the tibiotalar joint, rendering it ineffective as a stabilizer. When the foot dorsiflexes, the roles of the ATFL and CFL are reversed.[16,17]

CLINICAL BIOMECHANICS

At its most basic level, the foot can be conceptualized as a tripod. In stance, weight is distributed collectively between the head of the first metatarsal, the heel, and the four lesser metatarsal heads. Malalignment and alterations in biomechanics may disrupt this balance, resulting in painful conditions (**Figure 6**). For example, a cavus foot type is more prone to increased loading under the first metatarsal head and lateral aspect of the foot. A patient with a dorsiflexion malunion of a metatarsal fracture is at increased risk for a painful callus under another metatarsal head. A hallux valgus deformity may lead to second metatarsal phalangeal joint overload, plantar plate attenuation, and eventual crossover second toe

Chapter 1: Biomechanics of the Foot and Ankle

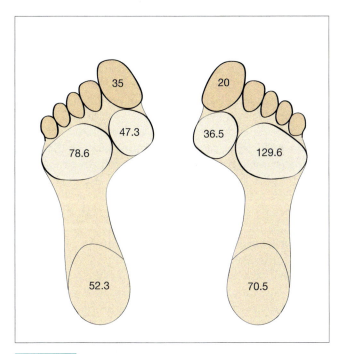

FIGURE 6 Illustration of peak forces, in newtons, measured on the plantar foot before and after silicone arthroplasty of the first metatarsophalangeal joint. (Adapted with permission from Springer Nature. Beverly MC, Horan FT, Hutton WC: Load cell analysis following silastic arthroplasty of the hallux. *Int Orthop* 1985;9[2]:101-104, Copyright 1985.)

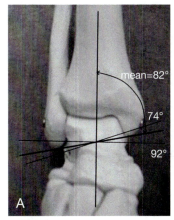
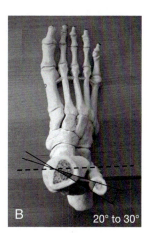

FIGURE 7 **A**, Ankle joint axis of rotation as viewed in the coronal plane. **B**, Ankle joint axis of rotation as viewed from the horizontal plane. (Reproduced with permission from de Asla RJ: Anatomy and biomechanics of the foot and ankle, in Thordarson DB, ed: *Orthopaedic Surgery Essentials: Foot and Ankle*, ed 2. Lippincott Williams & Wilkins, 2012.)

deformity.[18] In such cases, the extensor digitorum longus tendon is the greatest deforming force. Furthermore, foot deformity and position may ultimately affect more proximal joints, as seen in patients with planovalgus foot deformities. The rotational forces created by the planovalgus foot may eventually result in attenuation of the deltoid-spring ligament complex and valgus tilting of the talus. When a foot and ankle surgeon attempts to correct a deformity, the tripod concept must be kept in mind.

The true axis of rotation of the tibiotalar joint consists of a series of instant centers of rotation as the talus translates in the horizontal plane with dorsiflexion and plantar flexion. However, for most purposes, this axis can be estimated using a line that passes through the distal aspects of both malleoli. This empirical axis lies in approximately 20° to 30° of external rotation with respect to the coronal plane and is obliquely oriented at approximately 82° from the axis of the tibia (**Figure 7**). With the foot free and the leg in a fixed position, the oblique ankle joint axis causes the foot to externally rotate with dorsiflexion and internally rotate with plantar flexion (**Figure 8**). Conversely, when the foot is fixed to the floor, the oblique axis imposes an internal rotation force to the leg as the body passes over the foot, and the foot dorsiflexes. As the foot pushes off, ankle plantar flexion results in external rotation of the leg. Rotation of the tibia is coupled with the inversion and eversion motion of the subtalar joint. The normal coupling mechanism depends on the integrity of the deltoid and interosseous ligaments.[19] One study suggests that when tibiotalar motion is markedly reduced by arthritis, the normal motion coupling seen in healthy ankle joints breaks down.[20]

Motion of the subtalar joint has been compared with that of a mitered hinge. Its axis passes obliquely from

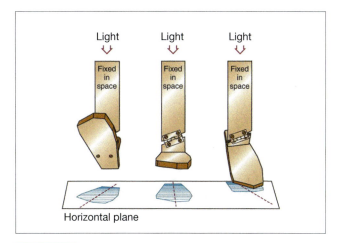

FIGURE 8 Illustration showing that, with the leg fixed in position and the foot free, the oblique ankle joint axis causes outward rotation with dorsiflexion and inward rotation with plantar flexion. (Reproduced with permission from Haskell A, Mann RA: Biomechanics of the foot and ankle, in Coughlin MJ, Saltzman CL, Anderson RB, eds: *Mann's Surgery of the Foot and Ankle*, ed 9. Saunders, 2014, pp 3-36.)

plantarlateral to dorsal medial, deviating from the horizontal plane by approximately 41° and from the sagittal plane by approximately 23°.[14,21] The subtalar axis of rotation is highly variable between patients. Using the model in **Figure 9** as a visual aid, a more horizontally oriented axis appears to translate to more rotation of the horizontal component with every degree of vertical component rotation. The reverse is true with a more vertically oriented axis. Clinically, it is recognized that patients with flatter feet (a more horizontal axis) have more subtalar motion, whereas patients with a cavus foot type (a more vertical axis) tend to experience stiffer motion.

The transverse tarsal joint allows for hindfoot motion while the forefoot remains plantigrade to the ground. This relationship is facilitated by the acetabulum pedis. The heel strikes the ground in varus and then quickly everts. Anatomically, the everted hindfoot places the axis of rotation of the calcaneal cuboid joint parallel to the axis of rotation of the talonavicular joint. This parallel configuration permits motion across the transverse tarsal joint, which accommodates uneven terrain and absorbs impact forces. As the body's center of mass moves forward over the foot, the tibia externally rotates, causing the hindfoot to rotate into varus through coupled motion. The changing position of the hindfoot causes the once-parallel axes of the transverse tarsal joints to converge. This convergence effectively locks the transverse tarsal joint, effectively changing the foot from an accommodating platform for stance into a rigid lever arm for efficient push-off.

Motions of the subtalar joint and transverse tarsal joint (also called the triple joint complex) are inextricably linked, with the talonavicular joint playing the key role. In conditions requiring arthrodesis of the talonavicular joint, motion through the remaining joints of the triple joint complex is virtually nonexistent.[22] Acting in conjunction with the bony architecture of the foot and ankle is a series of dynamic and static soft-tissue stabilizers. At heel strike, the tibialis anterior tendon eccentrically contracts to control foot descent, serving to dissipate forces and prevent slapping of the foot against the ground. The tibialis posterior tendon plays a vital role in producing hindfoot inversion during push-off through its action across the transverse tarsal joint. The pull of the tibialis posterior tendon adducts the navicular over the head of the talus, helping to invert the calcaneus, which follows the cuboid. The ability to perform an efficient heel rise depends on the tibialis posterior tendon's ability to secure the transverse tarsal joint in adduction. At heel rise, the triceps surae pulls the Achilles tendon to become the strongest hindfoot inverter. This ensures the midfoot will remain locked for toe-off.

When disease renders the posterior tibial tendon ineffective, the transverse tarsal midfoot locking mechanism is compromised. When the midfoot fails to lock, the stability of the medial longitudinal arch becomes solely dependent on plantar soft-tissue static stabilizers for support. Without dynamic stabilization and bony protection of the transverse tarsal joint, these stabilizers will attenuate and eventually fail under tension, resulting in progressive collapse of the medial longitudinal arch, abduction of the forefoot, and the eventual failure of the hindfoot to invert with toe rise. As a consequence, the Achilles tendon will pull on an everted hindfoot, ensuring that midfoot locking does not occur. In this scenario, the Achilles tendon becomes a deforming force that leads to an accelerated progressive collapsing foot deformity.

Traditional teaching and most literature concerning the topic of the progressive collapsing foot deformity (also referred to as an adult acquired flatfoot) suggest that an incompetent posterior tibial tendon serves as the initial catalyst preceding deformity. However, this concept is being challenged on a number of fronts. Using weight-bearing CT, investigators found that in patients with symptomatic flatfoot deformities the coronal orientation of the posterior facet was in significantly more valgus than in control patients. The investigators hypothesized that an excessively valgus subtalar joint leads to increased medial force vectors that, over time, lead to medial soft-tissue failure and progressive deformity.[23,24] More recent studies show the deltoid-spring ligament complex plays the primary role in maintaining the medial longitudinal arch while the posterior tibial tendon provides dynamic support of the ligaments function. In this secondary role, the posterior tibial tendon is incapable of preventing a progressive flatfoot deformity once the ligamentous structures have failed, as discussed in two studies published in 2019.[25,26]

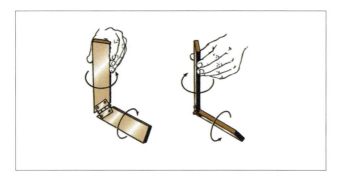

FIGURE 9 Illustration of a mitered joint hinge. (Reproduced with permission from Haskell A, Mann RA: Biomechanics of the foot and ankle, in Coughlin MJ, Saltzman CL, Anderson RB, eds: *Mann's Surgery of the Foot and Ankle*, ed 9. Saunders, 2014, pp 3-36.)

The medial longitudinal arch is a dynamic structure that aids in shock absorption and terrain accommodation on heel strike and in midstance, and then allows for efficient propulsion at toe-off. Two models have been proposed to help describe the biomechanics of the medial longitudinal arch.[27] In one model, the arch is conceptualized as a curved, segmented beam. The beam comprises the calcaneus, talus, navicular, cuneiforms, and the medial three metatarsals. The segments are stabilized by static plantar ligamentous connections. With weight bearing, compression forces develop on the dorsal aspect of the beam whereas tensile forces are created on the plantar aspect. The dorsal compression forces are resisted by the bony architecture of the arch, whereas plantar tensile forces are resisted by the ligaments (**Figure 10**).

The beam model of the medial longitudinal arch does not consider the role of the plantar fascia. This structure is incorporated in the truss model of the arch (**Figure 11**). In the truss model, the arch is conceptualized as a triangular structure composed of two oblique beams with a dorsal pivot connected plantarly by a tie rod. Anatomically, the plantar fascia functions as a tie rod, originating from the posterior calcaneal tuberosity and inserting onto the sesamoids and the bases of the proximal phalanges of the lesser toes. With loading, the plantar fascia resists the plantarly generated tensile forces.[28] Total or partial release of the plantar fascia may decrease arch height.[29]

During late midstance and toe-off, the hallux and lesser toes dorsiflex, which effectively tightens the plantar fascia and adds to the stability of the midfoot. The mechanism by which this occurs has been likened to a windlass device (**Figure 12**). A windlass is used to transport

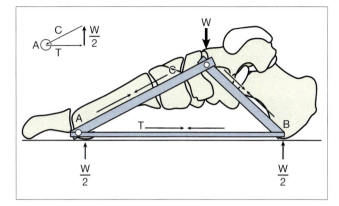

FIGURE 11 Illustration of the truss model of the medial longitudinal arch. The bony architecture of the foot is conceptualized as two beams connected by the plantar fascia, which functions as a tie rod. A = the insertion of the plantar fascia, B = the origin of the plantar fascia on the calcaneus, C = compressive force, T = tensile force, W = weight bearing force. (Redrawn with permission from Sarrafian SK: Functional characteristics of the foot and plantar aponeurosis under tibiotalar loading. *Foot Ankle* 1987;8[1]:9.)

or lift objects vertically. It makes use of a lever arm (the hallux and lesser toes) that is attached to a cable or rope (the plantar fascia) wound around a cylinder (the metatarsophalangeal joints), which acts as a fulcrum.

Weight-bearing CT is gaining prevalence in both research and clinical settings. This relatively new modality is changing how the normal foot configuration is defined and how deformity is measured and determined.[30,31] Weight-bearing CT is also creating new biometric tools such as the foot-ankle offset. Foot-ankle offset is a semiautomated software-driven calculation that uses biometric data to reconstruct the foot tripod to determine a virtual point where the ground reaction force is applied and find the center of the ankle where body weight is applied. The offset between the two represents

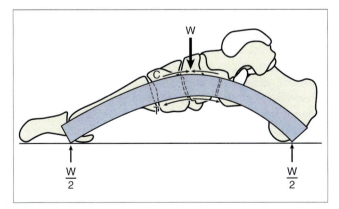

FIGURE 10 Illustration of the beam model of the medial longitudinal arch. Compression occurs through bony structures dorsally and tension occurs across plantar ligamentous structures. C = compressive force, T = tensile force, W = weight bearing force. (Redrawn with permission from Sarrafian SK: Functional characteristics of the foot and plantar aponeurosis under tibiotalar loading. *Foot Ankle* 1987;8[1]:9.)

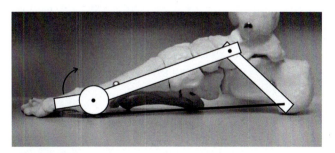

FIGURE 12 Windlass mechanism. A truss is shown superimposed over a skeletal model of the foot. As the toes dorsiflex, the drum (metatarsophalangeal joints) rotates, applying tension to the tie rod (plantar fascia) and effectively supporting the arch. (Reproduced with permission from de Asla RJ: Anatomy and biomechanics of the foot and ankle, in Thordarson DB, ed: *Orthopaedic Surgery Essentials: Foot and Ankle*, ed 2. Lippincott Williams & Wilkins, 2012.)

a coronal plane rotational torque lever arm.[32] The technique has been found to be reproducible with excellent correlation with pedobarographic data.[33] Foot-ankle offset may offer an entirely new way to assess normal and altered foot mechanics.

GAIT

Human gait is defined as the process by which the lower extremities are used for forward locomotion. Many biomechanical events unfold during human gait that simply occur too rapidly to evaluate clinically. Numerous techniques developed in the field of biomechanics can potentially quantitatively assess body segment motions and forces. Such techniques, however, usually necessitate the use of a formal gait laboratory and a dedicated team. Techniques include video gait analysis, force plates, fluoroscopic imaging, three-dimensional reconstruction software, electromyography, and a host of other technologies.

Despite the accuracy of certain gait analysis techniques, widespread clinical use has yet to occur and debate remains as to their clinical relevance. Criteria have been proposed regarding the inclusion of gait analysis as a routine part of an orthopaedic examination.[34,35]

Normal human gait is extremely efficient with regard to energy and oxygen consumption. The gait cycle is a pattern of recurring predefined events that can be analyzed in terms of stride. A single stride starts from the moment of heel strike to the moment the same heel strikes the ground again. Stride length is defined as the distance covered between these two consecutive heel strikes. A step is the distance between the heel strike of one foot and the heel strike of the opposite foot. Cadence is defined by the number of steps taken during a given unit of time. In walking, a single stride is divided into two phases: the stance phase and the swing phase. The stance phase begins when the foot strikes the ground and continues until the toes of the same foot leave the ground (or toe-off). This represents approximately 60% of the gait cycle. Swing phase is the remaining 40% of the cycle and extends from toe-off until the heel strikes the ground.

The stance phase is further divided into three intervals. The first interval starts at heel strike and ends at foot flat. This segment is characterized by weight acceptance and rapid ankle plantar flexion under eccentric control of the anterior leg musculature. The second interval extends from foot flat to opposite foot strike. During this interval, the body's center of gravity passes forward of the plantar foot. This controlled fall is halted when the contralateral heel strikes the ground. The final interval extends from the end of the second interval through toe-off. This interval is characterized by rapid ankle plantar flexion

and the cascade of biomechanical events that creates a rigid foot for efficient push-off.

Electromyographic measurements provide insight into muscle function during gait analysis. At heel strike, the anterior muscles of the leg actively control the descent of the foot to avoid slapping. This eccentric action also absorbs ground reaction forces. Activity of the extensor muscle group is followed by activity of the flexor groups. Flexor activity starts with the tibialis posterior tendon preparing the foot for heel rise. The peroneal tendons provide varus stability as the ankle rotates in dorsiflexion during single-limb stance. The triceps surae then activates, followed by recruitment of the toe flexors, causing heel rise, rapid plantar flexion, and eventual toe-off. In the early swing phase, the plantar muscles relax and the extensors act to dorsiflex the foot again, allowing for clearance and preparation for the next heel strike. As the foot progresses from foot strike to toe-off, the center of load progresses from the center of the heel through the hallux.

In the setting of gastrocnemius tightness, the risk of pain in the forefoot by increased plantar forefoot pressures appears when the muscle is maximally stretched. As a biarticular muscle this happens when both the knee is in extension and the ankle is in dorsiflexion.[36] Some studies have recommended stretching exercises to remedy this biomechanical disturbance, but others found no difference in gait analysis between stretched and nonstretched groups.[37]

Running alters the gait cycle in several important ways. During walking, one foot is always in contact with the ground. With running, however, there are two float phases where both feet are off the ground. In addition, there is no longer a period of double-limb support. Finally, with running, ground reaction force increases, the phasic activity of muscles is altered, and the range of motion of the lower extremity joints increases.

Alterations of normal gait can result in gait dysfunction. In general, a dysfunctional gait pattern leads to insufficiencies that cause increased energy and oxygen consumption. Pain is probably the most common cause of gait disturbance. One study demonstrated that patients with ankle arthritis who underwent either ankle arthroplasty or arthrodesis returned to a more normal gait pattern.[38] In another study, patients who underwent ankle arthrodesis had decreased stride length.[39] Among patients who have undergone amputation, the more proximal the amputation, the higher the required energy expenditure for gait.[40]

Many disorders of the foot and ankle result in discernible and characteristic patterns in human gait. An antalgic gait results from pain and is defined by the shortened stance phase of the affected limb. A steppage gait results from footdrop or weakness of the anterior musculature of the leg. It is characterized by lifting the affected limb higher during the swing phase so the foot adequately clears the ground. A calcaneal gait is characterized by exaggerated heel weight bearing and results from weakness or paralysis of the posterior compartment musculature. A waddling gait is the result of proximal myopathy and is characterized by a broad-based stance with the pelvis drooping toward the leg being raised during the swing phase. This gait abnormality is in contrast to a Trendelenburg gait, which is caused by weakness of the hip abductors and results in compensatory lurching of the trunk toward the weakened side during stance.

SUMMARY

With the advent of new technologies and techniques over the decades, the ability to measure foot and ankle biomechanics has substantially expanded. If surgeons are to create and optimize new treatment options for patients, the knowledge base must continue to expand.

KEY STUDY POINTS

- The foot is divided into three functional zones, the hindfoot, midfoot, and forefoot, each with its own functional role to play.
- At its most basic level, the foot can be likened to a tripod. Alterations in this balance can have biomechanical consequences.
- The transverse tarsal joint locking mechanism results from a complex interplay of both static and dynamic components and is critical for normal foot function.
- Motion coupling occurs between the tibia and the hindfoot through the ankle. Limitations in motion of one component affect the other.

ANNOTATED REFERENCES

1. Arndt A, Westblad P, Winson I, Hashimoto T, Lundberg A: Ankle and subtalar kinematics measured with intracortical pins during the stance phase of walking. *Foot Ankle Int* 2004;25(5):357-364.

2. de Asla RJ, Wan L, Rubash HE, Li G: Six DOF in vivo kinematics of the ankle joint complex: Application of a combined dual-orthogonal fluoroscopic and magnetic resonance imaging technique. *J Orthop Res* 2006;24(5):1019-1027.

3. Fassbind MJ, Rohr ES, Hu Y, et al: Evaluating foot kinematics using magnetic resonance imaging: From maximum plantar flexion, inversion, and internal rotation to maximum dorsiflexion, eversion, and external rotation. *J Biomech Eng* 2011;133(10):104502.

4. Kitaoka HB, Crevoisier XM, Hansen D, Katajarvi B, Harbst K, Kaufman KR: Foot and ankle kinematics and ground reaction forces during ambulation. *Foot Ankle Int* 2006;27(10):808-813.

5. Lundberg A: Kinematics of the ankle and foot. In vivo roentgen stereophotogrammetry. *Acta Orthop Scand Suppl* 1989;233:1-24.

6. Torg JS, Pavlov H, Cooley LH, et al: Stress fractures of the tarsal navicular. A retrospective review of twenty-one cases. *J Bone Joint Surg Am* 1982;64(5):700-712.

7. Harper MC: The lateral ligamentous support of the subtalar joint. *Foot Ankle* 1991;11(6):354-358.

8. Ringleb SI, Dhakal A, Anderson CD, Bawab S, Paranjape R: Effects of lateral ligament sectioning on the stability of the ankle and subtalar joint. *J Orthop Res* 2011;29(10):1459-1464.

9. Heilman AE, Braly WG, Bishop JO, Noble PC, Tullos HS: An anatomic study of subtalar instability. *Foot Ankle* 1990;10(4):224-228.

10. Beumer A, van Hemert WL, Swierstra BA, Jasper LE, Belkoff SM: A biomechanical evaluation of the tibiofibular and tibiotalar ligaments of the ankle. *Foot Ankle Int* 2003;24(5):426-429.

11. Hoefnagels EM, Waites MD, Wing ID, Belkoff SM, Swierstra BA: Biomechanical comparison of the interosseous tibiofibular ligament and the anterior tibiofibular ligament. *Foot Ankle Int* 2007;28(5):602-604.

12. Nester CJ, Findlow AF, Bowker P, Bowden PD: Transverse plane motion at the ankle joint. *Foot Ankle Int* 2003;24(2):164-168.

13. Tochigi Y, Rudert MJ, Saltzman CL, Amendola A, Brown TD: Contribution of articular surface geometry to ankle stabilization. *J Bone Joint Surg Am* 2006;88(12):2704-2713.

14. Inman VT: *The Joints of the Ankle*. Williams & Wilkins, 1976.

15. Takao M, Ozeki S, Olivia XM, et al: Strain pattern of each ligamentous band of the superficial deltoid ligament: A cadaver study. *BMC Musculoskelet Disord* 2020;21(1):289.

    This study aimed to measure the strain pattern of the deltoid ligament bands directly using miniaturization ligament performance probes. Level of evidence: IV.

16. Fujii T, Kitaoka HB, Luo ZP, Kura H, An KN: Analysis of ankle-hindfoot stability in multiple planes: An in vitro study. *Foot Ankle Int* 2005;26(8):633-637.

17. Ozeki S, Kitaoka H, Uchiyama E, Luo ZP, Kaufman K, An KN: Ankle ligament tensile forces at the end points of passive circumferential rotating motion of the ankle and subtalar joint complex. *Foot Ankle Int* 2006;27(11):965-969.

18. Coughlin MJ, Schutt SA, Hirose CB, et al: Metatarsophalangeal joint pathology in crossover second toe deformity: A cadaveric study. *Foot Ankle Int* 2012;33(2):133-140.

19. Hintermann B, Sommer C, Nigg BM: Influence of ankle ligament transection on tibial and calcaneal rotation with loading and dorsi-plantarflexion. *Foot Ankle Int* 1995;16(9):567-571.

20. Kozanek M, Rubash HE, Li G, de Asla RJ: Effect of post-traumatic tibiotalar osteoarthritis on kinematics of the ankle joint complex. *Foot Ankle Int* 2009;30(8):734-740.

21. Inman VT: *Human Walking*. Williams & Wilkins, 1981.

22. Astion DJ, Deland JT, Otis JC, Kenneally S: Motion of the hindfoot after simulated arthrodesis. *J Bone Joint Surg Am* 1997;79(2):241-246.

23. Apostle K, Coleman N, Sangeorzan BJ: Subtalar joint axis in patients with symptomatic peritalar subluxation compared to normal controls. *Foot Ankle Int* 2014;35:1153-1158.

24. Probasco W, Haleem A, Yu J, et al: Assessment of coronal plane subtalar joint alignment in peritalar subluxation via weight-bearing multiplanar imaging. *Foot Ankle Int* 2015;36:302-309.

25. Cifuentes-De la Portilla C, Larrainzar-Garijo R, Bayod J: Biomechanical stress analysis of the main soft tissues associated with the development of adult acquired flatfoot deformity. *Clin Biomech (Bristol, Avon)* 2019;61:163-171.

    In this study a finite element model of the foot was created, which included all bones, cartilages, and tissue related to the progressive collapsing foot deformity. The capacity of each soft tissue to support the plantar arch was measured. Level of evidence: IV.

26. Kelly M, Masqoodi N, Vasconcellos D, et al: Spring ligament tear decreases static stability of the ankle joint. *Clin Biomech (Bristol, Avon)* 2019;61:79-83.

    The aim of the study was to determine the effect of spring ligament injury and subsequent forked semitendinosis allograft reconstruction on static joint reactive force across the talonavicular and tibiotalar joints. Level of evidence: IV.

27. Sarrafian SK: Functional anatomy of the foot and ankle, in Sarafian SK, ed: *Anatomy of the Foot and Ankle: Descriptive, Topographic, Functional*, ed 2. Lippincott Williams & Wilkins, 1993.

28. Hicks JH: The mechanics of the foot. II: The plantar aponeurosis and the arch. *J Anat* 1954;88(1):25-30.

29. Cheung JT, An KN, Zhang M: Consequences of partial and total plantar fascia release: A finite element study. *Foot Ankle Int* 2006;27(2):125-132.

30. de Cesar Netto L, Schon LC, Thawait GK, et al: Flexible adult acquired flatfoot deformity: Comparison between weight-bearing and non-weight-bearing measurements using cone-beam computed tomography. *J Bone Joint Surg Am* 2017;99:e98.

31. de Cesar Netto L, Godoy-Santos AL, Saito GH, et al: Subluxation of the middle facet of the subtalar joint as a marker of peritalar subluxation in adult acquired flatfoot deformity: A case-control study. *J Bone Joint Surg Am* 2019;101:1838-1844.

    Using weight-bearing CT, the middle facet was investigated as an indicator of peritalar subluxation. The authors concluded that the degree of subluxation and incongruence of the middle facet represents an accurate diagnostic tool for symptomatic progressive collapsing foot deformity. Level of evidence: III.

32. Lintz F, Welck M, Bernasconi A, et al: 3D biometrics for hindfoot alignment using weightbearing CT. *Foot Ankle Int* 2017;38(6):684-689.

33. Richter M, Lintz F, Zech S, et al: Combination of PedCAT weightbearing CT with pedography assessment of the relationship between anatomy-based foot center and force/pressure-based center of gravity. *Foot Ankle Int* 2018;39:361-368.

34. Brand RA: Can biomechanics contribute to clinical orthopaedic assessments? *Iowa Orthop J* 1989;9:61-64.

35. Brand RA, Crowninshield RD: Comment on criteria for patient evaluation tools. *J Biomech* 1981;14(9):655.

36. Cazeau C, Stiglitz Y: Effects of gastrocnemius tightness on forefoot during gait. *Foot Ankle Clin* 2014;19(4):649-657.

37. Johanson MA, Cuda BJ, Koontz JE, et al: Effect of stretching on ankle and knee angles and gastrocnemius activity during the stance phase of gait. *J Sport Rehabil* 2009;18:521-534.

38. Flavin R, Coleman SC, Tenenbaum S, Brodsky JW: Comparison of gait after total ankle arthroplasty and ankle arthrodesis. *Foot Ankle Int* 2013;34(10):1340-1348.

39. Thomas R, Daniels TR, Parker K: Gait analysis and functional outcomes following ankle arthrodesis for isolated ankle arthritis. *J Bone Joint Surg Am* 2006;88(3):526-535.

40. Waters RL, Perry J, Antonelli D, Hislop H: Energy cost of walking of amputees: The influence of level of amputation. *J Bone Joint Surg Am* 1976;58(1):42-46.

CHAPTER 2

Shoes and Orthoses

JESSE F. DOTY, MD, FAAOS

ABSTRACT

An understanding of orthosis and bracing biomechanics will provide the foot and ankle clinician with opportunities to improve both surgical and nonsurgical outcomes. A team approach among the patient, physician, and orthotist will ensure success. A fundamental understanding of the basic elements of orthosis and shoe design will allow accurate assessment of contemporary footwear development and market trends. A multitude of commercially available shoes designed with sport-specific purpose or with therapeutic features incorporated into the engineering are now available for more purposeful application of footwear.

Keywords: brace; footwear; insole; orthosis; shoe

Dr. Doty or an immediate family member has received royalties from Arthrex, Inc., Globus Medical, and Wright Medical Technology, Inc.; is a member of a speakers' bureau or has made paid presentations on behalf of Arthrex, Inc., BoneSupport AB, Globus Medical, Immersive Tech, Inc., International Life Sciences, Novastep Inc., and Wright Medical Technology, Inc.; serves as a paid consultant to or is an employee of Arthrex, Inc., BoneSupport AB, Depuy/Synthes, Globus Medical, Immersive Tech, Inc., International Life Sciences, Novastep Inc., and Wright Medical Technology, Inc.; has stock or stock options held in Globus Medical; has received research or institutional support from Arthrex, Inc. and Wright Medical Technology, Inc.; and serves as a board member, owner, officer, or committee member of American Orthopaedic Foot and Ankle Society.

INTRODUCTION

The foot and ankle specialist should be familiar with bracing biomechanics and the effects of footwear components on the lower extremity. A successful bracing program for pathologic foot conditions is the result of history and physical examination characteristics coupled with feedback from both the patient and treating clinician. An orthotist may see the patient and modify the brace multiple times during the manufacturing and fitting process. It is important to discuss the fundamentals of shoe and insole design with updates on recent footwear trends. Knowledge of these topics will help clinicians more effectively communicate with orthotists regarding patient-specific clinical goals and anticipated outcomes.

SHOES

Shoes may protect the sole of the foot from the environment, but they also change the way one walks. A 2019 study showed that, when shod as opposed to walking barefoot, children demonstrated increased velocity, step length, and step time and decreased cadence.[1] Similarly, a 2021 study found that gait characteristics certainly affect shoe lifespan such as treadwear on the outsole.[2] Certain shoe modifications may offer protective advantages or enhance performance. A steel-toe, stiff-sole shoe may protect a manual laborer, whereas a soft-soled, cushioned shoe can prevent skin ulcers in patients with diabetes (**Figure 1**). Athletic shoes are now sport-specific and sometimes customizable. A survey of adolescent cross-country runners revealed that 73% identified arch-type compatibility with shoe design as the most important factor in choosing a shoe. Seventy-four percent reported not knowing how many miles they had logged before shoe replacement, even though loss of midsole cushion recoil is a risk factor for overuse injuries.[3] With injury prevention and playing surface type now being important topics in

© 2025 American Academy of Orthopaedic Surgeons

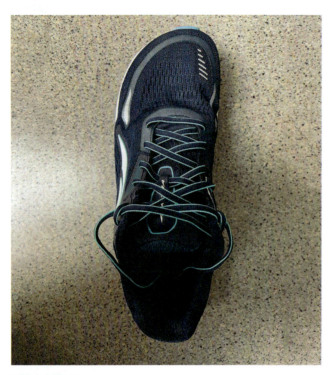

FIGURE 1 Photograph showing a shoe with a wide toe box that can be used to accommodate patients with hallux valgus or hammer toe deformities.

professional sports, organizations such as the National Football League have provided financial support for shoe research and development. Athletic footwear is now considered an integral piece of protective equipment rather than simply an extension of uniform apparel[4] (**Figure 2**). Some evidence suggests that artificial surfaces may increase the rate of injury by failing to release the shoe outsole from the playing surface. Some cleat designs tend to lose friction on natural grass surfaces and sheer more quickly, thereby decreasing torque transferred to the lower extremity.[5] New shoe designs with incorporation of inertial sensors, pressure sensors, and global positioning systems will allow temporospatial data analysis with application for athletics and everyday gait control mechanisms.[6]

Running sports have expanded with increasing popularity of barefoot-style running shoes and maximalist cushioned running shoes. Safety and efficacy of these design concepts are not completely backed by scientific validity. In the case of barefoot-style running, well-designed studies are necessary to prove whether this minimalist running style is beneficial or harmful to overall musculoskeletal health. There is some evidence that peak ground forces are reduced as a runner changes their gait pattern from a hindfoot strike, typical of shod runners, to a forefoot and midfoot strike described by minimalist runners.[7] When transitioning from running in cushioned shoes to minimalistic shoes, runners have increased pressures in the forefoot and may be at risk for stress fractures.[8] Proponents of minimalist running reference studies show decreased exertional compartment syndrome and anterior knee pain.[9] A study[10] evaluated barefoot runners, runners in a minimalist shoe, and runners in a cushioned running shoe. Runners could estimate direction and amplitude of terrain more accurately with a minimalist shoe model. No substantial differences were found between runners using the minimalist shoe model and those who ran completely barefoot. The authors suggested that cushioned shoes substantially impair foot position proprioception compared with less-structured shoes or barefoot conditions. Increased coordination and improved intrinsic muscle foot strength have also been suggested.[11] When comparing 18 runners transitioning to minimalist shoes with 19 control runners who did not switch, the abductor hallucis muscle cross-sectional area increased by 10.6%, but all other muscles tested did not change. Bone marrow edema developed in eight of the minimalist runners, whereas edema developed in only one control runner.[12] A prospective survey followed 107

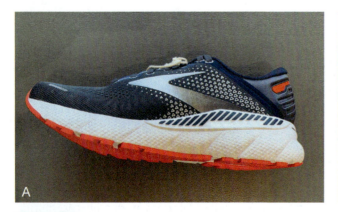 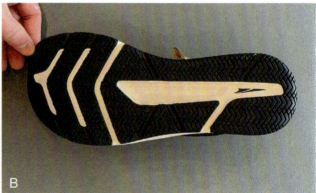

FIGURE 2 **A** and **B**, Photographs showing the design features of this shoe including extension of the midsole proximally to encompass hindfoot and enhance stability.

barefoot runners and 94 shod runners over the course of a 1-year period. Both groups had similar injury rates, although different types of injuries were seen depending on the running style.[13] Electromyographic studies have been used to evaluate the effects of habitual minimalist running on muscle activation. During stance phase, compared with shod runners, minimalist runners had greater muscle activity in the gastrocnemius medialis and gluteus maximus and lower activity in the tibialis anterior. During swing phase, minimalist running exhibited increased muscle activity in the vastus lateralis and medial gastrocnemius.[14]

Increasing variability of running sports has led to another popular alternative running shoe. Running in a thickly cushioned rocker sole has been termed maximalist running. Multiple maximalist running shoe companies such as HOKA and Altra have entered the global footwear market. Proponents of the maximalist running style suggest the extra cushion may prevent lower extremity injuries, particularly in long-distance running. Oxygen consumption with maximalist rocker shoes was found to be 4.5% higher than with standard shoes and 5.6% higher than with minimalist shoes, but this may be due to the larger mass effect of the rocker soles.[15] It has been reported that thicker soles evoke a stronger protective eversion response from the peroneal muscles to counter an increasing moment arm at the ankle-subtalar joint complex following sudden foot inversion.[16,17] Theoretically, thicker soles could increase risk of lateral ligament injury when the protective response of the peroneal tendons is overwhelmed (**Figures 3** and **4**).

Introduction of energy-storing mechanisms into athletic shoes has also seen a recent trend in running developmental technology. The Nike VaporFly shoe was introduced as a new concept in 2017 incorporating a lightweight upper with a new compliant and resilient foam sole providing energy return, and carbon fiber inserted in the midsole with the goal of improving longitudinal bending stiffness. Some evidence from a 2021 study suggested improved athletic performance in marathon runners shod with this new technology[18] (**Figure 5**).

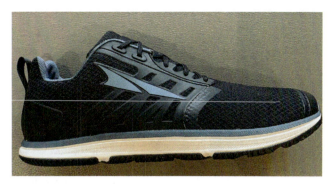

FIGURE 4 Photograph showing a zero-drop shoe with minimal cushioning to allow the foot to lie flat on the level surface of the outsole.

The influence of high-fashion footwear on foot and ankle pathoanatomy has long been a subject of concern. Some injuries, such as ankle sprains, are more likely to occur based on the positioning of the ankle mortise while in an extremely positive heel drop shoe. Habitual high-heeled shoe wearers have additionally been shown to have decreased range of motion in dorsiflexion and eversion compared with flat-shoe wearers.[19] The authors recommended ankle exercises and gastrocnemius stretching for habitual high-heeled shoe wearers. High heels also adversely affect muscle control and reduce loads in the quadriceps and spine musculature, and it has been suggested that the addition of a total-contact insert to a shoe might improve comfort rating and foot stability.[20] Despite continued evolution and specialization of footwear, many of the basic components that make up a shoe remain the same (**Table 1**).

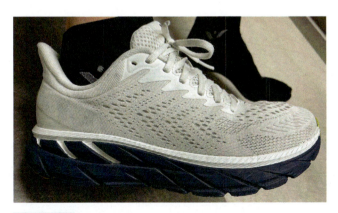

FIGURE 3 Photograph showing a maximally cushioned athletic shoe.

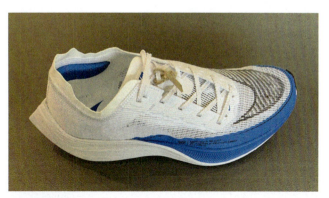

FIGURE 5 Photograph showing lightweight advanced foam incorporated with a carbon-fiber reinforcement to store energy and provide recoil.

Section 1: General Foot and Ankle Topics

Table 1

Basic Shoe Components

Upper	Encloses the dorsal foot above the insole; includes the toe box, vamp, and quarter
Lower	Plantar to the foot; includes the insole, midsole, and outsole
Toe box	Distal portion of the upper that provides space for the toes
Vamp	Midsection of the upper that covers the dorsum of the midfoot
Quarter	Posterior portion of the upper that covers the hindfoot; may have a reinforced area around the heel known as a heel counter
Insole	Portion of the lower that directly contacts the plantar surface of the foot and is frequently removable
Midsole	Cushioned area designed for shock absorption between the insole and outsole
Outsole	Portion of the lower that contacts the ground and provides traction

SHOE MODIFICATIONS

Historically, commercially available shoes were designed to protect the sole of the foot from the environment with few anatomic or pathologic considerations. Over the past few decades, consumer demand and industry marketing resulted in further shoe specification. Now patients with subtle anatomic deviations or chronic conditions may achieve pain relief through strategic footwear selection. For instance, forefoot malalignment can be accommodated by a shoe with a wide toe box to relieve pressure on the metatarsals and toes. Shoe companies market styles with varied degrees of arch support to accommodate runners with either planus or cavus alignment to increase comfort and stability. Patients with diabetes now have easier access to therapeutic in-depth shoes designed to relieve pressure over bony prominences by incorporating soft uppers with cushioned insoles. In-depth shoes feature an additional 0.25 to 0.375 inch of insole cushioning and can be modified by removing the factory inlay and inserting a custom orthosis without affecting the overall fit.[21]

Shoes can be modified to increase ambulation efficiency and compensate for decreased motion secondary to pain, fusion, arthritis, or deformity (**Table 2**). Typically, this is done by modifying the insole or midsole to increase stability or offload high-pressure areas.[21] Modifications may delay the need for surgical intervention or provide temporal relief for poor surgical candidates. The upper portion of a shoe can be stretched with a ball-and-ring stretcher to soften the material and make room for bony spurs, hallux valgus deformity, or a hammer toe. The vamp of the shoe may cause increased pain by compressing the sensory nerves over osteophytes in midfoot arthritis, and this can sometimes be relieved with simple alterations such as alternate lacing patterns or elastic laces. For plantar pain, a factory insole can be

Table 2

Shoe Types and Modifications

In-depth shoe	Additional 0.25- to 0.375-inch depth to accommodate deformity; may come with easily exchangeable insoles
Custom shoe	Fabricated from a mold or a CT scan to provide additional accommodation and protection
Relasting	Customization of a commercial shoe to accommodate deformity while maintaining the normal appearance. The outsole is removed and a cut is made through the remaining sole to add material, and then the outsole is reapplied
Flare	A firm strip of material added as an outrigger to provide a wider base of support on the sole for increased stability
Shank	Steel or carbon composite embedded in the sole to stiffen it from heel to toe; used to decrease bending forces
Rocker sole	Additional material generally added to the midsole to create a cam to allow rolling from heel strike to toe-off with decreased bending In general, the apex of the rocker is placed proximal to the area where pressure relief is desired

© 2025 American Academy of Orthopaedic Surgeons

Orthopaedic Knowledge Update®: Foot and Ankle 7

supplemented or removed and replaced with a commercially available insole or a custom insole. A metatarsal bar pad may additionally offload the metatarsal heads and relieve metatarsalgia during gait. Pads and insoles are manufactured in multiple sizes and shapes and are often commercially available.

Simply exchanging a thin, standard factory insole for a thick gel, foam, or air-cushioned insole may help relieve metatarsalgia, heel pain, or generalized foot discomfort. An orthosis redistributes forces by increasing support and contact area under the midfoot while decreasing pressure under the hindfoot and forefoot.[22] Some conditions may be relieved by retaining the cushioned insole and reducing shoe flexibility by adding a shank to the sole. A shank may stiffen the shoe enough to relieve pain from hallux rigidus, metatarsalgia, and midfoot arthritis by decreasing painful joint excursion. According to a 2019 study, some companies have engineered a carbon plate into insoles or into commercially available shoe midsoles to add recoil and propulsion for running.[23] Because of stress shielding, this carbon-fiber plate could also be therapeutic for the treatment of midfoot and forefoot stress syndromes or arthritis (Figure 6). Additionally, shoes should fit appropriately, which necessitates correct shape and depth with at least 0.375 inch of length past the longest toe to avoid impingement and to accommodate devices such as an orthosis.

A cobbler or pedorthist may add a rocker to the shoe by adding material to the midsole. This may decrease floor-reaction forces and bending forces on the foot. The rocker bottom may limit painful arthritic joint excursion, offload metatarsalgia, or improve gait in patients after arthrodesis procedures.[24] It may also be effective in reducing the windlass effect contributing to plantar fasciitis.[25] A negative heel rocker outsole design will alter the gait of a patient with diabetic neuropathy by reducing push-off power and thereby decrease ground reaction forces and peak forefoot pressures. However, a rocker sole can also compromise stability and gait symmetry, which may contribute to limited patient acceptance and limited use in clinical practice.[26]

Wedges or posts can be used to address varus or valgus deformities at the forefoot and hindfoot. A medial heel wedge provides a varus moment to the hindfoot, which may decrease lateral impingement or improve hindfoot position in patients with pes planus. Runners with pes planus have reported a decreased incidence of foot and knee pain when a medial heel wedge was added to their soft insole.[27] A lateral heel wedge provides a valgus moment to the hindfoot, which may relieve tension on the peroneal tendons and treat symptoms of lateral instability. Posting the forefoot can also indirectly alter hindfoot mechanics. Medial posting of a varus forefoot can decrease the valgus moment transferred to the hindfoot. Lateral posting of a valgus forefoot can decrease the varus moment transferred to the hindfoot.[28] A wedge insole also has the potential to affect other more proximal joints along the kinetic chain, such as a lateral wedge insole to unload medial knee osteoarthritis.[29]

ORTHOSES

An orthosis is a device used to support, align, prevent, or correct deformities or to improve functions of body motion. A basic understanding of the terminology and the clinical applications of orthoses ensures effective fabrication and biomechanical accuracy. Although much of this is based on clinical diagnosis and patient feedback, as discussed in a 2021 study new technology including computerized analysis with three-dimensional limb scanners has proved beneficial.[30] A foot orthosis extends from the heel to the forefoot area, whereas an ankle-foot orthosis (AFO) extends above the ankle joint. The goal is to alter the biomechanics or to achieve comfort and protection by offloading certain areas and distributing weight to a broader surface area. An orthosis can be designated as accommodative, supportive, or corrective. An accommodative orthosis is generally made of softer material shaped much like the patient's native anatomy to

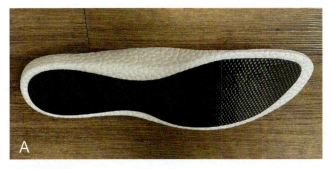
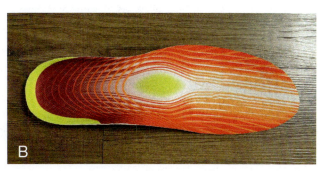

FIGURE 6 **A** and **B**, Photographs showing commercially available insoles that can be inserted into footwear for treatment of certain pathology or to enhance the exercise experience.

more evenly distribute weight along the plantar surface of the foot for cushioning and pressure relief. A supportive orthosis may be used to help stabilize a flexible deformity such as a flexible flatfoot treated with an arch support. A corrective orthosis is manufactured to intentionally alter alignment with anatomy deviation. Molded thermoplastic is a popular material used to provide and preserve the shape of an orthosis.

When writing an orthosis prescription, it also helps if the clinician designates the length of the desired orthosis. A full-length orthosis extends to the tip of the toes, a sulcus-length orthosis extends to the base of the toes, and a three-quarter–length orthosis ends proximal to the metatarsal heads. Ankle and hindfoot pathology may often be managed with a three-quarter–length orthosis. However, when forefoot pathology exists or when forefoot posting is desired, a full-length or sulcus-length orthosis is most effective. Sometimes when pathology is primarily localized to the midfoot

or hindfoot, it may be even more effective to extend the orthosis above the ankle. This can be done using an articulation, which allows sagittal ankle motion while decreasing varus and valgus forces. An articulated AFO may be beneficial for treatment of tendon pathology such as posterior tibial tendinitis or peroneal tendon dysfunction.[31]

A nonarticulated or solid-ankle AFO more completely immobilizes the ankle and can be used for ankle arthritis treatment. A dorsal wrap across the midfoot can be incorporated on the AFO to add rotational control for additional stability of the midfoot and hindfoot. An articulated AFO with a dorsal midfoot wrap will preserve ankle motion but also decrease rotational stresses contributing to pain from subtalar or midfoot arthritis. An AFO allows patient-specific customization, although noncustomized braces are readily available for some pathologies. Common AFO modifications are listed in **Table 3**.

Table 3

Ankle-Foot Orthosis Types and Modifications

Solid-ankle AFO	Trim lines fully enclose the malleoli to substantially decrease mobilization of the foot and ankle complex
Semisolid-ankle AFO	Trim lines enclose the posterior soft tissues but do not project anteriorly along the malleoli; allows limited ankle motion with weight bearing but dampens ground reaction forces
Posterior leaf spring AFO	Trim lines are narrow posteriorly and flexible to allow weight-bearing motion; retains shape memory to assist in dorsiflexion during swing phase
Articulated AFO	Foot and leg segments connected by an articulating mechanism aligned with the axis of the ankle to allow controlled sagittal motion. The hinge can be modified to restrict or assist in certain motions
Wrap-around AFO	Completely encloses the foot, ankle, and lower leg; maximizes skin contact area and may more effectively maintain desired alignment
Double upright AFO	Often attaches to the exterior of the shoe; skin contact is avoided; may be desirable for patients with swelling or skin breakdown
Carbon-fiber AFO	Many of the same designs and functions of plastic AFOs; carbon decreases bulk and returns recoil energy to the patient during gait
Post	Wedge under the medial or lateral forefoot to bring the floor up to a varus or valgus deformity or used in the hindfoot medially or laterally to tilt the heel
Cutout	Well, recess, or depression that can be used to unload a specific area
Lift	Generally used as a neutral heel wedge to lift the heel and relax the Achilles tendon
Cushion	Foam or other soft material used plantarly to relieve plantar pressure
Extension	Rigid lengthening of the sole to the tips of the toes to decrease bending forces of the midfoot and forefoot
Flange	Semirigid rim or lip extension on the orthosis to help support a certain area such as a collapsed arch
Metatarsal bar	Pad placed proximal to the metatarsal heads to unload plantar pressure at the area distal to the pad

AFO = ankle-foot orthosis

In a systematic review of 11 randomized controlled trials, it was reported that custom foot orthoses may produce clinically important improvements.[32] Custom foot orthoses appeared to be slightly beneficial in juvenile idiopathic arthritis, rheumatoid arthritis, pes cavus, and hallux valgus deformities. However, surgical treatment was reported to be more beneficial for hallux valgus deformities, and prefabricated orthoses were just as effective as custom orthoses for juvenile idiopathic arthritis.[32,33] A separate report found no difference in progression of the hallux valgus deformity with or without an orthosis.[34] A meta-analysis and a separate randomized controlled trial on the use of foot orthoses for the treatment of plantar fasciitis reported that custom and prefabricated orthoses were equally effective in diminishing pain.[35,36] When a foot orthosis is combined with a rocker bottom sole, it may be more effective in reducing plantar fasciitis pain.[37] A study on the use of nighttime AFOs in treating plantar fasciitis pain reported that an anterior orthosis was more comfortable and more effectively decreased pain than a posterior orthosis.[38]

A foot orthosis may have a positive effect on chronically unstable ankles because it influences multiple levels of somatosensory feedback and neuromuscular control.[39] A cavus foot orthosis that included a recess at the first metatarsal head and a ramp (post) at the lateral forefoot was effective in reducing ankle instability by decreasing forefoot-driven hindfoot varus. In an evaluation of flexible severe flatfoot treated with foot orthoses, the authors randomized 160 children to control, custom orthosis, and prefabricated orthosis treatment groups.[40] At 3- and 12-month follow-up, motor proficiency, self-perception, exercise efficiency, and pain were evaluated, and the authors found no evidence to justify the use of orthoses. The consideration of soft insoles with an elastic support orthosis in patients who find it comfortable and supportive may be the most practical, as discussed in a 2021 study.[41] In a meta-analysis of foot orthoses for lower limb overuse conditions,[42] no difference in custom versus prefabricated orthoses was seen. Although an orthosis appears to help prevent a first incidence of an overuse condition, little evidence supports therapeutic effectiveness after the overuse condition has developed.

Investigators looked at 25 feet and ankles with Charcot arthropathy in an attempt to identify an alternative to the Charcot Restraint Orthotic Walker and total-contact casting.[43] They reported that a prefabricated pneumatic removable walker brace (Aircast) fitted with a custom insole can successfully be used to manage Charcot arthropathy. The brace was an effective immobilizer during healing and was associated with a high satisfaction rate and safety profile.

Prefabricated walking boots or controlled ankle motion boots are often prescribed for foot and ankle patients in the immediate postinjury or postoperative period. Although therapeutic on the braced extremity, this may result in limb-length discrepancy, with gait deviations leading to pain in other joints or the lower back. The EVENup Shoe Lift was designed to eliminate the gait disturbance from the boot by applying more thickness to the shoe sole of the uninjured limb. In a group of patients undergoing unilateral lower extremity orthopaedic care, clinically relevant differences were found between the EVENup intervention group and the control group[44] (**Figure 7**).

Military combat injuries have been characterized by high-energy explosive wound patterns to the extremities. Surgical advances and rehabilitation programs have been developed to pursue limb salvage. The Intrepid Dynamic Exoskeletal Orthosis (IDEO, TechLink) was created to improve functional capabilities of the limb-salvage wounded warrior population and to be used in a high-intensity rehabilitation program known as the Return to Run clinical pathway. The IDEO is a custom AFO in which a proximal patella-bearing clamshell cuff helps offload the extremity and the foot-plate limits extremes of ankle motion. The IDEO's plantar flexion design shape and

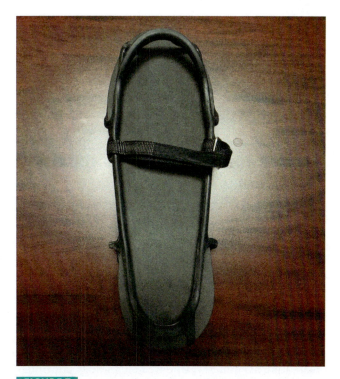

FIGURE 7 Photograph showing an orthotic shoe lift to provide equilibrium for patients wearing a boot on the contralateral extremity.

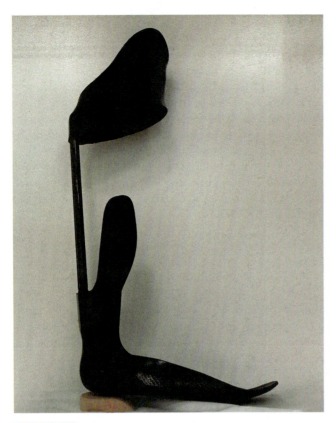

FIGURE 8 Photograph of an energy-storing orthosis commonly used in military veteran amputees.

carbon-fiber material store and deliver energy that simulates plantar flexion power. Researchers evaluated participants' functional performance in the IDEO and soldiers had improvements in multiple functional tests. After completion of the Return to Run clinical pathway with utilization of the IDEO, 70% of those who initially desired amputation chose to keep their limb, as discussed in a 2022 study[45] (Figure 8).

SUMMARY

Patients with painful lower extremity conditions and especially those who are poor surgical candidates may experience symptomatic relief with an orthosis, brace, or shoe modification. Basic knowledge of bracing treatment allows the clinician to accurately communicate goals to an orthotist. Some patients will inevitably opt for surgical intervention as wearing a brace can change walking speed, step length, and cadence and create limb asymmetry. Updated technology continues to be studied and incorporated into shoes and orthoses to further optimize safety, function, and patient satisfaction.

KEY STUDY POINTS

- A concerted effort including the patient, physician, and orthotist will ensure an effective bracing algorithm.
- Commercial footwear may be engineered with sport-specific purpose and therapeutic features incorporated into the overall design.
- Scientific evidence is limited and both risks and benefits exist to new running styles such as barefoot-style or maximalist cushioned running.
- An evolution to the final orthotic product is based on clinical examination and diagnosis coupled with feedback from the patient and global treatment team.
- Commercially available insoles, custom insoles, and orthoses extending above the ankle all have efficacy with purposeful utilization in the appropriate patient subsets.

ANNOTATED REFERENCES

1. Cranage S, Perraton L, Bowles KA, Williams C: The impact of shoe flexibility on gait, pressure and muscle activity of young children. A systematic review. *J Foot Ankle Res* 2019;12(1):55.

   Shod subjects showed increased step length and time in comparison with barefoot walkers. Level of evidence: II.

2. Hemler SL, Sider JR, Redfern MS, Beschorner KE: Gait kinetics impact shoe tread wear rate. *Gait Posture* 2021;86:157-161.

   A person's gait kinetics is related to the wear patterns on shoes. Level of evidence: I.

3. Enke RC, Laskowski ER, Thomsen KM: Running shoe selection criteria among adolescent cross-country runners. *PM R* 2009;1(9):816-819.

4. Jastifer J, Kent R, Crandall J, et al: The athletic shoe in football. *Sports Health* 2017;9(2):126-131.

5. Kent R, Forman JL, Lessley D, Crandall J: The mechanics of American football cleats on natural grass and infill-type artificial playing surfaces with loads relevant to elite athletes. *Sports Biomech* 2015;14(2):246-257.

6. Nagano H, Begg R: Shoe-insole technology for injury prevention in walking. *Sensors* 2018;18(5):1468.

7. Lieberman DE, Venkadesan M, Werbel WA, et al: Foot strike patterns and collision forces in habitually barefoot versus shod runners. *Nature* 2010;463(7280):531-535.

8. Szulc P, Waszak M, Bartkowiak M, et al: Distribution of plantar pressure during jogging barefoot or in minimalistic shoes in people who used to run in cushioned shoes. *J Sports Med Phys Fitness* 2017;57(5):565-571.

9. Roth J, Neumann J, Tao M: Orthopaedic perspective on barefoot and minimalist running. *J Am Acad Orthop Surg* 2016;24(3):180-187.

10. Squadrone R, Gallozzi C: Effect of a five-toed minimal protection shoe on static and dynamic ankle position sense. *J Sports Med Phys Fitness* 2011;51(3):401-408.

11. Hsu AR: Topical review: Barefoot running. *Foot Ankle Int* 2012;33(9):787-794.

12. Johnson AW, Myrer JW, Mitchell UH, Hunter I, Ridge ST: The effects of a transition to minimalist shoe running on intrinsic foot muscle size. *Int J Sports Med* 2016;37(2):154-158.

13. Altman AR, Davis IS: Prospective comparison of running injuries between shod and barefoot runners. *Br J Sports Med* 2016;50(8):476-480.

14. Snow NJ, Basset FA, Byrne J: An acute bout of barefoot running alters lower-limb muscle activation for minimalist shoe users. *Int J Sports Med* 2016;37(5):382-387.

15. Sobhani S, Bredeweg S, Dekker R, et al: Rocker shoe, minimalist shoe, and standard running shoe: A comparison of running economy. *J Sci Med Sport* 2014;17(3):312-316.

16. Ramanathan AK, Parish EJ, Arnold GP, Drew TS, Wang W, Abboud RJ: The influence of shoe sole's varying thickness on lower limb muscle activity. *Foot Ankle Surg* 2011;17(4):218-223.

17. Hannigan J, Pollard CD: Differences in running biomechanics between a maximal, traditional, and minimal running shoe. *J Sci Med Sport* 2020;23(1):15-19.

    Eversion mechanics in maximal shoes could place runners at increased risk for injury; however, more research is needed. Level of evidence: I.

18. Rodrigo-Carranza V, González-Mohíno F, Santos Del Cerro J, Santos-Concejero J, González-Ravé JM: Influence of advanced shoe technology on the top 100 annual performances in men's marathon from 2015 to 2019. *Sci Rep* 2021;11(1):22458.

    The new advanced shoe technology affected marathon runner's performances despite changes in environment, and runner orography, age, and birthplace. Level of evidence: I.

19. Kim Y, Lim JM, Yoon B: Changes in ankle range of motion and muscle strength in habitual wearers of high-heeled shoes. *Foot Ankle Int* 2013;34(3):414-419.

20. Hong WH, Lee YH, Lin YH, Tang SF, Chen HC: Effect of shoe heel height and total-contact insert on muscle loading and foot stability while walking. *Foot Ankle Int* 2013;34(2):273-281.

21. Janisse DJ, Janisse E: Shoe modification and the use of orthoses in the treatment of foot and ankle pathology. *J Am Acad Orthop Surg* 2008;16(3):152-158.

22. Chapman GJ, Halstead J, Redmond AC: Comparability of off the shelf foot orthoses in the redistribution of forces in midfoot osteoarthritis patients. *Gait Posture* 2016;49:235-240.

23. Flores N, Rao G, Berton E, Delattre N: The stiff plate location into the shoe influences the running biomechanics. *Sports Biomech* 2019;20(7):815-830.

    High stiff plate location decreased all the lower limb joint torques and work at the knee. Level of evidence: I.

24. Arazpour M, Hutchins SW, Ghomshe FT, Shaky F, Karami MV, Aksenov AY: Effects of the heel-to-toe rocker sole on walking in able-bodied persons. *Prosthet Orthot Int* 2013;37(6):429-435.

25. Lin SC, Chen CP, Tang SF, Wong AM, Hsieh JH, Chen WP: Changes in windlass effect in response to different shoe and insole designs during walking. *Gait Posture* 2013;37(2):235-241.

26. Bus SA, Maas JC, Otterman NM: Lower-extremity dynamics of walking in neuropathic diabetic patients who wear a forefoot-offloading shoe. *Clin Biomech (Bristol, Avon)* 2017;50:21-26.

27. Shih YF, Wen YK, Chen WY: Application of wedged foot orthosis effectively reduces pain in runners with pronated foot: A randomized clinical study. *Clin Rehabil* 2011;25(10):913-923.

28. LoPiccolo M, Chilvers M, Graham B, Manoli A II: Effectiveness of the cavus foot orthosis. *J Surg Orthop Adv* 2010;19(3):166-169.

29. Tezcan ME, Goker B, Lidtke R, Block JA: Long-term effects of lateral wedge orthotics on hip and ankle joint space widths. *Gait Posture* 2017;51:36-40.

30. Powers OA, Palmer JR, Wilken JM: Reliability and validity of 3D limb scanning for ankle-foot orthosis fitting. *Prosthet Orthot Int* 2021;46(1):84-90.

    Low-cost three-dimensional scanning can be used for reliable AFO fitting. Level of evidence: II.

31. Kulig K, Reischl SF, Pomrantz AB, et al: Nonsurgical management of posterior tibial tendon dysfunction with orthoses and resistive exercise: A randomized controlled trial. *Phys Ther* 2009;89(1):26-37.

32. Hawke F, Burns J, Radford JA, du Toit V: Custom-made foot orthoses for the treatment of foot pain. *Cochrane Database Syst Rev* 2008;(3):CD006801.

33. Hawke F, Burns J: Brief report: Custom foot orthoses for foot pain. What does the evidence say? *Foot Ankle Int* 2012;33(12):1161-1163.

34. Reina M, Lafuente G, Munuera PV: Effect of custom-made foot orthoses in female hallux valgus after one-year follow-up. *Prosthet Orthot Int* 2013;37(2):113-119.

35. Anderson J, Stanek J: Effect of foot orthoses as treatment for plantar fasciitis or heel pain. *J Sport Rehabil* 2013;22(2):130-136.

36. Baldassin V, Gomes CR, Beraldo PS: Effectiveness of prefabricated and customized foot orthoses made from low-cost foam for noncomplicated plantar fasciitis: A randomized controlled trial. *Arch Phys Med Rehabil* 2009;90(4):701-706.

37. Fong DT, Pang KY, Chung MM, Hung AS, Chan KM: Evaluation of combined prescription of rocker sole shoes and custom-made foot orthoses for the treatment of plantar fasciitis. *Clin Biomech (Bristol, Avon)* 2012;27(10):1072-1077.

38. Attard J, Singh D: A comparison of two night ankle-foot orthoses used in the treatment of inferior heel pain: A preliminary investigation. *Foot Ankle Surg* 2012;18(2):108-110.

39. Richie DH Jr: Effects of foot orthoses on patients with chronic ankle instability. *J Am Podiatr Med Assoc* 2007;97(1):19-30.

40. Whitford D, Esterman A: A randomized controlled trial of two types of in-shoe orthoses in children with flexible excess pronation of the feet. *Foot Ankle Int* 2007;28(6):715-723.

41. Hoyt BW, Nelson SY, Fay JG, Wade SM, Brooks DI, Potter BK: IDEO energy-storing orthosis: Effects on lower extremity function and preservation. *Injury* 2021;52(11):3505-3510.

    Patients with footdrop or weakness are more likely to continue IDEO brace use than those with a previous fusion. Level of evidence: III.

42. Collins N, Bisset L, McPoil T, Vicenzino B: Foot orthoses in lower limb overuse conditions: A systematic review and meta-analysis. *Foot Ankle Int* 2007;28(3):396-412.

43. Verity S, Sochocki M, Embil JM, Trepman E: Treatment of Charcot foot and ankle with a prefabricated removable walker brace and custom insole. *Foot Ankle Surg* 2008;14(1):26-31.

44. Kipp D, Village D, Edwards KJ: Effectiveness of Evenup™ shoe-lift use among individuals prescribed a walking boot. *J Allied Health* 2017;46(2):104-110.

45. Kudo S, Sakamoto K: Influence of a novel elastic foot orthosis in foot motion during locomotion in adults with mild flatfoot. *Gait Posture* 2022;93:59-63.

    The elastic foot orthosis brace decreased foot strain and may help support the arch during movement. Level of evidence: II.

CHAPTER 3

Imaging Studies of the Foot and Ankle

DANIEL J. FUCHS, MD, FAAOS • STEVEN M. RAIKIN, MD, FAAOS

ABSTRACT

Multiple imaging modalities are implemented to evaluate patients with foot and ankle pathology. The diagnostic imaging evaluation typically starts with weight-bearing radiographs of the foot and/or ankle if the patient is able to bear weight. Advanced imaging is obtained based on the specific anatomic region and pathologic condition being evaluated. Available modalities include MRI, CT, ultrasonography, tenography, and nuclear medicine studies. CT is often used to better evaluate osseous detail, whereas MRI is used to evaluate soft-tissue structures or to identify occult injuries. The most recent innovations of these advanced imaging methods include weight-bearing CT, single photon emission computed tomography, and cartilage mapping MRI. Clinical indications for these newer imaging methods are currently being defined.

Keywords: CT; MRI; radiography; SPECT-CT; weight bearing

INTRODUCTION

Imaging studies are an integral component of the clinical evaluation of a patient with a condition affecting the foot or ankle. After completion of a careful history and physical examination, imaging studies usually are

Neither of the following authors nor any immediate family member has received anything of value from or has stock or stock options held in a commercial company or institution related directly or indirectly to the subject of this chapter: Dr. Fuchs and Dr. Raikin.

performed as the next step in determining a diagnosis and treatment plan. Each of the available imaging modalities has appropriate indications and applications.

PLAIN RADIOGRAPHY

Plain radiography is the foundation of most diagnostic foot and ankle imaging. Bone anatomy, integrity, and alignment as well as joint congruency can be assessed through a routine set of radiographs, which usually can be obtained during the patient's initial office visit. Weight-bearing radiographs must be obtained whenever possible. Although a patient with an acute traumatic injury may only tolerate non–weight-bearing radiography to assess structural anatomy and rule out the presence of fracture, these radiographs do not show the foot or ankle in a loaded, physiologic position. They therefore may not facilitate detection of malalignment or some pathologic conditions.

The popularity of digital radiology has eclipsed that of printed radiographic studies. Radiographs are captured digitally in two ways.[1] CT is affordable, offers excellent image quality, and uses existing radiography systems. True digital radiography requires more expensive technology than traditional radiography or computerized modification but offers greater efficiency and the capacity for higher image quality and a lower radiation dosage. Images are stored in a picture archiving and communication system rather than on hard-copy radiograph. The most commonly used format for medical images is Digital Imaging and Communication in Medicine, which allows safe, high-quality off-site viewing and analysis of radiographs. Digital radiography also allows computer-assisted measurements of distances or angles to be generated for use in diagnosing pathologic foot and ankle conditions. An additional advantage is production of grayscale inverted images, which have been shown in a 2022 study to be useful in evaluating fractures about the ankle.[2]

The Foot

Routine radiography of the foot includes the AP, lateral, and oblique views. The internal (medial) oblique view usually is part of the routine three-view set and is useful for showing the lateral tarsometatarsal joints and detecting a possible calcaneonavicular coalition. The external (lateral) oblique view should be ordered to more clearly show perinavicular joints or identify an accessory navicular bone.

In specific circumstances, other views can be used to obtain additional information about the bony anatomy. The sesamoid axial projection can reveal sesamoid-metatarsal arthritis, fracture or osteonecrosis of the hallux sesamoids, or sesamoid alignment relative to the crista on the plantar aspect of the metatarsal head. The calcaneal axial (Harris-Beath) view is obtained at a 45° angle from posterior to proximal. This view allows analysis of the posterior and middle facet of the subtalar joint to detect arthritis or a tarsal coalition. The Broden views are a sequence of angled radiographs centered over the sinus tarsi and taken at 10° to 40° of cephalic tilt. These views reliably show the posterior facet of the subtalar joint in calcaneal fracture management or subtalar fusion. The talar neck view provides a true AP view and is useful in assessing talar neck fractures. This view is obtained with the foot internally rotated 15° and the beam angled 15° cephalad while centered over the talar neck.

The Ankle

A three-view weight-bearing set of radiographs is routinely recommended for analysis of the ankle, including the AP, lateral, and mortise views. For the AP view, the ankle mortise is aligned in approximately 20° of external rotation relative to the sagittal plane. A true mortise view, in which the x-ray beam is oriented perpendicular to the intermalleolar axis, is therefore obtained with the leg internally rotated. This view allows the best assessment of mortise congruity and the talar dome.

Several ankle-specific views also are used to evaluate the ankle joint. The 50° external rotation view is optimal for the detection of posterior malleolar fracture fragments. The hindfoot alignment view, often referred to as the Saltzman view, is obtained with the patient standing on a raised platform and the x-ray beam directed from behind and angled 20° caudally, with the cassette placed perpendicular to the beam.

Stress views are often used to assess ankle instability. While a lateral radiograph is being obtained, an anterior drawer test is performed (the evaluator's hands are protected by lead gloves, or a mechanical jig is used). Anterior displacement of the talus of more than 10 mm (or greater than 5 mm more than that seen when stressing the uninvolved ankle) is consistent with lateral ankle ligament dysfunction. Similarly, varus or valgus stress radiographs are used to assess the integrity of the lateral ligament complex or deltoid ligament, respectively. A 10° difference in the talar tilt of the injured and normal extremities is considered pathologic. However, the reliability and reproducibility of stress testing is questionable because of the wide variation in test findings in normal ankles and healthy patients, tester-dependent variation in forces applied against the ankle, and variation in patients' resistance to the force. Therefore, the results of stress testing alone should not determine the treatment of ankle instability.

Fluoroscopy has become a vital tool for assessing joint or bone alignment and positioning internal hardware during surgery. Technical advances have resulted in great improvement in fluoroscopic image quality as well as the size and ease of handling of the machine. The small C-arm units used by many foot and ankle surgeons expose the surgical team and patient to minimal radiation (outside of the direct path of the beam).[3] Multidimensional fluoroscopy has recently been evaluated in assessing intraoperative reduction and fixation of the ankle syndesmosis and calcaneus fractures. Use of this imaging modality results in adjustment of reduction or implants in approximately 50% of cases; however, as discussed in a 2021 study, surgical time is increased, and improved clinical outcomes have not been demonstrated.[4]

Radiographic Measurements

Many radiographic measurements have been described for evaluating the alignment of the foot and ankle, several of which are particularly important. Computer-assisted measurement of digital radiographs has resulted in improved accuracy. A smartphone goniometer application is extremely accurate for measuring certain angles.[5] All measurements are most accurate if based on weight-bearing radiographs.

The hallux valgus angle and the first–second intermetatarsal angles are the mainstay measurements for assessing the severity of hallux valgus deformity. These measurements have good intraobserver and interobserver reliability when standard methods are used. The first and second metatarsal axes are each drawn by connecting the midpoint of the shaft of the metatarsal 2 cm from the proximal and distal articular surfaces. The axis of the phalanx is drawn through the shaft midpoints 0.5 cm from each of its articulations. The hallux valgus interphalangeal angle is drawn between the phalangeal axis of the proximal and distal phalanges of the hallux. The distal metatarsal articular angle is the angle subtended by a line drawn perpendicular to the long axis of the first metatarsal and a line corresponding to the distal articular surface of the first metatarsal. Compared with the hallux valgus and first–second intermetatarsal angle, the distal metatarsal articular angle is less reliable and reproducible for determining joint congruency.[6] These measurements can be computer enhanced, but this step usually is not necessary.

The talus–first metatarsal angle, also called the Meary angle, is drawn through the long axes of the talus and the first metatarsal on the lateral radiograph. This angle is useful for assessing arch height and recently was found to be reliable for measuring adult flatfoot deformity.[7] The talonavicular coverage angle measures the lateral subluxation of the navicular at the talar head or the extent to which the talar head is uncovered, and it is useful for evaluating forefoot abduction in pes planovalgus deformities. On a weight-bearing AP radiograph of the foot, a line is created joining the two ends of the articular surface of the talar head, and another line joins the matching two ends of the joint surface of the navicular. The angle created by perpendicular lines drawn from the midpoints of each of these two lines is the talonavicular coverage angle; a normal value is less than 7°.

TENOGRAPHY

Plain radiographs can be used to observe secondary changes caused by tendon dysfunction but cannot be used to evaluate the tendons themselves. Tenography involves the injection of contrast material into the tendon sheath under fluoroscopy, often followed by a steroid injection. Tenosynovitis, stenosing tenosynovitis, and a tendon tear or rupture can be seen. Tenography can be particularly useful in a posttraumatic setting in which the value of other diagnostic modalities is limited by the presence of anatomic deformity or associated hardware (eg, in peroneal impingement after calcaneal fracture).[8] In the absence of a tendon tear, intrasheath steroid injection with tenography relieves symptoms in some patients with tenosynovitis around the foot and ankle.[9] This cost-effective but invasive technique is associated with a small risk of tendon rupture. Tenography has been less frequently used for diagnostic purposes since the widespread adoption of MRI.

ULTRASONOGRAPHY

Ultrasonographic evaluation of tendons around the foot and ankle offers several advantages over other modalities. Ultrasonography is cost effective, safe, noninvasive, and not based on radiation. Structures are evaluated in real time. Dynamic evaluation of tendon function allows conditions such as peroneal subluxation or dislocation to be directly visualized. The transducer can be manipulated to avoid interference from any metallic implant in the ankle. This ability is useful in evaluating tendon injury after hardware placement in the foot or ankle, which would create interference during MRI. Ultrasonography also avoids the possibility of the so-called magic angle phenomenon on MRI (artifact seen in tendons oriented 54.7° to the magnetic field), which can inaccurately suggest the presence of intratendinous pathology. Ultrasonography is slightly less sensitive than MRI for use in diagnosing tibialis posterior tendon pathology, but a study found that discrepancies did not result in altered clinical management.[10] Ultrasonography has high sensitivity and specificity for detecting peroneal tendon tears and 100% positive predictive value for detecting peroneal subluxation, as correlated with intraoperative findings.[11]

For evaluating tears in the lateral ankle ligaments, ultrasonography has sensitivity and specificity comparable to that of MRI. Morton neuroma, recurrent interdigital neuroma, and other soft-tissue masses or cysts can be detected on ultrasonography after an equivocal clinical evaluation.

Most modern ultrasonography machines are able to evaluate regional blood flow. The movement of blood cells within the vessels causes a change in the pitch of reflected sound waves called the Doppler effect. A computer converts the Doppler sounds into colors that are overlaid on the musculoskeletal ultrasonographic image. The presence of local hyperemia secondary to inflammation can confirm that the ultrasonographic findings are consistent with the pathology or symptoms.

The primary disadvantage of ultrasonography is that it is a technician-dependent modality. Many medical centers lack a radiologist trained and experienced in interpreting the results of musculoskeletal ultrasonographic studies. Additionally, ultrasonography offers only poor visualization of bone. Because direct skin contact and the application of gel are required, ultrasonography cannot be used through a cast or splint.

Recent advances in technology have led to improvements in the quality, portability, and cost of ultrasonography machines, and office-based ultrasonography is now feasible. To complement the clinical examination and standard radiographic evaluation, a diagnostic ultrasonographic examination can be performed during the patient's initial visit to the foot and ankle surgeon. Ultrasonography can be particularly useful in making a subtle diagnosis and planning treatment; for example, a determination that the patient has a Morton neuroma in the second web space rather than early plantar plate dysfunction precludes the use of a cortisone injection, which can cause metatarsophalangeal instability.[12] In-office ultrasonography also can be used to identify tendinosis, a tendon injury around the foot and ankle, a mass or tumor, or a nonradiopaque foreign body such as a wood splinter. Ultrasonography can be used to improve the accuracy of diagnostic injections in the foot or ankle, guide injections for a condition such as Morton neuroma or plantar fasciitis, and guide the aspiration of cysts. The use of ultrasonography was found to improve the accuracy and outcome of therapeutic injections and thereby reduce the need for additional procedures.[13]

COMPUTED TOMOGRAPHY

CT provides high-resolution thin-slice studies of the foot and ankle. The development and implementation of multidetector-row slip-ring technology has resulted in improved imaging of osseous structures. Source images acquired in the axial, coronal, or sagittal plane allow three-dimensional views of the bony anatomy for diagnosis and therapeutic planning. Relatively new computer software creates multiplane reconstructions without increasing the patient's exposure to ionizing radiation; for example, coronal images can be constructed from axial images, and three-dimensional reconstruction models can be created from the initial source images (**Figure 1**). Around the foot and ankle, studies with 3-mm or thinner slices are routinely recommended. The foot position in the scanner is important because the source image planes are obtained parallel to the osseous structures of the foot in each plane using a tomographic scout localizer image. The presence of cast or splinting material around the region does not interfere with CT but may create difficulty in positioning the foot. The advent of multidetector-row systems has permitted rapid image acquisition and high-quality three-dimensional reconstruction to be achieved with decreased radiation dosages.

In the foot and ankle, CT is most commonly used to assess bony abnormalities and is particularly useful in providing fine osseous detail not obtainable with plain radiography. Fracture, infection, osteochondral injury

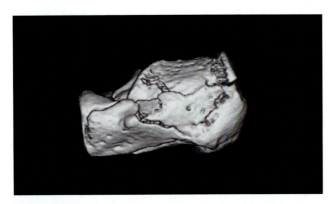

FIGURE 1 Three-dimensional CT showing a calcaneus fracture. Three-dimensional images are particularly useful in preoperative planning.

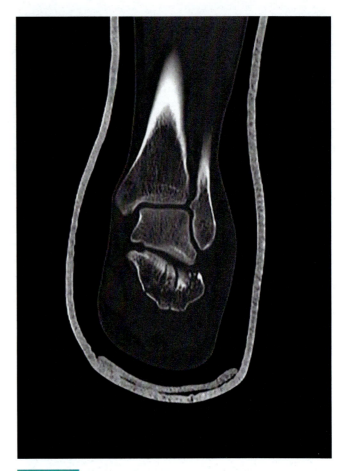

FIGURE 2 Coronal CT showing a comminuted intra-articular calcaneus fracture.

(requiring accurate assessment of the bony anatomy and lesion size), arthritis, osteonecrosis, and osseous tumor or congenital abnormality can be diagnosed using CT. This is particularly useful in suspected subtle fracture, joint diastasis, or articular incongruity not detectable on plain radiography, as in suspected Lisfranc injuries, syndesmotic injuries, and tibial plafond fractures. In addition, CT can be used to assess the extent of joint comminution in calcaneal or plafond fractures and to assist in preoperative planning (**Figure 2**).

CT has high accuracy and sensitivity for the detection of fracture nonunion and quantifying the percentage of bony union in certain fractures such as talus neck fractures. CT is more reliable than serial radiographic studies for assessing the extent of union after surgical arthrodesis[14] (**Figure 3**). The use of micro-CT and nano-CT technology is likely to further enhance the accuracy of this modality. The interpretation of postoperative CT can be negatively influenced by metallic artifact or scatter from internal hardware. Relatively new software uses metal deletion techniques to limit this effect and improve the accuracy of study interpretation.

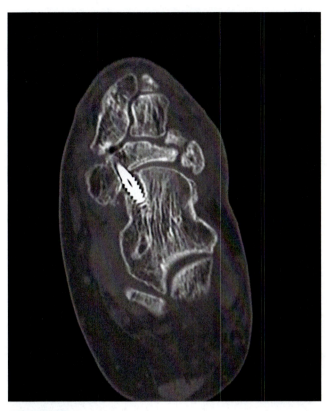

FIGURE 3 Axial CT showing nonunion after an attempted talonavicular arthrodesis.

Current CT scanners use multidetector configurations in which a narrow, fan-shaped x-ray beam and a detector rotate around the patient to quickly acquire multiple image sections. This technology cannot be used with the patient in a weight-bearing stance, as is needed to evaluate extremity alignment and deformity during physiologic loading. Axial loads can be applied to joints to simulate weight bearing when the patient is supine, but the resulting studies have questionable accuracy. The recently developed cone-beam CT technology uses a pyramid-shaped x-ray beam and a large-area detector to obtain volumetric data from multiple projections through a single rotation around the patient, who is in a standing, weight-bearing position.[15] The technique for image reconstruction is similar to that used for multidetector CT. The three-dimensional data obtained from cone-beam CT allow a much improved quantitative analysis of many pathologies. Other advantages of cone-beam CT over multidetector CT include more rapid acquisition of images, superior image quality, and lower radiation dosages (approximately 9 mGy compared with 27 to 40 mGy). The compact, portable design of the cone-beam CT machine has positive implications for workflow and storage. Cone-beam CT technology has the potential to be extremely valuable in musculoskeletal extremity imaging from both clinical and economic viewpoints.

Weight-bearing CT (WBCT) has recently become available for clinical use. This technology allows for three-dimensional imaging of the foot and ankle under the axial load of the patient's body weight. Various potential advantages of WBCT over non–weight-bearing CT have been proposed including the improved ability to evaluate deformity throughout the foot and ankle, determine the extent of joint space narrowing of arthritic joints, and assess for bony impingement that may only be radiographically apparent with weight bearing.[16] WBCT has been used as a research tool to define normal functional anatomic and physiologic relationships including the orientation of the subtalar joint, fibular rotation, and translation at the distal tibiofibular joint with tibiotalar motion and talus rotation within the ankle mortise with weight bearing.[17,18]

WBCT has produced interesting results on an investigational level. Although this technology has significant potential for clinical application, at this time those applications are still being defined. Few studies have shown clear benefit of WBCT over non–weight-bearing CT for specific indications. A systematic review of current literature on WBCT was performed and the utility of this technology for research as well as in clinical use to assist with assessment of foot alignment was acknowledged.[19] However, the authors of this study highlighted the need for standardization and validation of measurements performed using this technique. An updated 2020 review concluded that WBCT has useful clinical applications and is currently most applicable for assessment of adult-acquired flatfoot deformity and first metatarsal rotation in hallux valgus.[20] It was noted that at this time WBCT should not be used as a replacement for weight-bearing radiographs. An expert consensus statement on use of WBCT in progressive collapsing foot deformity also stated that WBCT should not replace weight-bearing radiographs but is strongly recommended if available.[21]

Algorithms have been developed to perform semiautomated measurements of WBCT data that reflect three-dimensional relationships. These may help define and enhance the clinical applicability of WBCT. Foremost among these is foot and ankle offset, which is used to measure the relationship between the weight-bearing tripod of the foot and the center of the ankle joint. Work has been done to prove high intraobserver and interobserver reliability of this measurement as well as correlation with two-dimensional manual WBCT measurements, physical examination, and clinical improvement in management of adult-acquired flatfoot deformity.[22-24]

NUCLEAR MEDICINE

Nuclear medicine studies involve the intravenous administration of a radioactive tracer and subsequent scanning with a gamma camera that detects a concentration of the tracer in the anatomic area of study. Conventional nuclear medicine studies of the musculoskeletal system (bone scans) involve the administration of technetium Tc-99m methylene diphosphonate, which binds to hydroxyapatite crystals during bone formation. Bone turnover caused by occult fracture, stress fracture, tumor, infection, or a metabolic disorder can be detected. Scanning is done in three phases. The first scan, the blood flow phase, is done within 1 minute of tracer administration to identify increased blood flow caused by inflammation. The second phase is obtained 5 minutes after tracer administration and detects blood pooling. The third, delayed phase is obtained 4 hours after injection of the tracer and detects bone turnover. The entire body can be scanned, or the scan can be restricted to pinhole views of the area of interest. Bone scans are highly sensitive but have poor specificity because many conditions affect blood flow and bone turnover. In some conditions, such as sympathetically mediated complex regional pain syndrome, increased tracer may appear in the affected area in all three phases of the study. It is important to note that bone scan results return to normal no earlier than 6 months after a fracture and that 10% of uncomplicated fractures still have increased local tracer uptake 2 years after the injury.[25]

Leukocyte labeling can be used to increase the specificity of bone scans for infection. Peripheral blood is aspirated from the patient, and the white blood cells are labeled with radioactive tracer several hours before scanning. The commonly used labels include technetium Tc-99m hexamethyl propylene amine oxide and indium-111 oxime. The advantages of labeling with technetium Tc-99m hexamethyl propylene amine oxide or technetium Tc-99m exametazime include a smaller radiation dosage and a shorter interval before scanning than required using indium-111 (4 hours compared with 24 hours). Delayed scanning identifies areas of increased leukocyte uptake, which signify inflammation or infection. Synchronous uptake in the same area on both a leukocyte-labeled and a standard three-phase bone scan specifically indicates bone activity caused by infection. To identify bone marrow infection, technetium Tc-99m sulfur colloid scanning is used. The addition of a leukocyte-labeled study increases the specificity of the study.

Positron emission tomography (PET) is a relatively new technique that usually involves intravenous injection of 18 fluorodeoxyglucose (FDG) followed by a scan for positron emission decay 1 hour later. In a study of patients with Charcot foot, FDG PET was found to exclude bone or soft-tissue infection in the presence of a foot ulcer with overall sensitivity of 100% and accuracy of 93.8%.[26] FDG PET also was found to be more accurate for diagnosing active chronic osteomyelitis than indium-111–labeled scanning.

Nuclear medicine imaging allows arterial limb perfusion to be assessed, particularly in the presence of calcified vessels that may have a spuriously elevated ankle-brachial index. Thallium-210 scanning detects deficiencies in muscle perfusion reserves and perfusion abnormalities in patients with asymptomatic diabetes who have clinically normal perfusion.[27] FDG PET accurately assesses the extent of atherosclerosis in the extremities of patients with diabetes.[28]

The combination of single photon emission computed tomography and CT (SPECT-CT) is a relatively new imaging modality in which highly detailed CT is analyzed with the functional information from a triple-phase radionuclide bone scan using a gamma camera.[29] SPECT-CT is not yet widely used but can enable detection of arthritis around the foot and particularly the differentiation of involved joints around the midfoot. In addition, SPECT-CT has potential in diagnosing clinically indeterminable soft-tissue impingement syndromes, excluding nonunion or arthritis seen on other radiographic modalities, and locating clinically relevant pathology in multifocal disease. Although some studies have supported the widespread use of SPECT-CT, most data do not justify its routine use.[29-31] Most recently, SPECT-CT has been used for the evaluation of painful

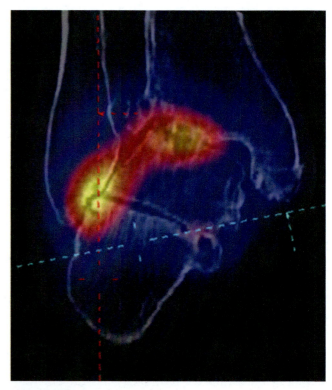

FIGURE 4 SPECT-CT demonstrating areas of lateral bony impingement in a valgus hindfoot.

total ankle arthroplasties. One study has shown that positive SPECT-CT uptake at the implant-bone interface is predictive of implant loosening; however, this study was a limited case series that included only eight patients with intraoperative findings to correlate with SPECT-CT.[32] In a 2020 study, SPECT-CT findings were confirmed by intraoperative evaluation in 26 of 28 cases of a painful total ankle arthroplasty, with aseptic loosening and impingement being the most frequent diagnoses.[33] Although larger series have been published in the knee and hip arthroplasty literature, the overall body of literature to support the routine use of SPECT-CT for painful total ankle arthroplasty or other conditions of the foot and ankle is lacking. SPECT-CT can also be useful in determining location of pain in both bone and soft tissue with higher anatomic locational accuracy than scintigraphy (**Figure 4**).

MAGNETIC RESONANCE IMAGING

Other than conventional radiography, MRI is the most frequently used modality for imaging the foot and ankle. MRI has the ability to evaluate bone, ligament, tendon, and muscle injuries about the foot and ankle, using a standard noncontrast protocol. Injury can be characterized based on known patterns of abnormal signal that indicate stress along a specific biomechanical axis. The advantages inherent to MRI in comparison with other imaging modalities include its multiplanar capabilities, sensitivity for both osseous and soft-tissue edema, and use of a magnetic field to generate images, without exposure of tissue to ionizing radiation. The disadvantages include its cost and the relatively long time period required for imaging. Some patients who have an implanted ferromagnetic device, such as a cardiac pacemaker, an automatic defibrillator, a biostimulator, an implanted infusion device, cerebral aneurysm clips, internal hearing aids, or metallic foreign bodies about the orbits, are not candidates for MRI. Many types of recently implanted medical devices and fixation hardware are nonferromagnetic, however, and thus are MRI compatible. Although the use of MRI in the foot and ankle has increased dramatically over the past decade, it is still not typically used as a first-line diagnostic modality. Most commonly, MRI of the foot and ankle is indicated if radiographic or CT findings are inconclusive or inconsistent with clinical symptoms, a primary soft-tissue process such as tendon or ligament dysfunction is suspected, or pain atypically persists during a treatment course.

MRI of the foot or ankle should include both fluid-sensitive (T2-weighted) and anatomy-specific (T1-weighted) sequences. Optimally, MRI of the foot or ankle should include at least two fat-suppressed sequences to maximize fluid sensitivity. MRI studies dedicated to the ankle should be distinct from those dedicated to the foot. Ankle MRI studies should begin proximal to the tibiotalar joint and proceed to the midfoot level, including the tibialis posterior and peroneus brevis insertions. In contrast, a foot MRI should begin at the talar head and proceed through the toes. All MRI protocols for imaging the ankle or foot should include three anatomic planes. At the ankle, the recommended protocols use two sagittal sequences, including one fluid-sensitive fat suppression sequence and one anatomy-specific sequence (T1-weighted spin-echo), as well as two axial sequences with similar parameters. A coronal fluid-sensitive sequence should be tailored to evaluate for potential osteochondral lesions at the tibiotalar joint. Acquisition of these five sequences can be accomplished on most systems in approximately 20 minutes. For MRI dedicated to the foot, optimal plane selection can be difficult because of varying definitions of terms such as coronal and axial; for this reason, descriptive terms are recommended for plane selection, including short axis, long axis, and sagittal. Both fluid-sensitive and anatomy-specific short-axis sequences (so-called bread slice sequences) should be acquired for showing metatarsal and intermetatarsal pathology. Inversion recovery sequences often provide the most homogeneous fat suppression in the sagittal plane, and a long axis fluid-sensitive sequence should be acquired along the metatarsals to simulate an AP radiographic view.

Intravenous gadolinium contrast occasionally is indicated in foot and ankle MRI. Precontrast and postcontrast imaging sequences are used in evaluating for a soft-tissue mass or osteomyelitis. Other relative indications for the use of intravenous contrast in foot or ankle MRI include inflammatory arthropathy, stenosing tenosynovitis, postoperative scarring, and intermetatarsal neuroma. Severe renal insufficiency is a relative contraindication for the use of a gadolinium-based contrast agent because of a suspected association with development of nephrogenic systemic fibrosis. An intra-articular contrast injection may prove useful as part of a dedicated arthrographic MRI protocol for a specific purpose, such as assessing the integrity of the lateral ankle ligaments or the stability of an osteochondral lesion.[34] The use of a circumferential receiver coil design, such as a head or an extremity coil, can be effective for generating adequate signal throughout the ankle or foot.

The use of one protocol with acquisition of images in a large field of view for both the foot and ankle is discouraged except for specific indications including complex regional pain syndrome. The patient history and clinical examination should allow the clinician to determine whether foot or ankle MRI is indicated. If injury affecting both the ankle and the forefoot is suspected, the use of two separate MRI protocols is recommended.

Numerous MRI system designs and field strengths are available, but some have limitations arising from patient characteristics such as claustrophobia and large body habitus. These factors usually do not need to be considered in imaging the foot or ankle. MRI should be acquired at standard or high field strength (1.5 or higher) to obtain adequate resolution of ligaments, tendons, and articular surfaces in the distal lower extremity. For the rare patient who cannot tolerate a standard closed 1.5-T MRI unit, a high-field-strength dedicated extremity system should be used in preference to a low-field-strength (0.2- or 0.3-T) open system.

Recent advances in ultra–high-field MRI, including 3-T units and high field strength, extremity-specific coils, have resulted in superior image quality and improvement in diagnostic accuracy.[35] Musculoskeletal structures exhibit a low signal-to-noise ratio at 1.5 T, but the ratio is almost doubled at 3 T. The application of relatively new techniques such as parallel acquisition improves both resolution and acquisition time; the decrease in imaging time is almost fourfold. Three-dimensional sequences obtained using a low-field scanner are characterized by a suboptimal signal-to-noise ratio and poor-contrast images that frequently are further degraded by artifacts. In comparison with 1.5-T imaging, 3-T imaging produces higher spatial resolution, smaller cut (almost halved) image thickness, and an increased contrast-to-noise ratio, which further improve the anatomic detail of the image.

Higher-Tesla MRI has the disadvantage of greater energy deposition, which can result in substantial artifacts, the most problematic of which are chemical shift and metal artifacts. Chemical shift artifact is noticeable at fat-water interfaces and particularly at bone-cartilage interfaces, where it may appear to represent abnormal cartilage thickness. Metal artifact is much more evident at 3 T than at 1.5 T, and it markedly degrades the image quality. Although techniques such as shortened echo time, parallel imaging with transmit-receive joint-specific multichannel coils, and widening of the receiver bandwidth can counteract the artifact effect, patients with implanted hardware in the field of view should undergo MRI with a 1.5-T magnet.

Some centers now offer 7-T MRI, which has been shown to further increase the signal-to-noise and contrast-to-noise ratios and thereby increase the accuracy of an ankle MRI evaluation.[36] These units are not yet widely available for clinical use, however. It is important to remember that regardless of field strength, MRI is limited by the quality and efficiency of the receiver coil. The use of a dedicated extremity coil or ankle coil is preferable for adequate MRI of the foot and ankle.

Osseous Injury

Displaced fractures most commonly are diagnosed using plain radiography or CT. In contrast, nondisplaced fractures and contusions about the foot and ankle can best be identified on MRI. Both types of fracture appear on fluid-sensitive, fat-suppressed MRI sequences as T2 hyperintense signal. The T2 hyperintense signal should be more focal and more intense in a fracture than in an osseous contusion, and it may have a linear morphology. Abnormal signal on T1-weighted sequences is characteristic of fractures and helps distinguish a fracture from a contusion. In a patient with known trauma, linear hypointense T1-weighted signal in the location of T2 hyperintensity can be interpreted as fracture with some certainty. Osteochondral impaction injury is characterized by abnormal T2 hyperintense and T1 hypointense signal extending in a sunburst pattern from an articular surface. The term osteochondral impaction injury is relatively nonspecific because in acute trauma a discrete osteochondral lesion can be difficult to distinguish from an osteochondral contusion.

MRI routinely is used for the diagnosis of osteochondral lesions or defects. Typical signal characteristics include a subchondral osseous T1 hypointense crescent (or a T2 hyperintense signal), which indicates fluid undercutting the bone fragment and implies instability (**Figure 5**). Osteochondral lesions on the talar dome are almost twice as likely to be medial (at the anterior to posterior equator) than lateral.[37] Medial talar dome lesions involve a larger surface area and tend to have deeper craniocaudal dimensions than their lateral counterparts. Less commonly, osteochondral lesions about the foot and ankle

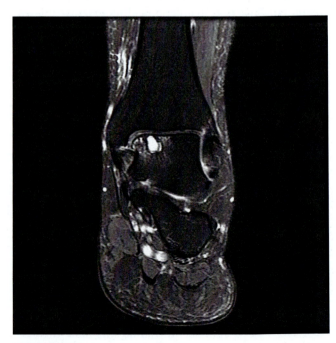

FIGURE 5 Coronal MRI of the ankle joint showing a type V osteochondral lesion of the medial talar dome (zone 4).

are located in the talar head, the tibial plafond, the calcaneocuboid joint, or the metatarsal heads. These lesions also can be effectively diagnosed with MRI.

Specific mechanisms of traumatic ankle and foot injuries often have a characteristic pattern of bony contusion on MRI. Analysis can result in a better understanding of the injury mechanism and diagnosis of associated soft-tissue injury. In an inversion ankle injury, the common locations of T2 hyperintense osseous contusions are the tip of the fibula, the entire medial malleolus, the anterior process and anterolateral body of the calcaneus, the talar neck or anteromedial talus extending to the middle subtalar joint, and the proximal cuboid at the calcaneocuboid articulation. An eversion injury causes bony contusion of the proximal aspect of the cuboid at the calcaneocuboid joint as well the malleoli. Bone marrow edema in the distal fibula tends to be diffuse and ill-defined, and bone marrow edema in the medial malleolus tends to be isolated to its tip, suggesting an avulsion injury.

MRI of the foot also is useful in assessing subtle bone injuries that can be difficult to detect with plain radiography alone. Bone contusion and osteochondral injury involving the distal articular surfaces of the cuneiforms and proximal articular surfaces of the metatarsals should increase suspicion for Lisfranc ligament injury. MRI is extremely sensitive for acute nondisplaced or stress fractures of the metatarsals, which are easily identified on short-axis sequences through the forefoot, where they appear as diffuse abnormal medullary T2 hyperintensity. Plantar plate injury can be diagnosed on MRI by identifying T2 hyperintensity within the metatarsal head and a breach in the soft-tissue structures intimately plantar to the plantar aspect of each metatarsal head. Osseous injury of the first metatarsophalangeal sesamoids can be identified on MRI and characterized as fracture, contusion, or osteonecrosis.

Ligamentous Injury

Normal ligaments should appear hypointense or dark on all MRI sequences. In an acute sprain, ligaments have poor definition as well as periligamentous fluid signal. Diffuse enlargement, attenuation, or complete disruption can indicate a subacute or chronic high-grade injury. It is difficult to establish the clinical competence of a sprained ligament solely on the basis of MRI.

Acute injury of the distal tibiofibular syndesmosis generally appears as focal enlargement and edema of ligamentous structures on axial MRI sequences. Although the anterior inferior tibiofibular ligament often is disrupted, the posterior syndesmosis rarely is abnormal on non–weight-bearing images. After injury, syndesmotic structures ossify over time and appear diffusely dark, thickened, and heterogenous on axial MRI.

MRI can help diagnose injuries of the lateral ligaments of the ankle. Because inversion injury and subsequent trauma are common, the anterior talofibular ligament rarely appears normal on MRI. Establishing a diagnosis of acute or subacute sprain of this ligament requires the ill-defined or enlarged ligament to be accompanied by bone contusions or edema within the lateral soft tissues. Chronic anterior talofibular ligament injury appears as diffuse ligament hypertrophy with scar tissue, as in anterolateral impingement, or as complete absence of the ligament, which suggests lateral instability. The calcaneofibular ligament is less frequently abnormal on MRI than the anterior talofibular ligament. The calcaneofibular ligament should appear as a thin, hypointense, linear structure that runs deep to the peroneal tendons in the subfibular region. This ligament is best assessed on sequential coronal sequences, and a normal insertion on the lateral calcaneus should be documented on every ankle MRI. Acute injury often appears as disruption of the ligament from the calcaneal periosteum with surrounding soft-tissue edema; chronic injury can appear as diffuse ligamentous enlargement. Although MRI has suboptimal sensitivity for diagnosing medial deltoid ligament injury, an osseous contusion pattern indicating eversion injury may be correlated with a sprain of the deltoid ligament. With a high-grade deltoid injury, the ligament can be seen on coronal MRI as entirely disrupted from its medial malleolus origin.

MRI is useful for diagnosing a ligament sprain in the foot, particularly a subtle or clinically confusing sprain. If a Lisfranc ligament injury is suspected, long axis sequences should be acquired in the plane of the Lisfranc (medial cuneiform–second and third metatarsal [C1-M2M3]) ligament to allow assessment of the morphology and signal pattern.[38] The Lisfranc ligament can be assessed from these sequences by directly identifying intraligamentous edema, partial tearing, or complete disruption. MRI detection of disruption of the plantar C1-M2M3 ligament portion of the Lisfranc ligamentous complex was found to be highly correlated with Lisfranc instability, as confirmed by gold-standard stress radiographs obtained under anesthesia.[39] In the forefoot, a sprain or tear of the plantar plate of the first metatarsophalangeal joint (turf toe) is recognizable on T2-weighted MRI sequences. MRI can differentiate ligamentous from osseous injury or complete tears from partial sprains.

Tendinous Injury

MRI is ideal for assessing the tendons of the foot and ankle. Structures are shown in the cross-sectional axial or sagittal plane, and normal tendons should appear hypointense with homogenous signal and smooth contours. Tenosynovitis appears as peritendinous high signal intensity consistent with fluid. An abnormal tendon appears heterogenous with intratendinous medium signal intensity as well as abnormal morphology such as hypertrophy, thickening, marked attenuation, or complete absence in a rupture. MRI can confirm a clinical diagnosis of tendon pathology and quantify the severity of disease.

MRI examination of the ankle can be used in assessing a degenerative tibialis posterior tendon.[40] Conventional non–weight-bearing MRI may show abnormal valgus alignment of the hindfoot on coronal images at the level of the middle subtalar joint. Sagittal MRI sequences may show midfoot sag, which is the analogue of an abnormal Meary angle. Axial sequences may show uncovering of the talar head by the navicular. Tibialis posterior tendon dysfunction is confirmed by the presence of this triad of malalignments. MRI is less sensitive for tendon degeneration relatively early in the course of tibialis posterior tendinopathy. On axial MRI sequences, the normal appearance of the distal insertion is characterized as resembling an inverted Hershey's Kiss candy. The navicular insertion of the tibialis posterior tendon blends with the medial bundle of the spring ligament to create a broad footprint. More proximally, the spring ligament is directed medially. The tibialis posterior tendon tapers quickly on axial sequences to an ovoid configuration that appears slightly larger than the adjacent flexor hallucis longus tendon. The absence of this rapid tapering and a broader configuration proximal to the navicular (a so-called Tootsie Roll configuration) can be the earliest clues to insertional tibialis posterior tendinopathy. Tibialis posterior tendinopathy also can develop more proximally behind the medial malleolus. Enlargement and intratendinous heterogeneity as well as subcortical malleolar marrow edema are hallmarks of advanced degeneration of the tendon. Tibialis posterior tendon pathology commonly is seen as a hypertrophic appearance or marked attenuation of the tendon; less commonly, a complete rupture appears as absence of the tendon within its sheath.

At the lateral ankle, numerous peroneal tendon pathologies can be reliably diagnosed using MRI (**Figure 6**). In the retrofibular or subfibular region, a peroneus brevis split tear can appear as a wishbone-shaped tendon on axial sequences or even as a splitting into two tendon bellies. At the level of the lateral malleolus, peroneal instability can be seen as redundancy or tearing of the superior peroneal retinaculum, stripping of the retinaculum off the periosteum of the malleolus, or frank dislocation of the peroneus longus tendon out of the groove and adjacent to the lateral malleolus itself. With degenerative peroneal tendon conditions, either tendon may show diffuse enlargement (in tendinosis) or longitudinal,

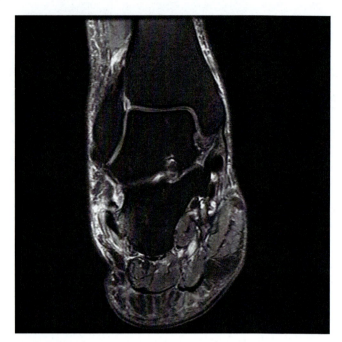

FIGURE 6 Coronal MRI of the ankle showing a degenerative tear of the peroneus brevis tendon.

intratendinous high signal on T2-weighted sequences (in interstitial tearing). A distal peroneus longus tendon tear can mimic other plantar soft-tissue injuries; to diagnose a dorsiflexion injury, it is important to follow the peroneus longus tendon under the calcaneocuboid joint and the midfoot to its insertion on the plantar surface of the first metatarsal. Accessory ossicles around the foot and ankle are prone to injury that may not be discernible on plain radiographs. With injury to the os trigonum posterior to the talus, MRI may show fluid collection on T2-weighted sequences or increased signal intensity within the synchondrosis. Similarly, painful os peroneum syndrome can be diagnosed on MRI by signal intensity change within the os peroneum, which lies within the peroneus longus tendon at the level of the calcaneal cuboid joint. Signal intensity changes indicate inflammatory changes, a stress fracture, or osteonecrosis of the ossicle.

Ankle MRI is an accurate diagnostic modality for traumatic and degenerative pathologies involving the Achilles and anterior tibial ankle tendons (**Figure 7**). Achilles tendon injury can be located in the critical zone or tendon insertion, or result in entheseal pathologies including retrocalcaneal bursitis, bone marrow edema in the dorsal calcaneus associated with Haglund exostosis, and insertional spurring, all of which can be detected and differentiated on MRI. Tendinosis can be seen on MRI as morphologic thickening of the tendon, signal change within the substance of the tendon itself, or linear splits within the tendon, which suggest degenerative tearing.

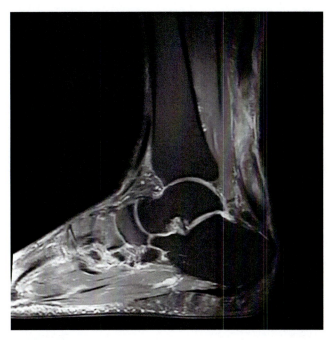

FIGURE 7 Sagittal MRI showing an acute-on-chronic tear of the Achilles tendon.

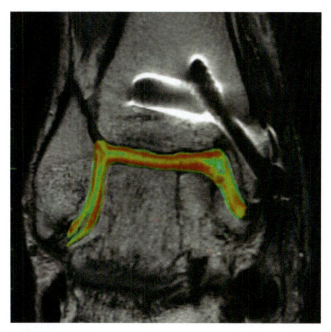

FIGURE 8 T2 mapping MRI demonstrating hyaline cartilage distribution following an osteochondral autograft transfer procedure.

In addition to diagnostic assistance, MRI can provide guidance in the management of insertional Achilles tendinopathy. A rupture in the tendon usually can be diagnosed by clinical evaluation alone, but MRI can be beneficial in confirming the rupture and quantifying any retraction gapping between the tendon ends.

Cartilage Injury

MRI has become the imaging study of choice for assessing the integrity of articular cartilage. Standard MRI studies do not evaluate the cartilage itself but instead detect decreased joint space (thinning of the articular cartilage) or periarticular bone marrow edema. The edema suggests abnormal biology of the adjacent cartilage, as occurs with osteochondral lesions and arthritis.

Routine MRI does not permit quantification of early degenerative changes. However, the T2 mapping technique has been used to assess the cartilage of the ankle joint in several foot and ankle pathologies. In the knee, T2 mapping was found to specifically quantify cartilage water content and collagen fiber orientation.[41]

T2 mapping is a color-coded method of quantifying the T2-weighted relaxation curve (**Figure 8**). T2 relaxation is an exponential decay function reflecting the loss of signal that occurs rapidly during the dephasing of the excited nuclei after a disturbing radiofrequency pulse is applied. The signal is influenced by the structural anisotropy of the collagen, where a well-defined relationship exists between the excited hydrogen atoms and the long axis of the magnetic field. When the angle between the external field and the spinning hydrogen atoms within the collagen reaches approximately 55°, there is an expected prolongation of T2 relaxation time, which is clinically manifested as increased signal intensity. Increased T2 relaxation time has been associated with the breakdown of the cartilage architecture, including loss of collagen fiber integrity, altered water content, and subsequent osteoarthritis. In the ankle, T2 mapping has been shown to identify very early cartilage injury in patients with chronic ankle instability. It has also been used as a research tool to evaluate success in restoring cartilage in the treatment of osteochondral lesions of the talus.[42]

Tissues that decay slowly can display a signal that is apparent on standard MRI. In contrast, some substances decay rapidly and thus have a very short T2 relaxation time that precludes their measurement on standard MRI sequences. To obtain a very short signal, as in the collagen found within tendons, ligaments, menisci, and cartilage, the use of a specialized pulse sequence is necessary. This ultrashort echo time can be obtained using the relatively new 3-T or higher magnet technology.[43]

Other Indications

MRI can be used to identify sources of ankle pain related to impingement of soft-tissue structures, including infiltration of the sinus tarsi, mass effect within the tarsal tunnel causing nerve compression, and intra-articular anterolateral or anteromedial ankle impingement. MRI can identify atraumatic osseous pathologies including os trigonum syndrome as well as patchy bone marrow edema related to altered biomechanics or stress response. MRI has an essential role in the workup of symptomatic midfoot or hindfoot coalition because of its ability to show osseous morphology as well as the sequelae of the resulting abnormal weight distribution.

MRI of the foot is a useful tool for patients with soft-tissue or osseous pathology and for those with acute injury or a degenerative condition. MRI is useful in the evaluation of refractory plantar fasciitis because of its ability to identify fascial tears and reactive bone marrow edema at the plantar calcaneus. MRI is the imaging modality of choice for many other common soft-tissue conditions of the foot, including plantar fibromatosis, intermetatarsal neuromas, ganglion cysts of tendon sheaths or joint capsules, and synovial chondromatosis of the ankle. With inflammatory arthropathies, MRI delineates the extent of both osseous erosion and periarticular synovitis. Finally, MRI has evolved into a modality of choice for imaging foot infections such as osteomyelitis because of its ability to accurately identify the presence and extent of osseous involvement as well as any soft-tissue abscess or phlegmon.

SUMMARY

Appropriate imaging of the foot and ankle is essential to the orthopaedic surgeon's ability to diagnose and guide the treatment of many lower extremity pathologies. An understanding of the available imaging modalities and their advantages and disadvantages contributes to an optimal outcome for patients with a foot or ankle disorder.

KEY STUDY POINTS

- Whenever possible, foot and ankle radiographs should be obtained as weight bearing while standing on the extremity to optimally evaluate alignment. Acute trauma is the exception to this rule.
- MRI is a usefully study to evaluate soft-tissue pathology and the bioactivity of bony involvement in the study area.
- CT scanning is useful to evaluate the bony anatomy and pathology of the involved area.
- Newer technology, including SPECT-CT, PET, WBCT, and tenography have demonstrated promising investigational results, but these have not translated into clinical mainstream use at this time.

ANNOTATED REFERENCES

1. Gallet J, Titus H: CR/DR systems: What each technology offers today; What is expected for the future. *Radiol Manage* 2005;27(6):30-36.

2. Eken G, Misir A: Comparison of computed tomography, traction, and inverted grayscale radiographs for understanding pilon fracture morphology. *Foot Ankle Int* 2022;43(3):398-403.

   Grayscale inversion radiographs improved detection of posterolateral fragments and lateral comminution in pilon fractures after ex-fix application, compared with normal radiographs. Level of evidence: III.

3. Giordano BD, Baumhauer JF, Morgan TL, Rechtine GR II: Patient and surgeon radiation exposure: Comparison of standard and mini-C-arm fluoroscopy. *J Bone Joint Surg Am* 2009;91(2):297-304.

4. Cunningham BA, Warner S, Berkes M, et al: Effect of intraoperative multidimensional fluoroscopy versus conventional fluoroscopy on syndesmotic reduction. *Foot Ankle Int* 2021;42(2):132-136.

   Of 30 patients, 14 required intraoperative adjustment following intraoperative multidimensional fluoroscopic imaging of syndesmosis. Of 30 patients, 3 still had malreduction of syndesmosis on postoperative CT. Level of evidence: II.

5. Ege T, Kose O, Koca K, Demiralp B, Basbozkurt M: Use of the iPhone for radiographic evaluation of hallux valgus. *Skeletal Radiol* 2013;42(2):269-273.

6. Chi TD, Davitt J, Younger A, Holt S, Sangeorzan BJ: Intra- and inter-observer reliability of the distal meta-tarsal articular angle in adult hallux valgus. *Foot Ankle Int* 2002;23(8):722-726.

7. Sensiba PR, Coffey MJ, Williams NE, Mariscalco M, Laughlin RT: Inter- and intraobserver reliability in the radiographic evaluation of adult flatfoot deformity. *Foot Ankle Int* 2010;31(2):141-145.

8. Chen W, Li X, Su Y, et al: Peroneal tenography to evaluate lateral hindfoot pain after calcaneal fracture. *Foot Ankle Int* 2011;32(8):789-795.

9. Schreibman KL: Ankle tenography: What, how, and why. *Semin Roentgenol* 2004;39(1):95-113.

10. Jain NB, Omar I, Kelikian AS, van Holsbeeck L, Grant TH: Prevalence of and factors associated with posterior tibial tendon pathology on sonographic assessment. *PM R* 2011;3(11):998-1004.

11. Neustadter J, Raikin SM, Nazarian LN: Dynamic sonographic evaluation of peroneal tendon subluxation. *AJR Am J Roentgenol* 2004;183(4):985-988.

12. Carlson RM, Dux K, Stuck RM: Ultrasound imaging for diagnosis of plantar plate ruptures of the lesser metatarsophalangeal joints: A retrospective case series. *J Foot Ankle Surg* 2013;52(6):786-788.

13. Reach JS, Easley ME, Chuckpaiwong B, Nunley JA II: Accuracy of ultrasound guided injections in the foot and ankle. *Foot Ankle Int* 2009;30(3):239-242.

14. Coughlin MJ, Grimes JS, Traughber PD, Jones CP: Comparison of radiographs and CT scans in the prospective evaluation of the fusion of hindfoot arthrodesis. *Foot Ankle Int* 2006;27(10):780-787.

15. Tuominen EKJ, Kankare J, Koskinen SK, Mattila KT: Weight-bearing CT imaging of the lower extremity. *AJR Am J Roentgenol* 2013;200(1):146-148.

16. Hirschmann A, Pfirrmann CWA, Klammer G, Espinosa N, Buck FM: Upright cone CT of the hindfoot: Comparison of the non-weight-bearing with the upright weight-bearing position. *Eur Radiol* 2014;24(3):553-558.

17. Colin F, Horn Lang T, Zwicky L, Hintermann B, Knupp M: Subtalar joint configuration on weightbearing CT scan. *Foot Ankle Int* 2014;35(10):1057-1062.

18. Lepojärvi S, Niinimäki J, Pakarinen H, Koskela L, Leskelä H-V: Rotational dynamics of the talus in a normal tibiotalar joint as shown by weight-bearing computed tomography. *J Bone Joint Surg Am* 2016;98(7):568-575.

19. Alexej B, Travis B, Martinus R, et al: Weightbearing computed tomography of the foot and ankle: Emerging technology topical review. *Foot Ankle Int* 2017;39(3):376-386.

20. Conti MS, Ellis SJ: Weight-bearing CT scans in foot and ankle surgery. *J Am Acad Orthop Surg* 2020;28(14):e595-e603.

    A review of WBCT in foot and ankle surgery was performed and it was concluded that the technology was useful but does not replace weight-bearing radiographs. The authors reported that the technology was most applicable for adult-acquired flatfoot deformity and assessment of first metatarsal rotation in hallux valgus. Level of evidence: V.

21. de Cesar Netto C, Myerson MS, Day J, et al: Consensus for the use of weightbearing CT in the assessment of progressive collapsing foot deformity. *Foot Ankle Int* 2020;41(10):1277-1282.

    Expert consensus states that weight-bearing plain radiographs are required in treatment of progressive collapsing flatfoot deformity. Hindfoot alignment view and WBCT are strongly recommended if available. WBCT should be used to evaluate for sinus tarsi impingement, subfibular impingement, increased valgus inclination of posterior facet of subtalar joint, and subluxation of the subtalar joint at the posterior and/or middle facet. Level of evidence: V.

22. Day J, de Cesar Netto C, Richter M, et al: Evaluation of a weightbearing CT artificial intelligence-based automatic measurement for the M1-M2 intermetatarsal angle in hallux valgus. *Foot Ankle Int* 2021;42(11):1502-1509.

    Automated two-dimensional and three-dimensional measurements obtained from WBCT were comparable to manual measurements of radiographs in measuring M1-M2 intermetatarsal angle in patients with symptomatic hallux valgus and normal control patiemts. Level of evidence: II.

23. de Cesar Netto C, Bang K, Mansur NS, et al: Multiplanar semi-automatic assessment of foot and ankle offset in adult acquired flatfoot deformity. *Foot Ankle Int* 2020;41(7):839-848.

    Foot and ankle offset, a semiautomated measurement using three-dimensional WBCT, is correlated with traditional manual measurements of two-dimensional WBCT images. Level of evidence: III.

24. Zhang JZ, Lintz F, Bernasconi A, Weight Bearing CT International Study Group, Zhang S: 3D biometrics for hindfoot alignment using weightbearing computed tomography. *Foot Ankle Int* 2019;40(6):720-726.

    WBCT was used to assess hindfoot alignment with foot and ankle offset and long-axis view. Both had good reliability. Foot and ankle offset was reproducible and correlated well with physical examination. Level of evidence: II.

25. Frater C, Emmett L, van Gaal W, Sungaran J, Deva-kumar D, Van der Wall H: A critical appraisal of pinhole scintigraphy of the ankle and foot. *Clin Nucl Med* 2002;27(10):707-710.

26. Basu S, Chryssikos T, Houseni M, et al: Potential role of FDG PET in the setting of diabetic neuro-osteoarthropathy: Can it differentiate uncomplicated Charcot's neuroarthropathy from osteomyelitis and soft-tissue infection? *Nucl Med Commun* 2007;28(6):465-472.

27. Lin CC, Ding HJ, Chen YW, Huang WT, Kao A: Usefulness of thallium-201 muscle perfusion scan to investigate perfusion reserve in the lower limbs of type 2 diabetic patients. *J Diabetes Complications* 2004;18(4):233-236.

28. Basu S, Zhuang H, Alavi A: Imaging of lower extremity artery atherosclerosis in diabetic foot: FDG-PET imaging and histopathological correlates. *Clin Nucl Med* 2007;32(7):567-568.

29. Singh VK, Javed S, Parthipun A, Sott AH: The diagnostic value of single photon-emission computed tomography bone scans combined with CT (SPECT-CT) in diseases of the foot and ankle. *Foot Ankle Surg* 2013;19(2):80-83.

30. Claassen L, Uden T, Ettinger M, Daniilidis K, Stukenborg-Colsman C, Plaass C: Influence on therapeutic decision making of SPECT-CT for different regions of the foot and ankle. *Biomed Res Int* 2014;2014:927576.

31. Chicklore S, Gnanasegaran G, Vijayanathan S, Fogelman I: Potential role of multislice SPECT/CT in impingement syndrome and soft-tissue pathology of the ankle and foot. *Nucl Med Commun* 2013;34(2):130-139.

32. Mason LW, Wyatt J, Butcher C, Wieshmann H, Molloy AP: Single-photon-emission computed tomography in painful total ankle replacements. *Foot Ankle Int* 2015;36(6):635-640.

33. Gurbani A, Demetracopoulos C, O'Malley M, et al: Correlation of single-photon emission computed tomography results with clinical and intraoperative findings in painful total ankle replacement. *Foot Ankle Int* 2020;41(6):639-646.

    Use of single photon emission computed tomography had 92.9% accuracy compared with intraoperative findings in making diagnosis for painful total ankle arthroplasty (in patients requiring return to operating room). Aseptic loosening and impingement were the most common diagnoses. Level of evidence: III.

34. Cerezal L, Abascal F, García-Valtuille R, Canga A: Ankle MR arthrography: How, why, when. *Radiol Clin North Am* 2005;43(4):693-707, viii.

35. Collins MS, Felmlee JP: 3T magnetic resonance imaging of ankle and hindfoot tendon pathology. *Top Magn Reson Imaging* 2009;20(3):175-188.

36. Juras V, Welsch G, Bär P, Kronnerwetter C, Fujita H, Trattnig S: Comparison of 3T and 7T MRI clinical sequences for ankle imaging. *Eur J Radiol* 2012;81(8):1846-1850.

37. Elias I, Zoga AC, Morrison WB, Besser MP, Schweitzer ME, Raikin SM: Osteochondral lesions of the talus: Localization and morphologic data from 424 patients using a novel anatomical grid scheme. *Foot Ankle Int* 2007;28(2):154-161.

38. Potter HG, Deland JT, Gusmer PB, Carson E, Warren RF: Magnetic resonance imaging of the Lisfranc ligament of the foot. *Foot Ankle Int* 1998;19(7):438-446.

39. Raikin SM, Elias I, Dheer S, Besser MP, Morrison WB, Zoga AC: Prediction of midfoot instability in the subtle Lisfranc injury: Comparison of magnetic resonance imaging with intraoperative findings. *J Bone Joint Surg Am* 2009;91(4):892-899.

40. Lim PS, Schweitzer ME, Deely DM, et al: Posterior tibial tendon dysfunction: Secondary MR signs. *Foot Ankle Int* 1997;18(10):658-663.

41. Potter HG, Black BR, Chong LR: New techniques in articular cartilage imaging. *Clin Sports Med* 2009;28(1):77-94.

42. Vira S, Ramme AJ, Chapman C, Xia D, Regatte RR, Chang G: Juvenile particulate osteochondral allograft for treatment of osteochondral lesions of the talus: Detection of altered repair tissue biochemical composition using 7 Tesla MRI and T2 mapping. *J Foot Ankle Surg* 2017;56(1):26-29.

43. Marik W, Apprich S, Welsch GH, Mamisch TC, Trattnig S: Biochemical evaluation of articular cartilage in patients with osteochondrosis dissecans by means of quantitative T2- and T2-mapping at 3T MRI: A feasibility study. *Eur J Radiol* 2012;81(5):923-927.

CHAPTER 4

Foot and Ankle Conditions in Children and Adolescents

ROBERT F. MURPHY, MD, FAAOS

ABSTRACT

The most common foot and ankle conditions in children and adolescents are accessory navicular, tarsal coalition, and flexible flatfoot. Painful symptoms associated with these conditions are usually self-limiting and can be successfully managed using nonsurgical modalities such as immobilization, activity modification, and physical therapy. Surgery is usually not necessary for these conditions, but can be effective for relieving pain and improving function in patients who have persistent symptoms and have exhausted nonsurgical treatments. To provide treatment, it is imperative to identify the location and character of the symptoms on history, as well as perform a comprehensive physical examination. The appropriate imaging modalities can help refine the diagnosis and guide the treatment plan.

Keywords: accessory navicular; flexible flatfoot; freiberg infraction; sever apophysitis; tarsal coalition

INTRODUCTION

Most foot and ankle conditions in children and adolescents are brought to the attention of the orthopaedic surgeon because of concerns regarding pain or cosmesis. The most frequent reasons for consultation include accessory navicular, tarsal coalition,

Dr. Murphy serves as a paid consultant to or is an employee of Globus Medical and Stryker and serves as a board member, owner, officer, or committee member of Pediatric Orthopaedic Society of North America and Scoliosis Research Society.

and flexible flatfoot. For patients with painful symptoms associated with accessory navicular, nonsurgical treatment is frequently satisfactory. In patients with a tarsal coalition, surgery can reliably restore hindfoot mechanics and alleviate pain. For flexible flatfoot, reassurance regarding the benign nature of the disorder is usually all that is necessary. Reconstruction with soft-tissue balancing and corrective osteotomies is indicated in recalcitrant painful cases, with reliably satisfactory results.

ACCESSORY NAVICULAR

An accessory navicular (os naviculare) is a common condition found in the pediatric and adolescent foot and ankle. It is usually identified incidentally and is often asymptomatic. Three types exist (**Figure 1**). A type I accessory navicular is a small, round ossicle of bone that lies completely separate from the native navicular within the substance of the tibialis posterior tendon at its insertion into the navicular. A type II accessory navicular is a larger bone that connects to the navicular tuberosity by a synchondrosis, and generally constitutes a large portion of the tibialis posterior tendon. Type III is similar to type II in appearance except for the absence of the synchondrosis; instead, the navicular is completely fused to the accessory ossicle.

Clinical Findings

An accessory navicular is typically diagnosed in adolescent patients with worsening medial midfoot pain. The symptoms typically begin with a sprain of the foot or ankle, and the pain is exacerbated by sports activities or shoe wear. A flexible pes planovalgus deformity is present in 50% of patients. The patient typically reports tenderness to palpation over the medial prominence, which can be reproduced by resisted tibialis posterior tendon contraction by asking the patient to plantarflex

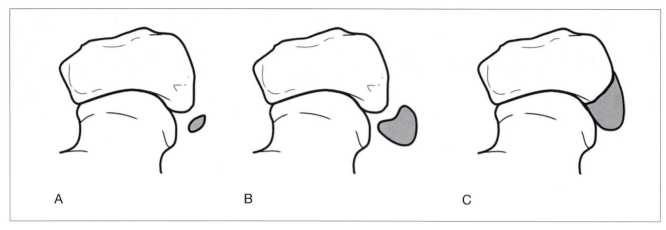

FIGURE 1 Illustrations showing the classification of the accessory navicular. **A**, Type I, in which a small, round ossicle is completely separate from the navicular. **B**, Type II, in which a larger ossicle is connected to the navicular by a synchondrosis. **C**, Type III, which is similar to type II except for the absence of a synchondrosis.

and invert the foot. The patient and parents may be concerned about the size and appearance of the bump on the medial arch (**Figure 2**).

Radiographic Evaluation

Standing AP, internal oblique, and lateral radiographic views usually are sufficient for detecting the accessory bone although a reverse (external) oblique radiograph of the foot may be helpful (**Figure 3**). It is important to identify any associated abnormalities, such as pes planus or a tarsal coalition. Advanced imaging such as CT or MRI is unnecessary unless there are concerns for additional pathology based on history or physical examination. However, MRI is excellent for defining the soft-tissue anatomy of the tibialis posterior tendon insertion and identifying a synchondrosis, and often reveals edema in the synchondrosis and nearby bony structures.[1] Although rarely indicated, a bone scan is likely to show signal intensity at the site of the ossicle in a type II deformity.

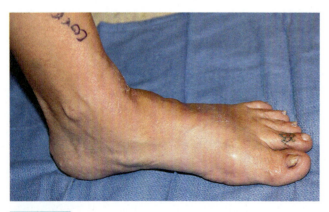

FIGURE 2 Clinical photograph showing a foot with an accessory navicular.

Nonsurgical Treatment

Patients with an insidious onset of symptoms often can achieve pain relief with activity modifications, wearing an over-the-counter soft orthosis, and/or using NSAIDs. A rigid arch-support orthosis can be painful because of increased contact pressure over the prominent accessory navicular. Patients with associated flatfoot deformity and a contracture of the gastrocnemius or Achilles tendon may benefit from a stretching program. A period of immobilization in a walking cast or boot may help relieve symptoms. A 2019 review demonstrated that most patients (68%) can be successfully treated using nonsurgical measures, with an average treatment time of 8 months.[2]

Surgical Treatment

Surgical treatment is an option if an extended course of nonsurgical treatment does not result in relief of symptoms. The original Kidner procedure involved excision of the accessory ossicle and advancement of the tibialis posterior tendon. Satisfactory results have been reported with a modified Kidner procedure that entails simple excision of the ossicle and side-to-side repair, rather than advancement, of the tibialis posterior tendon.[3,4]

The type of accessory navicular dictates the surgical plan. A type I accessory navicular ossicle can be simply excised through a longitudinal split in the tibialis posterior tendon. A type II or III deformity requires subperiosteal dissection from the tibialis posterior tendon insertion, and bony decompression. Resection of a large type II or III deformity may require nearly complete detachment of the tibialis posterior tendon insertion to achieve adequate bony decompression, and care should be taken to avoid violating the talonavicular joint capsule. Depending on the magnitude of tibialis posterior dissection, the tendon can be repaired in a side-to-side

Chapter 4: Foot and Ankle Conditions in Children and Adolescents

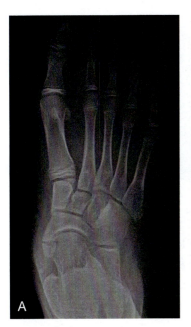
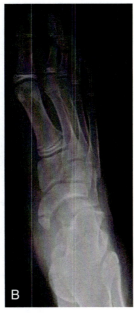

FIGURE 3 **A**, AP radiograph showing an accessory navicular. **B**, An external oblique view sometimes helps detect or fully delineate the accessory bone.

fashion or reattached to the residual navicular using bone tunnels or suture anchors (**Figure 4**). Recent literature has found no significant difference in outcomes or complications after simple excision with or without advancement of the tibialis posterior tendon.[4,5]

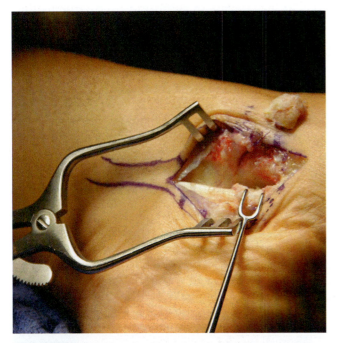

FIGURE 4 Intraoperative photograph showing disruption of the tibialis posterior tendon insertion after excision of an accessory navicular. Reattachment with suture anchors is required.

Some studies have reported arthrodesis of an accessory ossicle to the native navicular with screw fixation, which has the apparent advantage of avoiding disruption of the insertion of the tibialis posterior tendon. Although a 20% rate of nonunion was reported in one study, overall patient satisfaction was high.[6,7] Studies with larger numbers of patients and lengthy follow-up are necessary to determine the role of this technique.

Surgical treatment of associated flatfoot deformity and a gastrocnemius or Achilles contracture at the time of accessory navicular excision remains controversial. Furthermore, some studies have reported concomitant subtalar arthroereisis,[8] calcaneocuboid-cuneiform osteotomies,[9] and medial displacement calcaneal osteotomies[10] at the time of symptomatic accessory navicular treatment. It is unclear whether these additional procedures result in better long-term outcomes than simple excision.

TARSAL COALITION

Tarsal coalition is an abnormal connection between the bones of the hindfoot or midfoot and is caused by failure of mesenchymal segmentation. A coalition can be fibrous, cartilaginous, or bony, and can occur in isolation or as a component of a genetic syndrome. Progression from fibrous to cartilaginous tissue and ultimately to bone occurs during skeletal maturation, coinciding with a gradual onset of symptoms. This process explains why a symptomatic coalition is rare in young children. An association between rigid pes planus and tarsal coalition has been described, commonly referred to as peroneal spastic flatfoot.

A 2021 population-based database reported the annual incidence of a symptomatic tarsal coalition is 3.5 per 100,000 children with calcaneonavicular and talocalcaneal coalitions as the most common.[11] Coalitions between other tarsal bones occur less often. Fifty percent of coalitions are bilateral. Although multiple coalitions are rare, it is essential to consider this possibility before undertaking surgical treatment.[12]

Clinical Findings

A tarsal coalition is usually identified in a juvenile or adolescent patient, often after an ankle sprain or another minor trauma caused by impaired subtalar mobility. Patients report lateral hindfoot pain and tenderness in the sinus tarsi and often have peroneal muscle spasm secondary to pain. Hindfoot motion is limited, especially in patients with a complete bony coalition. Pes planovalgus deformity is typical and often is associated with an Achilles tendon or gastrocnemius muscle contracture.

On single-limb heel rise test, the foot has poor restoration of the medial longitudinal arch and persistence of hindfoot eversion.

Radiographic Evaluation
The initial radiographic evaluation includes the weight-bearing AP, lateral, and 45° internal oblique views of the foot as well as an axial (Harris) view of the hindfoot. Talar beaking (a dorsal osteophyte) at the talonavicular joint often is seen in a talocalcaneal or calcaneonavicular coalition and is not typically associated with true talonavicular arthritis. A calcaneonavicular coalition is best seen on an internal oblique radiograph. A lateral radiograph may reveal prominence of the anterior process of the calcaneus toward the navicular (the so-called anteater's nose sign; **Figure 5**). A talocalcaneal coalition is best seen on the axial view as an irregularity and an oblique orientation of the middle subtalar facet. A talocalcaneal coalition is less consistently seen on the lateral view, usually because the valgus obliquity of the subtalar joint causes it to be poorly defined.

The difficulty of diagnosing a tarsal coalition using plain radiographs, especially a talocalcaneal coalition, has resulted in the increased use of CT and MRI. CT can be used to identify the coalition, determine its extent, differentiate a bony from a fibrous coalition, and identify degenerative changes or additional coalitions in other parts of the foot (**Figure 6**). CT also is useful for evaluating other structural abnormalities that are difficult to see on plain radiographs such as an accessory anterior facet or a calcaneofibular impingement, which often accompanies a talocalcaneal coalition.[13] MRI is the preferred modality for evaluating young children, who are more likely to have a fibrous coalition because ossification is incomplete.[14,15]

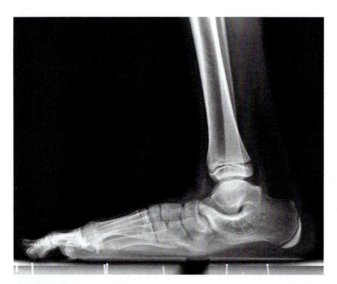

FIGURE 5 Lateral radiograph showing a calcaneonavicular coalition and an anteater's nose sign.

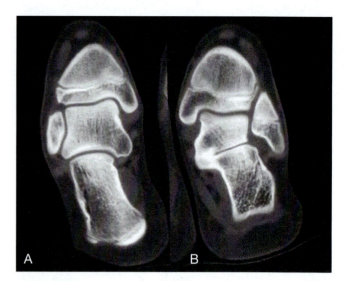

FIGURE 6 Coronal CT images showing a normal foot (**A**) and a foot with a middle facet coalition and arthrosis (**B**).

Nonsurgical Treatment
Initial nonsurgical treatment is recommended for all patients with a tarsal coalition. The modalities include rest, activity modification, and a period of immobilization in a cast, boot, or brace. After the symptoms subside, the patient can progress to using a custom orthosis and slowly resume activities. A stretching program for the Achilles tendon and gastrocnemius should be considered for patients with a contracture. Subsequent treatment may include the use of an orthosis to control hindfoot eversion.

Surgical Treatment
Calcaneonavicular coalitions are excised through a longitudinal Ollier incision over the sinus tarsi. The adequacy of the excision is assessed both clinically and radiographically; full hindfoot motion should be obtained intraoperatively. An associated gastrocnemius-soleus complex contracture should be treated at the time of surgical resection. Care must be taken not to injure the talonavicular joint or the talar head. In an effort to prevent recurrence, it is recommended to interpose soft tissue into the coalition site. The extensor digitorum brevis muscle belly and fascia can be advanced and interposed into the excision site. The use of fat graft is effective and may avoid skin cosmesis issues or inadequate coverage of the resection site associated with extensor digitorum brevis interposition.[16] Additionally, fat graft has been shown to have lower rates of reossification when compared with extensor digitorum brevis interposition.[17]

Surgical procedures for treating talocalcaneal coalitions include arthrodesis, coalition resection, and osteotomy without resection. The long-held criteria for determining whether a coalition should be resected include size of less than 30% to 50% of the posterior facet, hindfoot valgus of 16° to 21°, and little or no narrowing or degeneration of the posterior facet of the subtalar joint. The site of pain and the severity of the valgus deformity may be at least as important as the size of the coalition, however. Calcaneal lengthening osteotomy is preferred over arthrodesis for a painful talocalcaneal coalition and advanced hindfoot valgus.[18]

Talocalcaneal coalitions are excised through a medial approach between the flexor digitorum longus and flexor hallucis longus tendons. Care must be taken to avoid the medial neurovascular bundle. It is crucial that the coalition be adequately resected, particularly from anterior to posterior. Careful inspection of the anterior and posterior subtalar facets is necessary after removal of the coalition. Most surgeons prefer to interpose bone wax and local fat in the resected coalition site, although other interpositional materials have been used. Fat graft can be obtained from the buttocks or locally anterior to the Achilles tendon. A study of a large number of patients treated with resection and fat interposition reported good deformity correction and high American Orthopaedic Foot and Ankle Society ankle and hindfoot scale scores.[19] Most experts recommend single-stage coalition resection and flatfoot reconstruction rather than arthrodesis as an initial treatment of moderate to severe coalitions.[18,20]

Correction of calcaneofibular impingement is another potential advantage of deformity correction and calcaneal lengthening. Calcaneofibular impingement often is present in patients with a talocalcaneal coalition, and further investigation is needed to determine the relationship between impingement and symptoms. Arthroscopic resection of talocalcaneal coalitions has been described, but further evaluation of its safety and efficacy is needed, compared with well-established open techniques.[21,22]

Surgical treatment of a tarsal coalition usually results in improvement in pain and function, as evidenced by recent data demonstrating over 70% patient satisfaction at an average of 4.5 years following surgery.[23] Emerging data demonstrate remarkable improvement in American Orthopaedic Foot and Ankle Society and University of California Los Angeles scores at 6 months, 1 year, and 2 years in surgically treated patients when compared with preoperative scores.[24] However, some long-term results demonstrate that normal kinematics and pedobarographic parameters are not fully restored.[25,26] One study found no association between the size of a talocalcaneal coalition or a hindfoot valgus angle and the long-term functional outcome.[27] A 2020 population-based database reported a revision surgery rate in tarsal coalitions of 8.7%.[28] A decision on surgical reconstruction with subtalar fusion or triple arthrodesis should be based on the presence of arthritic changes, hindfoot rigidity,

and the severity of planovalgus deformity. Although triple arthrodesis is a reliable salvage procedure, isolated hindfoot fusion generally is preferable in adults to avoid stress transfer to the ankle joint and the development of degenerative arthritis.[18]

FLEXIBLE PEDIATRIC FLATFOOT

Flexible pes planovalgus (flatfoot) deformity is found in as many as 80% of young children, but its prevalence decreases with age to approximately 9% to 12% in older adolescents.[29] Children and adolescents with obesity are at increased risk for pain as well as worsening of the deformity.[29,30] Children with flexible flatfoot deformity, especially when it is painful, often have an associated Achilles tendon or gastrocnemius contracture.[31] Muscle activity appears to have minimal influence on the development or persistence of flexible flatfoot deformity.

Clinical Findings

Most children with flexible flatfoot deformity do not have symptoms. The parents often seek an orthopaedic evaluation because of concern about the appearance of the child's feet. The supple deformity consists of loss of the normal medial longitudinal arch and hindfoot valgus. The talar head often is palpable medially, secondary to navicular uncovering. On examination, the deformity is easily reducible. With heel rise, the arch is restored and the hindfoot inverts. The arch is also restored in the foot's resting gravity position, or with passive dorsiflexion of the first metatarsophalangeal joint. Patients with symptoms have tenderness along the talonavicular joint or medial longitudinal arch in the midsubstance of the plantar fascia. Skin changes such as calluses may be present over the uncovered talar head. The patient may have night pain in the medial leg, gastrocnemius-soleus complex, and plantar foot.[32] In a patient with severe deformity, sinus tarsi pain can develop secondary to calcaneofibular abutment. Furthermore, it is important to assess the patient's entire lower extremity for rotational malalignment.

Radiographic Evaluation

Although radiographic differences appear in children with flexible flatfoot, little evidence supports the routine use of radiography in the absence of symptoms. When radiographic evaluation is necessary, it includes the weight-bearing AP, 45° internal oblique, and lateral views. Weight-bearing AP ankle and axial hindfoot views occasionally are used to evaluate for other potential sources of the valgus appearance of the foot. Patients with pes planovalgus have an increased talar declination and an increased convex-downward Meary (talar–first metatarsal) angle on the lateral radiograph (**Figure 7**). The weight-bearing AP view shows uncovering of the talar head with abduction of the navicular and forefoot. Patients with an Achilles tendon or gastrocnemius contracture have a decreased calcaneal pitch. Considerable interobserver and intraobserver error in radiographic measurements of pes planus is associated with the number of measurement steps.[33] The amount of talar head coverage is the only clinically relevant measurement that differs based on the presence or absence of symptoms.[34] In a 2022 series of 81 feet with flatfoot, MRI was found to identify additional relevant diagnostic information in 23.5% of cases, especially in patients with a rigid flatfoot.[35]

Nonsurgical Treatment

Counseling and education as to the benign nature of flexible flatfoot are the mainstay responses to the condition. No high-level evidence supports any form of nonsurgical intervention in the absence of symptoms.[36,37] In a patient with an Achilles tendon or gastrocnemius contracture, a stretching program may be useful for relief of symptoms, but no long-term studies have proved the benefit of such a program. A prescription orthosis or medial midfoot pad can be used, but there are no long-term studies documenting the benefit of a custom orthosis for treating the condition. Orthoses, braces, or corrective shoes have not been shown to correct the deformity or prevent its progression in patients without symptoms. In a 2020 prospective study of 31 children in whom flatfoot was diagnosed, 18 were treated with orthoses, compared with 13 control patients. At mean 4-year follow-up, there were no significant differences in radiographic parameters between the two groups.[38]

Surgical Treatment

Surgical treatment should be considered for the few patients who have persistent pain after exhausting nonsurgical treatment. Arthroereisis (insertion of an implant into the sinus tarsi) has had some success. A foreign body reaction to the original polymeric silicone implants in the sinus tarsi necessitated the development of metallic implants. Radiographic parameters have improved with the use of relatively new implants, and patient satisfaction rates now range from 79% to 100%.[39] However, rates of complications and unplanned revision surgery have been high. Improved outcomes were reported when arthroereisis was performed in conjunction with gastrocnemius recession.[40] After unsuccessful subtalar arthroereisis, revision with a lateral column calcaneal lengthening osteotomy can be considered at the time of implant removal or can be performed in a staged fashion. Talonavicular fusion at one time was considered an option for treating flexible pediatric planus, but now is reserved for patients with painful neuromuscular pes planus.[41]

A study compared arthroereisis with lateral column lengthening in adolescent patients with symptomatic flatfoot. These authors found comparable patient outcomes and rates of complications between the two procedures, and suggested the further study with long-term outcomes is warranted to determine if less invasive methods may be satisfactory for this condition.[42] Isolated gastrocnemius/soleus recession has also been reported to provide satisfactory outcomes for the treatment of flatfoot deformity and associated equinus contracture.[43]

After unsuccessful nonsurgical treatment, many patients can be treated with a lateral column-lengthening osteotomy. Care must be taken to protect the sural nerve and peroneal tendons during lateral dissection of the calcaneal wall. A saw or osteotome is used under fluoroscopic guidance for a lateral-to-medial calcaneal osteotomy between the anterior and middle facets of the subtalar joint. The medial wall can be left intact. In this technique, it has been suggested to pin the calcaneocuboid joint before correction, so as to avoid joint subluxation with osteotomy distraction. A study has demonstrated that some dorsal calcaneocuboid subluxation occurs with this procedure immediately postoperatively, but this improves over time, and no evidence of calcaneocuboid joint arthritis is observed up to 2 years out from the procedure.[44] However, a 2021 study demonstrated that maintenance of the pin in the calcaneocuboid joint during the postoperative period was associated with an increased risk of radiographic signs of calcaneocuboid arthritis, as opposed to removing it intraoperatively after the graft has been secured.[45] An 8- to 10-mm wedge-shaped autograft or allograft is inserted (**Figure 8**). Graft placement and foot positioning are crucial for correction of midfoot abduction as well as any residual supination. Compression screws, staples, lateral plating, or threaded Kirschner wires are chosen for fixation depending on the size and bone quality of the patient. Excessive dorsal graft within the sinus tarsi must be trimmed to prevent

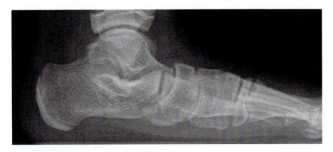

FIGURE 7 Lateral radiograph showing talar declination and disruption of the talar-first metatarsal angle (Meary angle) in a juvenile patient with a painful flatfoot.

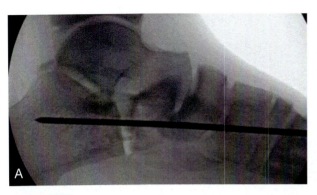 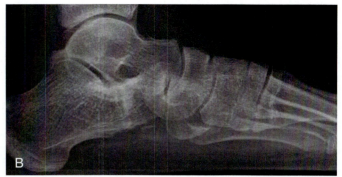

FIGURE 8 Lateral intraoperative fluoroscopic image (**A**) from the patient mentioned in Figure 7 showing improvement in Meary angle following a calcaneal lengthening osteotomy with fibular strut allograft. At 1-year follow-up, lateral weight-bearing radiograph (**B**) demonstrates maintenance of correction with graft incorporation.

impingement. Although use of allograft for this procedure is acceptable and avoids autograft-related complications, recent literature has demonstrated a rate of 4% failure with allograft.[46]

A comparison of outcomes at midterm follow-up after a calcaneal lengthening osteotomy or combined calcaneal-cuboid-cuneiform osteotomies found good clinical and radiographic results after both procedures.[16] Patients who underwent lateral column lengthening had greater postoperative talar head coverage but also had a slightly higher complication rate. A talonavicular capsulotomy, spring ligament repair, and flexor digitorum longus transfer can be added to improve deformity correction and inversion strength in patients who are skeletally mature and have severe deformity and weak inversion. A 2020 medium-term report on 20 feet found that 13 patients (65%) had good clinical and radiographic results, with residual forefoot supination as the strongest predictor of persistent pain.[47]

APOPHYSITIS

Sever Disease

Sever disease, or calcaneal apophysitis, is most common in children age 9 to 12 years, seen more frequently in overweight and taller children.[48] Symptoms often are exacerbated by aggressive sports activities but can occur with simple walking, and symptom severity is linked to chronicity.[48] Patients report pain at the Achilles tendon insertion into the calcaneus, in the calcaneal apophysis itself, or near the origin of the plantar fascia. They may be tender to palpation over the calcaneal tuberosity on examination. Associated Achilles tendon or gastrocnemius contracture is common. Pedobarographic analysis found an association between high plantar pressures, hindfoot equinus, and symptoms of calcaneal apophysitis. Sever disease has no classic radiographic findings, and as such, the diagnosis is primarily clinical. Imaging can be useful for ruling out other causes of heel pain, such as a stress fracture or benign bone lesion, with rates of abnormal findings on radiographs around 1% to 5%.[49,50]

Symptoms typically resolve with closure of the calcaneal apophysis. Treatment options include activity modification, silicone heel wedges, ice, NSAIDs, and a stretching program for the gastrocnemius-soleus complex. A brief period of cast or boot immobilization is helpful if other treatments have been unsuccessful. The waxing and waning course of Sever disease can be frustrating for patients and their families, who must be instructed about the natural history of the disease and the treatment options. Frequent reassurance may be necessary until the child reaches skeletal maturity. A prospective trial compared observation, orthoses, and physical therapy exercise regimen as three treatment modalities for Sever apophysitis. Although all three groups demonstrated improved patient outcomes at 3-month follow-up, no significant difference was identified between any of the modalities.[51]

Iselin Disease

Iselin disease is a traction apophysitis at the base of the fifth metatarsal (**Figure 9**). Chronic symptoms can result from overuse, and acute symptoms can be the result of an inversion injury. Although the pain is located at the base of the fifth metatarsal, it can radiate up the lateral border of the foot along the course of the peroneus brevis. Examination reveals tenderness to palpation over the fifth metatarsal base apophysis at the insertion of the peroneus brevis tendon. This pain can be reproduced by eversion of the foot against resistance. Radiographic evaluation may be necessary to rule out a fracture, but the fifth metatarsal base apophysis can be confused with an avulsion fracture, particularly after an acute injury. Contralateral comparison radiographs can be useful in this instance. The treatment of Iselin disease includes rest (often with a short period of immobilization), ice, and NSAIDs.

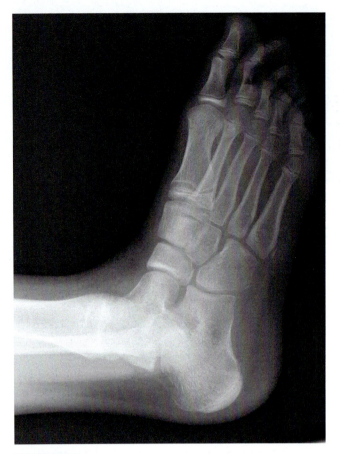

FIGURE 9 Internal oblique radiograph showing a fifth metatarsal base apophysis.

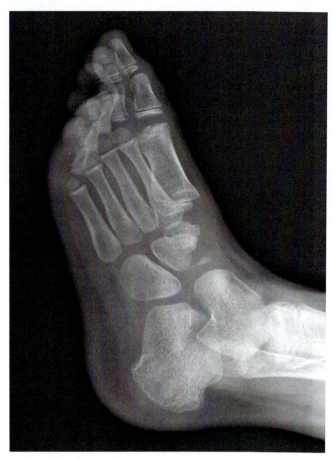

FIGURE 10 Lateral radiograph showing sclerosis and fragmentation of the navicular in a patient with Köhler disease.

OSTEOCHONDROSIS

Symptomatic necrosis can occur in almost any bone of the foot during childhood or adolescence. The etiology of these avascular events or osteochondroses remains a mystery. The two most common types of osteochondrosis in pediatric patients involve the navicular and the metatarsal head.

Köhler Disease

Köhler disease is the eponym for navicular osteochondrosis. Patients can have pain in the medial midfoot, occasionally have swelling over the navicular, and often walk with a limp. Boys are more commonly affected than girls. The symptoms and abnormal radiographic appearance typically resolve within 6 months to 1 year (**Figure 10**). Patients with mild symptoms can be treated with activity modification and NSAIDs. Patients with more severe pain may require a period of cast or boot immobilization for adequate relief of pain. Scheduling longitudinal follow-up with serial radiographs is helpful to reassure parents regarding the benign natural history of this condition.

Freiberg Infraction

Freiberg infraction is radiographic osteonecrosis in the second metatarsal head. The second ray is most commonly affected, but changes also may be seen in any of the other metatarsal heads. Freiberg infraction is most common in adolescent girls who are athletes. Patients often report pain and swelling over the affected metatarsophalangeal joint or point tenderness over the plantar aspect of the metatarsal head during weight bearing. Radiographic evaluation may reveal sclerosis, metatarsal head flattening, and enlargement of the metatarsal epiphysis. The etiology is unknown, but seems to be related to repetitive trauma resulting in vascular insult to the metatarsal epiphysis. Symptoms usually resolve after treatment with activity modification, NSAIDs, and soft shoe inserts. Patients who have severe symptoms may require a brief period of immobilization. Symptoms and radiographic changes typically spontaneously resolve over the course of 2 years. Surgery may be undertaken if the patient has residual pain or mechanical symptoms from a malformed metatarsal head or loose bodies. Surgical procedures include removal of loose bodies, local synovectomy, and débridement of osteophytes or necrotic bone. A dorsal wedge osteotomy of the metatarsal neck can be used to move normal plantar cartilage into a position of articulation with the proximal phalanx.[52] Metatarsal head resection is avoided if possible, as it can result in continued pain, transfer metatarsalgia, and joint instability. If necessary in advanced cases, only the distal portion of the head is removed, leaving the more proximal weight-bearing portion of the bone intact. An excellent systematic review details the existing literature and outcomes on Freiberg infraction.[53]

SUMMARY

Disorders of the foot and ankle affecting children and adolescents usually improve and are frequently treated with observation, activity modification, and physical therapy. If surgical treatment is undertaken, a favorable outcome usually can be expected. Understanding the anatomy of the skeletally immature foot and establishing the correct diagnosis are key to choosing the appropriate treatment.

KEY STUDY POINTS

- Symptomatic painful accessory navicular in children and adolescents can be treated with simple excision of the accessory bone without posterior tibial tendon advancement
- For recalcitrant pain associated with tarsal coalition, satisfactory results can be obtained with coalition resection and soft-tissue interposition. Reconstruction of any associated flatfoot deformity is preferred to initial arthrodesis in this patient population.
- Although some data are emerging that arthroereisis may provide satisfactory results for pediatric and adolescent flatfoot deformity, the preferred treatment is reconstruction with calcaneal lengthening osteotomy.

ANNOTATED REFERENCES

1. Sizensky JA, Marks RM: Imaging of the navicular. *Foot Ankle Clin* 2004;9(1):181-209.

2. Wynn M, Brady C, Cola K, Rice-Denning J: Effectiveness of nonoperative treatment of the symptomatic accessory navicular in pediatric patients. *Iowa Orthop J* 2019;39(1):45-49.

   In this series of 228 symptomatic accessory naviculae, 70% of patients achieved partial or complete pain relief with nonsurgical therapy. Average time in nonsurgical treatment was 8 months. Level of evidence: III.

3. Lee KT, Kim KC, Park YU, Park SM, Lee YK, Deland JT: Midterm outcome of modified Kidner procedure. *Foot Ankle Int* 2012;33(2):122-127.

4. Cha SM, Shin HD, Kim KC, Lee JK: Simple excision vs the Kidner procedure for type 2 accessory navicular associated with flatfoot in pediatric population. *Foot Ankle Int* 2013;34(2):167-172.

5. Pretell-Mazzini J, Murphy RF, Sawyer JR, et al: Surgical treatment of symptomatic accessory navicular in children and adolescents. *Am J Orthop* 2014;43(3):110-113.

6. Chung JW, Chu IT: Outcome of fusion of a painful accessory navicular to the primary navicular. *Foot Ankle Int* 2009;30(2):106-109.

7. Scott AT, Sabesan VJ, Saluta JR, Wilson MA, Easley ME: Fusion versus excision of the symptomatic type II accessory navicular: A prospective study. *Foot Ankle Int* 2009;30(1):10-15.

8. Garras DN, Hansen PL, Miller AG, Raikin SM: Outcome of modified Kidner procedure with subtalar arthroereisis for painful accessory navicular associated with planovalgus deformity. *Foot Ankle Int* 2012;33(11):934-939.

9. Kim JR, Park CI, Moon YJ, Wang SI, Kwon KS: Concomitant calcaneo-cuboid-cuneiform osteotomies and the modified Kidner procedure for severe flatfoot associated with symptomatic accessory navicular in children and adolescents. *J Orthop Surg Res* 2014;9:131.

10. Cao HH, Tang KL, Lu WZ, Xu JZ: Medial displacement calcaneal osteotomy with posterior tibial tendon reconstruction for the flexible flatfoot with symptomatic accessory navicular. *J Foot Ankle Surg* 2014;53(5):539-543.

11. Jackson TJ, Larson AN, Mathew SE, Milbrandt TA: Incidence of symptomatic pediatric tarsal coalition in olmsted county: A population-based study. *J Bone Joint Surg Am* 2021;103(2):155-161.

    This 50+ year population-based study from a single county in Minnesota demonstrated the annual incidence of symptomatic tarsal coalition in children, at a rate of 3.5 per 100,000. The most common was calcaneonavicular, followed by talocalcaneal. Level of evidence: IV.

12. Masquijo JJ, Jarvis J: Associated talocalcaneal and calcaneonavicular coalitions in the same foot. *J Pediatr Orthop B* 2010;19(6):507-510.

13. Kernbach KJ, Blitz NM: The presence of calcaneal fibular remodeling associated with middle facet talocalcaneal coalition: A retrospective CT review of 35 feet. Investigations involving middle facet coalitions – Part II. *J Foot Ankle Surg* 2008;47(4):288-294.

14. Guignand D, Journeau P, Mainard-Simard L, Popkov D, Haumont T, Lascombes P: Child calcaneonavicular coalitions: MRI diagnostic value in a 19-case series. *Orthop Traumatol Surg Res* 2011;97(1):67-72.

15. Nalaboff KM, Schweitzer ME: MRI of tarsal coalition: Frequency, distribution, and innovative signs. *Bull NYU Hosp Jt Dis* 2008;66(1):14-21.

16. Mubarak SJ, Patel PN, Upasani VV, Moor MA, Wenger DR: Calcaneonavicular coalition: Treatment by excision and fat graft. *J Pediatr Orthop* 2009;29(5):418-426.

17. Masquijo J, Allende V, Torres-Gomez A, Dobbs MB: Fat graft and bone wax interposition provides better functional outcomes and lower reossification rates than extensor digitorum brevis after calcaneonavicular coalition resection. *J Pediatr Orthop* 2017;37(7):e427-e431.

18. Mosca VS, Bevan WP: Talocalcaneal tarsal coalitions and the calcaneal lengthening osteotomy: The role of deformity correction. *J Bone Joint Surg Am* 2012;94(17):1584-1594.

19. Gantsoudes GD, Roocroft JH, Mubarak SJ: Treatment of talocalcaneal coalitions. *J Pediatr Orthop* 2012;32(3):301-307.

20. Lisella JM, Bellapianta JM, Manoli A II: Tarsal coalition resection with pes planovalgus hindfoot reconstruction. *J Surg Orthop Adv* 2011;20(2):102-105.

21. Singh AK, Parsons SW: Arthroscopic resection of calcaneonavicular coalition/malunion via a modified sinus tarsi approach: An early case series. *Foot Ankle Surg* 2012;18(4):266-269.

22. Knorr J, Soldado F, Menendez ME, Domenech P, Sanchez M, Sales de Gauzy J: Arthroscopic talocalcaneal coalition resection in children. *Arthroscopy* 2015;31(12):2417-2423.

23. Mahan ST, Spencer SA, Vezeridis PS, Kasser JR: Patient-reported outcomes of tarsal coalitions treated with surgical excision. *J Pediatr Orthop* 2015;35(6):583-588.

24. Mahan ST, Miller PE, Kasser JR, Spencer SA: Prospective evaluation of tarsal coalition excision show significant improvements in pain and function. *J Pediatr Orthop* 2021;41(9):e828-e832.

    Compared with preoperative levels, children and adolescents who undergo surgical treatment for tarsal coalition demonstrate marked improvement in patient-reported outcomes (including Modified American Orthopaedic Foot and Ankle Society scores and University of California Los Angeles activity scores) at 6 months, 1 year, and 2 years postoperatively. Level of evidence: II.

25. Skwara A, Zounta V, Tibesku CO, Fuchs-Winkelmann S, Rosenbaum D: Plantar contact stress and gait analysis after resection of tarsal coalition. *Acta Orthop Belg* 2009;75(5):654-660.

26. Hetsroni I, Nyska M, Mann G, Rozenfeld G, Ayalon M: Subtalar kinematics following resection of tarsal coalition. *Foot Ankle Int* 2008;29(11):1088-1094.

27. Khoshbin A, Law PW, Caspi L, Wright JG: Long-term functional outcomes of resected tarsal coalitions. *Foot Ankle Int* 2013;34(10):1370-1375.

28. Jackson TJ, Mathew SE, Larson AN, Stans AA, Milbrandt TA: Characteristics and reoperation rates of paediatric tarsal coalitions: A population-based study. *J Child Orthop* 2020;14(6):537-543.

    This population-based review found that at median 14.4-year follow-up, risk of revision surgery in children who undergo surgical treatment for tarsal coalition is 8.7%. Level of evidence: III.

29. Tenenbaum S, Hershkovich O, Gordon B, et al: Flexible pes planus in adolescents: Body mass index, body height, and gender – An epidemiological study. *Foot Ankle Int* 2013;34(6):811-817.

30. Chen KC, Yeh CJ, Tung LC, Yang JF, Yang SF, Wang CH: Relevant factors influencing flatfoot in preschool-aged children. *Eur J Pediatr* 2011;170(7):931-936.

31. Mosca VS: Flexible flatfoot in children and adolescents. *J Child Orthop* 2010;4(2):107-121.

32. Benedetti MG, Ceccarelli F, Berti L, et al: Diagnosis of flexible flatfoot in children: A systematic clinical approach. *Orthopedics* 2011;34(2):94.

33. Metcalfe SA, Bowling FL, Baltzopoulos V, Maganaris C, Reeves ND: The reliability of measurements taken from radiographs in the assessment of paediatric flat foot deformity. *Foot (Edinb)* 2012;22(3):156-162.

34. Moraleda L, Mubarak SJ: Flexible flatfoot: Differences in the relative alignment of each segment of the foot between symptomatic and asymptomatic patients. *J Pediatr Orthop* 2011;31(4):421-428.

35. Bagley C, McIlhone S, Singla N, et al: MRI for paediatric flatfoot: Is it necessary? *Br J Radiol* 2022;95(1132):20210784.

    In a cohort of 81 patients with flatfoot, MRI identified additional diagnostic information in 23.5% of patients, with the highest yield in rigid flatfoot patients. Level of evidence: IV.

36. Rome K, Ashford RL, Evans A: Non-surgical interventions for paediatric pes planus. *Cochrane Database Syst Rev* 2010;7:CD006311.

37. Jane MacKenzie A, Rome K, Evans AM: The efficacy of nonsurgical interventions for pediatric flexible flat foot: A critical review. *J Pediatr Orthop* 2012;32(8):830-834.

38. Choi JY, Lee DJ, Kim SJ, Suh JS: Does the long-term use of medial arch support insole induce the radiographic structural changes for pediatric flexible flat foot? – A prospective comparative study. *Foot Ankle Surg* 2020;26(4):449-456.

    In a group of 18 patients with pediatric flexible flatfoot, medial arch supports worn from age 10 to 11 years until physeal closure resulted in improvement in radiographic annotations. However, an untreated comparative control also demonstrated radiographic improvements during the same time frame. Level of evidence: III.

39. Metcalfe SA, Bowling FL, Reeves ND: Subtalar joint arthroereisis in the management of pediatric flexible flatfoot: A critical review of the literature. *Foot Ankle Int* 2011;32(12):1127-1139.

40. Jay RM, Din N: Correcting pediatric flatfoot with subtalar arthroereisis and gastrocnemius recession: A retrospective study. *Foot Ankle Spec* 2013;6(2):101-107.

41. de Coulon G, Turcot K, Canavese F, Dayer R, Kaelin A, Ceroni D: Talonavicular arthrodesis for the treatment of neurological flat foot deformity in pediatric patients: Clinical and radiographic evaluation of 29 feet. *J Pediatr Orthop* 2011;31(5):557-563.

42. Chong DY, Macwilliams BA, Hennessey TA, Teske N, Stevens PM: Prospective comparison of subtalar arthroereisis with lateral column lengthening for painful flatfeet. *J Pediatr Orthop B* 2015;24(4):345-353.

43. Rong K, Ge WT, Li XC, Xu XY: Mid-term results of intramuscular lengthening of gastrocnemius and/or soleus to correct equinus deformity in flatfoot. *Foot Ankle Int* 2015;36(10):1223-1228.

44. Ahn JY, Lee HS, Kim CH, Yang JP, Park SS: Calcaneocuboid joint subluxation after the calcaneal lengthening procedure in children. *Foot Ankle Int* 2014;35(7):677-682.

45. Attia E, Heldt B, Roepe IG, Shenava VR, Hill JF: Does the stabilization of the calcaneocuboid joint with Steinmann pin in Evans osteotomy affect its incidence of arthritis? *Foot (Edinb)* 2021;49:101846.

    After a calcaneal lengthening osteotomy and stabilization of the calcaneocuboid joint with a Steinmann pin, rates of radiographic evidence of calcaneocuboid joint arthritis are high in patients with maintenance of the pin postoperatively, compared with patients who undergo pin removal intraoperatively. Level of evidence: III.

46. Lee IH, Chung CY, Lee KM, et al: Incidence and risk factors of allograft bone failure after calcaneal lengthening. *Clin Orthop Relat Res* 2015;473(5):1765-1774.

47. Nejib K, Delpont M: Medium-term results of calcaneus lengthening in idiopathic symptomatic flat foot in children and adolescents. *J Child Orthop* 2020;14(4):286-292.

This review of 20 patients with mean follow-up of 8.3 years found good results in 13 patients. In the 35% with continued pain, residual deformity was most commonly supination of the forefoot. Level of evidence: IV.

48. James AM, Williams CM, Luscombe M, Hunter R, Haines TP: Factors associated with pain severity in children with calcaneal apophysitis (sever disease). *J Pediatr* 2015;167(2):455-459.

49. Kose O: Do we really need radiographic assessment for the diagnosis of non-specific heel pain (calcaneal apophysitis) in children? *Skeletal Radiol* 2010;39(4):359-361.

50. Rachel JN, Williams JB, Sawyer JR, Warner WC, Kelly DM: Is radiographic evaluation necessary in children with a clinical diagnosis of calcaneal apophysitis (sever disease)? *J Pediatr Orthop* 2011;31(5):548-550.

51. Wiegerinck JI, Zwiers R, Sierevelt IN, van Weert HCPM, van Dijk CN, Struijs PAA: Treatment of calcaneal apophysitis: Wait and see versus orthotic device versus physical therapy – A pragmatic therapeutic randomized clinical trial. *J Pediatr Orthop* 2016;36(2):152-157.

52. Pereira BS, Frada T, Freitas D, et al: Long-term follow-up of dorsal wedge osteotomy for pediatric Freiberg disease. *Foot Ankle Int* 2016;37(1):90-95.

53. Schade VL: Surgical management of Freiberg's infraction: A systematic review. *Foot Ankle Spec* 2015;8(6):498-519.

SECTION 2

Neuromuscular Disease

Section Editor:
Rebecca A. Cerrato, MD, FAAOS

CHAPTER 5

Cavovarus Deformity

AMIETHAB AIYER, MD, FAAOS, FAOA • NIGEL HSU, MD, FAAOS • NIALL SMYTH, MD

ABSTRACT

The cavovarus foot is characterized by hindfoot varus, a high medial longitudinal arch, a plantar-flexed first ray, and toe clawing. Hereditary sensory motor neuropathies or other causes of muscle imbalance often lead to deformities seen clinically. Clinical findings vary depending on the etiology and the severity of the deformity. Treatment is based on the symptoms, physical findings, deformity flexibility, and patient goals. Nonsurgical measures may involve bracing, orthotic devices, alterations in shoe wear, and physical therapy. Surgical intervention may involve soft-tissue releases, tendon transfers, osteotomies, and sometimes fusion with joint arthrodesis as indicated.

Keywords: calcaneal osteotomy; cavovarus; Charcot-Marie-Tooth (CMT) disease; pes cavus

Dr. Aiyer or an immediate family member serves as a paid consultant to or is an employee of Bioventus, KCI, Novastep, Smith & Nephew, and Vilex and serves as a board member, owner, officer, or committee member of American Orthopaedic Foot and Ankle Society. Dr. Hsu or an immediate family member is a member of a speakers' bureau or has made paid presentations on behalf of Arthrex, Inc. Neither Dr. Smyth nor any immediate family member has received anything of value from or has stock or stock options held in a commercial company or institution related directly or indirectly to the subject of this chapter.

INTRODUCTION

The cavovarus foot involves a complex array of deformities of the hindfoot, midfoot, and forefoot. The elevated medial longitudinal arch is caused by hyperplantar flexion of the first ray (forefoot equinus) and relative dorsiflexion of the calcaneus (calcaneocavus, elevated calcaneal pitch). The hindfoot is in varus, and the forefoot is pronated. Claw toes develop, and the plantar metatarsal fat pad migrates distally. These characteristic deformities result from muscle imbalance secondary to neurologic (commonly hereditary motor sensory neuropathy), traumatic, or other causes. Altered foot and ankle mechanics and the resulting abnormal gait can cause a multitude of issues, including lateral instability, lateral column bony overload, stress fracture, loss of motion, and possibly a fixed arthritic limb. Treatment is guided by the relative flexibility of the foot, the extent of deformity, and subsequent symptoms.

ETIOLOGY

Cavovarus foot deformities have several etiologies. Previously, approximately one-third of incidences were classified as idiopathic, but improved diagnostic methods demonstrate that neurologic conditions are responsible for most of these cases.[1] Charcot-Marie-Tooth (CMT) disease is the most common cause of pes cavovarus, but other etiologies also have been identified[2,3] (**Table 1**).

Hereditary motor sensory neuropathies, which are responsible for CMT disease (and other less common syndromes and diseases), are the most common cause of the cavovarus foot. CMT disease encompasses several genotypically different syndromes with similar clinical

Section 2: Neuromuscular Disease

This chapter is adapted from Johnson AH: Cavovarus deformity, in Chou LB, ed: *Orthopaedic Knowledge Update®: Foot and Ankle 6*. American Academy of Orthopaedic Surgeons, 2020, pp 51-64.

Table 1

Causes of Adult Cavovarus Foot

Congenital
- Arthrogryposis
- Talipes equinovarus (clubfoot)

Idiopathic

Neurologic
- Cerebral palsy
- Cerebrovascular accident (stroke)
- Charcot-Marie-Tooth disease (hereditary motor sensory neuropathy)
- Friedreich ataxia
- Poliomyelitis
- Spinal cord lesion (eg, myelomeningocele, syringomyelia, tumor)
- Spinal muscular atrophy

Traumatic
- Burn injury
- Compartment syndrome
- Crush injury
- Peroneal nerve injury
- Peroneal tendon insufficiency, severe chronic ankle instability
- Talus fracture nonunion

phenotypes. Jean-Martin Charcot, a French neurologist and anatomist, described the disease with Pierre Marie in 1886. In the same year, Dr. Howard Tooth, an English physician, described the same disorder as peroneal muscular atrophy.[4]

CMT neuropathies result from a mutation in one of more than 40 genes that affect Schwann cells and neurons. The disease has demyelinating (CMT1 and CMT4), axonal (CMT2 and CMT4), and intermediate (CMTX, CMT2E, and CMT) forms.[5-7] The classic phenotype of the most common form, CMT1, results from an abnormality in the peripheral myelin protein-22 (*PMP22*) gene; it is characterized by axonal demyelination that causes distal sensory loss, muscle weakness, and skeletal deformity.[5] Patients with CMT disease typically have abnormalities before they reach age 20 years and often before age 10 years. The peripheral neuropathy leads to distal muscle weakness, with intrinsic muscle degeneration. Over time this degeneration moves proximally to larger muscle groups, resulting in the myotendinous imbalances in the foot/ankle that lead to the characteristic cavovarus deformity.[8]

There are multiple other neurologic conditions, including other hereditary motor sensory neuropathies unrelated to CMT disease, that can result in the cavovarus foot, including amyotrophic lateral sclerosis, Huntington disease, cerebral palsy, spinal cord lesions, and other cerebral injuries. In a child with pes cavus, the clinician must consider a spinal cord anomaly, especially if the deformities are unilateral.[9] Congenital causes of pes cavovarus, such as congenital talipes equinovarus (clubfoot) and arthrogryposis, can be identified from birth. Arthrogryposis typically causes early rigid deformity, but other causes of rigid cavovarus in adolescence or young adulthood can be avoided if they are treated effectively during childhood.[10] In the past, poliomyelitis, which affects the anterior horn cells of the spinal cord, was a common cause of foot and ankle deformity.

Trauma to the lower extremity can cause cavovarus deformity. Malunion of a talar neck fracture can lead to medial column shortening, adduction of the talonavicular joint from overpull of the posterior tibial tendon, subtalar inversion, and a fixed hindfoot. An untreated calcaneus fracture can heal in a varus malunion. Superficial peroneal nerve injury can cause footdrop and posterior tibial tendon overdrive. Any isolated tendon injury can leave the strength of the opposing tendon unchecked, causing deformity over time. A burn injury or a compartment syndrome causing muscle contraction and neurologic injury can lead to cavovarus deformity. Some cases of cavovarus deformity have no obvious etiology and may be the result of an undetected peripheral neuropathy.

ANATOMY AND PATHOMECHANICS

Pes cavovarus can be seen as the product of any of several different etiologies arising in an imbalance of both the intrinsic and extrinsic musculature of the foot.[11] Depending on the muscles involved and the etiology of the disorder, the appearance of the deformity varies. Many deformities continue to progress over time.

In the normal foot, proper function is maintained by pairs of muscles working in opposition to each other. These agonist-antagonist pairs keep the foot balanced to facilitate weight bearing on the tripod of the foot (first and fifth metatarsal heads and the calcaneus). If one muscle is disturbed, relative overdrive of the opposing muscle results and a deformity develops. Understanding the normal anatomy and function of the muscle groups is essential to comprehending the pathologic cavovarus foot (**Table 2**).

The tibialis anterior inserts on the plantarmedial aspects of the first metatarsal and medial cuneiform. This facilitates primary dorsiflexion and secondary inversion of the ankle. The antagonist of the tibialis anterior

Chapter 5: Cavovarus Deformity

Table 2

Muscles of the Foot and Ankle

Muscle	Insertion	Function	Antagonist
Tibialis anterior	Navicular, medial cuneiform	Strong dorsiflexion, weak inversion	Peroneus longus
Tibialis posterior	Medial column (wide insertion at medial and plantar midfoot and forefoot)	Strong inversion, weak plantar flexion	Peroneus brevis
Peroneus longus	First metatarsal base, medial cuneiform	Strong plantar flexion of the first metatarsal, weak eversion	Tibialis anterior
Peroneus brevis	Fifth metatarsal base	Eversion	Tibialis posterior
Intrinsics (lumbricals, interossei)	Proximal phalanges (extensor expansions)	Flexion of metatarsophalangeal joints, extension of proximal and distal interphalangeal joints	Extrinsic long extensors and flexors
Extrinsic long extensors (extensor digitorum longus, extensor hallucis longus, extensor digitorum brevis, extensor hallucis brevis)	Extensor hood at metatarsophalangeal joint, distal phalanges	Extension of metatarsophalangeal joints, proximal and distal interphalangeal joints	Intrinsics, extrinsic long flexors
Extrinsic long flexors (flexor digitorum longus, flexor hallucis longus, flexor digitorum brevis, flexor hallucis brevis)	Flexor sheath, plantar aspect of distal phalanges	Toe flexion at proximal and distal interphalangeal joints	Extrinsic long extensors

is the peroneus longus, which acts as a plantar flexor of the first ray and weak evertor (relative to peroneus brevis); it inserts on the plantarlateral aspect of the medial cuneiform and the first metatarsal base. The tibialis posterior, with its wide insertion along the medial and plantarmedial aspect of the medial column (primarily the navicular), is a primary inverter of the foot and a secondary plantarflexor. The tibialis posterior is opposed by the peroneus brevis, a strong evertor that inserts at the base of the fifth metatarsal.

The intrinsic muscles, including the lumbricals and the interossei, insert into the extensor mechanism at the proximal phalanx; they flex the metatarsophalangeal (MTP) joints and extend the proximal and distal interphalangeal joints. The extrinsic extensor muscles, including the extensor digitorum longus, extensor hallucis longus, extensor digitorum brevis, and extensor hallucis brevis, extend the toes through the MTP, proximal interphalangeal, and distal interphalangeal joints. The extrinsic long flexors (including the flexor digitorum longus and flexor hallucis longus) and the short flexors (including the flexor digitorum brevis) flex the toes at the proximal and distal interphalangeal joints; the flexor hallucis brevis attaches to the base of the proximal phalanx and flexes the hallux MTP joint.

CMT disease is the most commonly used clinical example of cavovarus deformity. In the most widely accepted etiology, weakness in the peroneus brevis and tibialis anterior is primarily responsible for the deformity. As these two muscle groups deteriorate, there is overpull of the opposing posterior tibial tendon and peroneus longus; this leads to inversion of the foot through the talonavicular joint and plantar flexion of the first ray, respectively. Given that the pull of the tibialis posterior is unopposed by the peroneus brevis, this leads to inversion of the hindfoot and locks the subtalar joint in supination.[4] As the tibialis anterior becomes unable to dorsiflex the ankle, the long toe extensors attempt to act as a substitute, and they hyperextend the toes at the MTP joints. Weakness of the intrinsic muscles leads to loss of flexion of the lesser MTP joints and the unopposed long/short flexors flex the proximal/distal interphalangeal joints, all of which contribute to the clawing of the toes and distal migration of the plantar fat pad. Dorsiflexion of the lesser MTP joints drive the metatarsal heads plantarly and leads to an equinus deformity of the midfoot. This

Section 2: Neuromuscular Disease

© 2025 American Academy of Orthopaedic Surgeons

Orthopaedic Knowledge Update®: Foot and Ankle 7

53

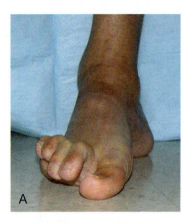 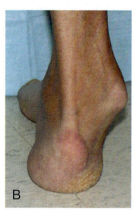

FIGURE 1 Photographs show a cavovarus foot in a patient with Charcot-Marie-Tooth disease. **A**, Anterolateral view shows the high medial longitudinal arch and clawing of the toes. **B**, Posterior view shows the varus position of the hindfoot. (Reproduced from Johnson AH, May CJ: Adult cavovarus foot. *Orthop Knowl Online J* 2012;10[4].)

can lead to contracture of the plantar fascia, accentuation of the cavus deformity, and subsequent plantar flexion of the metatarsal heads. Furthermore, contracture of the Achilles tendon from medial displacement of the hindfoot can worsen contracture of the plantar fascia.[12,13] Forefoot/midfoot equinus and plantar flexion of the first ray cause forefoot pronation. As the forefoot deformity becomes fixed, the balance of deformity between the plantarflexed first ray and varus hindfoot facilitates keeping the foot plantigrade[10,14] (Figure 1).

The mechanism of development may be different in cavovarus stemming from other etiologies. In poliomyelitis, triceps surae involvement causes weak push-off strength. The long toe flexors are recruited, leading to forefoot plantar flexion and the development of cavus. A deep posterior compartment syndrome with subsequent muscle contracture can lead to tibialis posterior overpull with equinus and cavovarus. Identification of the etiology of the disorder and the affected nerves and muscles allows further understanding of the pathomechanics manifested by the patient over time.

DIAGNOSIS

Patients typically present with foot pain and/or lateral instability in the ankle; lateral foot pain from bony overload at the base of the fifth metatarsal may result in a stress reaction or fracture at the fifth metatarsal base; recurrent stress fracture can occur in a subtle cavovarus foot or with a fixed deformity.[15] Forefoot pain at the sesamoid bones with hyperplantar flexion of the first ray may also be a presenting symptom. Pain beneath the metatarsal heads may be caused by distal migration of the plantar fat pad associated with subluxated or dislocated MTP joints and claw toes. Late in the disease, when the deformities are fixed, the cause of pain may be secondary to degenerative changes in the joints (particularly the hindfoot, midfoot, and ankle joints). Lateral ankle and subtalar instability typically results from loss of dynamic lateral ankle stability (peroneal brevis eversion weakness), lateral ligament insufficiency, and the mechanical contribution of hindfoot varus. Patients may report history of recurrent ankle sprains.

History and Physical Examination

A careful history is an important first step in diagnosing the cause of a cavovarus deformity. The family history can be useful because the patient often describes a sibling or parent with similar physical characteristics. Identification of a family member with pes cavovarus may suggest a hereditary sensorimotor neuropathy. Unilateral deformity, especially if it is severe or accompanied by other neurologic abnormalities, may be indicative of a spinal cord abnormality.[9] Children with minimal symptoms of pes cavus are often referred for evaluation. The presence of clinical features such as weakness, unsteady gait, family history, or other neurologic deficits can obviate the need for further testing if the diagnosis of CMT seems clear.[16]

The patient should be examined standing and walking, with the limbs unclothed. During the swing phase of gait, footdrop or recruitment of the toe extensors indicates tibialis anterior weakness. The lower extremities should be compared with one another while the patient is standing. From behind, the position of the heel is noted relative to the midfoot and forefoot; hindfoot varus is more apparent from this viewpoint. The Coleman block test can be useful to understand the relative flexibility of the hindfoot and if the hindfoot deformity is driven by the forefoot. A rectangular block 0.5 to 1 inch thick is placed under the lateral border of the foot; if the heel is corrected to neutral or a few degrees of valgus, the hindfoot is considered flexible, and correction of the forefoot deformity should correct the hindfoot deformity. If the hindfoot remains in varus, the deformity is considered rigid, and a hindfoot and forefoot procedure probably will be necessary to achieve full deformity correction[17] (Figure 2).

Tibiotalar joint motion is examined to identify an equinus contracture. While holding the subtalar joint in neutral, if dorsiflexion of the ankle increases when the knee is bent, the gastrocnemius is contracted. If the contracture is not corrected with the knee flexed, the cause may be an Achilles tendon contracture or it may be a mechanical block to dorsiflexion (bone spurs, capsular contracture, or a medialized talus). A thorough neurologic examination is critical. Vibration, position, sensation, and reflexes should be checked, and any muscle

Chapter 5: Cavovarus Deformity

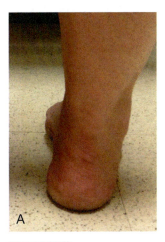 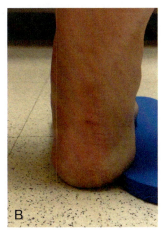

FIGURE 2 Posterior photographs show a cavovarus deformity before (**A**) and during (**B**) the Coleman block test. With the Coleman block in place, the hindfoot is corrected to neutral, and the hindfoot deformity is found to be flexible.

atrophy or weakness, noted. Pediatric patients should be examined to detect spinal skin dimples, a hair patch, or another sign of occult spinal disease.

Any patient presenting with lateral instability (including recurrent sprains) or peroneal weakness, peroneal tendinopathy/tear, or fifth metatarsal fracture must be evaluated for a cavovarus deformity. Even a subtle hindfoot varus deformity can lead to lateral overload and further deformity. Overall alignment must always be considered in addition to the acute diagnosis.[18]

The diagnosis of CMT disease is based on physical examination findings, neurologic testing, family history, and genetic testing. A physician may be alerted to the presence of pes cavus by physical examination findings consistent with the disorder, such as a high arch, weak extensors, claw toes, and even footdrop.

Electromyography and nerve conduction studies can be used to identify patterns of deficiency often seen with CMT disease. If a familial link appears to be present, genetic testing is indicated for purposes of determining the prognosis, a need for family planning, and eligibility for a clinical study.[16,19] Algorithms for neurologic and genetic testing have been developed and published.[20] Nerve biopsies typically are unnecessary for diagnosis.

Imaging Studies

AP, oblique, and lateral weight-bearing radiographs of the foot and ankle are the essential initial imaging studies. An axial heel view, a Canale view of the talar neck, and a Cobey-Saltzman view to evaluate hindfoot alignment may also be useful.[21] CT further assesses the extent of joint degeneration and helps to further demonstrate three-dimensional bony alignment. Weight-bearing CT (WBCT) is a newer modality that is growing in utility. Recent studies demonstrate its ability to differentiate CMT from idiopathic forms of cavovarus, differences in articular surface interactions in cavovarus deformity, and the correlation between WBCT measurements and clinical examination findings in this patient population as well. Additionally, WBCT has been able to evaluate the rotational/adduction through the transverse tarsal joints of patients with CMT.[22-24] MRI is used to determine the ligamentous and tendinous integrity of the foot and ankle.

The weight-bearing lateral radiograph is perhaps the most useful study for evaluating and understanding a cavovarus deformity. A thorough understanding of the normal lateral radiographic landmarks and the commonly measured angles (Meary, Hibb, and calcaneal pitch) is essential to identify radiographic anomalies and variations[25] (**Figure 3**). Subtle abnormalities, such as a

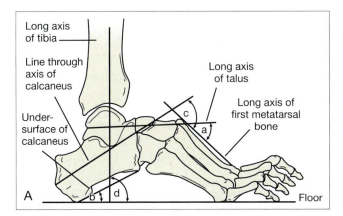 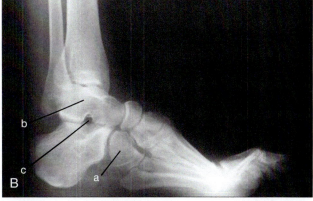

FIGURE 3 **A**, Schematic drawing shows the angles used to evaluate the cavovarus foot. a, Meary angle; b, calcaneal pitch angle; c, Hibb angle; d, tibioplantar angle. **B**, Lateral weight-bearing radiograph demonstrates characteristic findings. a, bell-shaped cuboid; b, double talar dome; c, open sinus tarsi. (Panel B reproduced and adapted from Johnson AH, May CJ: Adult cavovarus foot. *Orthop Knowl Online J* 2012;10[4].)

bell-shaped cuboid, a double talar dome, or an open sinus tarsi, can be seen on a weight-bearing lateral radiograph and help guide the formation of the pes cavus diagnosis. If a spinal cord abnormality is suspected, imaging of the hips and spine may be indicated.

NONSURGICAL TREATMENT

The goal of treating a cavovarus foot is to improve function and allow the patient to ambulate with a painless plantigrade foot. The treatment varies with the extent of the deformity and its relative flexibility. Stable or slowly progressive deformity may be managed with nonsurgical treatment, but surgical treatment should be considered early in progressive deformity while the foot is still supple.

Initial nonsurgical treatment includes the use of orthotic devices and bracing treatment. An off-the-shelf insert may be beneficial for a foot with mild hindfoot varus, but a custom-molded semirigid orthotic device with a lateral post is more often necessary for any clinical effects. A recess under the first metatarsal is helpful to accommodate the plantarflexed first ray. Metatarsal pads can be added to off-load painful lesser metatarsal heads. Lace-up ankle brace can be used to treat ankle instability. A custom Arizona brace can be used for pain from degenerative joint changes. A custom-molded ankle-foot orthosis is useful for treating severe ankle and/or subtalar instability, rigid deformity, arthritic pes cavus, or footdrop. Care must be taken to avoid skin breakdown and ulceration, especially in a patient with neuropathy.

Shoe modifications and the use of extra-depth shoes may be necessary to accommodate the high arch and claw toes of a cavovarus foot and to allow sufficient room to seat an ankle brace or other orthotic device.

Physical therapy and a stretching program are important to maintain range of motion, particularly eversion and dorsiflexion.

SURGICAL TREATMENT PLANNING

Surgical intervention is chosen based on the extent, etiology, and rigidity of the deformity as well as other variables.

Careful preoperative planning is crucial. Flexible joints should be preserved when possible, and rigid and/or arthritic joints may require fusion. Osseous corrections alone do not correct the underlying cause of the deformity. Tendon transfers act to remove deformity forces and augment a lack of function; tendon transfers also lead to a loss of a grade of strength. In a patient with muscle imbalance, tendon transfers and realigning osteotomies lead to better outcomes than fusion.[26,27]

Myotendinous imbalances related to CMT include peroneus longus overpowering the weak tibialis anterior, and the posterior tibialis tendon overpowering the weak peroneus brevis. Contracted tendons should be released or lengthened, and contracted joints should be released or fused.[2] Some surgeons prefer early surgical intervention to prevent progressive deformity in patients with identified muscle imbalance.

Preoperative planning must include thorough imaging and diagnostic studies. Standard radiographs including three weight-bearing views of the foot and ankle are mandatory. CT may be necessary for understanding the three-dimensional anatomy of the foot and gauging the extent of joint degeneration. WBCT enables images to be obtained under physiologic load in the standing position. It can highlight the deformity severity in the standing position.[28] MRI is useful for evaluating ligament and tendon integrity and assessing the cartilaginous surface of the joints to determine whether fusion or joint salvage is preferable. If tendon transfers are being considered and physical examination findings are equivocal, electromyography may be needed to assess tendon strength and viability.

SOFT-TISSUE PROCEDURES

Plantar Fascia Release

The plantar fascia in a cavovarus foot is contracted as a result of the calcaneovarus and the first ray plantar flexion. Plantar fascia release can reduce the height of the arch. A plantar fascia release (Steindler procedure) often is the first step in cavovarus reconstruction.[29] An oblique incision of approximately 2 to 3 cm is made at the glabrous fold at the level of the medial insertion point of the plantar fascia. Meticulous dissection through the fat will expose the fascia of the abductor hallucis for release and plantar retraction. The contracted plantar fascia is then identified and isolated with retractors or elevators and released sharply transversely. As discussed in a 2020 study, endoscopic plantar fascia release is a newer technique that can reduce pain from surgical dissection while still offers clear visualization of the anatomy.[30]

Gastrocnemius Recession

Depending on the extent of the equinus component, an Achilles tendon lengthening is likely to be part of any cavovarus foot reconstruction. Gastrocnemius or Achilles contracture may limit the capability of other procedures, such as calcaneal osteotomy, to correct the deformity.[31,32] If the hindfoot is in varus, the Achilles tendon is effectively shortened, and the type of lengthening depends on the extent of Achilles tendon involvement. A preoperative Silfverskiöld test helps determine whether the contracture is coming from the gastrocnemius or the Achilles tendon.[33] Ankle dorsiflexion is assessed with the knee first held straight and then flexed 90°. If the gastrocnemius is tight, dorsiflexion is limited with the knee extended (the gastrocnemius is stretched) and is improved with the knee flexed (the gastrocnemius is relaxed). If ankle dorsiflexion is limited with the knee either flexed or extended, the Achilles tendon is tight.

Gastrocnemius recession is most easily performed with the patient supine and the medial aspect of the calf exposed. A 2- to 3-cm longitudinal incision is made midcalf, with dissection carried down to the fascia while protecting the saphenous nerve and vein. The fascia is incised, and blunt dissection is used to identify the gastrocnemius muscle just proximal to the aponeurosis at the Achilles tendon. The gastrocnemius is isolated with retractors or a small speculum, and the gastrocnemius fascia is released medially to laterally as the ankle is held in dorsiflexion. Care should be taken to identify and protect the sural nerve, which often is just posterior to the fascia. After the release, the ankle is gently stretched in dorsiflexion. The fascia should be reapproximated to avoid muscle herniation.

Achilles Tendon Lengthening

If Achilles tendon contracture is responsible for the equinus component of the cavovarus deformity, the tendon itself will require lengthening. Percutaneous lengthening is usually adequate, and only rarely an open lengthening is necessary to gain adequate length. In the percutaneous approach, through three small, sequential stab incisions 1.5 cm apart, starting 1.5 cm proximal to the tendon insertion, one-half of the tendon is sharply released horizontally alternating laterally, medially, and laterally again. The ankle is gently tensioned in dorsiflexion, and the tendon is Z-lengthened. Open lengthening usually is done through a medial incision.

Modified Jones Procedure

With loss of tibialis anterior strength, the extensor hallucis longus overcompensates to aid in ankle dorsiflexion. The result is hyperdorsiflexion of the first MTP joint and clawing of the big toe. The pulling of the peroneus longus to plantarflex the first ray contributes to the deformity. Traditionally, this deformity has been treated using the modified Jones procedure.[34] Fusing the interphalangeal joint and transferring the extensor hallucis longus to the metatarsal head largely corrects the deformity.[35] The interphalangeal joint is fused first. Through a small dorsal incision, the interphalangeal joint is prepared, compressed, and fixed with crossing screws or a single 4.0-mm screw across the joint. The extensor hallucis longus is released from its insertion. The distal metatarsal is exposed, and a transverse drill hole is made across the level of the distal third of the joint. The extensor hallucis longus is threaded through the hole and sewn back onto itself while the ankle is held in 10° of dorsiflexion.

An alternative to the Jones procedure involves harvesting the flexor hallucis longus, which is released through a medial incision at the MTP joint as far distally as possible. The tendon is passed plantar to dorsal through a 2.5-mm drill hole in the plantar base of the proximal phalanx and then sewn back to itself or to the periosteum. The extensor hallucis longus may need to be lengthened, and the MTP joint capsule may need to be released.[36,37]

Peroneus Brevis–to–Peroneus Longus Tenodesis and Lateral Ligament Reconstruction

Lateral instability with peroneus brevis weakness and relative peroneus longus overdrive is seen in CMT disease. In other disorders causing pes cavovarus, such as peroneal nerve injury, traumatic tendon rupture, and chronic ankle instability, hindfoot varus and peroneal deficiency can lead to mechanical lateral instability.

If the peroneus longus remains intact and functional, it can be tenodesed to the brevis to act as an evertor. In this situation, the peroneal tendons are exposed laterally at the ankle and hindfoot. The peroneus longus is sewn adjacent to the peroneus brevis at the level of the ankle joint, posterior to the fibula, using a strong nonabsorbable suture. An intact peroneus brevis can remain, and tenodesis of the peroneus longus can be done distally, close to its insertion on the fifth metatarsal. If the peroneus brevis tendon is damaged as well, further augmentation will likely be necessary. If the muscle is still viable, free autograft or allograft hamstring tendon can be used to bridge the damaged portion of tendon or secured proximally and then attached to the base of the fifth metatarsal using a biotenodesis screw or suture anchors. If the peroneus brevis muscle is deficient, a flexor hallucis longus transfer may be considered.

Torn but viable lateral ligaments should be imbricated and reattached to their footprints on the distal fibula using suture anchors. The extensor retinaculum can be mobilized and oversewn to reinforce the repair (the Broström-Gould technique).[38] If the lateral ligament complex is severely deficient, further augmentation may be required using tendon autograft, allograft, and/or synthetic suture tapes.

Posterior Tibial Tendon Transfer

The posterior tibial tendon often contributes to cavovarus deformity as it inverts and plantarflexes the foot unopposed in the setting of peroneus brevis and tibialis anterior weakness. By transferring the tendon to the dorsal aspect of the midfoot, this robust tendon becomes a dorsiflexion

Section 2: Neuromuscular Disease

checkrein. The tendon is harvested through a medial incision from its broad insertion along the navicular and medial column. Another small incision is made 8 to 10 cm above the ankle joint adjacent to the medial tibia, through which the tendon is pulled proximally. A lateral incision is made 3 to 4 cm distal to this, and the tendon is tunneled through the interosseous membrane, exiting in the anterior compartment. Finally, the tendon is tunneled under the soft tissue, under the retinaculum to the middle or lateral cuneiform, and is fixed with a biotenodesis screw; this technique facilitates improved excursion. To maximize tension on the repair the transfer is routed superficial to the inferior extensor retinaculum. Care is taken to fix the tendon while the ankle is held in a neutral position to provide adequate tension. Final fixation of the tendon should be delayed until the end of the surgery, after any concomitant procedures are completed. An alternative method would be transferring the posterior tibialis tendon to the cuboid to not only improve dorsiflexion but also eversion strength.[39]

Other Tendon Transfers

Other tendon transfers may be considered, depending on the etiology of the deformity and the extent of weakness, even though these transfers may not be traditional for cavovarus deformity. For example, there may be a need to transfer an anterior tibial tendon laterally to the middle or lateral cuneiform so that it will not continue to contribute to inversion. The extensor digitorum longus can be used for dorsiflexion of the foot if the posterior tibial tendon is weak. The tendon slips can be released distally and sutured together and then routed to the dorsal midfoot at the middle or lateral cuneiform and secured with a biotenodesis screw or through a bone tunnel. Claw toe deformity is common in pes cavus. Releasing the long extensors distally helps to correct toe clawing.[36] Flexor tendon transfer can be used for flexible claw toe deformities. For rigid deformities, MTP joint capsule release, extensor tendon release, and proximal interphalangeal arthrodesis may be necessary to correct the deformity.

BONY PROCEDURES

First Metatarsal Dorsiflexion Osteotomy

If the primary cause of a cavovarus deformity is forefoot driven, confirmed with a Coleman block test demonstrating hindfoot correction, a first metatarsal dorsiflexion osteotomy is needed for correction. With a hyperplantarflexed first ray in CMT disease or another disorder, the patient may report plantar forefoot pain and have clawing of the first MTP joint. A longitudinal incision is made over the dorsum of the base of the first metatarsal. The osteotomy is made 1 cm distal to the first tarsometatarsal joint, and a 4- to 5-mm dorsal

wedge is removed. Closing more than a 7- to 8-mm gap may compromise the integrity of the plantar cortex. The gap is closed and fixed with a small, low-profile plate or with 2.7- or 3.5-mm screws. If additional correction is needed, a further dorsiflexion osteotomy can be performed through the medial cuneiform. This can be either a dorsal closing wedge or plantar opening wedge depending on surgeon preference. As discussed in a 2020 study, a consensus group did conclude that a dorsal closing-wedge osteotomy of the first metatarsal is needed in almost all cases of CMT.[40] Alternatively, the first tarsometatarsal joint can be fused in dorsiflexion, with similar results. It is important to note that WBCT has highlighted the role of first metatarsal rotation with regard to hindfoot alignment. According to a 2022 study, although a dorsiflexion osteotomy may correct sagittal plane deformity, rotational deformity may also be addressed with a first tarsometatarsal fusion.[41]

Calcaneal Osteotomy

A lateralizing calcaneal osteotomy should be considered in a patient with a hindfoot varus deformity that is not correctable passively or with the Coleman block test. The osteotomy moves the heel into a physiologically neutral or slightly valgus position. The Achilles tendon should typically be concomitantly lengthened through a gastrocnemius recession or direct tendon lengthening to allow the tuber to shift laterally and thereby shift the Achilles tendon moment arm laterally. A calcaneal osteotomy not only corrects hindfoot varus but also shifts the center of force laterally at the ankle joint.[42]

Multiple osteotomies have been described to correct heel alignment from varus to a more physiologic position in 2° to 5° of valgus. A lateral slide osteotomy can achieve a powerful correction without shortening the calcaneus (**Figure 4**). The Dwyer closing-wedge osteotomy, modified with lateralization of the tuber, has been shown to achieve significant correction of the varus heel. Historically, the Dwyer had been reported to undercorrect the hindfoot, shorten the calcaneus, and therefore weaken the Achilles. However, when modified with lateralization of the tuber, it has been shown in cadaver and in vivo studies to be a powerful tool for correction.[43-48] In this procedure, the incision is made laterally on the heel extending from the anterior aspect of the Achilles tendon insertion to the anterior edge of the calcaneal tuber. The cut should be perpendicular to the long axis of the calcaneus. Two 1.25-mm guide-wires can be used superiorly and inferiorly to mark the intended location of the osteotomy, which can be confirmed on lateral fluoroscopy. A sagittal saw is used to make the cut, and a wide osteotome or laminar spreader is used to spread the periosteum medially to allow the

Chapter 5: Cavovarus Deformity

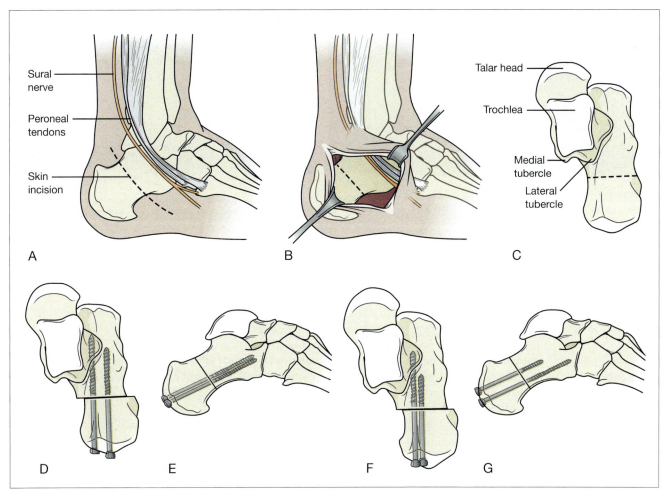

FIGURE 4 Schematic drawings show the procedure for a lateral slide calcaneal osteotomy. **A**, Lateral view shows the posterior lateral incision. **B**, Lateral view shows placement of the calcaneus cut with a saw after the soft tissues have been retracted. **C**, Oblique coronal view of the osteotomy, which avoids penetrating close to the sustentaculum tali. **D** and **E** show the osteotomy held with two side-by-side transcalcaneal screws. **F** and **G** show alternative screw positioning with superior and inferior screws. Dashed line, incision; solid line, osteotomy. (Adapted with permission from Hansen ST Jr, ed: *Functional Reconstruction of the Foot and Ankle*. Lippincott Williams & Wilkins, 2000, p 369.)

heel to slide up to 1 cm laterally. A lateral wedge can be removed to finish the correction. The posterior fragment can also be moved superiorly to decrease the calcaneal pitch. The osteotomy is fixed with one or two screws placed through the posterior tuber anteriorly. Overhanging lateral bone is tamped down or resected for bone graft (**Figure 5**). Further correction of plantar pressure and weight bearing has been shown to be achieved when incorporating internal rotation of the posterior calcaneus.[47]

The Z-shaped osteotomy is another powerful procedure to correct hindfoot varus and may actually achieve the most correction.[43,49] This version of the calcaneal lateral slide allows multiplanar correction[35] (**Figure 6**). A Z-shaped cut is made laterally into the calcaneus. The superior vertical limb is cut about 1.5 cm anterior to the Achilles insertion at the slope of the superior calcaneal cortex. The inferior vertical limb is cut at the posterior extent of the posterior facet. A horizontal saw cut joins the cut limbs, and a lateral-based wedge is removed to increase the valgus correction. The heel is moved laterally and may also be externally rotated. One or two screws are used for fixation (**Figure 7**). Because of the degree of correction that can be achieved, care should be taken to avoid overcorrection.[39]

A calcaneal osteotomy through a minimally invasive approach has been described as well. Through a 0.5- to 1-cm lateral incision centered over the lateral calcaneal tuber, a 2 × 30–mm Shannon burr is used to make a straight lateral or chevron-shaped osteotomy.[50] Regardless of the approach, care must be taken to avoid the sural nerve during the exposure to the lateral

Section 2: Neuromuscular Disease

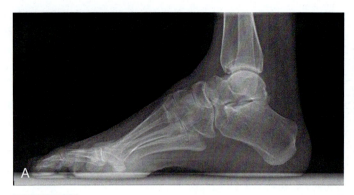 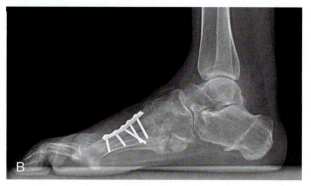

FIGURE 5 Lateral radiographs show a forefoot-driven cavovarus foot before (**A**) and after (**B**) first metatarsal dorsiflexion osteotomy, lateral ligament reconstruction with peroneus longus-to-peroneus brevis tenodesis, calcaneal osteotomy, and gastrocnemius recession.

calcaneus. In addition, lateral translation of the calcaneus has the potential to compress the tarsal tunnel, resulting in an iatrogenic tarsal tunnel syndrome.[51] The surgeon needs to be aware that any postoperative tibial nerve deficit or acute nerve pain could represent acute tarsal tunnel syndrome. Some authors even advocate prophylactic tarsal tunnel decompression during the procedure.[52]

In light of the numerous methods for performing a calcaneal osteotomy, it is important to highlight that a consensus group of experts did not reach a unanimous opinion regarding a single optimal technique.[40]

Fusion

Fusion is indicated if the deformities are rigid or arthritic and symptomatic, and a plantigrade, stable foot cannot be achieved through osteotomy, tissue releases, and tendon transfers alone. Arthrodesis cannot be used in isolation in the presence of deforming muscular forces, however, or further deformity may occur. Muscle balancing must be used in conjunction with fusion to maintain the neutral position achieved at the time of surgery.[2,40]

Subtalar fusion is used if rigid hindfoot varus coexists with degenerative changes in the joint. The varus can be corrected through the joint by removing lateral bone or adding a bone block to the medial side of the joint. The approach to the subtalar joint depends on the other procedures to be done on the lateral side of the foot at the same time. After preparing the joint and adding bone graft, if necessary, the joint is stabilized with internal fixation and is assessed clinically and radiographically. If residual varus remains, a calcaneal slide osteotomy can be added before final screw fixation from the heel into the talar dome and neck.

A triple arthrodesis is indicated if degenerative changes are seen at the talonavicular, calcaneocuboid, and/or subtalar joint. Often the medial capsule, spring ligament, and a portion of the posterior tibial tendon must be released to rotate the talus medially in relation to the navicular joint. The joints are prepared and fixed in the standard fashion, and concomitant forefoot procedures are done as needed.

The Siffert beak triple arthrodesis combines osteotomy and triple arthrodesis to correct varus and cavus in severe, rigid deformity.[53,54] This correction is technically challenging but can provide substantial correction. The subtalar and calcaneocuboid joints are prepared through a lateral approach. Through a medial approach, the capsule over the talonavicular joint is elevated without stripping the blood supply to the talus. Step cuts are made in the plantar aspect of the talar head and in the adjacent dorsal navicular, with more bone taken dorsally, and the two bones are linked into each other. The lateral side is shortened through the calcaneocuboid joint. The joints are fixed with screws and/or plates.[53]

Midfoot osteotomies with fusion can be useful for correcting cavus. In the Jahss[55] osteotomy, dorsal bone wedges are resected at the tarsometatarsal joints, and the joints are fused. The Cole and Japas osteotomies correct cavus with dorsal closing-wedge osteotomies and navicular cuneiform fusion.[4] The Siffert beak triple arthrodesis incorporates closing-wedge osteotomies at the talonavicular, calcaneocuboid, and subtalar joints as part of a triple arthrodesis to correct severe rigid deformity.[48] These procedures can be challenging, and fusion may be difficult to achieve. Newer procedures including navicular excision and cuboid closing-wedge osteotomies for severe deformity attempt to salvage some motion and avoid fusion in relatively young patients.[56] Again, there is no consensus regarding the optimal choice of osteotomy.[40]

The options are limited if the foot deformity is rigid and the ankle is arthritic, in varus, and symptomatic. Pantalar fusion may be the only viable option

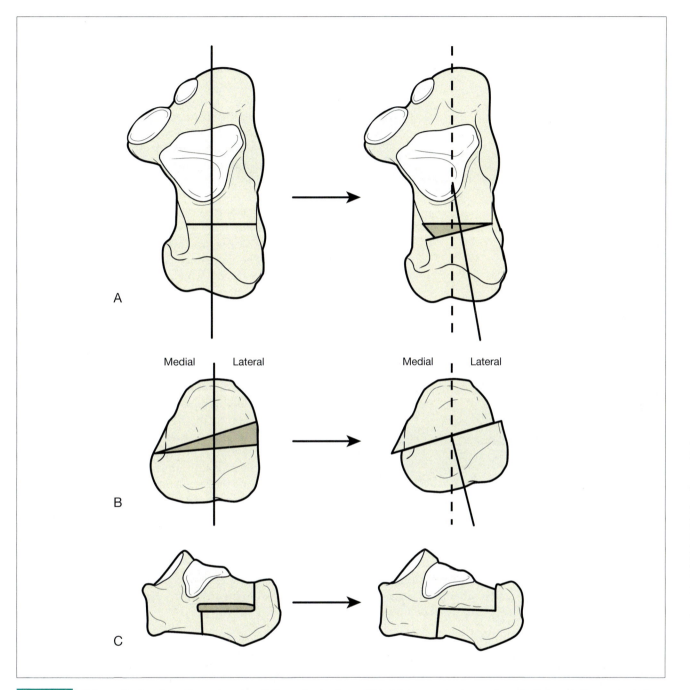

FIGURE 6 Schematic drawings show steps in a Z-shaped osteotomy. This triplanar osteotomy allows both translation and rotation for a more powerful correction of the hindfoot varus. The solid vertical lines on the left drawings and the dashed lines on the right drawings represent the central axis of the calcaneus in each plane. **A**, Axial view of the calcaneal osteotomy (left) and the lateral rotation of the osteotomy with medial gapping (right). **B**, Posterior view of the calcaneus shows the lateral wedge cut (left), which is then removed and closed down creating valgus through the cut (right). **C**, Lateral view of the calcaneus shows the lateral wedge cut (left), and then the wedge is removed and closed down creating valgus through the cut (right).

to straighten the foot and ankle, although the results are poor with low patient satisfaction (**Figure 8**). Experienced foot and ankle surgeons use total ankle arthroplasty in combination with triple arthrodesis or foot reconstruction in select patients with cavovarus and ankle arthritis[42] (**Figure 9**). Although in the past ankle replacement in patients with coronal plane deformity was contraindicated, improvements in technique, instrumentation, and implants have made arthroplasty a viable option for some patients with

Section 2: Neuromuscular Disease

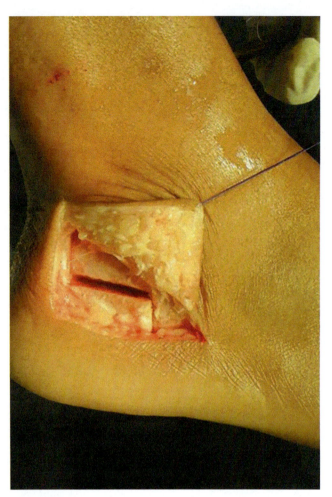

FIGURE 7 Intraoperative photograph shows a Z-shaped calcaneal osteotomy. (Courtesy of Ruth L. Thomas, MD, Little Rock, AR.)

pes cavus and ankle varus. Total ankle arthroplasty should be selected with caution as any remaining varus deformity in the ankle can lead to abnormal patterns of wear on the prosthesis and early failure of components.

Correcting the hindfoot deformity and plantar flexion of the first ray is imperative to create a stable platform for the ankle.[57,58] Identifying the site of maximum deformity is important when deciding the surgical plan to achieve appropriate correction. As an example, in CMT maximal rotational and abduction deformity occurs through the transverse tarsal joints.[24] The surgeon must also always be aware that the deformity is three dimensional and any surgical technique chosen must address the deformity in both the sagittal and transverse planes.[40]

Claw Toe Correction

Claw toes result from extensor overload at the MTP joints and flexor overload at the proximal interphalangeal joints. The deformity is worsened by contracture of the plantar fascia, which leads to increased plantar flexion of the metatarsals. Dynamic deformities can be resolved with correction of the deforming forces after a cavovarus reconstruction of the foot.[6] Flexor-to-extensor transfer can be useful for flexible deformities that persist. The Girdlestone-Taylor flexor-to-extensor tendon transfer and its various iterations involve transferring the flexor digitorum longus to the extensor digitorum longus dorsally at the MTP joint.[59,60] Through a plantar incision at the MTP joint, the long flexor is carefully dissected and then released as far distally as possible. The tendon is brought up on the lateral side of the joint or split and sutured, each end to the medial and the lateral side of the extensor expansion. Alternatively, a simple flexor tenotomy may be sufficient. Rigid claw toes require formal correction with MTP joint releases, proximal interphalangeal resections, and pinning or internal fixation to fuse and straighten the toes. With regard to the great toe, fusion of the interphalangeal joint with a retrograde screw and transfer of the extensor hallucis longus to the first metatarsal is commonly performed.[40]

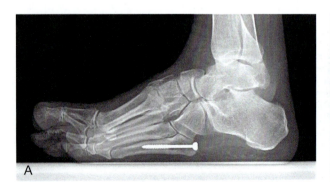
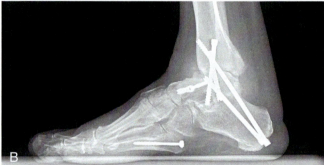

FIGURE 8 Lateral radiographs show severe, rigid cavovarus in a patient with multiple sclerosis. **A,** The patient had a prior fifth metatarsal stress fracture from lateral overload fixated with a screw. **B,** Image taken after a pantalar fusion to reestablish a plantigrade, stable weight-bearing foot.

Chapter 5: Cavovarus Deformity

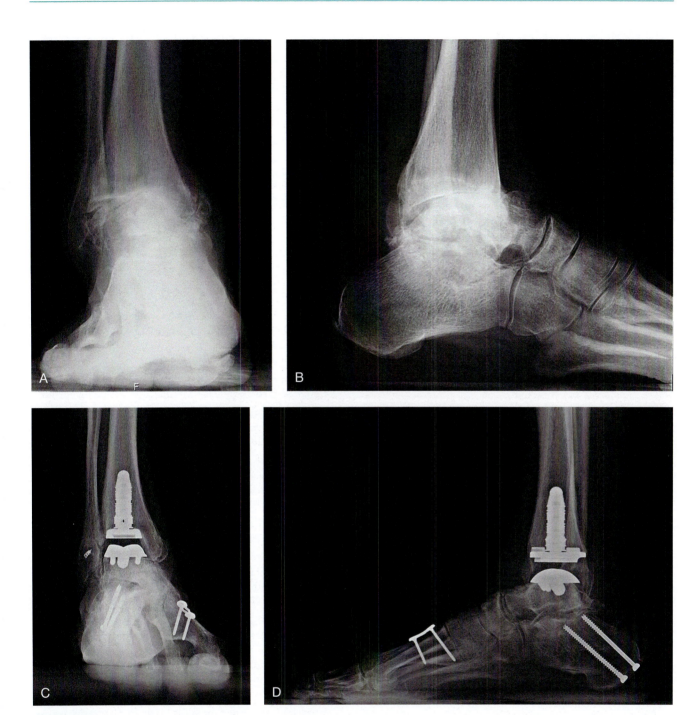

FIGURE 9 **A** and **B**, Radiographs of cavovarus foot with concomitant varus ankle arthritis. **C** and **D**, Radiographs of corrected cavovarus foot after calcaneal Z-type osteotomy and first metatarsal dorsiflexion osteotomy with total ankle arthroplasty. (Courtesy of Constantine Demetracopoulos, MD, Hospital for Special Surgery, New York, NY.)

SUMMARY

The cavovarus foot is characterized by hindfoot varus, a high medial longitudinal arch, and claw toes caused by muscle imbalances. The clinical findings vary depending on the etiology and severity of the deformity. Cavovarus foot can be caused by a neurologic disorder, trauma, a congenital deformity, or an unknown cause. A neurologic workup should be considered if the cause is unknown or the deformity is bilateral. The treatment is based on the extent of deformity and the flexibility of the foot, with the goal to preserve motion, if possible, and to establish a plantigrade, pain-free foot. Surgical treatment may be indicated if nonsurgical treatment is unsuccessful or the deformity progresses. Soft-tissue and bony procedures including tendon transfers and osteotomies should be tailored to the characteristics of the foot. Arthrodesis can be used to treat arthritic or rigid deformity, and in some cases, ankle arthroplasty may be an option. The surgical plan must be individualized to reestablish function and preserve motion with careful consideration given to the patient's needs and the possibility of future interventions.

KEY STUDY POINTS

- Cavovarus foot deformity is characterized by hindfoot varus, a high arch, plantarflexed first ray, and claw toes.
- Etiology of cavovarus deformities is typically neurologic, with CMT being the most common cause.
- Treatment of the cavovarus foot is based on the severity and flexibility of the deformities, with the goal of maintaining function and reestablishing a plantigrade foot.

ANNOTATED REFERENCES

1. Piazza S, Ricci G, Caldarazzo Ienco E, et al: Pes cavus and hereditary neuropathies: When a relationship should be suspected. *J Orthop Traumatol* 2010;11(4):195-201.

2. Younger AS, Hansen ST Jr: Adult cavovarus foot. *J Am Acad Orthop Surg* 2005;13(5):302-315.

3. Lovell WW, Morrissy RT, Winter RB, eds: *Lovell and Winter's Pediatric Orthopaedics*, ed 3. Lippincott Williams & Wilkins, 1990.

4. Wenz W, Dreher T: Charcot-Marie-Tooth disease and the cavovarus foot, in Pinzur MS, ed: *Orthopaedic Knowledge Update®: Foot and Ankle 4.* American Academy of Orthopaedic Surgeons, 2008, pp 291-306.

5. Patzkó A, Shy ME: Update on Charcot-Marie-Tooth disease. *Curr Neurol Neurosci Rep* 2011;11(1):78-88.

6. Thomas PK, Griffin JW, Low P, Poduslo J, Dyck PJ, eds: *Peripheral Neuropathy*, ed 3. WB Saunders, 1993.

7. Bird TD, Ott J, Giblett ER, Chance PF, Sumi SM, Kraft GH: Genetic linkage evidence for heterogeneity in Charcot-Marie-Tooth neuropathy (HMSN type I). *Ann Neurol* 1983;14(6):679-684.

8. Holmes JR, Hansen ST Jr: Foot and ankle manifestations of Charcot-Marie-Tooth disease. *Foot Ankle* 1993;14(8):476-486.

9. Miller A, Guille JT, Bowen JR: Evaluation and treatment of diastematomyelia. *J Bone Joint Surg Am* 1993;75(9):1308-1317.

10. Alexander IJ, Johnson KA: Assessment and management of pes cavus in Charcot-Marie-Tooth disease. *Clin Orthop Relat Res* 1989;246:273-281.

11. Samilson RL, Dillin W: Cavus, cavovarus, and calcaneocavus: An update. *Clin Orthop Relat Res* 1983;177:125-132.

12. Maynou C, Szymanski C, Thiounn A: The adult cavus foot. *EFORT Open Rev* 2017;2(5):221-229.

13. Stecco C, Corradin M, Macchi V, et al: Plantar fascia anatomy and its relationship with Achilles tendon and paratenon. *J Anat* 2013;223(6):665-676.

14. McCluskey WP, Lovell WW, Cummings RJ: The cavovarus foot deformity: Etiology and management. *Clin Orthop Relat Res* 1989;247:27-37.

15. Bluth B, Eagan M, Otsuka NY: Stress fractures of the lateral rays in the cavovarus foot: Indication for surgical intervention. *Orthopedics* 2011;34(10):e696-e699.

16. Karakis I, Gregas M, Darras BT, Kang PB, Jones HR: Clinical correlates of Charcot-Marie-Tooth disease in patients with pes cavus deformities. *Muscle Nerve* 2013;47(4):488-492.

17. Coleman SS, Chesnut WJ: A simple test for hindfoot flexibility in the cavovarus foot. *Clin Orthop Relat Res* 1977;123:60-62.

18. Maskill MP, Maskill JD, Pomeroy GC: Surgical management and treatment algorithm for the subtle cavovarus foot. *Foot Ankle Int* 2010;31(12):1057-1063.

19. Miller LJ, Saporta AS, Sottile SL, Siskind CE, Feely SM, Shy ME: Strategy for genetic testing in Charcot-Marie disease. *Acta Myol* 2011;30(2):109-116.

20. Murphy SM, Laura M, Fawcett K, et al: Charcot-Marie-Tooth disease: Frequency of genetic subtypes and guidelines for genetic testing. *J Neurol Neurosurg Psychiatry* 2012;83(7):706-710.

21. Saltzman CL, el-Khoury GY: The hindfoot alignment view. *Foot Ankle Int* 1995;16(9):572-576.

22. Lintz F, Jepsen M, De Cesar Netto C, Bernasconi A, Ruiz M, Siegler S: Distance mapping of the foot and ankle joints using weightbearing CT: The cavovarus configuration. *Foot Ankle Surg* 2021;27(4):412-420.

    This is a case-control study of 10 cavovarus feet using WBCT. Three-dimensional models were used to generate articular surface distance maps. There were significant differences compared with control subjects, including changes at the ankle, hindfoot, and midfoot joints. Level of evidence: III.

23. Foran IM, Mehraban N, Jacobsen SK, et al: Impact of Coleman block test on adult hindfoot alignment assessed by clinical examination, radiography, and weight-bearing computed tomography. *Foot Ankle Orthop* 2020;5(3):2473011420933264.

    This is a retrospective review of six patients undergoing clinical evaluation for cavovarus foot. WBCT was completed with and without a Coleman block test, in addition to clinical photographs. The Coleman block test was found to correct deformity (clinically/radiographically) albeit incompletely. Clinical examination findings and WBCT measurements were strongly correlated. Level of evidence: IV.

24. An T, Haupt E, Michalski M, Salo J, Pfeffer G: Cavovarus with a twist: Midfoot coronal and axial plane rotational deformity in Charcot-Marie-Tooth disease. *Foot Ankle Int* 2022;43(5):676-682.

    This is a retrospective case-control study of 27 WBCT scans from 21 patients with CMT. Maximal rotational (supination) deformity was found in the talonavicular/calcaneocuboid joints; the talonavicular joint was the location of greatest adduction. These findings support that soft-tissue release at the talonavicular joint is important for cavovarus deformity correction. Level of evidence: III.

25. Schwend RM, Drennan JC: Cavus foot deformity in children. *J Am Acad Orthop Surg* 2003;11(3):201-211.

26. Ward CM, Dolan LA, Bennett DL, Morcuende JA, Cooper RR: Long-term results of reconstruction for treatment of a flexible cavovarus foot in Charcot-Marie-Tooth disease. *J Bone Joint Surg Am* 2008;90(12):2631-2642.

27. Leeuwesteijn AE, de Visser E, Louwerens JW: Flexible cavovarus feet in Charcot-Marie-Tooth disease treated with first ray proximal dorsiflexion osteotomy combined with soft tissue surgery: A short-term to mid-term outcome study. *Foot Ankle Surg* 2010;16(3):142-147.

28. Bernasconi A, Cooper L, Lyle S, et al: Pes cavovarus in Charcot-Marie-Tooth compared to the idiopathic cavovarus foot: A preliminary weightbearing CT analysis. *Foot Ankle Surg* 2021;27(2):186-195.

    This is a retrospective case-control review of patients with cavovarus deformity (CMT and idiopathic) who underwent WBCT. Significant differences were seen in comparison with control subjects. There was greater three-dimensional evidence of varus of the hindfoot in cavovarus associated with CMT patients compared idiopathic cavovarus. Two-dimensional measurements were similar among patients with cavovarus deformity (with the exception of the forefoot arch angle). Level of evidence: III.

29. Steindler A: The treatment of pes cavus (hollow claw foot). *Arch Surg* 1921;2(2):325-337.

30. Malahias MA, Cantiller EB, Kadu VV, Müller S: The clinical outcome of endoscopic plantar fascia release: A current concept review. *Foot Ankle Surg* 2020;26(1):19-24.

    A systematic review of 15 studies was completed to evaluate the outcomes of endoscopic plantar fascia release. Overall quality of studies was low. Studies demonstrated that postoperative clinical and functional outcomes improved after endoscopic plantar fascia release. Level of evidence: V.

31. Strayer LM Jr: Recession of the gastrocnemius: An operation to relieve spastic contracture of the calf muscles. *J Bone Joint Surg Am* 1950;32(3):671-676.

32. Strayer LM Jr: Gastrocnemius recession: Five-year report of cases. *J Bone Joint Surg Am* 1958;40(5):1019-1030.

33. Silfverskiol DN: Reduction of the uncrossed two-joints muscles of the leg to one-joint muscles in spastic conditions. *Acta Chir Scand* 1924;56:315-328.

34. Breusch SJ, Wenz W, Döderlein L: Function after correction of a clawed great toe by a modified Robert Jones transfer. *J Bone Joint Surg Br* 2000;82(2):250-254.

35. Tynan MC, Klenerman L: The modified Robert Jones tendon transfer in cases of pes cavus and clawed hallux. *Foot Ankle Int* 1994;15(2):68-71.

36. Ryssman DB, Myerson MS: Tendon transfers for the adult flexible cavovarus foot. *Foot Ankle Clin* 2011;16(3):435-450.

37. Myerson MS: Cavus foot correction and tendon transfers for management of paralytic deformity, in Myerson MS, ed: *Reconstructive Foot and Ankle Surgery: Management of Complications*, ed 2. Elsevier, 2010, pp 155-189.

38. Gould N, Seligson D, Gassman J: Early and late repair of lateral ligament of the ankle. *Foot Ankle* 1980;1(2):84-89.

39. Kaplan JRM, Aiyer A, Cerrato RA, Jeng CL, Campbell JT: Operative treatment of the cavovarus foot. *Foot Ankle Int* 2018;39(11):1370-1382.

40. Pfeffer GB, Gonzalez T, Brodsky J, et al: A consensus statement on the surgical treatment of Charcot-Marie-Tooth disease. *Foot Ankle Int* 2020;41(7):870-880.

    This is a consensus statement from 13 board-certified orthopaedic foot and ankle surgeons and one neurologist to review clinical and surgical facets of care of patients with CMT disease. The group defined history/physical examination considerations and provided recommendations for approach surgical management of these patients. Level of evidence: V.

41. Bakshi N, Steadman J, Philippi M, et al: Association between hindfoot alignment and first metatarsal rotation. *Foot Ankle Int* 2022;43(1):105-112.

    This is a retrospective cohort study of 196 patients evaluating weight-bearing plain radiographs and WBCT scans. Hindfoot alignment (calcaneal moment arm) and metatarsal rotation were evaluated. Hindfoot alignment was associated with metatarsal rotation. Level of evidence: III.

42. Krause FG, Sutter D, Waehnert D, Windolf M, Schwieger K, Weber M: Ankle joint pressure changes in a pes cavovarus model after lateralizing calcaneal osteotomies. *Foot Ankle Int* 2010;31(9):741-746.

43. Knupp M, Horisberger M, Hintermann B: A new Z-shaped calcaneal osteotomy for 3-plane correction of severe varus deformity of the hindfoot. *Tech Foot Ankle Surg* 2008;7(2):90-95.

44. Malerba F, De Marchi F: Calcaneal osteotomies. *Foot Ankle Clin* 2005;10(3):523-540, vii.

45. Dwyer FC: Osteotomy of the calcaneum for pes cavus. *J Bone Joint Surg Br* 1959;41(1):80-86.

46. Dwyer FC: The present status of the problem of pes cavus. *Clin Orthop Relat Res* 1975;106:254-275.

47. An TW, Michalski M, Jansson K, Pfeffer G: Comparison of lateralizing calcaneal osteotomies for varus hindfoot correction. *Foot Ankle Int* 2018;39(10):1229-1236.

48. Cody EA, Kraszewski AP, Conti MS, Ellis SJ: Lateralizing calcaneal osteotomies and their effect on calcaneal alignment: A three-dimensional digital model analysis. *Foot Ankle Int* 2018;39(8):970-977.

49. Pfeffer GB, Michalski MP, Basak T, Giaconi JC: Use of 3D prints to compare the efficacy of three different calcaneal osteotomies for the correction of heel varus. *Foot Ankle Int* 2018;39(5):591-597.

50. Sherman TI, Guyton G: Minimal incision/minimally invasive medializing displacement calcaneal osteotomy. *Foot Ankle Int* 2018;39(1):119-128.

51. VanVulkenberg S, Hsu RY, Palmer DS, Blankernhorn B, Den Hartog BD, DiGiovanni CW: Neurologic deficit with lateralizing calcaneal osteotomy for cavovarus foot correction. *Foot Ankle Int* 2016;37(10):1106-1112.

52. Bruce BG, Bariteau JT, Evangelista PE, Arcuri D, Sandusky M, DiGiovanni CW: The effect of medial and lateral calcaneal osteotomies on the tarsal tunnel. *Foot Ankle Int* 2014;35(4):383-388.

53. Siffert RS, Forster RI, Nachamie B: "Beak" triple arthrodesis for correction of severe cavus deformity. *Clin Orthop Relat Res* 1966;45:101-106.

54. Siffert RS, del Torto U: "Beak" triple arthrodesis for severe cavus deformity. *Clin Orthop Relat Res* 1983;181:64-67.

55. Jahss MH: Tarsometatarsal truncated-wedge arthrodesis for pes cavus and equinovarus deformity of the fore part of the foot. *J Bone Joint Surg Am* 1980;62(5):713-722.

56. Mubarak SJ, Dimeglio A: Navicular excision and cuboid closing wedge for severe cavovarus foot deformities: A salvage procedure. *J Pediatr Orthop* 2011;31(5):551-556.

57. Krause FG, Henning J, Pfander G, Weber M: Cavovarus foot realignment to treat anteromedial ankle arthrosis. *Foot Ankle Int* 2013;34(1):54-64.

58. Jung HG, Jeon SH, Kim TH, Park JT: Total ankle arthroplasty with combined calcaneal and metatarsal osteotomies for treatment of ankle osteoarthritis with accompanying cavovarus deformities: Early results. *Foot Ankle Int* 2013;34(1):140-147.

59. Taylor RG: The treatment of claw toes by multiple transfers of flexor into extensor tendons. *J Bone Joint Surg Br* 1951;33(4):539-542.

60. Barbari SG, Brevig K: Correction of clawtoes by the Girdlestone-Taylor flexor-extensor transfer procedure. *Foot Ankle* 1984;5(2):67-73.

CHAPTER 6

Diabetic Foot Disease

BOPHA CHREA, MD • LARA C. ATWATER, MD, FAAOS

ABSTRACT

Diabetes is a growing global problem with a number of associated health consequences. Foot and ankle surgeons must recognize and be able to treat the myriad of often devastating diabetic complications, including infection, Charcot neuroarthopathy, ulceration, and amputation. A multidisciplinary approach to treatment of patients with diabetes is essential in caring for the complex needs of these individuals.

Keywords: amputation; Charcot; diabetes; neuropathy; ulcer

INTRODUCTION

Diabetes mellitus first was recognized and described approximately 1,500 years ago, but the course of the disease dramatically changed with the discovery of insulin in 1922. Diabetes causes comorbidities affecting multiple systems. Foot morbidity is the most common reason for hospitalization of patients with diabetes in the United States and is responsible for substantial consumption of health care resources.

Dr. Chrea or an immediate family member serves as a paid consultant to or is an employee of Novastep. Neither Dr. Atwater nor any immediate family member has received anything of value from or has stock or stock options held in a commercial company or institution related directly or indirectly to the subject of this chapter.

Diabetic foot disease is associated with the risk of ulceration, infection, foot deformity, amputation, vasculopathy, and neuroarthropathy. The success of orthopaedic care depends on the vascularity of the limb as well as patient cooperation in glycemic control and foot care. Care should be coordinated by a comprehensive team that includes an orthopaedic surgeon, an endocrinologist, an infectious disease specialist, a vascular surgeon, a plastic surgeon, a physical therapist, and a pedorthotist.

EPIDEMIOLOGY

Diabetes is increasing at alarming rates worldwide with more than half of people with diabetes unaware that they have it. Approximately 1 in 10 (537 million) of the world's adult population is living with diabetes. This is expected to increase to 783 million people by 2045.[1] The increasing incidence in the United States is a direct reflection of the increasing rate of obesity.[2] The number of individuals in the United States in whom diabetes was diagnosed is 37.3 million (11.3% of the population). In addition, an estimated 8.5 million individuals have diabetes, but the disease has not been diagnosed. More than 96 million people in the United States aged 18 years and older are considered to be in the prediabetes stage. Thirty-five percent of the American population younger than 20 years, approximately 283,000 individuals, are now estimated to have diabetes.[1] Diabetes is a risk factor for severe SARS-CoV-2 (COVID-19) outcomes, hospitalization, and mortality. Specifically, 40% of COVID-19 deaths were in patients with diabetes.[3] The direct medical cost of caring for patients with diabetes in the United States was $237 billion in 2017. This figure represents a 35% increase over the

This chapter is adapted from Gross CE, Huh J: Diabetic foot disease, in Chou LB, ed: *Orthopaedic Knowledge Update®: Foot and Ankle 6*. American Academy of Orthopaedic Surgeons, 2020, 65-82.

© 2025 American Academy of Orthopaedic Surgeons

preceding 5 years and amounts to 12.5% of all expenditures for direct medical care in the United States.[4] The estimated global and direct health expenditure on diabetes in 2019 is $760 billion and is expected to grow to a projected $825 billion by 2030 and $845 billion by 2045.[5]

Complications associated with diabetic foot disease are the most common reason patients with diabetes are admitted to the hospital. The global incidence of diabetic foot ulcers is estimated to be 6.3%, with higher regional incidences in North America as high as 15%. A 2021 study estimated that 19% to 34% of patients with diabetes will experience a diabetic foot ulcer within their lifetime.[6]

ETIOLOGY

Diabetic neuropathy is the most important factor in the development of diabetic foot disease. As the severity of neuropathy increases, so does the risk of ulceration, amputation, and death. With increasing neuropathy, the patient's functional ability, balance, and coordination decline. Neuropathy probably is the result of both metabolic and vascular factors. Sensation, motor control, and autonomic function are disturbed with diabetic neuropathy, and these changes occur simultaneously. The risk of neuropathy in a patient with diabetes increases over time. The prevalence of peripheral neuropathy is estimated to be between 6% and 51% among adults with diabetes depending on age, duration of diabetes, glucose control, and type (1 versus 2).[7] It eventually affects 75% of patients with diabetes.[8,9]

Neuropathy begins distally and progresses proximally in a stocking-glove pattern. It can herald diabetes because those with impaired glucose tolerance can also be affected.[9] Somatic sensory neuropathy affects the large-fiber nerves and is length dependent; it affects the longest nerves and is related to the patient's height (a tall patient is at greatest risk). Disturbance of large sensory fibers is reflected in a decreased awareness of light touch and diminished proprioception with diminished or absent reflexes. Disturbance of small sensory fibers is reflected in a loss of pain and temperature perception. Almost one-third of patients with neuropathy report pain that is worse in the evening. The pain commonly is bilateral and symmetric, and it may be characterized in terms of burning, paresthesias, allodynia, electric shock, deep shooting pain, cramping, or aching. Over time, vibratory sensation is lost, and deep tendon reflexes disappear. It is commonly associated with development of retinopathy and nephropathy. Surgical decompression can be helpful if identifiable nerve compression is present, but only limited research supports this recommendation.[10,11] A meta-analysis has shown the efficacy of surgical decompression in relieving neurologic symptoms and restoring some of the sensory deficits in diabetic neuropathy.[12] Pharmacologic treatment includes gabapentin, pregabalin, tricyclic antidepressants, venlafaxine, and duloxetine. Topical medications such as capsaicin cream or gel may also benefit patients.

Autonomic neuropathy occurs in 20% to 40% of patients with diabetes. It rarely occurs in isolation because it frequently is accompanied by sensory neuropathy.[9] Symptoms are usually mild until the late stages of diabetes. The major clinical manifestations of autonomic neuropathy include resting tachycardia, exercise intolerance, orthostatic hypotension, constipation, gastroparesis, erectile dysfunction, cutaneous sudomotor dysfunction, impaired neurovascular function, so-called brittle diabetes, and hypoglycemic autonomic failure.[13] Autonomic dysfunction affects control of sweat glands, blood vessel tone, and thermoregulation. The normal hyperemic response, which is necessary to fight infection, is lost. The skin becomes dry and scaly, cracks and fissures develop, and bacteria are able to invade, causing infection.

While standing, foot pressures can become very high. In the absence of sufficient blood flow to the underlying skin and tissue, cell oxygenation is inadequate and tissue dies. The result is ulceration beneath the points of greatest pressure. Ulceration can occur during less than 1 hour of constant standing. Repetitive mild trauma, as in walking, can cause preulcerative conditions that over time progress to complete ulceration. The triad of neuropathy, foot deformity, and repetitive trauma creates a high risk of ulcer formation.

EVALUATION OF THE DIABETIC FOOT AND ANKLE

Obtaining a thorough history is crucial in a patient with diabetes. The identification of peripheral neuropathy and vascular disease, followed by appropriate intervention, can decrease the risk of subsequent infection and ulceration.

Examination of the foot and ankle should begin with an evaluation of the patient's gait, posture, range of motion, muscle strength, and skin coverage. Limited joint mobility can increase plantar pressures, resulting in foot ulceration. Thin, shiny, atrophic, and hairless skin is indicative of diminished vascularity. Any corns, calluses, or ulcerations should be documented by size, location, margins, and depth. Areas with intradermal hemorrhage or blistering represent preulceration. It is also important to observe any exposure of a tendon and to determine whether an ulceration can be probed to bone. Thick toenails indicate vascular or fungal disease. Any deformities of the foot and ankle should be noted, and the presence or absence of protective sensation should be documented. The accepted threshold for normal sensation is the ability to perceive a Semmes-Weinstein size 5.07 nylon monofilament wire applied perpendicular to the skin. This should ideally be performed in conjunction with at least one other assessment (pinprick, temperature, vibration sensation using a 128-Hz tuning fork or ankle reflexes).[14] Previous studies have shown vibration perception threshold testing to have greater sensitivity for detecting impaired sensation.[15,16] However, this requires a biothesiometer, which is an instrument that is not readily available in most offices. Alternatively, a 128-Hz tuning fork can be used. Guidelines for 2021 suggest that the absence of monofilament sensation is highly suggestive of a loss of protective sensation, while at least two normal tests (and no abnormal tests) rule out loss of protective sensation.[14] One should be wary of flexion contractures of the toes because they could increase distal pressure, leading to ulceration and ultimately osteomyelitis. The fit and material of the patient's shoes also should be evaluated. The interior of the shoes should be checked for foreign objects, and the insole removed to look for blood or other fluid discharge. Examination of the sole of the shoe may reveal an abnormal wear pattern related to deformity.

Often, an examiner must distinguish between an acute episode of Charcot neuroarthropathy and foot infection. The rubor in Charcot is more pronounced in a dependent position. A diagnostic strategy is for a physician to elevate the leg for 5 minutes. If the redness dissipates, then the diagnosis is likely an acute Charcot attack.

It is important for the examiner to determine the patient's palpable tibialis posterior pulse, dorsalis pedis pulse, and capillary filling time. Any evidence of ischemia or a nonhealing wound warrants a vascular evaluation. Arterial Doppler ultrasonography is effective in assessing the adequacy of circulation. This test is reproducible and is not operator dependent. The results are reported in terms of toe pressures and the ratio of ankle pressure to arm Doppler arterial pressure. An acceptable level for healing is toe pressures higher than 40 mm Hg or an ankle-brachial index higher than 45 mm Hg. Absolute toe pressures are a better predictor of healing than the ankle-brachial index.[17] A triphasic waveform is present within normal vessels. When the vessel is calcified, the waveform is monophasic, and the reading can be falsely elevated. Transcutaneous oxygen tension values higher than 30 mm Hg indicate an acceptable potential for healing; this technique does not produce false readings with calcified vessels. If screening reveals limb ischemia, arteriography can identify the site of occlusion. This test is expensive, however, and has possible complications including allergic dye reaction, pseudoaneurysm, and acute renal failure in patients with compromised renal function or dehydration.

Vascular disease is 30 times more common in patients with diabetes than in other individuals.[18] Heart disease continues to be the leading cause of death in patients with diabetes; approximately 74% of patients with diabetes have concurrent hypertension.[19] The risk of cerebrovascular accident is as much as four times greater in patients with diabetes than in the general population.[19] The typical lower extremity atherosclerotic findings in patients with diabetes include bilateral, diffuse, circumferential, with plaque formation in the medial layer of blood vessels. Atherosclerosis in the population who do not have diabetes usually is patchy, with plaque formation occurring in the intimal layer of blood vessels. Patients with diabetes are affected by atherosclerosis at a younger age, and the disease progression is more rapid. The iliac and femoral vessels often are affected. Involvement typically occurs at or just distal to the popliteal trifurcation involving the anterior tibialis, posterior tibialis, and peroneal arteries. Compromised blood flow to either lower extremity, combined with neuropathy, dramatically increases the risk for subsequent foot ulceration.

When evaluating vascular supply to the foot, no screening tool is completely accurate. When vascular compromise is of concern, a vascular consultation should be obtained to determine whether revascularization (transluminal angioplasty and vascular bypass) is an option. 2021 standard-of-care guidelines suggest vascular imaging and revascularization should be considered in a patient with a diabetic foot ulcer and ankle-brachial index less than 50 mm Hg, toe pressure less than 30 mm Hg, or transcutaneous oxygen pressure less than 25 mm Hg.[20]

Imaging

The imaging of the diabetic foot begins with plain weight-bearing radiographs of the foot and ankle, which are primarily used to evaluate major structural changes, joint alignment, soft-tissue gas, vascular calcifications, foreign bodies, and osteomyelitis. Focal demineralization, a reflection of underlying marrow changes, is the earliest radiographic change related to neuroarthropathy or osteomyelitis. In diabetic neuroarthropathy, localized osteopenia increases the risk of fracture with continued weight bearing. Excessive osteoclastic activity has been identified in Charcot-reactive bone, with cytokine mediators inciting bone resorption.[21] The classic triad of osteomyelitis, which includes periosteal reaction, osteolysis, and bone destruction, may not be evident during the early stages of the disease (within the first 20 days).[22]

Charcot Neuroarthropathy and Infectious Radiographic Characteristics

CT is preferable to plain radiography for identifying osteomyelitic cortical erosions, but it has limited value in diagnosing early osteomyelitis. CT also is unable to distinguish between the changes of chronic infection and neuroarthropathy. CT is most useful for assessment of deformity and bone stock during surgical planning.

MRI has a high sensitivity for the detection of early soft-tissue and bone marrow edema associated with both Charcot neuroarthropathy and osteomyelitis; however, in isolation, MRI is unable to differentiate between these two pathologic processes.[23,24] The basis of diagnosis of osteomyelitis by MRI includes abnormal bone marrow signals typified by confluent hypointensity on T1-weighted images, which reflect infiltration of the infectious process.[25] Gadolinium contrast injection can improve the ability to detect the abscess or necrosis associated with osteomyelitis. MRI can be used to differentiate a sterile joint effusion from septic arthritis.[25,26] Secondary findings such as direct spread from an ulcer or the presence of a sinus tract can contribute to the diagnosis. Because of its multiplanar capability and high spatial and contrast resolution, MRI is considered the best modality when the diagnosis of infection has already been confirmed for defining the extent of soft-tissue and bone marrow involvement for surgical planning.[24-28] The role of MRI in determining disease resolution and guiding management is also important and remains under investigation.[29]

In isolation, triple-phase bone scanning using technetium Tc-99m (^{99}Tc) phosphonates has 94% sensitivity and 95% specificity for the diagnosis of osteomyelitis, in the absence of another abnormality.[24,30] However, specificity is reduced to 33% in the presence of neuroarthropathy, trauma, recent surgical procedure, or malignancy. ^{99}Tc bone scanning is advantageous because its high sensitivity has a high negative predictive value; therefore, a negative bone scan essentially rules out infection. Indium-111 white blood cell (WBC) scintigraphy is even more accurate than ^{99}Tc bone scanning for diagnosing osteomyelitis, and a negative result strongly supports the absence of infection. If trying to differentiate between Charcot neuroarthropathy and osteomyelitis, the best diagnostic test is a combination of nuclear medicine scans (ie, ^{99}Tc bone scan and indium-111–labeled WBC scan).[23,29,31] Positron emission tomography–CT with 18-fluorodeoxyglucose, which indicates an increase in glucose metabolism, also has high accuracy and specificity for the differentiation of osteomyelitis from neuroarthropathy and is superior to leukocyte-labeled studies for the diagnosis of chronic osteomyelitis.[32,33]

Ultrasonography has a limited role in diabetic imaging, although it can help identify a foreign body or with identifying and aspirating an abscess. If there is a need to differentiate between infected and uninfected fluid surrounding a tendon sheath, ultrasonography can reveal the abnormal internal echogenicity characteristic of an infected fluid collection.[24]

Laboratory Studies and Vital Signs

If cellulitis or a deeper infection is suspected, appropriate laboratory testing should be done. An elevated WBC count indicates infection, but the WBC count can be normal even if an infection is present, because of an impaired immune response.[34] Leukocytosis higher than 11×10^9/L is associated with a 2.6-fold increase in the risk of amputation, and fever higher than 100.5°F (38°C) is associated with a 1.3-fold increase in the risk of amputation.[35] Interestingly, more than 50% of patients with acute osteomyelitis of the foot had a normal WBC count, and 82% had a normal oral body temperature.[36] An evaluation of 400 patients with moderate or severe diabetic foot infection found a mean WBC count of 8.24 $\times 10^9$/L; those whose treatment was unsuccessful had a mean WBC count of 9.98×10^9/L, and those who favorably responded to treatment had a mean WBC count of 7.93×10^9/L.[37]

A total lymphocyte count lower than 1.5×10^9/L is correlated with immunocompetence in wound healing. Albumin levels above 30 g/dL support a nutritional status satisfactory for healing; healing can occur but is less predictable with lower levels.[38] Patients requiring transtibial amputation have substantially lower serum albumin levels than patients who underwent successful limb salvage.[39]

An elevated erythrocyte sedimentation rate often is correlated with inflammation or infection; usually, a level less than 40 is more common with cellulitis or a local soft-tissue infection. A level higher than 67 (mm/hr) suggests underlying osteomyelitis. The C-reactive protein level is highly sensitive but not specific for inflammation. When it is greater than 14 mg/L, the sensitivity and specificity are 0.85 and 0.83.[34] C-reactive protein level is a better parameter than WBC count or neutrophil count for diagnosis and monitoring of treatment in deep diabetic foot infections.[40] The erythrocyte sedimentation rate can remain elevated 3 months after initiation of infection treatment, although it still can be used to monitor efficacy of treatment.[34] Worsening glycemic control may be one of the earliest signs of diabetic foot infection.

COMPLICATIONS AND TREATMENT

Diabetic Foot Ulcer

Diabetic foot ulceration is a devastating complication of diabetes mellitus and is a major source of morbidity and mortality. Foot ulcers and infections are the most common reason for hospital admission in people with diabetes in the United States.[14] The prevalence of diabetic ulcers is 7% to 8%; however, the incidence of diabetic foot ulcers is up to 25% in a patient's lifetime.[41] Fifty-six percent of ulcers become infected and one in five of these will require some level of amputation.[14]

Diabetic foot ulcers are the leading cause of lower extremity amputation in these patients,[40] and more than half of all diabetic foot ulcers become infected.[42] The risk of death at 5 years is over twice as high in patients with diabetes and foot ulcers compared with patients with diabetes and no foot ulcers.[43] In conjunction with its heavy morbidity and mortality burden, the cost of care for those with foot ulcers is five times higher than in those without ulcers.[44] Management of diabetic foot ulcers accounts for approximately one-third the total cost of diabetic care, which in the United States was estimated to be $348 billion in direct health care expenditures in 2017.[44] The causes of diabetic foot ulceration are multifactorial and include autonomic, sensory, and motor neuropathy; foot deformity; decreased vascularity; loss of skin integrity; poor glucose regulation; impaired leukocyte function; and repetitive trauma.

Autonomic neuropathy leads to decreased sweating with resultant dry, cracked skin, vulnerable to open wounds. Sensory neuropathy leads to loss of protective sensation. Motor neuropathy can result in clawing and hammering of the toes secondary to loss of intrinsic muscle balance. Fixed toe deformities often result in pressure over the proximal interphalangeal joints and beneath the metatarsal heads, which are common sites for ulcer development. Progressive Achilles tendon contracture further increases forefoot pressures. In a comparison of 32 patients with diabetes and 32 healthy control patients, patients with diabetes had a thicker Achilles tendon and stiffer plantar soft tissue than the control patients.[45] As much as a fivefold increase in the mechanical stiffness of the plantar soft tissues has been reported in patients with diabetic foot disease.[46] This results in increased tissue hydrostatic pressure in the loaded foot, effectively reducing the blood supply to the areas of highest pressure.[45]

Risk factors for development of a diabetic ulcer include loss of sensation, diminished pulses, foot deformity, abnormal reflexes, advanced age, history of a foot ulcer, and an abnormal neuropathy disability score.[47] The most common reasons a diabetic ulcer does not heal include decreased vascular supply, deep infection, and failure to mechanically unload the affected area. Wound size, wound duration, and wound grade are directly associated with the likelihood of wound healing by the 20th week of care.[48] The Brodsky classification system, which is based on ulcer depth and ischemia, helps determine the need for hospitalization and possible surgical management[49] (**Figure 1**).

In 2020, a validated clinical prediction model was developed as a tool to more accurately assess the risk of foot ulceration within 2 years. The foundation for the Prediction Of Diabetic foot UlcerationS (PODUS) Clinical Prediction Rule came from data obtained through four international cohort studies identified by systematic review, comprising 8,255 total patients.[50,51] Three simple clinical indicators were found to be predictive of ulceration: a previous history of ulceration or amputation, insensitivity to a 10-g monofilament, and at least one absent pedal pulse. These three factors comprise a score from 0 to 4, with previous ulcer/amputation worth two points and absence of pulses or sensation worth one point, respectively. The risk of ulceration at 2 years with scores ranging from 0 to 4 is 2.4%, 6.0%, 14%, 29%, and 51%, respectively.[51]

Ulcer Management Strategies

The principles of diabetic foot ulcer treatment begin with pressure offloading and ulcer protection. It is imperative to offload plantar pressures and any shear stress from the ulcer by distributing both over a larger surface area, thus reducing mechanical stress and promoting an environment conducive to healing. Although offloading can be accomplished by avoiding weight bearing on the involved extremity, patient compliance is problematic. Total contact casting (TCC) has historically been considered the benchmark method of pressure offloading for diabetic foot ulcers based on shorter healing times and better healing rates compared with a half shoe or removable cast walker.[52] Despite its effectiveness in ulcer healing, the application of a TCC requires technical skill, and the reported complication rates are as high as 17%.[13] Alternatively, there has been growing evidence that other nonremovable knee-high device options, in the form of commercially available walking devices rendered irremovable by overwrapping with plaster, can achieve similar results as TCC.[53-55] More recently, some studies have also reported positive outcomes with removable walker devices compared with TCC and removable walker devices.[55] In the setting of infection or ischemia, offloading is still important. The removable option is attractive in patients who are unable to tolerate a nonremovable device or in situations where they are contraindicated, such as significant peripheral artery disease and infection.

Surgical management may be used as a method of offloading. Metatarsal offloading can be performed through lengthening of the gastrocnemius or Achilles tendon in the setting of an equinus contracture to decrease plantar pressure and allow forefoot ulcers to heal.[56,57] However, overcorrection can lead to an increase in peak pressure under the heel, a calcaneal gait, and a subsequent heel ulcer that eventually may require partial calcanectomy or transtibial amputation.[56] Plantar fascia release has been shown to result in healing of forefoot ulcers.[58] More recently, minimally invasive metatarsal osteotomies, that is, distal metatarsal diaphyseal osteotomy, have been found to be equal or more effective than traditional open techniques in offloading metatarsal head pressures.[59,60]

Section 2: Neuromuscular Disease

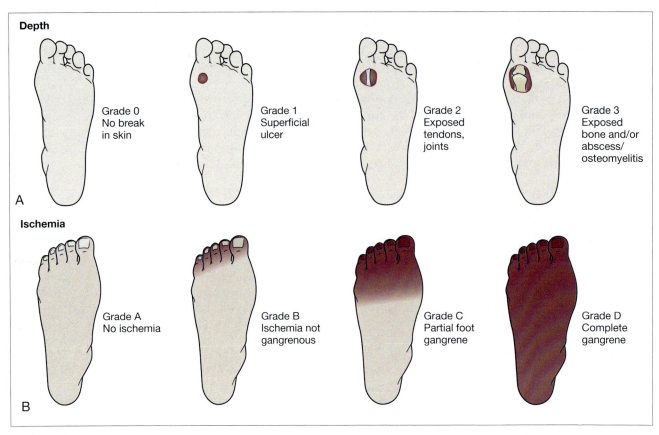

FIGURE 1 Schematic drawings showing a classification system for diabetic foot lesions based on ulcer depth (**A**) and ischemia (**B**). (Adapted and redrawn with permission from Brodsky JW: The diabetic foot, in Coughlin MJ, Mann RA, Saltzman CL, eds: *Surgery of the Foot and Ankle*, ed 8. Mosby, 2007, vol 2, pp 1281-1368.)

Next, restoration of tissue perfusion is a core principle in ulcer management principle. Revascularization should be considered if the toe pressure is less than 30 mm Hg or transcutaneous oxygen pressure is less than 25 mm Hg. For ulcers that fail to demonstrate improvement by greater than 50% wound area reduction after a minimum of 4 weeks of standard wound therapy, the International Diabetes Federation recommends adjunctive wound therapy options.[44] Multiple adjuvant therapies are available and being studied for the care of diabetic foot ulcers. These include nonsurgical débridement agents, dressings and topical products, oxygen therapies, negative-pressure wound therapy (NPWT), acellular bioproducts, human growth factors, skin grafts and bioengineered skin, energy-based therapies, and systemic therapies. Although systematic reviews of various wound dressings have found no evidence that any specific type is better than others, for foot ulcers with heavy exudate, the International Diabetes Federation recommends a dressing that absorbs moisture, whereas dry wounds need topical treatments that add moisture. Hyperbaric oxygen therapy is among the adjuvant therapies for diabetic foot ulcers that has been available and studied for multiple decades. Despite this, evidence remains mixed with inconclusive data regarding clinical and cost effectiveness.[20] A Cochrane review showed a significant increase in healing rate with hyperbaric oxygen therapy at 6 weeks, but no difference at 1-year follow-up, and no statistically significant difference in major amputation rate.[61] A double-blind randomized controlled trial concluded that 12 weeks of hyperbaric oxygen therapy does not reduce indication for amputations in patients with Wagner grade 2 to 4 diabetic foot ulcers.[62] NPWT is another well-studied adjuvant therapy. A systematic review of 11 randomized controlled trials comparing NPWT with standard dressing changes showed that NPWT had a higher rate of healing, shorter healing time, and fewer amputations, with no difference in incidence of treatment-related adverse effects.[63]

The treatment of any active infection is also imperative. Surgical ulcer management involves removing all necrotic tissue and surrounding callus. This step converts a chronic wound into an acute wound and encourages healing with granulation tissue formation and reepithelialization. Débridement also contributes to infection control, because devitalized tissue may provide a nidus for bacterial proliferation. Elliptical wounds usually heal better than circular wounds. The wound should be débrided weekly or more frequently.

Approximately 77% of diabetic foot ulcers heal within 1 year,[42] and of those that heal, approximately 40% have recurrence within 1 year after ulcer healing, almost 60% within 3 years, and 65% within 5 years.[36] It is well known that the strongest predictor of a diabetic foot ulcer is a prior foot ulcer. In addition to glycemic control and diabetic foot education, identification of preulcerative lesions, including abundant callus, blistering, or hemorrhage, and treatment in a timely manner can prevent many ulcer recurrences. Early diagnosis and treatment of Charcot neuropathy is essential in preventing deformities that increase the risk for ulceration and amputation. The American Diabetes Association 2021 guidelines recommend wide and square toe boxes, laces with three or four eyes per side, padded tongues, and extra depth to accommodate a cushioned insole. Routine prescription of therapeutic footwear is not recommended.[20]

Infection

When compared with individuals without diabetes, those with diabetes are at greater risk for cellulitis, osteomyelitis, sepsis, and death resulting from infection.[19] The use of antibiotics should be considered if infection is present. An infection that does not threaten the limb can be treated with oral antibiotics. Oral antibiotics have been used to keep osteomyelitis in remission under certain circumstances, but have not been uniformly successful.[63] An infection that does not respond to wound management and the use of oral antibiotics is limb-threatening and can be life-threatening. Surgical management should be the primary focus for these patients, with adjunctive intravenous antibiotic therapy. The authors and their institutional infectious disease consultants prefer to use empiric intravenous vancomycin and piperacillin/tazobactam antibiotics until the results of surgically obtained tissue cultures are available to dictate subsequent antibiotic therapy.

The isolated use of topical antibiotics is not recommended for treating an infected ulcer. Multiple Cochrane reviews have concluded that randomized controlled trial data on safety and effectiveness of topical antimicrobials are limited by small, poorly designed trials.[64-66] A Cochrane review suggests topical antimicrobials do increase diabetic ulcer healing, though with low certainty evidence.[66] Bacterial biofilm production can interfere with ulcer healing, and removal of this biofilm is an extremely important aspect of wound management. Surgical irrigation using detergents improves the efficacy of débridement; topical agents to facilitate biofilm removal are available for clinical use.[67,68]

The risk of ulcer infection is increased with hyperglycemia, which has a deleterious effect on neutrophils and granulocytes.[69] Poor glycemic control is associated with ulcer cluster, and very poor glycemic control is associated with an increase in the concentration of *Staphylococcus*-rich and *Streptococcus*-rich ulcer clusters.[70] Swab culturing is notoriously inaccurate because of the risk of contamination and is thus not recommended. Culture specimens can be most accurately obtained in the operating room after surgical preparation. Deep tissue, including bone or granulation tissue, should be obtained, rather than the tissue exposed to the outside environment. Most diabetic foot ulcers have polymicrobial contamination; 75% were found to have a mean 2.4 organisms per wound.[68] Aerobic gram-positive cocci, especially staphylococci, are the most common causative organisms.[68] Aerobic gram-negative bacilli often are copathogens in infections that are chronic or occur after antibiotic treatment. Obligate anaerobes can be copathogens in ischemic or necrotic wounds. With increasing ulcer depth, anaerobic bacteria become more abundant than staphylococci. Bacterial diversity, species richness, and relative abundance of proteobacteria increase as the age of the ulcer increases.[70] The risk of multidrug-resistant bacteria in diabetic foot ulcers increases with deep and recurrent ulcers, history of previous hospitalization, elevated hemoglobin (Hb)A1c level, nephropathy, and retinopathy.[62]

It is important to initially determine the type and severity of infection. The International Working Group on the Diabetic Foot and Infectious Diseases Society of America continually update a classification system with four grades of severity, called the PEDIS classification (**Table 1**). It is useful to help identify patients who require hospital admission for intravenous antibiotics.[71] It has also been validated to predict risk of both minor and major amputation.[72] Other groups have established different guidelines for severe diabetic foot infection.

Wet gangrene or soft-tissue emphysema represents severe infection. The most commonly isolated pathogens in osteomyelitis are gram-positive organisms, especially *Staphylococcus aureus*. However, a review of 341 patients found that 44% of bone cultures contained gram-negative pathogens alone or in combination with a gram-positive organism.[73] Infections with gram-negative pathogens more often were associated with a fetid odor, necrotic tissue, and clinical signs of severe infection than those with gram-positive pathogens.[73]

Weight bearing on an infected foot should be discouraged because the infection will spread from an area of high pressure (the infection site) to areas of lower pressure (uninfected sites), most commonly from the plantar foot to the dorsal foot. Infections spread through the foot along tendons and their sheaths. Infection spread is observed when purulent drainage is expressed through the ulcer during palpation at a distant location. Each compartment that becomes infected is associated with

Table 1

International Working Group on the Diabetic Foot/Infectious Diseases Society of America System

Clinical Manifestation	Infection Severity	PEDIS Grade
Wound lacking purulence or any manifestations of inflammation	Uninfected	1
Presence of ≥2 manifestations of inflammation (purulence, erythema, tenderness, warmth, or induration), but any cellulitis/erythema extends ≤2 cm around the ulcer, and infection is limited to the skin or superficial subcutaneous tissues; no other local complications or systemic illness	Mild	2
Infection (as above) in a patient who is systemically well and metabolically stable but which has ≥1 of the following characteristics: Cellulitis extending >2 cm, lymphangitic streaking, spread beneath the superficial fascia, deep-tissue abscess, gangrene, and involvement of muscle, tendon, joint, or bone	Moderate	3
Infection in a patient with systemic toxicity or metabolic instability (eg, fever, chills, tachycardia, hypotension, confusion, vomiting, leukocytosis, acidosis, severe hyperglycemia, or azotemia)	Severe	4

PEDIS = perfusion, extent/size, depth/tissue loss, infection and sensation

Reprinted with permission from Monteiro-Soares M, Russell D, Boyko EJ, et al: Guidelines on the classification of diabetic foot ulcers (IWGDF 2019). *Diabetes Metab Res Rev* 2020;36(suppl 1):e3273.

increased compartment pressure, which can result in extensive tissue damage. As part of the surgical débridement, the involved compartment must be opened and all necrotic tissue removed.

Simple surgical intervention may include abscess drainage, aggressive débridement of ulcers, and application of NPWT with mechanical offloading. NPWT is more effective than topical moist wound dressings and can be safely applied after an infected diabetic ulcer is débrided.[40] More aggressive surgical intervention can include exostectomy, deformity correction, muscle or microvascular free flaps, or amputation. Staged reconstructive surgical procedures sometimes are necessary.

Amputation

Every 30 seconds, a lower limb amputation is performed in the world as a consequence of diabetes.[44] Nonhealing foot wounds are a factor in 85% of lower extremity amputations. Even minor trauma can result in amputation.[74] A strong correlation exists between morbid obesity and diabetes-associated morbidity.[75] The risk of amputation is highest in patients who live in poverty, belong to a racial or ethnic minority group, are older than 50 years, are men rather than women, or smoke tobacco.[76-78] Thirty percent of patients with a unilateral amputation undergo amputation of the contralateral limb within 3 years.[17] Two-thirds of patients die within 5 years of the amputation. A retrospective control cohort study[39] of 100 patients with diabetes found that those admitted for a severe foot infection had an increased hospital stay by 60% and a risk of amputation of 55%.

The levels of amputation are identified as partial digital, digital, ray resection, transmetatarsal, Chopart, Syme, transtibial, and transfemoral. In choosing the level of amputation, the surgeon must consider both the optimal level for healing (the vascular supply) and optimal residual limb function. The factors contributing to the decision include the quality of the tissue, the extent of the infection, the vascularity of the limb, and the patient's nutritional, immune, and ambulatory status. Osteomyelitis of the heel is more likely to require transtibial amputation than osteomyelitis of the forefoot or midfoot.[79] Midfoot amputation may require tendon lengthening or releases and possibly tendon transfers to balance the foot. After metatarsal head resection, the greatest risk of reulceration is at the first metatarsal head, and the lowest risk is at the fifth metatarsal head.[80] An 84.5% healing rate was reported after a first Syme amputation.[39] The risk of major reamputation after minor foot amputation in patients with diabetes is strongly associated with the presence of peripheral vascular disease.[81] Transtibial amputation is associated with high rates of morbidity and mortality. Nonetheless, a comparison with partial foot amputation found that after 1 and 3 years only transmetatarsal amputation resulted in a statistically lower mortality rate than transtibial amputation.[82]

After amputation, an inverse relationship exists between the amount of energy consumption and the length of the residual limb; more energy is consumed if the patient has a shorter residual limb. Transmetatarsal and Chopart amputations resulted in better ambulatory ability and longer durability than other partial foot amputations. Amputation rates among patients with diabetes with Medicare decreased by one-half between 2000 and 2009, but actually increased slightly between 2009 and 2017. Overall increase in rates was driven by more foot and toe amputations, whereas transfemoral and transtibial rates continue a gradual decline.[83] Simultaneously, the use of orthopaedic interventions such as TCC and Achilles tendon lengthening has increased.

Charcot Neuroarthropathy

Charcot neuroarthropathy involves progressive destruction of the joints, most commonly in the feet and ankles. The reported incidence of this complication is less than 1% in the general population of patients with diabetes and is as high as 13% in high-risk patients with diabetes. Men and women are at equal risk. Contralateral Charcot develops in approximately 20% of patients at a mean of 2.5 years, and a contralateral ulcer develops in nearly half of them.[84]

Two theories are proposed to explain the development of Charcot neuroarthropathy. The theory of neurotraumatic destruction states that joint destruction is the result of cumulative trauma unrecognized by an insensate foot. In contrast, the theory of neurovascular destruction states that bone resorption and ligament laxity are secondary to a neurally controlled vascular reflex. Most experts believe that a combination of these pathways is responsible for the destruction seen in the affected diabetic foot or ankle.

Increased expression of nuclear transcription factor NF-κB results in increased osteoclastogenesis, thus confirming the role of inflammatory cytokines.[77] These findings suggest the possibility of using pharmacologic agents to limit cytokine activation and osteoclastic resorption. The severity of diabetes is not correlated with the risk of Charcot neuroarthropathy. Charcot neuroarthropathy can develop in patients with mild diabetes who are being treated with oral hypoglycemic medications or diet control.

Charcot neuroarthropathy was first described in three classic stages[85] in 1966, based on the natural history of the condition. Stage I, the development or fragmentation phase, is clinically characterized by hyperemia, edema, increased warmth, and erythema around the affected joint. Stage I is radiographically characterized by fragmentation of bone associated with fracture and joint subluxation. In stage II, the coalescence or subacute phase, the acute inflammatory findings decrease. Radiographs show evidence of bone debris and new bone formation. Stage III is the reconstruction and reconstitution or consolidation phase. Swelling and warmth surrounding the joint resolves, and the joint will seem stable, but there may be considerable residual deformity. On radiographs, the fragmentation is seen to have consolidated, but residual joint deformity and bone loss are evident. In 1990, stage 0, or the prodromal phase, was added to the classification because clinical signs often precede any radiographic changes, resulting in normal radiographs.[86,87]

Charcot involvement of the foot and ankle is described in terms of the four commonly affected anatomic areas[49] (**Figure 2**). Type I, which occurs in 60% of patients, affects the midfoot, tarsometatarsal, and naviculocuneiform joints. The subsequent collapse most commonly results in a residual deformity involving a plantarmedial bony exostosis that places the foot at risk of pressure ulceration. Type II, which affects 30% to 35% of patients, involves the hindfoot, with subsequent instability resulting in foot subluxation and ulcer formation. Type IIIA, which affects 5% of patients, involves the ankle joint and is the most unstable pattern. Type IIIB involves fracture of the calcaneal tuberosity and results in weak push-off, pes planus, and risk of ulceration associated with the avulsed bony prominence. In general, the more proximal the Charcot joint involvement, the higher the risk of subsequent joint instability.

In a second classification, type I is described as destruction of the metatarsophalangeal joint, with medial plantar prominence and abduction deformity[88] (**Figure 3**). Type II involves the naviculocuneiform joint, with residual plantarlateral prominence under the fourth and fifth tarsometatarsal joints. Type III affects the navicular and the medial column, with collapse resulting in an adducted-supinated deformity and a plantarlateral prominence under the cuboid. Type IV involves the transverse tarsal joints with associated prominence under the calcaneocuboid and talonavicular joints. Substage A, B, or C is assigned based on the severity of the rocker-bottom sole (**Figure 4**).

Regardless of the classification system, the goal of treatment after stage III (the consolidation phase) is for the foot to be stable, plantigrade, and amenable to bracing treatment or accommodative orthotic devices and shoes. Any residual deformity should be treated to enable these goals to be reached and to keep the foot free of ulceration and infection. The nonsurgical treatment of a foot at stage I includes rest, elevation, and protection. A total-contact cast with weekly cast changes and minimal to protected weight bearing can be useful until the acute process begins to resolve. As the foot improves, the cast can be changed every 2 weeks. During the transition to stage II, the swelling and temperature begin to stabilize. A removable boot walker or ankle-foot orthosis can be substituted for the total-contact cast, with continued limitation of forefoot and midfoot pressures. During stage III, the use of accommodative shoes with a custom-molded protective orthotic device can be initiated.

Section 2: Neuromuscular Disease

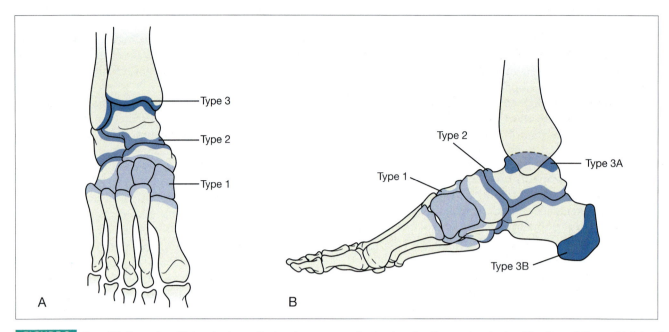

FIGURE 2 **A** and **B**, Dorsal and lateral schematic drawings, respectively, showing the anatomic classification of Charcot joints of the tarsus. Type 1 (midfoot) involves the tarsometatarsal and naviculocuneiform joints. Type 2 (hindfoot) involves the subtalar, talonavicular, and calcaneocuboid joints. Type 3A (ankle) involves the tibiotalar joint. Type 3B (calcaneus) involves a pathologic fracture of the tubercle of the calcaneus. (Adapted and redrawn with permission from Brodsky JW: The diabetic foot, in Coughlin MJ, Mann RA, Saltzman CL, eds: *Surgery of the Foot and Ankle*, ed 8. Mosby, 2007, vol 2, pp 1281-1368.)

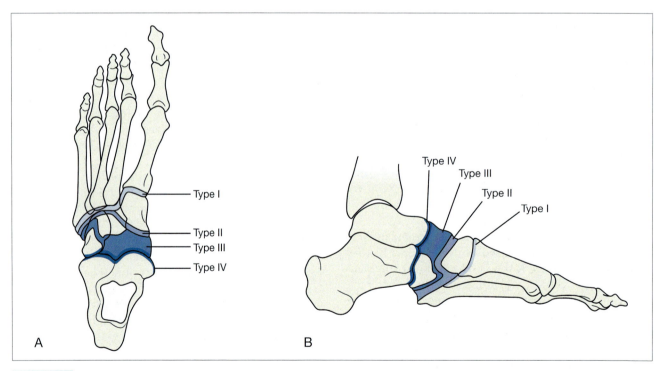

FIGURE 3 Schematic drawings showing the four types of chronic Charcot rocker-bottom deformity. **A**, AP view. **B**, Lateral view. (Redrawn with permission from Schon LC, Weinfeld SB, Horton GA, Resch S: Radiographic and clinical classification of acquired midfoot tarsus. *Foot Ankle Int* 1998;19:394-404.)

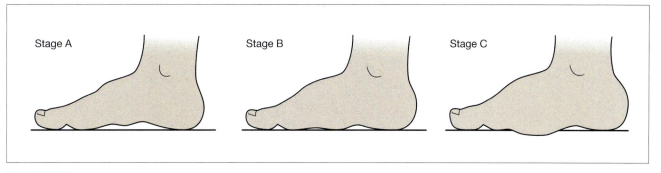

FIGURE 4 Schematics showing the three stages of chronic Charcot rocker-bottom deformity. (Redrawn with permission from Schon LC, Weinfeld SB, Horton GA, Resch S: Radiographic and clinical classification of acquired midfoot tarsus. *Foot Ankle Int* 1998;19:394-404.)

Residual deformity can result in chronic pressure and subsequent ulceration. If shoe wear modification and bracing treatment do not prevent recurrent episodes of ulceration, surgical intervention is required. Orthopaedic foot and ankle surgeons have a growing interest in the correction of acquired deformities to improve the patient's walking independence and quality of life. Internal fixation, external fixation, or a combination can be used to achieve this goal.

Surgical Complications

After an ankle fracture, patients with diabetes are at increased risk of complications including failure of wound healing, infection, malunion, delayed union, nonunion, and Charcot neuroarthropathy.[89,90] Charcot ankle neuroarthropathy most commonly occurs in patients with diabetes who have a delayed diagnosis and/or delayed immobilization or who have a nonsurgically treated displaced ankle fracture.[88] In a review of 160,000 patients with ankle fracture, the incidence of diabetes was 5.7%.[91] Those with diabetes were found to have a significantly longer hospital length of stay, in-hospital mortality, in-hospital postoperative complications, and nonroutine discharge ($P < 0.001$ for all factors).

Glycemic control is important in the perioperative management of diabetes in patients undergoing foot and ankle surgical treatment.[92,93] In a study of 21,845 Veterans Administration Hospital patients with diabetes undergoing elective foot and ankle surgical procedures,[92] for each 1% increase in HbA1c, the odds of developing a complication increased by 5%. In a 2021 study of 19,547 patients treated for ankle fracture, 5.06% had insulin-dependent diabetes. Compared with people without diabetes, patients with insulin-dependent diabetes mellitus had significantly greater adjusted odds of osteomyelitis (OR, 10.27) and wound dehiscence (OR, 2.47), among other risks.[93] Peripheral neuropathy, Charcot neuroarthropathy, current or past smoking, and increased surgical time were significantly associated with surgical site infections. To assess the risk factors associated with nonunion, delayed union, and malunion, the outcomes of 165 patients with diabetes who had undergone arthrodesis, osteotomy, or fracture reduction were reviewed. Peripheral neuropathy, surgical time, and HbA1c levels higher than 7% were found to be significant for bone-healing complications, with peripheral neuropathy having the strongest association. Surgical treatment of these patients at high risk should emphasize optimal glycemic control, maximization of limb vascularity, meticulous soft-tissue care, and prolonged avoidance of weight bearing after surgical treatment.[89,90]

ESTABLISHING RISK AND PREVENTIVE CARE

Amputation rates can be reduced by 45% to 85% if patients participate in a comprehensive foot care program that includes risk assessment, foot care education, and preventive therapy, with treatment of foot problems and referral to a specialist when indicated.[94] All patients with diabetes should undergo an annual foot examination.[95] These patients should be taught the importance of blood glucose monitoring and daily self-examination of the feet (**Table 2**). The risk of future foot complications can be predicted based on the patient's history and physical examination.

The risk of foot complications is scored from 0 to 3[17] (**Table 3**). A normal-appearing foot with normal sensation and no more than minor deformity is assigned to risk category 0. The patient should have basic knowledge of foot care, receive an annual examination, and wear ordinary footwear. In contrast, an insensate foot with deformity and a history of ulceration is assigned to risk category 3. The patient requires foot risk education

Table 2

Foot Care Instructions for Patients With Diabetes

Washing your feet	Wash your feet daily. Dry them carefully, especially between the toes. Do not soak your feet (unless instructed to do so by your clinician). If your feet are dry, apply a very thin coat of lubricant (oil or cream) after bathing and drying them. Don't put oil or cream between your toes.
Inspecting your feet	Inspect your feet daily. Use an unbreakable mirror to help see the bottom of your feet. Check for scratches, cuts, or blisters. Always check between your toes. If your vision is impaired, ask someone to check your feet for you.
Cutting your toenails	Cut your toenails by following the contour of the nail. Smooth the corners with an emery board. Don't trim into the corners of your toenails or cut ingrown toenails. If redness appears around your toenails, see your clinician immediately.
Treating corns and calluses	Do not cut corns or calluses. Do not use corn plasters or chemicals for removing corns or calluses. Do not use strong antiseptic solutions or adhesive tape on your feet.
Avoiding heat and cold	Avoid extreme temperatures. Test water with your hand or elbow before bathing. Don't walk on hot surfaces, such as sand at the beach or cement around a swimming pool. In winter, wear wool socks and protective footgear such as fleece-lined boots. Do not apply a hot water bottle or heating pad to your feet. If your feet are cold at night, wear socks.
Choosing shoes	Don't walk barefoot, even indoors. Don't wear sandals with thongs between your toes. Don't wear shoes without stockings or socks. Inspect the inside of your shoes every day for foreign objects, nail points, torn linings, and rough areas. Shoes should be comfortable at the time of purchase. Don't buy shoes that are too tight and depend on them to stretch out. Break in new shoes before wearing them regularly. Ask your podiatrist or other clinician about the types of shoes most appropriate for you.
Avoiding harm to your legs	Don't wear restrictive clothing on your legs (such as leg garters). Avoid crossing your legs. Doing so can cause pressure on the nerves and blood vessels in the legs.
Avoiding tobacco and alcohol	Do not smoke. Do not drink alcohol excessively.
Talking to your clinicians	See your clinician regularly, and be sure your feet are examined at least four times a year. Tell your podiatrist or other clinician at once if you develop a blister or sore on your foot. Be sure to tell your podiatrist that you have diabetes.

and should perform a foot self-examination several times daily. Protective shoes should be worn during walking and while standing. Cross-sectional studies support the use of rocker sole footwear and custom orthotic devices to reduce plantar pressure, but longitudinal studies are needed to confirm this benefit.[96] Most centers that care for patients with diabetic foot disease recommend extra-depth shoes constructed of soft leather or another accommodative material, with minimal seams, adjustable lacing, and custom-fabricated, pressure-dissipating insoles. Rigid orthotic devices should be avoided. For some patients, a brace or CROW (Charcot Restraint Orthotic Walker) boot is necessary to provide stability, limit motion, unload pressure, distribute forces evenly throughout the foot, and accommodate deformities.

Patients at high risk should undergo a foot examination by a physician every 2 months and a visual inspection of the feet during every encounter with a clinician. In addition, any new skin or nail issue should immediately be clinically evaluated. Foot infection in patients with diabetes almost always follows trauma, and it is associated with a high risk of hospitalization and possible amputation. Accordingly, patients with diabetes who have foot trauma, especially those with peripheral vascular disease, should be targeted for rapid intervention to prevent infection.

Racial, ethnic, and sex disparities in preventive diabetes care have been well documented.[97-102] These preventive care disparities affect outcomes. After enactment of the Affordable Care Act, states with early Medicaid expansion (before 2014) demonstrated lower rates of

Table 3

Categories of Risk for Foot Complications

Category	Risk Factors	Treatment Recommendations
0	No history of ulceration No deformity No previous amputation Pedal pulses present No sensory loss	Instruction in basic foot care Annual foot examination Regular footwear
1	No history of ulceration No deformity No previous amputation Pedal pulses present Sensory loss	Daily foot self-examination Instruction in diabetic foot care Foot examination by physician every 6 months Depth shoes or running shoes Nonmolded, soft inlays Possible total-contact orthotic devices
2	No history of ulceration Moderate (prelesion) deformity (eg, hallux rigidus, metatarsal head prominence, claw toes or hammer toes, callus, plantar bony prominence, hallux valgus, dorsal exostosis) Pedal pulses present Single lesser ray amputation Sensory loss	Daily foot self-examination Instruction in diabetic foot care Foot examination by physician every 4 months Depth shoes or running shoes Custom-molded orthotic devices Possible adjuncts including silicon toe sleeves, lamb's wool, foam toe separators, hammer toe crests, metatarsal pads External shoe modifications including metatarsal bars, rocker-bottom soles, extended steel shanks, medial or lateral heel wedges
3	History of ulceration Presence of deformity (eg, charcot neuroarthropathy, hallux rigidus, metatarsal head prominence, claw toes, hammer toes, callus, plantar bony prominence, hallux valgus, dorsal exostosis) Previous amputation (multiple ray, first ray, transmetatarsal, Chopart) Pedal pulses present or absent sensory loss	Daily foot self-examination Instruction in diabetic foot care for at-risk patients Foot examination by physician every 2 months Custom-fabricated, pressure-dissipating accommodative foot orthotic devices Inlay-depth, soft-leather, adjustable-lacing shoes External shoe modifications including rocker-bottom soles, extended steel shanks, solid ankle-cushion heels well filled with low-density material Offloading orthotic devices including patellar tendon–bearing brace, ankle-foot orthoses Immediate clinical evaluation of any new skin or nail issue Possible evaluation by orthopaedic foot and ankle surgeon

Adapted from Philbin TM: The diabetic foot, in Pinzur MS, ed: *Orthopaedic Knowledge Update® Foot and Ankle 4*. American Academy of Orthopaedic Surgeons, 2008, pp 273-290.

lower extremity amputation among racial and ethnic minorities.[103] Prevention programs should concentrate on patient compliance with medications and clinical follow-up, especially in patients who are members of a racial or ethnic minority. A multidisciplinary team approach to the management of diabetic foot disease has repeatedly been shown to improve clinical outcomes.[33,100-102]

SUMMARY

The global health burden of diabetic foot disease is steadily increasing. Continuing research into effective management strategies remains critical. Patient education and early intervention are most likely to result in a successful outcome when a multidisciplinary team approach is used.

KEY STUDY POINTS

- Diabetic care should be coordinated by a team that includes an orthopaedic surgeon, an endocrinologist, an infectious disease specialist, a vascular surgeon, a plastic surgeon, a physical therapist, and a pedorthotist.
- Diabetic neuropathy is the most important factor in the development of diabetic foot disease. As the severity of neuropathy increases, so does the risk of ulceration, amputation, and death. It can herald true diabetes as those with impaired glucose tolerance can be affected.
- Charcot neuroarthropathy has three classic stages. Stage I, the fragmentation phase, is clinically characterized by hyperemia, edema, increased warmth, and erythema around the affected joint. In stage II, the subacute or coalescence phase, the acute inflammatory findings decrease. Stage III is the chronic or consolidation phase.
- The goal of nonsurgical and surgical treatment of Charcot neuroarthropathy is to obtain a stable, plantigrade foot that is free from ulcerations. The primary indications for surgical treatment in Charcot neuroarthropathy of the foot and ankle are recurrent ulceration, significant deformity, deep infection, and pain.
- Glycemic control is important in perioperative management of patients with diabetes undergoing foot and ankle surgical treatment. For each 1% increase in HbA1c, the odds of developing a complication increases by 5%.

ANNOTATED REFERENCES

1. International Diabetes Federation IDF Diabetes Atlas, ed 10. 2021. Available at: https://www.diabetesatlas.org. Accessed April 30, 2022.

   The International Diabetes Federation Diabetes Atlas is the authoritative resource on the global burden of diabetes. First published in 2000, it is produced by the International Diabetes Federation biennially in collaboration with experts from around the world and contains data on diabetes cases, prevalence, mortality, and expenditure on the global, regional, and national level. Level of evidence: I.

2. Hebert JR, Allison DB, Archer E, Lavie CJ, Blair SN: Scientific decision making, policy decisions, and the obesity pandemic. *Mayo Clin Proc* 2013;88(6):593-604.

3. American Diabetes Association 2020 Annual Report. Available at: https://diabetes.org/sites/default/files/2021-08/ADA-2020-AnnualReport-FINAL.pdf. Accessed April 30, 2022.

   American Diabetes Association annual review details statistics, research, and COVID-19 response in 2020. Level of evidence: I.

4. American Diabetes Association: Economic costs of diabetes in the U.S. in 2017. *Diabetes Care* 2018;41(5):917-928.

5. Williams R, Karuranga S, Malanda B, et al: Global and regional estimates and projections of diabetes-related health expenditure: Results from the International Diabetes Federation Diabetes Atlas, 9th edition. *Diabetes Res Clin Pract* 2020;162;108072-108076.

   The International Diabetes Federation highlights the direct health expenditure of diabetes and diabetes prevalence estimates globally. Level of evidence: VI.

6. Sorber R, Abularrage CJ: Diabetic foot ulcers: Epidemiology and the role of multidisciplinary care teams. *Semin Vasc Surg* 2021;34(1):47-53.

   This study reviews the epidemiology, clinical care of diabetic foot ulcers, and role of multidisciplinary team in the treatment of diabetic foot disease. Level of evidence: V.

7. Hicks CW, Selvin E: Epidemiology of peripheral neuropathy and lower extremity disease in diabetes. *Curr Diab Rep* 2019;19(10):86.

   This review summarizes the epidemiology, risk factors, and management of diabetic peripheral neuropathy and related lower extremity complications. Level of evidence: V.

8. Berlet GC, Philbin TM: The diabetic foot and ankle, in Lieberman JR, ed: *AAOS Comprehensive Orthopaedic Review.* American Academy of Orthopaedic Surgeons, 2009, pp 1217-1224.

9. Albers JW, Pop-Busui R: Diabetic neuropathy: Mechanisms, emerging treatments, and subtypes. *Curr Neurol Neurosci Rep* 2014;14(8):473.

10. Dellon AL, Muse VL, Scott ND, et al: A positive Tinel sign as predictor of pain relief or sensory recovery after decompression of chronic tibial nerve compression in patients with diabetic neuropathy. *J Reconstr Microsurg* 2012;28(4):235-240.

11. Valdivia Valdivia JM, Weinand M, Maloney CT Jr, Blount AL, Dellon AL: Surgical treatment of superimposed, lower extremity, peripheral nerve entrapments with diabetic and idiopathic neuropathy. *Ann Plast Surg* 2013;70(6):675-679.

12. Zhu CL, Zhao WY, Qiu XD, Zhao SW, Zhong LZ, He N: A meta-analysis of surgical decompression in the treatment of diabetic peripheral neuropathy. *Medicine* 2018;97(37):12399.

13. Vinik AI, Maser RE, Mitchell BD, Freeman R: Diabetic autonomic neuropathy. *Diabetes Care* 2003;26(5):1553-1579.

14. International Diabetes Federation Clinical Practice Recommendations on the Diabetic Foot. 2017. Available at: https://www.idf.org/e-library/guidlines/119.idf-clinical-practice-recommendations-on-diabetic-foot-2017.html.

15. Wienemann T, Chantelau EA: The diagnostic value of measuring pressure pain perception in patients with diabetes mellitus. *Swiss Med Wkly* 2012;142:w13682.

16. Richard JL, Reilhes L, Buvry S, Goletto M, Faillie JL: Screening patients at risk for diabetic foot ulceration: A comparison between measurement of vibration perception threshold and 10-g monofilament test. *Int Wound J* 2014;11(2):147-151.

17. Apelqvist J, Castenfors J, Larsson J, Stenström A, Agardh CD: Prognostic value of systolic ankle and toe blood pressure levels in outcome of diabetic foot ulcer. *Diabetes Care* 1989;12(6):373-378.

18. Philbin TM: The diabetic foot, in Pinzur MS, ed: *Orthopaedic Knowledge Update® Foot and Ankle*, ed 4. American Academy of Orthopaedic Surgeons, 2008, pp 273-290.

19. American Diabetes Association: Statistics About Diabetes: Diabetes From the National Diabetes Statistics Report. 2017. Available at: htttp://www.diabetes.org/diabetes-basics/statistics/. Accessed May 27, 2018.

20. American Diabetes Association: 11. Microvascular complications and foot care: Standards of medical care in diabetes-2021. *Diabetes Care* 2021;44(suppl 1):S151-S167.

    The American Diabetes Association provides updated standards-of-care practices in the treatment of microvascular-related foot complications in diabetic feet. These recommendations, treatment goals, and guidelines are meant to guide clinical practice. Level of evidence: I.

21. Baumhauer JF, O'Keefe RJ, Schon LC, Pinzur MS: Cytokine-induced osteoclastic bone resorption in Charcot arthropathy: An immunohistochemical study. *Foot Ankle Int* 2006;27(10):797-800.

22. Donovan A, Schweitzer ME: Current concepts in imaging diabetic pedal osteomyelitis. *Radiol Clin North Am* 2008;46(6):1105-1124, vii.

23. Gandsman EJ, Deutsch SD, Kahn CB, McCullough RW: Differentiation of Charcot joint from osteomyelitis through dynamic bone imaging. *Nucl Med Commun* 1990;11(1):45-53.

24. Loredo R, Rahal A, Garcia G, Metter D: Imaging of the diabetic foot: Diagnostic dilemmas. *Foot Ankle Spec* 2010;3(5):249-264.

25. Kapoor A, Page S, Lavalley M, Gale DR, Felson DT: Magnetic resonance imaging for diagnosing foot osteomyelitis: A meta-analysis. *Arch Intern Med* 2007;167(2):125-132.

26. Toledano TR, Fatone EA, Weis A, Cotten A, Beltran J: MRI evaluation of bone marrow changes in the diabetic foot: A practical approach. *Semin Musculoskelet Radiol* 2011;15(3):257-268.

27. Schweitzer ME, Daffner RH, Weissman BN, et al: ACR appropriateness criteria on suspected osteomyelitis in patients with diabetes mellitus. *J Am Coll Radiol* 2008;5(8):881-886.

28. Rozzanigo U, Tagliani A, Vittorini E, Pacchioni R, Brivio LR, Caudana R: Role of magnetic resonance imaging in the evaluation of diabetic foot with suspected osteomyelitis. *Radiol Med* 2009;114(1):121-132.

29. Dodd A, Daniels TR: Current concepts review: Charcot neuroarthropathy of the foot and ankle. *J Bone Joint Surg Am* 2018;100(8):696-711.

30. Ranachowska C, Lass P, Korzon-Burakowska A, Dobosz M: Diagnostic imaging of the diabetic foot. *Nucl Med Rev Cent East Eur* 2010;13(1):18-22.

31. Poirier JY, Garin E, Derrien C, et al: Diagnosis of osteomyelitis in the diabetic foot with a 99mTc-HMPAO leucocyte scintigraphy combined with a 99mTc-MDP bone scintigraphy. *Diabetes Metab* 2002;28(6 pt 1):485-490.

32. Kumar R, Basu S, Torigian D, Anand V, Zhuang H, Alavi A: Role of modern imaging techniques for diagnosis of infection in the era of 18F-fluorodeoxyglucose positron emission tomography. *Clin Microbiol Rev* 2008;21(1):209-224.

33. Nawaz A, Torigian DA, Siegelman ES, Basu S, Chryssikos T, Alavi A: Diagnostic performance of FDG-PET, MRI, and plain film radiography (PFR) for the diagnosis of osteomyelitis in the diabetic foot. *Mol Imaging Biol* 2010;12(3):335-342.

34. Michail M, Jude E, Liaskos C, et al: The performance of serum inflammatory markers for the diagnosis and follow-up of patients with osteomyelitis. *Int J Low Extrem Wounds* 2013;12(2):94-99.

35. Bone RC, Sibbald WJ, Sprung CL: The ACCP-SCCM consensus conference on sepsis and organ failure. *Chest* 1992;101(6):1481-1483.

36. Armstrong DG, Lavery LA, Sariaya M, Ashry H: Leukocytosis is a poor indicator of acute osteomyelitis of the foot in diabetes mellitus. *J Foot Ankle Surg* 1996;35(4):280-283.

37. Lipsky BA, Sheehan P, Armstrong DG, Tice AD, Polis AB, Abramson MA: Clinical predictors of treatment failure for diabetic foot infections: Data from a prospective trial. *Int Wound J* 2007;4(1):30-38.

38. Pinzur MS, Stuck RM, Sage R, Hunt N, Rabinovich Z: Syme ankle disarticulation in patients with diabetes. *J Bone Joint Surg Am* 2003;85(9):1667-1672.

39. Wukich DK, Hobizal KB, Brooks MM: Severity of diabetic foot infection and rate of limb salvage. *Foot Ankle Int* 2013;34(3):351-358.

40. Dzieciuchowicz Ł, Kruszyna Ł, Krasiski Z, Espinosa G: Monitoring of systemic inflammatory response in diabetic patients with deep foot infection treated with negative pressure wound therapy. *Foot Ankle Int* 2012;33(10):832-837.

41. Guven MF, Karabiber A, Kaynak G, Ogut T: Conservative and surgical treatment of the chronic Charcot foot and ankle. *Diabet Foot Ankle* 2013; August 2 [Epub ahead of print].

42. Prompers L, Huijberts M, Apelqvist J, et al: High prevalence of ischaemia, infection and serious comorbidity in patients with diabetic foot disease in Europe: Baseline results from the Eurodiale study. *Diabetologia* 2007;50(1):18-25.

43. Boyko EJ, Ahroni JH, Smith DG, Davignon D: Increased mortality associated with diabetic foot ulcer. *Diabet Med* 1996;13(11):967-972.

44. International Diabetes Federation (IDF): *Diabetes Atlas*, ed 8. International Diabetes Federation, 2017.

45. Cheing GLY, Chau RMW, Kwan RLC, Choi CH, Zheng YP: Do the biomechanical properties of the ankle-foot complex influence postural control for people with type 2 diabetes? *Clin Biomech (Bristol, Avon)* 2013;28(1):88-92.

46. Sun JH, Cheng BK, Zheng YP, Huang YP, Leung JY, Cheing GL: Changes in the thickness and stiffness of plantar soft tissues in people with diabetic peripheral neuropathy. *Arch Phys Med Rehabil* 2011;92(9):1484-1489.

47. Noor S, Zubair M, Ahmad J: Diabetic foot ulcer – A review on pathophysiology, classification and microbial etiology. *Diabetes Metab Syndr* 2015;9(3):192-199.

48. Margolis DJ, Gupta J, Hoffstad O, et al: Lack of effectiveness of hyperbaric oxygen therapy for the treatment of diabetic foot ulcer and the prevention of amputation: A cohort study. *Diabetes Care* 2013;36(7):1961-1966.

49. Brodsky JW: The diabetic foot, in Coughlin MJ, Mann RA, Saltzman CL, eds: *Surgery of the Foot and Ankle*, ed 8. Mosby, 2007, pp 1281-1368.

50. Leese G, Schofield C, McMurray B, et al: Scottish foot ulcer risk score predicts foot ulcer healing in a regional specialist foot clinic. *Diabetes Care* 2007;30(8):2064-2069.

51. Chappell FM, Crawford F, Horne M, et al: Development and validation of a clinical prediction rule for development of diabetic foot ulceration: An analysis of data from five cohort studies. *BMJ Open Diabetes Res Care* 2021;9(1):e002150.

    This study highlights a novel clinical prediction rule for diabetic foot ulceration that is user-friendly in the clinical setting and designed based on previously published literature from four international cohort studies, identified by systematic review. A fifth study was published focusing on validation of the clinical prediction rule. Level of evidence: V.

52. Armstrong DG, Nguyen HC, Lavery LA, van Schie CH, Boulton AJ, Harkless LB: Off-loading the diabetic foot wound: A randomized clinical trial. *Diabetes Care* 2001;24(6):1019-1022.

53. Katz IA, Harlan A, Miranda-Palma B, et al: A randomized trial of two irremovable off-loading devices in the management of plantar neuropathic diabetic foot ulcers. *Diabetes Care* 2005;28(3):555-559.

54. Lewis J, Lipp A: Pressure-relieving interventions for treating diabetic foot ulcers. *Cochrane Database Syst Rev* 2013;1:CD002302.

55. Piaggesi A, Macchiarini S, Rizzo L, et al: An off-the-shelf instant contact casting device for the management of diabetic foot ulcers: A randomized prospective trial versus traditional fiberglass cast. *Diabetes Care* 2007;30(3):586-590.

56. Colen LB, Kim CJ, Grant WP, Yeh JT, Hind B: Achilles tendon lengthening: Friend or foe in the diabetic foot? *Plast Reconstr Surg* 2013;131(1):37e-43e.

57. Mueller MJ, Sinacore DR, Hastings MK, Strube MJ, Johnson JE: Effect of Achilles tendon lengthening on neuropathic plantar ulcers: A randomized clinical trial. *J Bone Joint Surg Am* 2003;85(8):1436-1445.

58. Kim JY, Hwang S, Lee Y: Selective plantar fascia release for nonhealing diabetic plantar ulcerations. *J Bone Joint Surg Am* 2012;94(14):1297-1302.

59. Biz C, Gastaldo S, Dalmau-Pastor M, Corradin M, Volpin A, Ruggieri P: Minimally invasive distal metatarsal diaphyseal osteotomy (DMDO) for chronic plantar diabetic foot ulcers. *Foot Ankle Int* 2018;39(1):83-92.

60. Tamir E, Finestone AS, Avisar E, Agar G: Mini-invasive floating metatarsal osteotomy for resistant or recurrent neuropathic plantar metatarsal head ulcers. *J Orthop Surg Res* 2016;11(1):78.

61. Kranke P, Bennett MH, Martyn-St James M, Schnabel A, Debus SE, Weibel S: Hyperbaric oxygen therapy for chronic wounds. *Cochrane Database Syst Rev* 2015;2015(6):CD004123.

62. Liu S, He CZ, Cai YT, et al: Evaluation of negative-pressure wound therapy for patients with diabetic foot ulcers: Systematic review and meta-analysis. *Ther Clin Risk Manag* 2017;13:533-544.

63. Embil JM, Rose G, Trepman E, et al: Oral antimicrobial therapy for diabetic foot osteomyelitis. *Foot Ankle Int* 2006;27(10):771-779.

64. Bergin SM, Wraight P: Silver based wound dressings and topical agents for treating diabetic foot ulcers. *Cochrane Database Syst Rev* 2006;1:CD005082.

65. Vermeulen H, van Hattem JM, Storm-Versloot MN, Ubbink DT: Topical silver for treating infected wounds. *Cochrane Database Syst Rev* 2007;1:CD005486.

66. Dumville JC, Lipsky BA, Hoey C, Cruciani M, Fiscon M, Xia J: Topical antimicrobial agents for treating foot ulcers in people with diabetes. *Cochrane Database Syst Rev* 2017;6(6):CD011038.

67. Lipsky BA, Hoey C: Topical antimicrobial therapy for treating chronic wounds. *Clin Infect Dis* 2009;49(10):1541-1549.

68. Pinzur MS, Gil J, Belmares J: Treatment of osteomyelitis in Charcot foot with single-stage resection of infection, correction of deformity, and maintenance with ring fixation. *Foot Ankle Int* 2012;33(12):1069-1074.

69. Wilson RM: Neutrophil function in diabetes. *Diabet Med* 1986;3(6):509-512.

70. Gardner SE, Hillis SL, Heilmann K, Segre JA, Grice EA: The neuropathic diabetic foot ulcer microbiome is associated with clinical factors. *Diabetes* 2013;62(3):923-930.

71. Monteiro-Soares M, Russell D, Boyko EJ, et al: Guidelines on the classification of diabetic foot ulcers (IWGDF 2019). *Diabetes Metab Res Rev* 2020;36(suppl 1):e3273.

    The International Working Group on the Diabetic Foot publishes multiple evidence-based guidelines on the classification and management of diabetic ulcers. Their focus is optimizing treatment rather than predicting future ulceration. The International Working Group on the Diabetic Foot/Infectious Diseases Society of America classification is incorporated into the Wound, Ischemia, and foot Infection system (WIfI), which incorporates ischemia and gangrenous changes. Level of evidence: V.

72. Bravo-Molina A, Linares-Palomino JP, Vera-Arroyo B, SalmerónFebres LM, Ros-Díe E: Inter-observer agreement of the Wagner, University of Texas and PEDIS classification systems for the diabetic foot syndrome. *Foot Ankle Surg* 2018;24(1):60-64.

73. Aragón-Sánchez J, Lipsky BA, Lázaro-Martínez JL: Gram-negative diabetic foot osteomyelitis: Risk factors and clinical presentation. *Int J Low Extrem Wounds* 2013;12(1):63-68.

74. Smith DG, Assal M, Reiber GE, Vath C, LeMaster J, Wallace C: Minor environmental trauma and lower extremity amputation in high-risk patients with diabetes: Incidence, pivotal events, etiology, and amputation level in a prospectively followed cohort. *Foot Ankle Int* 2003;24(9):690-695.

75. Pinzur M, Freeland R, Juknelis D: The association between body mass index and foot disorders in diabetic patients. *Foot Ankle Int* 2005;26(5):375-377.

76. Wachtel MS: Family poverty accounts for differences in lower-extremity amputation rates of minorities 50 years old or more with diabetes. *J Natl Med Assoc* 2005;97(3):334-338.

77. Moura Neto A, Zantut-Wittmann DE, Fernandes TD, Nery M, Parisi MCR: Risk factors for ulceration and amputation in diabetic foot: Study in a cohort of 496 patients. *Endocrine* 2013;44(1):119-124.

78. Anderson JJ, Boone J, Hansen M, Spencer L, Fowler Z: A comparison of diabetic smokers and non-smokers who undergo lower extremity amputation: A retrospective review of 112 patients. *Diabet Foot Ankle* 2012; October 16 [Epub ahead of print].

79. Faglia E, Clerici G, Caminiti M, Curci V, Somalvico F: Influence of osteomyelitis location in the foot of diabetic patients with transtibial amputation. *Foot Ankle Int* 2013;34(2):222-227.

80. Molines-Barroso RJ, Lázaro-Martínez JL, Aragón-Sánchez J, García-Morales E, Beneit-Montesinos JV, Álvaro-Afonso FJ: Analysis of transfer lesions in patients who underwent surgery for diabetic foot ulcers located on the plantar aspect of the metatarsal heads. *Diabet Med* 2013;30(8):973-976.

81. Nerone VS, Springer KD, Woodruff DM, Atway SA: Reamputation after minor foot amputation in diabetic patients: Risk factors leading to limb loss. *J Foot Ankle Surg* 2013;52(2):184-187.

82. Brown ML, Tang W, Patel A, Baumhauer JF: Partial foot amputation in patients with diabetic foot ulcers. *Foot Ankle Int* 2012;33(9):707-716.

83. Harding JL, Andes LJ, Rolka DB, et al: National and State-level trends in nontraumatic lower-extremity amputation among U.S. Medicare Beneficiaries with diabetes, 2000-2017. *Diabetes Care* 2020;43(10):2453-2459.

    Medicare fee-for-service claims were obtained from Centers for Medicare and Medicaid Services for 2000 to 2017. Nontraumatic lower extremity amputation decreased from 8.5 (per 1,000 people with diabetes) in 2000 to 4.4 in 2009. This increased slightly to 4.8 by 2017 as a result of more foot and toe amputations. Rates were highest in the oldest patients, Blacks, and men. Level of evidence: III.

84. Waibel FWA, Berli MC, Gratwohl V, et al: Midterm fate of the contralateral foot in Charcot arthropathy. *Foot Ankle Int* 2020;41(10):1181-1189.

    Records of 130 consecutive patients were retrospectively studied. At a mean of 2.5 years, 19.2% had contralateral Charcot, with females at higher risk (OR, 3.13; CI, 1.21 to 7.7). A contralateral ulcer developed in 46.2% of patients, with the most contralateral ulcers (57.1%) developing in patients with Sanders type 2 feet (midfoot) Charcot arthropathy. Level of evidence: IV.

85. Eichenholtz SN: *Charcot Joints*. Thomas, 1966.

86. Rosenbaum AJ, Dipreta JA: Classifications in brief: Eichenholtz classification of Charcot arthropathy. *Clin Orthop Relat Res* 2015;473(3):1168-1171.

87. Shibata T, Tada K, Hashizume C: The results of arthrodesis of the ankle for leprotic neuroarthropathy. *J Bone Joint Surg Am* 1990;72(5):749-756.

88. Schon LC, Marks RM: The management of neuroarthropathic fracture-dislocations in the diabetic patient. *Orthop Clin North Am* 1995;26(2):375-392.

89. Bibbo C, Lin SS, Beam HA, Behrens FF: Complications of ankle fractures in diabetic patients. *Orthop Clin North Am* 2001;32(1):113-133.

90. McCormack RG, Leith JM: Ankle fractures in diabetics: Complications of surgical management. *J Bone Joint Surg Br* 1998;80(4):689-692.

91. Ganesh SP, Pietrobon R, Cecílio WA, Pan D, Light-dale N, Nunley JA: The impact of diabetes on patient outcomes after ankle fracture. *J Bone Joint Surg Am* 2005;87(8):1712-1718.

92. Domek N, Dux K, Pinzur M, Weaver F, Rogers T: Association between hemoglobin A1c and surgical morbidity in elective foot and ankle surgery. *J Foot Ankle Surg* 2016;55(5):939-943.

93. Liu JW, Ahn J, Nakonezny PA, et al: Insulin dependence increases the risk of 30-day postoperative complications following ankle fracture surgery in patients with diabetes mellitus. *J Foot Ankle Surg* 2021;60(5):917-922.

    A retrospective observational study of 19,547 patients undergoing ankle surgery between 2012 and 2016 identified by the ACS-NSQIP database was performed. 989 patients (5.05%) had insulin-dependent diabetes and 1,256 patients (6.43%) had non–insulin-dependent diabetes. Compared with people without diabetes, patients with insulin-dependent diabetes had higher rates of infection, intubation, sepsis, readmission, and death (among other outcomes). Patients with non–insulin-dependent diabetes had higher rates of pneumonia and longer hospital length of stay. Level of evidence: III.

94. Singh N, Armstrong DG, Lipsky BA: Preventing foot ulcers in patients with diabetes. *J Am Med Assoc* 2005;293(2):217-228.

95. Healy A, Naemi R, Chockalingam N: The effectiveness of footwear as an intervention to prevent or to reduce biomechanical risk factors associated with diabetic foot ulceration: A systematic review. *J Diabetes Complications* 2013;27(4):391-400.

96. Blumberg SN, Warren SM: Disparities in initial presentation and treatment outcomes of diabetic foot ulcers in a public, private, and Veterans Administration hospital. *J Diabetes* 2014;6(1):68-75.

97. Pu J, Chewning B: Racial difference in diabetes preventive care. *Res Social Adm Pharm* 2013;9(6):790-796.

98. Kim G, Ford KL, Chiriboga DA, Sorkin DH: Racial and ethnic disparities in healthcare use, delayed care, and management of diabetes mellitus in older adults in California. *J Am Geriatr Soc* 2012;60(12):2319-2325.

99. Yu MK, Lyles CR, Bent-Shaw LA, Young BA: Sex disparities in diabetes process of care measures and self-care in high-risk patients. *J Diabetes Res* 2013;2013:575814.

100. Kuehn BM: Prompt response, multidisciplinary care key to reducing diabetic foot amputation. *J Am Med Assoc* 2012;308(1):19-20.

101. Maderal AD, Vivas AC, Zwick TG, Kirsner RS: Diabetic foot ulcers: Evaluation and management. *Hosp Pract (1995)* 2012;40(3):102-115.

102. Pickwell KM, Siersma VD, Kars M, Holstein PE, Schaper NC, Eurodiale consortium: Diabetic foot disease: Impact of ulcer location on ulcer healing. *Diabetes Metab Res Rev* 2013;29(5):377-383.

103. Tan TW, Calhoun EA, Knapp SM, et al: Rates of diabetes-related major amputations among racial and ethnic minority adults following medicaid expansion under the patient protection and affordable care Act. *JAMA Netw Open* 2022;5(3):e223991.

Diabetes-related amputations were studied in states that expanded Medicaid access within 2 years of passage of the Affordable Care Act. Compared with states without early Medicaid expansion, there was a relative improvement in the major amputation rate among African American, Hispanic, and other racial and ethnic minority adults. Level of evidence: II.

CHAPTER 7

Peripheral Nerve Disorders

DAVID E. OJI, MD, FAAOS

ABSTRACT

Diagnosis of nerve entrapment at various sites in the foot and ankle can be difficult. It is important to discuss appropriate clinical examination, diagnostic tests, and relevant investigations, along with pathophysiology and treatment.

Keywords: interdigital neuralgia; nerve compression; tarsal tunnel syndrome

INTRODUCTION

Peripheral nerve disorders caused by entrapments in the foot and ankle are less common than in the upper limb and can be difficult to diagnose. It is important to discuss the most common peripheral nerve disorders in the foot and ankle. These disorders can be more difficult to manage, and the response to intervention may be limited. It is important to diagnose and initiate early treatment to help prevent long-term effects. A comprehensive history, physical examination, and proper use of diagnostic tests can lead to early diagnosis.

Dr. Oji or an immediate family member is a member of a speakers' bureau or has made paid presentations on behalf of CrossRoads Extremity and Stryker; serves as a paid consultant to or is an employee of CrossRoads Extremity Solutions; and serves as a board member, owner, officer, or committee member of American Orthopaedic Foot and Ankle Society.

INTERDIGITAL PLANTAR NEURALGIA

Interdigital plantar neuralgia was first described as early as 1845 for pain in relation to the third interspace. This entity, commonly referred to as Morton neuroma and first described in 1876, was reported as a peculiar and painful affliction of the fourth metatarsophalangeal (MTP) joint that was treated by resection of that joint with the additional removal of soft tissue surrounding the joint including digital branches of the third and fourth web space nerves. The swollen portion of the tissue that was removed was thought to be a neuroma. It is now known that the term neuroma is a misnomer, as the nerve enlargement is not a tumor. The histologic findings include interstitial sclerohyalinosis, degeneration of nerve fibers without wallerian degeneration, intraneural and perineural fibrosis, and stromal changes with increased elastic fibers.[1,2] This condition has also been referred to as compression neuropathy.

Anatomy and Pathophysiology

There is no clear explanation of the etiology of this condition. Multiple theories have been suggested. The plantar aspect of the foot is innervated by the medial plantar nerve (MPN), which branches into the first, second, and third digital nerves, and the lateral plantar nerve (LPN), which provides the common digital nerve to the fourth interspace and a proper digital branch to the lateral side of the fifth toe. The common digital nerve to each web space passes beneath the deep transverse metatarsal ligament (DTML). This ligament has been implicated as the site and cause of the nerve compression. The pathologic findings of intraneural fibrosis and degeneration occur distal to the DTML supporting this theory.[2] It has also been shown that during heel-off and midstance phases of

This chapter is adapted from Sathe VM: Peripheral nerve disease, in Chou LB, ed: *Orthopaedic Knowledge Update®: Foot and Ankle 6*. American Academy of Orthopaedic Surgeons, 2020, pp 83-102.

gait, the area of pathology is always distal to the DTML.[3] Nerve biopsies performed on patients with interdigital neuralgia (IDN) compared with asymptomatic nerves at autopsy failed to show any significant difference between specimens.[4]

It has been previously postulated that the nerve in the third web space composed of communicating branches from the MPN and LPN is thicker and consequently more prone to injury,[5] but this has not been supported clinically. Another study observed that the second and third intermetatarsal spaces are narrower than the first and fourth spaces. It has been theorized that this could be the reason for the more common entrapment of the nerves in these interspaces.[6] A communicating branch between the third and fourth common digital nerves is present in up to 28% of feet, and an injury to one of these communicating branches could lead to pain and might be responsible for recurrent pain after neuroma resection.[7]

Another proposed contributing factor is the difference in mobility between the medial three rays compared with the lateral two rays. The first, second, and third metatarsals are more firmly fixed to the corresponding cuneiforms, compared with the fourth and fifth metatarsals, which have more movement with their cuboid articulation. This difference may expose the common digital nerve to trauma. Although this theory can be argued for the third web space, it is negated by the presence of neuromas in the second interspace.[8]

Other causes of interdigital plantar neuralgia include direct injuries to the interdigital nerve such as stepping on sharp objects, crush injuries, or traction injuries. It has also been proposed that repetitive activities such as prolonged standing or walking on hard surfaces with noncushioned shoes might lead to IDN. In runners, dancers, or athletes, high forefoot forces during cutting, twisting, spinning, or jumping activities might lead to overuse injury of the interdigital nerve. Similarly, modern footwear can promote excessive dorsiflexion of the MTP joint, causing forced plantar flexion of the metatarsals and subsequent trauma to the nerves.[9] Fat pad atrophy can also make the nerve more vulnerable. Rarely, the transverse metatarsal ligament may become thickened or have an aberrant band, which when released will resolve the symptoms of IDN.[9] Other extrinsic causes of nerve injury include the presence of ganglion, lipoma, or MTP joint instability. In approximately 10% to 15% of patients, MTP joint capsule attenuation allows medial deviation of the third toe and consequent lateral shifting of the third metatarsal, reducing the third intermetatarsal space and causing interdigital plantar neuralgia.[9] Injury to the plantar plate with subluxation or dislocation of the MTP joint may put additional strain on the nerve. Patients with proximal nerve compression may experience double-crush syndrome whereby the distal nerve

becomes more sensitive to any pressure. Arthritis and synovitis of the MTP joints due to various causes and fracture sequelae such as malunion may also result in interdigital plantar neuralgia.

History and Physical Examination

The most common age for presentation of interdigital plantar neuralgia is reportedly 55 years (age range 29 to 81 years). Interdigital plantar neuralgia is 4 to 15 times more likely to be diagnosed in women than in men.[8,10] Typically, the presenting symptoms are in the second or third interspace. The occurrence of symptoms in the first or fourth interspace is rare and atypical. Unilateral involvement is more common, but there is a 15% incidence of bilateral neuromas. A 3% incidence of two neuromas in the same foot has been reported.[11] Patients report burning, stabbing, tingling, electric-type shooting pain radiating into the corresponding affected toes. Removing tight-fitting shoes often relieves the symptoms. Walking barefoot on soft surfaces also helps to ease the pain. Some patients may describe fullness under the toes. The normal gait pattern of heel strike then rolling onto the ball of the foot may be lost as patients try to curl the toes during stance to reduce the pain.

Physical examination begins with observation of standing foot alignment to detect deviations in the toes, clawing, and swelling or fullness in the interspace compared with the contralateral side. The skin on both the dorsal and plantar aspect is examined closely for the presence of corns, calluses, or erythema. It is also important to inspect the patient's shoes because tight-fitting footwear is common. Careful palpation of the foot should be performed, noting any areas of tenderness and/or fullness. Each MTP joint is evaluated for synovitis, range of motion, laxity, and instability. The MTP joint drawer test assesses stability. It is important to rule out pathology in the MTP joints as responsible for the painful symptoms. The intermetatarsal spaces are then examined individually, using compression to identify the origin of pain.

Various tests and examination techniques have been described for interdigital plantar neuralgia. The most commonly reported clinical findings include plantar tenderness in 95%, radiation of pain into the toes in 46%, a palpable mass in 12%, and numbness and widening of the interspace in 3%.[9] Another study showed that web space tenderness was positive in 95%, foot squeeze test positive in 88%, plantar percussion positive in 61%, and toe tip sensation deficit present in 67%.[12] A digital nerve stretch test has also been described, with 100% sensitivity and 95% positive predictive value. To perform this test, both ankles are held in full dorsiflexion and the lesser toes on either side of the suspected web space are passively fully extended on both feet. The test is positive if the patient reports discomfort in the web space of the affected foot.[13] The Mulder test is performed by using compression with mediolateral pressure to the corresponding metatarsal heads while palpating the plantar web space. A palpable click or clunk that reproduces patient symptoms is considered to be indicative of interdigital plantar neuralgia.[14] Palpation of the affected toes rarely shows loss of sensation.

A gross motor examination, including motor function and reflexes, is performed to rule out lumbar radiculopathy. Sensation in the sural, saphenous, and superficial peroneal nerves (SPNs) is tested.

Diagnostic Studies

AP, lateral, and oblique radiographs are obtained to evaluate for dislocation, subluxation, arthritis, foreign bodies, or other abnormalities. A study failed to show any relationship between metatarsal length and angular measurements in symptomatic IDN.[15] Additional modalities that have been used for diagnosis of interdigital plantar neuralgia include ultrasonography and MRI. Both are controversial with routine use in diagnosing interdigital plantar neuralgia. The size of the lesion is very important in detecting IDN using these modalities. In one study, both ultrasonography and MRI were found to be inaccurate. Specifically, ultrasonography was shown to have inaccuracies for lesions smaller than 5 mm.[16] This study concluded that relying on ultrasonography or MRI would have led to inaccurate diagnosis in 18 of 19 cases. A detailed clinical examination was found to be the most sensitive and specific diagnostic modality. Another report found ultrasonography to be very good at detecting intermetatarsal interdigital plantar neuralgia, with 92% accuracy.[17]

No reliable electrodiagnostic studies are available to document the evidence of an interdigital plantar neuralgia. In one study using near-nerve needle sensory nerve conduction, an abnormal dip phenomenon was the most characteristic electrophysiologic diagnostic marker for interdigital plantar neuralgia.[18] Overall, electrodiagnostic studies are mainly used for detection of more proximal nerve compression or if there is suspicion for radiculopathy.

Selective injections into the painful intermetatarsal space can be used as a diagnostic tool. Although complete relief may be obtained, it is not advised to interpret this as a confirmation of interdigital plantar neuralgia without further support from the physical examination.

Nonsurgical Treatment

Early treatment involves fitting the patient with a wide, soft, laced shoe, preferably with a low heel. This type of shoe wear allows the toes to spread, thereby relieving local pressure and also eliminating chronic hyperextension of the MTP joints. A soft metatarsal support pad just proximal to the metatarsal heads may provide relief from pressure in the area and offload the forefoot, reducing painful symptoms.

The use of corticosteroid injections may be helpful but usually does not provide long-lasting pain relief. Significant relief can be obtained after local injection in 60% to 82% of patients.[19-24] In many instances, the effect of steroid injection can wane after several months.[21,22,24,25] A 2021 systematic review of corticosteroid injections in the treatment of Morton interdigital neuroma demonstrated that up to 30% of patients eventually underwent surgical excision after steroid injection.[26] In a blind randomized trial, patients received an injection of 40 mg methylprednisolone with 1% lidocaine under ultrasonographic control by a radiologist. Compared with the control group, global assessment of foot health was better in the corticosteroid group at 3 months. The authors concluded that corticosteroid injections for interdigital plantar neuralgia can often provide symptomatic benefit for at least 3 months.[24] In a separate randomized controlled trial with patients treated with steroid injection versus placebo with anesthetic only, a larger number of patients reported early pain improvement with steroid injection although the effect decreased over time. At 6 months after injection, there was no statistical difference between the two groups, although both did have a 33% reduction from baseline pain values. At the conclusion of the study, there was no statistical difference between the two groups in requesting neuroma excision or adding steroid to the injection.[25]

Corticosteroid injections can be associated with serious side effects, especially if the injection is given at the wrong site. Injections should be used with some degree of caution. Atrophy of the subcutaneous fat pad and skin discoloration have been reported.[27] Disruption of the joint capsule with resultant damage to the collateral ligaments and subsequent deviation of the toe medially or laterally can also be a serious problem.

Many studies have evaluated the efficacy of neurolysis using alcohol sclerosing therapy, with 69% to 90% of patients having improvement after the injection.[28-30] Moreover, the injections may decrease the size of the neuroma by 20% to 30%.[28,31] However, a 5-year prospective cohort study demonstrated that only 29% of patients were pain free at 5 years after injection and that 36% of patients underwent neurectomy.[32] Although alcohol injections can be seen as a less traumatic treatment option, many patients observed significant pain with the injection along with dysesthesia and recurrence. Other risks of the injection can include scar formation and infection. Furthermore, a study on rats receiving sciatic nerve injection showed no demonstrable effect on cellular histology, apoptosis, or cell survival after dehydrated alcohol injection, raising questions about efficacy of using alcohol injection in humans.[33]

Injections with either botulinum toxin or capsaicin have been proposed as nonsurgical treatment options. Botulinum toxin demonstrates an analgesic effect and has been used for treatment of refractory pain in many conditions including plantar fasciitis, low back pain, allodynia, and chronic migraines.[34] A small cohort study of 17 patients demonstrated significant reduction in pain scores after the injection, although the follow-up period was only 12 weeks.[35] Further studies are needed to evaluate the long-term efficacy of botulinum toxin. A prospective randomized controlled trial evaluated the use of capsaicin in neuromas to test its efficacy, tolerability, and safety. The results indicated significant reduction in average pain scores in their cohort of 58 patients at 4 weeks after injection.[36] However, further studies are lacking, along with long-term results.

Of note, injections done with the use of ultrasonographic guidance have not been shown to demonstrate improved results.[20]

As discussed in a 2020 study, radiofrequency ablation showed a reduction in pain scores following treatment, with an overall satisfaction rate of 81%.[37] However, follow-up on average was limited to 9 months and in some of the studies steroids were injected at the time of treatment, leading to a large confounding factor.[38-40] Postablation complications include difficulty wearing footwear and severe pain.[39,40] Given the confounding factors and lack of long-term results, the evidence to support its use is limited.

Other nonsurgical treatments include extracorporeal shock wave therapy, laser therapy, and cryoablation. Similar to botulinum and capsaicin injection, all three treatments demonstrate reduction in pain scores; however, results are based on studies with low levels of evidence and limited follow-up.[41-44]

Other treatment options include NSAIDs, oral vitamin B$_6$ (200 mg daily for 3 months and then 100 mg daily), off-label use of tricyclic antidepressants, serotonin uptake inhibitors, and antiseizure medications.

Overall, between 60% and 70% of patients in whom interdigital plantar neuralgia is diagnosed eventually undergo surgical intervention after failure of nonsurgical treatment.[12] A retrospective review attempted to identify factors predicting the need for further intervention following a single corticosteroid injection. Fifty-one percent required further treatment within 2 years. Neuromas with an average size of 10 mm or larger and younger age predicted a greater chance of surgical intervention. This study suggests surgical treatment for larger neuromas and younger patients rather than repeat injections.[45]

Surgical Treatment

If nonsurgical treatment fails, then surgical intervention is indicated. Successful results after surgery have been reported to be between 51% and 93%.[1,8,46-49] Surgical excision of the nerve is the most frequent technique used to relieve pain from interdigital plantar neuralgia. Other options include neurectomy combined with burying the nerve residuum into nearby nerve or muscle, nerve transposition, transverse intermetatarsal ligament (IML) release with or without neurolysis, and endoscopic decompression of the transverse metatarsal ligament. An isolated IML release as primary surgical management has been described. In a retrospective study, 11 patients with isolated IML release with previous failed nonsurgical treatment were followed after surgery. Visual analog scale (VAS) scores preoperatively and postoperatively were compared and showed improvement down from 6.4 to 1.5 at final follow-up. All patients reported significant pain improvement and overall satisfaction. The study concluded that isolated IML release of chronic Morton neuroma showed promising short-term results.[50] In a 2020 study, neurectomy was compared with IML release with dorsal translocation of the nerve. The IML release group with dorsal translocation of the nerve was more effective in pain reduction among patients (92% versus 82%), and patients had earlier return to work, earlier return to routine footwear, and better resolution of symptoms postsurgery.[51] A retrospective 2019 study evaluated neurectomy versus neurolysis and dorsal translocation showing equivocal functional outcome scores between the two but higher satisfaction scores with the translocation group.[52]

Endoscopic decompression has been reported to provide excellent pain relief with low rate of complications.[53] An alternate technique without endoscopy was performed in 14 patients (17 nerve decompressions) using instrumentation designed for carpal tunnel release. The authors of this study reported complete pain relief in 11 of 14 patients, 26 months after surgery.[54] A 2020 study evaluated the role of ultrasonography in identification and percutaneous release of the IML. Results indicated 54 of the 56 participants had significant pain reduction.[55] In another 2020 study, minimally invasive neurolysis was done using a proprietary system to release the IML. Results indicated significant pain reduction in patients without a Mulder click preoperatively (83%) and higher rates of continued pain (40%) in those with a Mulder click. It was concluded that minimally invasive nerve decompression may not be as effective as previously reported and it may be more appropriate for patients with smaller or nascent neuromas.[56]

Typically, a dorsal incision is used for primary surgery, but plantar incision also has been described. A level I prospective randomized controlled study of plantar and dorsal incisions for surgical treatment of primary Morton neuroma demonstrated clinically good outcomes with both approaches, with no difference in regard to pain, restrictions of daily activities, and scar tenderness.

Chapter 7: Peripheral Nerve Disorders

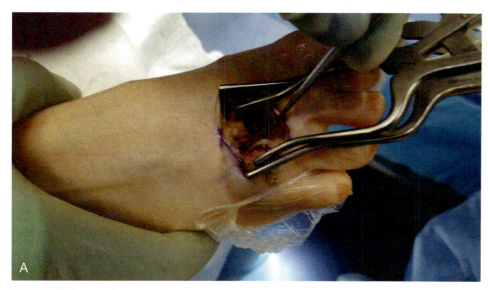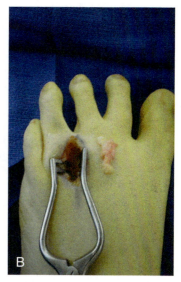

FIGURE 1 **A**, Intraoperative photograph showing dorsal approach for neuroma excision. **B**, Intraoperative photograph of floor of the foot seen after neuroma excision.

Scar complications were more commonly reported in the plantar group, whereas resection of artery rather than nerve, wound infection and dehiscence, and pain after neurectomy were more commonly reported in the dorsal group[57] (Figure 1).

In revision cases, a plantar approach improves visualization of the residual plantar nerve (Figures 2 and 3). It is important to place the incision between the metatarsal heads to prevent a tender scar on the weight-bearing surface of the foot.

Regardless of the approach, care must be taken to identify and resect all plantar nerve branches, which might tether the interdigital nerve and prevent its proximal retraction off the weight-bearing area of the forefoot. The nerve should be transected proximal to the level of the metatarsal heads. An uncut retained branch that originates proximally may be a conduit for persistent neuritic symptoms. Adjacent web space nerve resection should be avoided whenever possible because it may lead to dense sensory loss in the central toe.[58] A retrospective analysis of 674 consecutive primary neuroma excision surgeries showed that 38.9% of pathology specimens included a digital artery.[59]

Multiple outcome studies after interdigital nerve excision have been done. In one study of 56 patients with 76 interdigital plantar neuralgias, 71% became

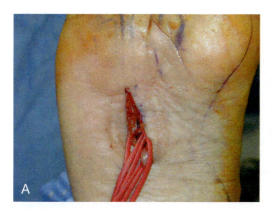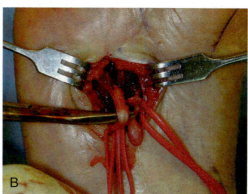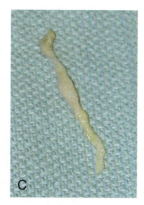

FIGURE 2 **A**, Intraoperative photograph demonstrates vessel loops being placed beneath three nerves that were found in the area immediately deep to the plantar fascia within the adipose tissue between the flexor digitorum longus tendons. **B**, Intraoperative photograph of retraction that enables excellent visualization of these structures. **C**, Photograph of the resected plantar nerve from a patient with suspected recurrent and adjacent neuroma. (Panels A and B reproduced from Title CI, Schon LC: Morton's neuroma. *Orthopaedic Knowledge Online Journal*. American Academy of Orthopaedic Surgeons, 2005; 3[3]. Panel C reproduced from Title CI, Schon LC: Morton neuroma: Primary and secondary neurectomy. *J Am Acad Orthop Surg* 2008;16: 550-557. Copyright 2008, by American Academy of Orthopaedic Surgeons.)

Section 2: Neuromuscular Disease

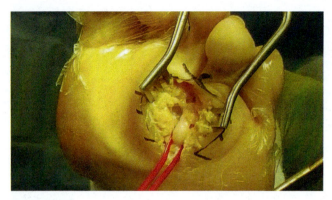

FIGURE 3 Intraoperative photograph showing plantar approach to neuroma excision.

asymptomatic, 9% had substantial improvement, 6% had marginal improvement, and treatment failed in 14%. Still, 65% of the satisfied patients had residual plantar pain and 32% reported normal sensation in the web space.[8] Another study on 66 patients with 5.8 years follow-up reported an 85% satisfaction rate. Approximately 70% of these patients needed some modification in their shoe wear to remain pain free.[32] Another study of 120 patients with an average follow-up of 5.6 years used the Giannini neuroma score to evaluate results. Fifty-one percent had good to excellent results, 10% had fair results, and 40% had poor results. The average VAS score was 2.5. A second web space interdigital plantar neuralgia was a prognostic indicator of poor outcome. It was concluded that long-term outcomes are not as good as previously reported, possibly secondary to residual toe numbness.[47]

A retrospective study compared simple neurectomy (66 patients) with neurectomy with intramuscular implantation (33 patients) with a minimum follow-up of 6 months. This study concluded that both simple neurectomy and neurectomy with intramuscular implantation demonstrated significant improvement in terms of functional outcomes as measured with the Foot Function Index, Short Form 36, and VAS score in patients with interdigital neuroma. It was concluded that although requiring a longer surgical time, neurectomy with intramuscular implantation technique might offer superior pain relief with comparable complications to the simple neurectomy technique.[60]

Recurrent neuromas may occur, and the presenting symptoms are often identical to those of the initial presentation. The symptoms can result from inadequate proximal nerve resection or incomplete resection of tethering plantar nerve branches.[61-63] The bulb neuroma, which forms at the end of the cut nerve, takes approximately 12 months to become large enough to cause pain. Accordingly, patients may present with recurrence of symptoms several months to even years after the index surgery. Usually, patients with persistent or recurrent neuromas have a well-localized area of plantar tenderness. Palpation produces a Tinel sign with electric-like pain. Adjacent metatarsal head tenderness may be caused by the regenerating nerve innervations of the skin over the metatarsal heads. An option for revision surgery is the implantation of the nerve residuum into the intrinsic muscles of the foot, which has been reported to provide pain relief in 80% of patients.[64]

Revision surgery should be undertaken with caution because the results are not as predictable as primary surgery. When evaluating these patients with recurrent symptoms of interdigital plantar neuralgia, the clinician should be suspicious of various causes including inadequate initial resection, formation of a true residual neuroma, misdiagnosis of correct web space, adjacent web space neuroma, and a proximal tarsal tunnel syndrome (TTS) or nerve entrapment resulting from spine pathology.

TARSAL TUNNEL SYNDROME

TTS is an entrapment neuropathy of the tibial nerve or one of its branches as it passes through the tarsal tunnel. Originally described in 1960, the condition became known as TTS in 1962.[65] This syndrome can result from space-occupying lesions or constriction of the posterior tibial nerve. In addition, talocalcaneal coalitions have been described as a risk factor for TTS[66] and venous dilatation in a 2022 study.[67] It has been compared with carpal tunnel syndrome in the hand because of name similarity, but in reality, these two entities have little in common.

Anatomy

At the level of the ankle, the flexor retinaculum or laciniate ligament is composed of the deep and superficial aponeuroses of the leg and creates a fibro-osseous tunnel posterior to the medial malleolus. Contents passing through this tunnel include the posterior tibial tendon, flexor digitorum longus tendon, flexor hallucis longus tendon, the posterior tibial artery, nerve, and vein. The floor of the tunnel is formed by the superior aspect of the calcaneus, the medial wall of the talus, and the distal-medial aspect of the tibia. The proximal and inferior borders of the tunnel are delineated by the inferior and superior margins of the flexor retinaculum. Within this tunnel, the posterior tibial nerve lies between the tendons of the flexor digitorum longus and flexor hallucis longus.

The tibial nerve ends by bifurcating into the MPN and LPN. This usually occurs within the tarsal tunnel (93% to 96%), with the remaining 4% to 7% occurring more proximally. Proximal division is considered a risk factor for TTS because of the increased volume of two nerves entering the canal, causing narrowing of the canal.[68] The

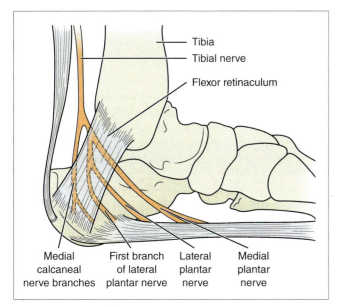

FIGURE 4 Illustration showing the contents of the tarsal tunnel. The flexor retinaculum passes posteriorly over the tarsal tunnel. The medial calcaneal nerve may originate from the tibial nerve proximal to the tarsal tunnel and may have multiple branches. The first branch of the lateral plantar nerve may originate within the tarsal tunnel. The medial plantar nerve frequently provides one or more calcaneal branches.

medial calcaneal nerve usually branches off the tibial nerve. This nerve pierces the flexor retinaculum to provide sensory innervations to the medial and posterior heel (**Figure 4**). Variations include the nerve running superficial to the retinaculum[69] or arising from the LPN.[68]

History and Physical Examination

Patients with TTS typically report burning pain and sometimes paresthesias along the medial and plantar aspects of the foot. Alternatively, radiating, diffuse, or poorly defined pain can be the presenting symptom. Typically, the pain increases with activity and improves with rest. It may also occur at night because of abnormal posture or pressure during sleep. Up to one-third of patients also report pain radiating proximally into the midcalf.[9] Valleix points are seen as tenderness along the course of the nerve.

Precise and careful questioning is required to evaluate other potential sources of nerve pain. Differential diagnoses include rheumatologic conditions leading to chronic tenosynovitis, lumbar spine issues leading to radicular pain, and double-crush syndrome. With double-crush syndrome, proximal compression renders the nerve more susceptible for distal entrapment. Diabetes, vitamin deficiency, and alcoholism also can contribute to double-crush syndrome.

Physical examination may also provide insight into TTS etiology. The patient should be examined in standing position to assess hindfoot alignment. Heel valgus puts the nerve under tension, whereas varus may result in nerve compression. While the patient is seated, the medial aspect of the leg, ankle, and foot is examined for any masses, inflammation, or swelling. Evaluation for the Tinel sign should be performed in the heel both in neutral and heel valgus to assess sensitivity of the tibial nerve. Percussion along the course of the nerve may produce paresthesias. Inversion and eversion of the hindfoot can also influence tarsal canal pressure and affect symptoms.[70] Another provocative maneuver is a dorsiflexion eversion test, which can induce symptoms quickly.[71] Sensory testing to touch and use of a Semmes-Weinstein monofilament may help to isolate terminal branches responsible for creating symptoms. Demonstration of plantar numbness and intrinsic motor weakness can be difficult, but loss of small toe abduction compared with the opposite, normal foot is more easily measurable and indicates loss of innervation of the abductor digiti quinti muscle.

Diagnostic Studies

Routine radiographs of the foot and ankle are obtained to rule out bony abnormalities, such as malunited fractures or bone spurs. If a space-occupying lesion is suspected, MRI can be performed.

In one study of 35 feet in which TTS is suspected, MRI showed abnormality in 85%.[72] MRI studies have shown changes in the volume of the tarsal tunnel in inversion and eversion thereby increasing pressure on the nerve.[73] Ultrasonography is operator dependent but can be used as an adjunct to diagnosis of TTS. Electrodiagnostic studies are performed in most patients in whom TTS is suspected, but literature reports differ as to which test is more reliable. Electrodiagnostic studies have been reported as 90% accurate in identifying tarsal tunnel entrapment.[74] These studies do play an important role in helping to differentiate TTS from radiculopathy or peripheral neuropathy. An evaluation of use of nerve conduction velocity (NCV) studies and electromyography at the ankle concluded that NCV may be useful, but the consensus was that there are no reliable studies available to evaluate reliability and reproducibility of electrodiagnostic studies in TTS.[75]

Nonsurgical Treatment

In the absence of a space-occupying lesion, nonsurgical treatment is indicated and includes NSAIDs, oral vitamin B, and tricyclic antidepressants. Temporary immobilization in a cast, walking boot, or an orthotic device to correct foot alignment may benefit some patients. In cases of tenosynovitis of the flexor digitorum longus tendon, a steroid injection may be indicated. However, some authors caution against the use of injections because of possible tendon rupture and intravascular injection,[76] although intravascular injections can be minimized by injecting under ultrasound guidance. Modalities such as heat, cold, and vibration are not recommended because they may irritate the sensitive nerves.[77] Instead, physical therapy may incorporate topical anti-inflammatory agents, nerve reliever socks, and iontophoresis.

Surgical Treatment

For good surgical results, correct patient selection is important. A positive physical examination with appropriate studies such as NCV, electromyography, or MRI is helpful in making the decision for surgical intervention.

Surgical intervention has been advocated when nonsurgical modalities fail. Space-occupying lesions in TTS, including lipoma, ganglion, and varicose veins, should be removed to reduce pressure on the nerve. If there is an underlying cause of TTS such as hindfoot instability, talocalcaneal coalition, or calcaneal malunion with bone spurs, these need to be addressed during surgical treatment.

Four separate medial ankle tunnels have been described.[78] Careful anatomic analysis demonstrates that the tarsal tunnel is not the equivalent of the carpal tunnel, rather, it is more closely the equivalent of the forearm. Hence, the flexor retinaculum is equivalent to distal forearm fascia. The MPN tunnel, lateral plantar tunnel, and the calcaneal tunnel have been described as three additional tunnels within the tarsal tunnel. Cadaver and surgical studies support pressure changes in the medial, lateral, and tarsal tunnels with different ankle and subtalar positions.[79,80] Pronation and plantar flexion significantly increase pressures within the medial and lateral tunnels leading to nerve compression. Surgical release of each tunnel including excision of the septum between medial and lateral tunnels significantly reduces pressure within the tarsal tunnel.

A large study of 87 legs that underwent neurolysis of the tibial nerve within the tarsal tunnel, which included release of the medial plantar tunnel, lateral plantar tunnel, and calcaneal tunnel, reported 82% excellent results at mean follow-up of 3.6 years.[81]

Endoscopic tarsal tunnel release has been described. A report with short-term follow-up on a small number of patients has shown good results.[82]

More recently, ultrasound-guided tarsal tunnel release has been reported as an alternative to open surgery with potentially decrease wound complications, infection, and fibrosis.[55,83,84] The technique has been shown in a 2021 study decrease tarsal tunnel in addition to medial and lateral plantar tunnels.[85] A 2020 retrospective 18-month follow-up study reported 77% of patients had excellent results and 14% with good results. The 10% of patients with poor results were those who had the longest course of symptoms. Complications included superficial hematoma

and decreased sensation in the medial calcaneal branch. Both conditions resolved spontaneously over time.[86]

Clinical Outcomes

Surgical treatment is generally successful when a space-occupying lesion is identified in the tarsal tunnel.[87,88] A short-term outcome study was performed on a series of patients who underwent tarsal tunnel release for benign space-occupying lesions. Only 13 of 20 patients were available for follow-up. The average age of the patients was 51.3 years, with average duration of symptoms of 16.5 months. The most common lesion identified was ganglion cyst in 10 patients, but other identified lesions included synovial chondromatosis, schwannoma, and tarsal coalition. VAS and American Orthopaedic Foot and Ankle Society scores were measured preoperatively and postoperatively. Seven patients were satisfied, three had fair results, and three were dissatisfied.[89]

In the absence of space-occupying lesions, tunnel decompression may provide relief of symptoms in up to 75% of patients.[9] A 2022 study reported 93% improvement in patients with a space-occupying lesion versus only 26.7% improvement in idiopathic TTS cases.[67]

Timing of surgery may also be important. Chronic compression can lead to intraneural fibrosis resulting in muscle wasting and poorer outcomes after surgery.[90] Furthermore, improved American Orthopaedic Foot and Ankle Society scores were reported at 12 months after decompression if it was performed less than 1 year from the onset of symptoms.[91]

In a prospective evaluation of 46 patients (56 feet) who underwent nonsurgical and surgical treatment of TTS, pain intensity was documented before and after treatment with the Wong-Baker FACES Pain Rating Scale applied to anatomic regions of the plantar aspect of the foot. The results of the study showed that pretreatment motor nerve conduction latency was substantially greater in patients who needed surgical treatment than those receiving nonsurgical treatment. The study concluded that anatomic pain intensity rating models may be useful in the pretreatment and follow-up evaluation of TTS. Predictors of failed nonsurgical treatment included longer motor nerve conduction latency (7.4 m/s or greater) and greater predominance of foot comorbidities.[92]

Other independent predictors of favorable outcomes after decompression include a positive Tinel sign and space-occupying lesion. Sensory deficit in the absence of a Tinel sign is a negative predictor.[93,94] In addition, evidence of neuropathy on ultrasonography has been found to be associated with decreased outcomes after surgery. In the same study, in patients with possible venous dilatation as an etiology of TTS, patients with constant compression had better outcomes compared with those with intermittent compression.[67]

A retrospective review of 74 primary and 5 revision surgeries was done with medium-term outcomes and complications. The study concluded that tarsal tunnel release demonstrated significant improvement of functional outcomes and pain relief in medium-term follow-up as measured with Short Form 36, Foot Function Index, and VAS. Revision surgery demonstrated less favorable outcomes, whereas preoperative Tinel test and duration of symptoms more than 12 months did not affect outcome. Overall the procedure was effective and feasible for TTS with minor complications.[95]

Recurrence and Revision

Some patients have had recurrences even up to 5 years after index surgery, and a small number have reported an increase in symptoms after the release. Generally, outcomes for revision surgeries are worse than for primary procedures. The most common causes of failure of surgical release are inadequate release because of lack of understanding of the anatomy, failure to properly execute the release, bleeding with scarring, damage to the nerve or its branches during release, persistent hypersensitivity of the nerve, and initial intrinsic damage to the nerve. Each cause of failure should be evaluated and treated accordingly.[96] The concept of barrier wrapping of nerves to prevent adhesions to surrounding tissue has also been recommended. Autogenous vein grafts, free fat grafts, and collagen tubes have been used. If the nerve has intrinsic damage, sural nerve grafts and collagen conduits or wandering vein conduits have been suggested. Finally, complex regional pain syndrome (CRPS) type 2 should be considered for intractable pain with recurring or persistent symptoms.

MPN ENTRAPMENT

MPN entrapment, or jogger's foot, was first described in 1978.[97] The condition is thought to be secondary to local entrapment of the MPN at the fibromuscular tunnel formed by the abductor hallucis muscle and its border with the navicular tuberosity. It is often associated with a valgus foot deformity and in long-distance running. It is characterized by neuritic pain at the medial arch radiating into the toes along the distribution of the MPN. Rarely, a crush injury or transection of the nerve may occur, leading to severe symptoms.

Anatomy

The MPN typically branches from the tibial nerve under the abductor hallucis muscle and travels with the medial plantar artery and veins. It innervates the abductor hallucis and terminates under the plantar fascia into the intermetatarsal nerves to the first and second, second and third, and third and fourth intermetatarsal spaces.

It also provides motor branches to the intrinsic muscles of the foot. In the longitudinal arch, the nerve lies medial and adjacent to the flexor digitorum and flexor hallucis longus tendons close to the knot of Henry.

Etiology

MPN entrapment is seen in joggers with a history of repetitive impact and trauma during running, which leads to inflammation of the nerve. This clinical presentation is more common in planovalgus feet, whereby more pressure and stretch is placed on the nerve. An excessively high-arch insert may also put pressure on this nerve. MPN entrapment has also been seen in ballet dancers.

Clinical Symptoms and Diagnosis

A high index of suspicion and awareness is required for diagnosing MPN entrapment. In many cases, symptoms may be present for more than 1 year before diagnosis. The runner often describes chronic pain on the inside of the middle portion of the foot. In addition, pain, aching, or a burning sensation over the arch of the foot is described and a giving-away sensation in the foot may occur while running. Rarely, the pain may radiate proximally into the ankle.

A detailed foot examination should be performed, specifically looking for hindfoot valgus. Shoes and orthotics should be examined. A stress test can be done by asking the patient to go for a run before the clinical examination. With MPN entrapment, tenderness is noted posterior to the navicular bone on the medial surface of the arch. A Tinel sign may be elicited to indicate the hypersensitive nerve. Local injection of lidocaine with subsequent relief of symptoms can also be a diagnostic tool.

Treatment

Initial treatment involves rest and shoe modifications including inserts. Oral anti-inflammatory agents and a trial of steroid injection may be considered. If nonsurgical measures fail, then surgical decompression is indicated. Decompression of the MPN is done by releasing the fascia over the abductor hallucis and around the knot of Henry. In addition, part of the naviculocalcaneal ligament is released to provide more space for the MPN. Most runners with MPN entrapment improve without surgical treatment. Because of the rarity of this condition, large-scale reporting in the literature is not seen.

LPN ENTRAPMENT

Entrapment of the first branch of the LPN (Baxter nerve) can present as plantar heel pain. Because this nerve is in close vicinity to the inflammation associated with plantar fasciitis, it is thought that some degree

Section 2: Neuromuscular Disease

of nerve entrapment may be a contributing factor in up to 20% of patients with chronic heel pain. Hence, an accurate diagnosis is difficult because of overlap of symptoms.

Anatomy

The first branch of the LPN is located posteriorly just under the upper edge of the abductor hallucis. Rarely, it may branch directly from the lateral portion of the main tibial nerve. The first branch travels under the abductor hallucis and its deep fascia and over the medial fascia of the quadratus plantae. It then passes over the quadratus fascia and under the medial edge of the plantar fascia, then continues transversely across the heel under the flexor digitorum brevis muscle and sends a sensory branch to the central heel. It then terminates in the muscle of abductor digiti quinti.

Etiology

Entrapment of the first branch occurs between the abductor hallucis and quadratus plantae muscle. Direct heel trauma and calcaneal fractures can also lead to symptoms. Usually, it is a traction neuritis of the LPN and its first branch. Other causes of LPN entrapment include hypertrophy of the abductor hallucis or quadratus plantae, the presence of accessory muscles or bursae, and phlebitis in the calcaneal venous plexus. In addition, hypermobile flatfeet can also put traction on the nerve causing pain.

Clinical Symptoms

This condition most commonly occurs in the age group of 19 to 67 years (average age: 43 years).[98] Patients present with chronic heel pain that is increased while walking or running. Pain can radiate proximally to the medial ankle or to the lateral aspect of the foot. It is worse when the patient takes their first step in the morning and may not remit with continued walking or rest.

Diagnosis

Classically, there is distinct tenderness at the origin of the abductor hallucis muscle that can radiate both proximally and distally with paresthesias. Pain often exacerbates with hyperpronation or Phalen maneuver (forced inversion and plantar flexion). In advanced cases, patients may lose the ability to abduct the fifth toe when compared with the opposite foot. Potential proximal nerve lesions should be excluded by palpating the nerve proximally. It is equally important to exclude other sources of heel pain. Injury or entrapment of the superficial calcaneal sensory nerve branches may also produce similar symptoms.

Treatment

Nonsurgical treatment includes orthoses to limit foot pronation and local corticosteroid injection. A custom total-contact orthosis with a posteromedial nerve relief channel may be helpful.[99] The channel is placed in the medial wall of the heel component and up to the midline in the plantar area corresponding with the anatomy of the LPN and its first branch. Surgical treatment should be considered if nonsurgical treatment fails. The nerve is typically decompressed by releasing the deep fascia beneath the abductor hallucis and a portion of the plantar fascia.

DEEP PERONEAL NERVE ENTRAPMENT (ANTERIOR TTS)

This entity was first described in 1960 and later referred to as anterior TTS in 1968.[100] It is a rare condition, with patients reporting a burning sensation across the dorsum of the foot with paresthesia in the first web space. There may be wasting and weakness of the extensor digitorum brevis muscle.

Anatomy

The deep peroneal nerve in the proximal one-third of the leg is a mixed motor and sensory nerve located between tibialis anterior and extensor digitorum longus. It travels with the anterior tibial artery and descends into the leg between the extensor digitorum and hallucis longus 5 cm proximal to the ankle joint. At approximately 1 cm above the ankle joint, the nerve branches to form a mixed branch that courses laterally to innervate extensor digitorum brevis and provide sensation to the lateral tarsal joints. The other branch is sensory only and runs distally with the dorsalis pedis artery between the extensor hallucis longus and brevis tendons to innervate the skin in the first web space.

The extensor retinaculum has a superior band located 5 cm above the ankle joint. The inferior Y-shaped band splits into two bands: the superomedial and inferomedial. The anterior tarsal tunnel is a fibro-osseous canal located just distal to the inferior medial band. The canal is in a 1.5-cm confined space formed superficially by the inferior extensor retinaculum, deep by the capsule of the talonavicular joint, laterally by the lateral malleolus, and medially by the medial malleolus. It contains the dorsalis pedis artery and vein, deep peroneal nerve, tendons of extensor hallucis longus, extensor digitorum longus, tibialis anterior, and peroneus tertius.

Etiology and Physical Examination

There are several potential sites of deep peroneal nerve entrapment that result in slightly different clinical presentations. The causes are varied and can be due to intrinsic or extrinsic mechanisms. Causes of intrinsic compression include space-occupying lesions, osteophytes, bony fragments, hypertrophic muscle bellies, and peripheral edema. Extrinsic compression can be associated with tight shoe laces and trauma, including single or repetitive events such as multiple ankle sprains.

A rare and very proximal entrapment can occur under the superior extensor retinaculum and involves the motor branch to the extensor digitorum brevis muscle. Referred pain to the sinus tarsi or atrophy and weakness of short toe extensors may develop. The most common site of entrapment occurs at the inferior edge of the extensor retinaculum. This results in sensory deficit only, as the motor portion of the nerve has already branched out. These patients have deep, aching pain in the dorsal midfoot along with tingling, numbness, and burning in the area between the first and second toes. The pain is worse with activity and better with rest. Patients may be awakened at night by increased nerve pressure as the foot goes into plantar flexion. Tight-fitting or high lace-up shoes worsen the pain, which improves after removal of those shoes. Hypertrophy of the extensor digitorum brevis muscle may lead to more distal and sensory symptoms only.

Clinical examination should begin with palpation of the deep peroneal nerve along its entire course. The proximal course of the nerve near the fibular neck is examined for tenderness, along with the Tinel sign, and on percussion of the nerve. Forceful plantar flexion and inversion of the ankle puts the nerve under stretch and reduces available space in the anterior tarsal tunnel compressing the nerve against its floor. This maneuver may clinically produce the symptoms of nerve compression.[101]

Diagnosis

Plain radiographs may play an important role. A lateral foot and ankle radiograph may reveal osteophytes, particularly near the talonavicular joint, and old fractures with bone fragments. CT could be used for detailed bony anatomy of the tarsal canal, whereas MRI is important if a mass is suspected of causing compression. Electrodiagnostic studies may show a proximal source of nerve compression such as lumbar radiculopathy. It also determines if there is involvement of the extensor digitorum brevis muscle, which is suggestive of a lesion proximal to the inferior retinaculum. The results should be correlated with clinical findings because abnormal fasciculations have been found in up to 76% of normal subjects and decreased motor recruitment in 38% of normal adults.[102] Electrodiagnostic data are technically difficult to obtain, and anatomic variations further complicate the interpretation.

Treatment

Nonsurgical treatment begins with identification of the source of compression. Shoe wear accommodations may decrease the pressure over the nerve. Orthotics may improve biomechanical alignment and help reduce symptoms.[100] Physical therapy is helpful in patients with ankle instability. NSAIDs and other anti-inflammatory agents can also be used. Local injection of anesthetic and corticosteroid is a useful technique for evaluating and treating many patients. Resolution of pain and paresthesias may be obtained with serial injections into the anterior tarsal tunnel.[100]

When nonsurgical treatment fails, surgery should be considered. A slightly curved S-shaped incision is made over the dorsum of the foot, starting at the bases of the first and second metatarsals and extending proximally to the ankle joint. Care is taken to preserve branches of the SPN. The extensor retinaculum is released enough to free up the deep peroneal nerve. Any osteophytes or other structures present on the dorsal edge of the talonavicular joint are removed. A hypertrophied extensor hallucis brevis may be resected. Simple closure and soft dressings are applied. Noncompressive shoe wear in the postoperative period is encouraged before gradual resumption of activity over 4 to 6 weeks.

SUPERFICIAL PERONEAL NERVE

Entrapment of the SPN is a relatively uncommon finding and is referred as mononeuralgia of the peroneal nerve. In a study of 480 patients with chronic leg pain, only 3.5% had pain attributable to SPN entrapment.[103]

Anatomy

The SPN branches off the common peroneal nerve (CPN) laterally at the level of the neck of fibula. It supplies motor innervations to the lateral compartment of the leg including peroneus longus and brevis. It then continues as a sensory nerve. Proximally, it passes deep to the peroneus longus, traveling between this muscle and the fibula in the lateral compartment. It then becomes superficial as it courses distally between the peroneus longus and brevis piercing the deep fascia approximately 10 to 12 cm proximal to the tip of lateral malleolus as it leaves the lateral compartment. Significant variation in the course of this nerve has been reported. In one anatomic study, the SPN was identified in the lateral compartment immediately adjacent to the fascial septum in 72% of specimens, with a branch in the anterior and lateral compartment in 5% of specimens and located in the anterior compartment only in 23%. The clinical implication of this study is that the surgeon must be aware that the SPN may be located in the lateral compartment and may also exhibit branches in both the anterior and lateral compartment.[104] Approximately 6 cm proximal to the lateral malleolus the nerve divides into the intermediate dorsal cutaneous nerve (IDCN) and the medial dorsal cutaneous nerve (MDCN). Variations have also been described in the sensory branches of SPN. In one cadaver dissection study, three distinct branching patterns were identified. In type I (63.3%), the SPN penetrated the crural fascia 8.1 ± 1.78 cm proximal to the intermalleolar line and then divided into the IDCN and MDCN (classic type). In type II (26.7%), the IDCN and MDCN arose independently from the SPN. In type III (10%), the SPN penetrated the crural fascia 10.1 ± 7 cm proximal to the intermalleolar line as a single branch. This single branch had a course similar to the MDCN.[105]

Etiology

The most common site of entrapment is usually 8 to 12 cm proximal to the tip of the fibula where the nerve exits from the deep fascia of the lateral compartment. The sharp fascial edge entraps the nerve as it pierces through the lateral fascia. This impingement could also be part of chronic exertional compartment syndrome of the leg. The classically described SPN injury occurs in the setting of repeated ankle inversion sprains resulting in traction injury to the nerve. This injury has also been described in dancers and other athletes with ankle instability and lateral ligament deficiency. These individuals are also at increased risk secondary to their often hypertrophied peroneal musculature that can result in entrapment of the nerve in its short fibrous tunnel as it pierces the fascia.[106] Iatrogenic injuries can occur as a consequence of procedures approaching the ankle anteriorly. Ankle arthroscopy is a common foot and ankle surgical procedure in which these injuries have been reported. In one study of 294 cases reporting on complications of ankle arthroscopy using contemporary noninvasive distraction technique, 6 cases (2%) had neurologic complications related to the anterolateral portal. This study suggested an injury to the IDCN branch of the SPN.[107]

One of the most common causes of SPN injury is direct trauma. Compartment fasciotomy with resultant shifting of the peroneal tunnel can result in stretching and impingement of the nerve. Other causes include ganglion, fibular fracture, syndesmotic sprains, and chemotherapy causing neuropathy and edema.

Incidence and Clinical Presentation

SPN entrapment was reported in 17 of 480 patients (3.5%) with chronic leg pain.[103] It occurs equally in men and women, usually between ages of 28 to 36 years. It is frequent in runners but has also been reported in hockey, soccer, and racquetball players.[9]

Clinical presentation can be variable. Classically, pain is located over the middle to distal third of the leg, often intense over the anterior aspect with radiation to the dorsal aspect of the foot. Patients also describe numbness or tingling from the lateral side of the ankle with radiation and extending into the sinus tarsi or dorsum of the foot. Night pain and rest pain are rare symptoms usually aggravated with increased activity. Typically, clinical examination of the foot reveals no specific motor weakness, and approximately two-thirds of patients will have no sensory loss in the foot.

Diagnosis

Low back pathology and CPN impingement should be evaluated to rule out a proximal etiology for the symptoms. SPN irritability is identified by percussion along the course of the nerve 8 to 12 cm above the distal tip of the fibula. Three provocative maneuvers designed to place the nerve on stretch can be used to assist in the diagnosis. First, the foot is palpated and pressure is applied over the site of entrapment while the patient actively dorsiflexes and everts the foot against resistance. In the second maneuver, the patient's foot is passively plantarflexed and the ankle inverted without pressure on the nerve. In the third maneuver, the examiner percusses the foot while passively maintaining stretch with the ankle inverted. A positive result is pain/paresthesia in two out of the three maneuvers.[108] A fourth toe flexion sign has also been described accentuating the subcutaneous course of the SPN. The ankle is held in plantar flexion and then further flexion of the fourth toe accentuates the subcutaneous course of the cutaneous branches of SPN. This was confirmed on local infiltration of the nerve with 1% lidocaine and then mapping the area of hypoesthesia on the dorsum of the foot.[109]

Imaging/Tests

Standard weight-bearing radiographs of the ankle are obtained to rule out bony impingement by fibular fracture callus, exostoses, or osteochondromas. CT and MRI are used only if specifically indicated. NCV studies are used as adjuncts for diagnosis. One study found an insignificant decrease in conduction velocity from 49 m/s in unaffected nerves to 28 m/s on average on the affected side.[103] It is important to remember that normal NCV studies do not rule out SPN entrapment and thus must be used only as a tool to assist in diagnosis.

Nonsurgical Treatment

Localized injection of anesthetic at the site of maximal tenderness can serve as both a diagnostic and therapeutic intervention. SPN impingement is thought to respond less well to nonsurgical treatment compared with impingement of the DPN. Lateral shoe wedges may help reduce varus stress on the ankle and the nerve. Use of NSAIDs, neuropathic drugs such as gabapentin and serotonin reuptake inhibitors, adequate rest, and physical therapy for ankle strengthening may also be helpful.

Surgical Treatment

After nonsurgical treatment has failed, surgical intervention may be indicated. If ankle instability coexists, then lateral ligament reconstruction should be done. The SPN is released from the surrounding fascia at the point where it exits the crural fascia. Before surgery, the site of nerve compression is identified and marked. The SPN is decompressed at its entrance into the peroneal fibrous tunnel, which varies from 3 to 11 cm in length. If exertional compartment syndrome coexists, the fascia of the lateral compartment should be released completely. Complete opening of the peroneal tunnel close to the anterior intermuscular septum is advocated. In one study, 80% of patients reported relief of symptoms with this approach.[103] Other studies support more limited decompression centered 5 to 8 cm proximal to the lateral malleolus.[110] Specific recommendations for limited release depend on clinical symptoms, sites of compression, and the presence or absence of exertional compartment syndrome. More research is needed for long-term outcomes after various types of release or decompression are performed.

SURAL NERVE

Entrapment of the sural nerve is rare but has been extensively studied in humans because of its status as a purely sensory nerve. This nerve is frequently used as a nerve graft.

Anatomy

The sural nerve is a pure sensory nerve that is derived from the S1 and S2 nerve roots. A cadaver study and literature review detail the various branches and the names given to them.[111] The sural nerve anatomy adheres to basic principles. It is typically made up of two components merging: a medial component from the tibial nerve (medial sural cutaneous nerve or tibial nerve component) and a lateral component from the lateral sural cutaneous nerve (LSCN or CPN component). However, it may consist of just a single component, either tibial or CPN. In 73% of patients studied, tibial and peroneal nerve components merge to form the sural nerve (Pattern I). The peroneal communicating branch (PCB) may branch off the LSCN (pattern Ia) or directly originate from the CPN (pattern Ib).

In 24%, medial sural cutaneous nerve alone represented the sural nerve, whereas LSCN coursed independently (pattern II) or the LSCN was absent (pattern III).

In 3%, the LSCN represented the sural nerve, whereas medial sural cutaneous nerve terminated distally in the calf (pattern IV) or is absent (pattern V).

A PCB was present in 63% with three types of origin—In type A: 74% PCB branches off LSCN; in type B: 16% PCB and LSCN originate as a common trunk from CPN; and in type C: 10% PCB and LSCN originate independently from CPN, with the PCB always medial and proximal to LSCN.

In general, the sural nerve begins distal to the popliteus fossa traveling between the two heads of the gastrocnemius muscle and pierces the deep fascia in the middle third of the posterior surface of the leg. At this point, it is typically joined by the PCB. Approximately 10 cm from the calcaneus, the sural nerve passes over the lateral edge of the Achilles tendon and continues distally posterior and then inferior to the lateral malleolus. It then passes plantar to the lateral malleolus and posterior to the peroneal tendons, curving anteriorly traveling on the lateral border of the foot where it becomes the lateral dorsal cutaneous nerve. It then divides at the base of the fifth metatarsal to form dorsal and plantar branches. The dorsal branch gives rise to the dorsal digital nerve to the lateral side of the fifth toe and may communicate with other digital branches of the fourth and fifth toe. The plantar branch provides sensibility along the lateral border distally and may join distal branches of LPN. The sural nerve supplies sensation to the posterior lateral lower leg and ankle, the lateral heel and foot, and the fifth toe with or without the fourth toe.

Etiology

Entrapment of the sural nerve in trauma situations can result from direct traumatic contusions or from fractures of the calcaneus, fifth metatarsal, posterolateral process of the talus, or os peroneum. Traction injury can occur with ankle sprains. Rarely, posterolateral or hindfoot arthroscopy portals are associated with injury to the nerve.

Clinical Presentation

The clinical findings of sural nerve entrapment are similar to those encountered with entrapment at other sites in the foot. Patients often report chronic burning, numbness, or aching along the posterolateral aspect of the leg, which frequently becomes worse at night and with physical exertion. Often, there is mild to moderate tenderness to palpation posterior and lateral to the myotendinous junction of the Achilles tendon. This represents the location of the fibrous arcade and the most common site of sural nerve entrapment. Some patients may report recurrent ankle sprains or instability. Percussion may elicit a Tinel sign along the course of the nerve. Pain can be poorly localized but a focal area of tenderness is occasionally noted along the course of the nerve.[9] Provocative maneuvers such as plantar flexion of the foot and inversion may reproduce symptoms.

A history of direct injury, Achilles tendon surgery, ankle arthroscopy, or calcaneal fracture surgery suggests that the sural nerve could be involved. Concerns about possible referral pain caused by S1 nerve root radiculopathy must be assessed. Reflex and motor function in the leg should be normal if only the sural nerve is involved.

Diagnostic Studies

The diagnosis is primarily based on history, symptoms, and physical examination. Plain radiographs help rule out fractures, callus, subtalar arthritis, and other abnormalities. Stress views of the ankle should be obtained if underlying ankle instability is suspected. Electrodiagnostic and NCV studies may be useful but have limited benefit because of difficulty in interpretation of the study and due to anatomic variations in the nerve. MRI may be helpful to identify space-occupying lesions compressing the nerve. CT can be used if bony compression of the nerve is suspected. Diagnostic injection of local lidocaine in specific areas may assist in isolating the origin of symptoms.

Treatment

Nonsurgical treatment can be tried if ankle instability is the underlying cause. An ankle brace for support and physical therapy to improve strength and proprioception may help relieve some of the symptoms. Treatment of underlying conditions such as edema may alleviate symptoms. Topical medication with capsaicin or lidocaine patches can also be helpful along with oral tricyclic antidepressants.

If nonsurgical treatment has failed and there is well-localized entrapment, then surgery should be considered. Nerve compression due to bony fragments, callus, or ganglion can be managed with surgical excision. A thorough nerve decompression should be done with minimal nerve handling. Other procedures such as peroneal tendon stabilization, lateral ligament repair, and lateral calcaneal wall decompression should be done as indicated. Nerve injury resulting in neuromas should either be resected or transposed to an area of less vulnerable injury.

MEDIAL PLANTAR PROPER DIGITAL NERVE SYNDROME

Medial plantar proper digital nerve (MPPDN) syndrome was first described in 1971 as a traumatic perineural fibrosis of the MPPDN.[112] This injury occurs either where the nerve crosses the first MTP joint or on the medial aspect of the great toe. Repetitive trauma is seen as a cause in sports involving repetitive pivoting, impact, and motion such as running, basketball, skiing, and ballet. Chronic compression is caused by inadequate or tight shoe wear.

Anatomy

The MPPDN arises from the MPN, which is the medial branch of the posterior tibial nerve. The MPPDN bifurcates into two terminal branches at the base of the first metatarsal bone: the medial branch, which forms the first common digital nerve, and the lateral branch, which forms the second and third common digital nerves. As the MPPDN courses distally through the subcutaneous tissue, it supplies sensation to the skin on the medial plantar aspect of the first MTP joint, hallux, and the tip of the toe.

Clinical Presentation

Typically, the patient reports pain and paresthesia on the medial side of the big toe when walking and wearing tight footwear. There can be an area of local sensory disturbance on the toe or an enlarged cord-like nerve immediately proximal to the interphalangeal joint, which is painful to touch. Hypoesthesia or hyperesthesia can be present with a positive Tinel sign in some cases. Forefoot valgus or a plantarflexed first ray can be a contributing factor. Abnormal pronation of the great toe leads to increased shearing forces between soft tissue and bone leading to the symptoms.

Diagnosis

A thorough history and clinical examination is important in diagnosing MPPDN compression. A new method to perform MPPDN NCV studies has been described.[113] This technique records the sensory nerve action potential of the MPPDN. It was concluded that antidromic stimulation of the MPPDN at a distance of 8 to 10 cm from the medial side of the first metatarsal head of the great toe yields reliable sensory nerve action potential responses. This type of NCV study is done to evaluate impulse along sensory nerve fibers. It is also useful in localizing a nerve lesion in relation to dorsal root ganglion. The dorsal root ganglion is located in the neural foramen and contains the sensory cell body. Lesions proximal to it (root, spinal cord) preserve the sensory nerve action potential despite clinical sensory abnormalities. This is because axonal transport from the cell body to the axon continues to remain intact. Sensory nerve action potentials are typically considered more sensitive than compound motor action potential in the detection of an incomplete peripheral nerve injury.

Treatment

Initial treatment should be nonsurgical with footwear modification, protective or accommodative padding, and orthotics. Local corticosteroid injection can be helpful, but because the site is very superficial, subcutaneous atrophy and increased symptoms can occur. Surgical treatment may involve surgical neurolysis and transposition of the nerve away from the sesamoid or shaving a portion of the sesamoid to assist in decompressing the nerve.

COMPLEX REGIONAL PAIN SYNDROME

CRPS is a neuropathic pain disorder with significant autonomic features. It is one of the most difficult and challenging conditions both for the physician and the patient. It can lead to significant disability with chronicity and relapses. In 1864, a civil war surgeon used the term causalgia to describe the condition. Since then, it has been known by different names including Sudeck dystrophy, CRPS, posttraumatic dystrophy, painful osteoporosis, and sympathalgia. In an attempt to reduce confusion over naming the condition, the International Association for the Study of Pain prefers the phrase complex regional pain syndrome. The word complex describes the various clinical presentations and regional describes the distribution of different symptoms and findings.

Early diagnosis and treatment is required to prevent long-standing or permanent disability. Very few types of treatments have proven effective, in part, because of the historically poor understanding of the mechanisms underlying the disorder. Research conducted largely in the past 10 years has substantially increased knowledge regarding its pathophysiologic mechanisms, indicating that they are multifactorial. Both the peripheral and central nervous system mechanisms are involved. Relative contributions of the mechanisms underlying CRPS may differ across patients and even an individual patient over time, particularly in the transition from warm or acute CRPS to cold or chronic CRPS.

CRPS typically develops after acute tissue trauma. It is an exaggerated response with classic neuropathic pain characteristics including intense burning pain, hyperalgesia, and allodynia. It is also associated with autonomic changes including altered sweating, and skin color and skin temperature changes. Trophic changes in the skin, hair, and nails are seen. Altered function including loss of strength, decreased active range of motion, and tremor may also occur. If central nervous mechanisms are affected because of repeated stimulus, then neuronal pathways undergo plastic modification and acute pain is converted to chronic pain.

Classification

The International Association for the Study of Pain classification system divides CRPS into two types. The clinical presentation is similar in both with two exceptions: type I may have an orthostatic component that worsens with pain with limb dependency, and type II is associated with nerve injury.

Complex Regional Pain Syndrome Type I

1. After the inciting event, sensory, motor, and autonomic responses occur throughout the extremity.
2. Spontaneous pain, allodynia (perception of pain from a nonpainful stimulus), or hyperalgesia (an exaggerated sense of pain) occur throughout the entire extremity and are not limited to the territory of a single peripheral nerve.
3. Sudomotor activity (abnormal skin blood flow) leads to extremity swelling, vasodilation, and skin warming in the area of pain.
4. There are no other coexisting conditions accounting for these changes.

Complex Regional Pain Syndrome Type II

1. A peripheral nerve injury is present and is often the trigger.
2. The sensory, motor, and autonomic changes may or may not be limited in the specific distribution of the peripheral nerve.
3. Motor changes, including deficits, are caused by direct injury to motor axons.
4. Swelling and trophic changes are discrete.

Epidemiology

CRPS can affect all ages, but diagnosis in the pediatric population is often delayed in comparison with that in adults. In one population-based study, the incidence was found to be 5.46 per 100,000 person-years. Female to male ratio was 4:1, with median age of 46 years at onset. The upper limb was affected twice as commonly as the lower limb. In almost 46% of cases, fracture was the trigger event.[114] At least, 50,000 new cases of CRPS type I occur annually in the United States alone.[115] Occurrence is strongly associated with cigarette smoking.

Pathophysiology

The factors leading to CRPS are multifactorial. Although pathogenesis remains unclear, various hypotheses have been suggested. It has now been accepted that different mechanisms are involved simultaneously. CRPS is not only sympathetically mediated but is also a disease of the central nervous system.[116] Various mechanisms include central and peripheral sensitization, impaired sympathetic function, inflammatory factors, genetic factors, brain plasticity, and psychological factors.[117]

A report found an association between psychological factors and developing CRPS in patients with ankle fractures. A total of 163,529 patients were identified who sustained an ankle fracture, and CRPS was identified in 10,127 of these (6.2%). Patients with psychological disorders, such as delirium (OR, 5.60, $P < 0.001$), bipolar disorder (OR, 5.64, $P < 0.001$), and anxiety disorder (OR, 5.08, $P < 0.001$), were five times more likely to have CRPS after sustaining an ankle fracture. Surgical management did not increase this risk.[118]

History and Clinical Examination

The patient may recall specific trauma, but in other cases with no history of trauma the patient may be viewed with suspicion as they report continuing pain. The typical features of spontaneous pain, hyperalgesia, allodynia, and abnormal vasomotor and motor activity may remain beyond the normal time of expected healing. These symptoms may worsen and psychological changes may occur during the course of developing CRPS.

The patient may guard and protect the extremity with overzealous care and attention. They may adopt a protective posture, and in some cases, the patient may not allow anyone to touch or examine the affected extremity.

Skin changes will vary from dry, warm, and erythematous to cold, blue, and mottled. The skin temperature difference between both extremities usually exceeds 1°C. Motor dysfunction includes tremors, dystonia, and spasms with loss of strength and endurance. Muscle wasting and joint contractures may be seen at later stages. Exaggerated tendon reflexes may also be present. In addition, there may be trophic changes in the skin with loss of subcutaneous fat, and nails may become hypertrophic.

Diagnosis

CRPS cannot be proven by any diagnostic test and is essentially a clinical diagnosis. Differential diagnostic tools may help eliminate other possible causes. Infection and other systemic conditions can be evaluated with complete blood count, C-reactive protein, erythrocyte sedimentation rate, antinuclear antibodies, serum calcium and alkaline phosphatase levels, and thyroid function tests.

Plain radiographs of the foot, ankle, and lower extremity typically show spotty osteoporotic changes after 4 to 8 weeks.[119] Disuse osteopenia develops secondary to decreased use and mobility of the affected extremity. Other tests that may be helpful include sweat test, thermography, and electromyography. Diagnostic sympathetic blocks with local anesthetics may help if vasomotor or sudomotor dysfunction is present. A block is considered successful if there is more than 50% pain reduction.

A three-phase bone scan with technetium Tc 99m is used to confirm CRPS. It is usually helpful in early stages where increased uptake in the delayed phase 3 is seen.

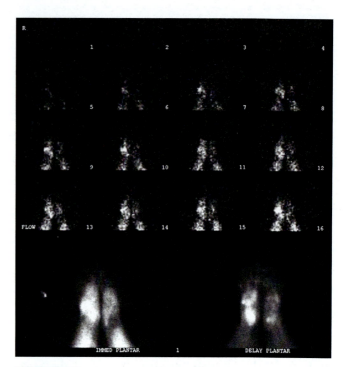

FIGURE 5 Three-phase bone scan showing increased uptake in complex regional pain syndrome. (Courtesy of Tarun Pandy, MD.)

In later stages, the accuracy of the scan is variable. In early stages, 44% to 96% sensitivity and 75% to 98% specificity has been reported[120] (**Figure 5**).

Treatment

A multidisciplinary approach is used to treat CRPS, addressing both the physical and psychological elements. Patients may present to the orthopaedic surgeon, neurologist, or primary care physician. In some cases, the physical therapist treating the patient may make the diagnosis. The main goals of treatment are pain control, restoration of limb function, and physical and psychological rehabilitation. The treatment is focused on the severity of pain and presentation. Psychiatric evaluation is helpful to address anxiety, depression, and sleep disturbances.

Physical therapy is an important part of the treatment because it can help in edema reduction, avoiding joint contractures and muscle wasting, maintaining limb function, and desensitization of the limb. In a systematic review of physiotherapy management in patients with CRPS, there is level II evidence supporting pain management physiotherapy/medical management.[121]

Various pharmacologic agents have been tried in the treatment of CRPS. Gabapentin and pregabalin are commonly prescribed. Antidepressants, NSAIDs, opioids, and corticosteroids are used by the pain management and psychiatric teams. Diphosphonates have been used to inhibit bone resorption. Free radical scavengers such as dimethyl sulfoxide, *N*-acetylcysteine, and mannitol have been tried with limited benefits.

A preliminary study investigated the use of immunoglobulin in the management of CRPS with positive results.[122] However, a larger randomized controlled trial with 6 weeks of immunoglobulin treatment was not effective in decreasing pain in patients with moderate to severe CRPS.[123]

A 2021 systematic literature review was done to evaluate the use of naltrexone in the treatment of CRPS.[124] Prior studies found the use of naltrexone to be promising in decreasing symptoms from CRPS.[125-127] Although there was evidence of pain reduction with naltrexone, a definitive recommendation could not be made without further prospective studies evaluating its efficacy in treating CRPS.[124]

The beneficial effect of vitamin C to prevent CRPS in wrist fractures has already been noted. The effect of 1 g vitamin C daily on prevention of CRPS type I in elective foot and ankle surgery has been evaluated. It was shown that vitamin C is effective in preventing CRPS type I of the foot and ankle, and vitamin C was recommended for preventive management.[128,129]

Topical agents such as lidocaine patch, fentanyl patch, transdermal clonidine, and capsaicin have been used increasingly by the pain management team.

Pain control is essential for management of CRPS. If pain is not adequately controlled by medications, then regional anesthetic blocks can be considered. Sympathetic blocks have been used for many years and are effective if performed early, before central pathways for pain are set.[130] Spinal cord and peripheral nerve stimulation have been used with limited benefits.

Surgical intervention is needed only if there are pain generators such as TTS or fractures. Surgery can also exacerbate CRPS and hence should be done sparingly. Amputation of the limb has been tried, but CRPS can recur in the residual limb, especially if the amputation level was symptomatic at the time of surgery.

SUMMARY

Interdigital plantar neuralgias usually respond to shoe wear modifications and local injections. Surgical excision through a dorsal approach can lead to significant pain relief. Peripheral nerve entrapments in the foot and ankle are relatively uncommon. Physician knowledge of specific nerve anatomy aids in diagnosis as can the judicial use of imaging modalities and electrodiagnostic tests. Nerve entrapment usually responds to nonsurgical management, but for patients who do not respond and in whom a proper diagnosis has been made, surgical intervention has shown good success in relieving symptoms.

CRPS remains a difficult condition to diagnose and treat, although significant advances have recently been made in diagnosis and treatment.

KEY STUDY POINTS

- Morton neuroma (interdigital plantar neuralgia) is not a true tumor of interdigital nerve but rather enlargement of the nerve secondary to histologic and degenerative changes within the nerve. Nonsurgical measures will fail in 60% to 70% of patients with interdigital plantar neuralgia and eventually these patients undergo surgical intervention.
- TTS is an entrapment neuropathy of the tibial nerve. Typical symptoms include plantar paresthesias, with one-third experiencing proximal radiating pain (Valleix phenomenon). Surgical results are improved with release of the individual tunnels including the septum between the medial and lateral plantar tunnels.
- Jogger's foot is entrapment of the MPN at the level of the navicular tuberosity. Most patients improve with nonsurgical measures.
- Twenty percent of patients with chronic medial heel pain have some degree of entrapment of the first branch of the LPN (Baxter nerve). Classically, patients have distinct tenderness at the origin of the abductor hallucis without sensory loss.
- Entrapment of the SPN occurs most frequently where the nerve exits the deep fascia of the lateral compartment.
- The factors leading to CRPS are multifactorial. Early diagnosis and treatment are important to prevent permanent disability.

ANNOTATED REFERENCES

1. Giannini S, Bacchini P, Ceccarelli F, Vannini F: Interdigital neuroma: Clinical examination and histopathologic results in 63 cases treated with excision. *Foot Ankle Int* 2004;25(2):79-84.

2. Graham CE, Graham DM: Morton's neuroma: A microscopic evaluation. *Foot Ankle* 1984;5(3):150-153.

3. Kim JY, Choi JH, Park J, Wang J, Lee I: An anatomical study of Morton's interdigital neuroma: The relationship between the occurring site and the deep transverse metatarsal ligament (DTML). *Foot Ankle Int* 2007;28(9):1007-1010.

4. Morscher E, Ulrich J, Dick W: Morton's intermetatarsal neuroma: Morphology and histological substrate. *Foot Ankle Int* 2000;21(7):558-562.

5. Jones JR, Klenerman L: A study of the communicating branch between the medial and lateral plantar nerves. *Foot Ankle* 1984;4(6):313-315.

6. Levitsky KA, Alman BA, Jevsevar DS, Morehead J: Digital nerves of the foot: Anatomic variations and implications regarding the pathogenesis of interdigital neuroma. *Foot Ankle* 1993;14(4):208-214.

7. Govsa F, Bilge O, Ozer MA: Anatomical study of the communicating branches between the medial and lateral plantar nerves. *Surg Radiol Anat* 2005;27(5):377-381.

8. Mann RA, Reynolds JC: Interdigital neuroma – A critical clinical analysis. *Foot Ankle* 1983;3(4):238-243.

9. Schon LC, Mann R: Diseases of the nerves, in Coughlin MM, MR , Saltzmann C, eds: *Surgery of the Foot and Ankle*, ed 8. Mosby, 2007, pp 613-686.

10. Bradley N, Miller WA, Evans JP: Plantar neuroma: Analysis of results following surgical excision in 145 patients. *South Med J* 1976;69(7):853-854.

11. Thompson FM, Deland JT: Occurrence of two interdigital neuromas in one foot. *Foot Ankle* 1993;14(1):15-17.

12. Owens R, Gougoulias N, Guthrie H, Sakellariou A: Morton's neuroma: Clinical testing and imaging in 76 feet, compared to a control group. *Foot Ankle Surg* 2011;17(3):197-200.

13. Cloke DJ, Greiss ME: The digital nerve stretch test: A sensitive indicator of Morton's neuroma and neuritis. *Foot Ankle Surg* 2006;12(4):201-203.

14. Mulder JD: The causative mechanism in Morton's metatarsalgia. *J Bone Joint Surg Br* 1951;33-B(1):94-95.

15. Naraghi R, Bremner A, Slack-Smith L, Bryant A: Radiographic analysis of feet with and without Morton's neuroma. *Foot Ankle Int* 2017;38(3):310-317.

16. Sharp RJ, Wade CM, Hennessy MS, Saxby TS: The role of MRI and ultrasound imaging in Morton's neuroma and the effect of size of lesion on symptoms. *J Bone Joint Surg Br* 2003;85(7):999-1005.

17. Oliver TB, Beggs I: Ultrasound in the assessment of metatarsalgia: A surgical and histological correlation. *Clin Radiol* 1998;53(4):287-289.

18. Almeida DFd, Kurokawa K, Hatanaka Y, Hemmi S, Claussen GC, Oh SJ: Abnormal dip phenomenon: A characteristic electrophysiological marker in interdigital neuropathy of the foot. *Arq Neuropsiquiatr* 2007;65(3B):771-778.

19. Greenfield J, Rea J Jr. Ilfeld FW: Morton's interdigital neuroma. Indications for treatment by local injections versus surgery. *Clin Orthop Relat Res* 1984;185:142-144.

20. Mahadevan D, Attwal M, Bhatt R, Bhatia M: Corticosteroid injection for Morton's neuroma with or without ultrasound guidance: A randomised controlled trial. *Bone Joint J* 2016;98-B(4):498-503.

21. Makki D, Haddad BZ, Mahmood Z, Shahid MS, Pathak S, Garnham I: Efficacy of corticosteroid injection versus size of plantar interdigital neuroma. *Foot Ankle Int* 2012;33(9):722-726.

22. Markovic M, Crichton K, Read JW, Lam P, Slater HK: Effectiveness of ultrasound-guided corticosteroid injection in the treatment of Morton's neuroma. *Foot Ankle Int* 2008;29(5):483-487.

23. Saygi B, Yildirim Y, Saygi EK, Kara H, Esemenli T: Morton neuroma: Comparative results of two conservative methods. *Foot Ankle Int* 2005;26(7):556-559.

24. Thomson CE, Beggs I, Martin DJ, et al: Methylprednisolone injections for the treatment of Morton neuroma: A patient-blinded randomized trial. *J Bone Joint Surg Am* 2013;95(9):790-798, S1.

25. Lizano-Diez X, Gines-Cespedosa A, Alentorn-Geli E, et al: Corticosteroid injection for the treatment of Morton's neuroma: A prospective, double-blinded, randomized, placebo-controlled trial. *Foot Ankle Int* 2017;38(9):944-951.

26. Choi JY, Lee HI, Hong WH, Suh JS, Hur JW: Corticosteroid injection for Morton's interdigital neuroma: A systematic review. *Clin Orthop Surg* 2021;13(2):266-277.

This is a systematic review of steroid injection for neuroma treatment. Satisfactory results are seen with steroid injection although 30% of patients eventually underwent surgical treatment. The authors recommended additional studies were needed to evaluate multiple injections along with using outcomes scores to determine the true efficacy of steroid injections for neuroma treatment. Level of evidence: IV.

27. van Vendeloo SN, Ettema HB: Skin depigmentation along lymph vessels of the lower leg following local corticosteroid injection for interdigital neuroma. *Foot Ankle Surg* 2016;22(2):139-141.

28. Fanucci E, Masala S, Fabiano S, et al: Treatment of intermetatarsal Morton's neuroma with alcohol injection under US guide: 10-month follow-up. *Eur Radiol* 2004;14(3):514-518.

29. Musson RE, Sawhney JS, Lamb L, Wilkinson A, Obaid H: Ultrasound guided alcohol ablation of Morton's neuroma. *Foot Ankle Int* 2012;33(3):196-201.

30. Pasquali C, Vulcano E, Novario R, Varotto D, Montoli C, Volpe A: Ultrasound-guided alcohol injection for Morton's neuroma. *Foot Ankle Int* 2015;36(1):55-59.

31. Hughes RJ, Ali K, Jones H, Kendall S, Connell DA: Treatment of Morton's neuroma with alcohol injection under sonographic guidance: Follow-up of 101 cases. *AJR Am J Roentgenol* 2007;188(6):1535-1539.

32. Gurdezi S, White T, Ramesh P: Alcohol injection for Morton's neuroma: A five-year follow-up. *Foot Ankle Int* 2013;34(8):1064-1067.

33. Mazoch MJ, Cheema GA, Suva LJ, Thomas RL: Effects of alcohol injection in rat sciatic nerve as a model for Morton's neuroma treatment. *Foot Ankle Int* 2014;35(11):1187-1191.

34. Jabbari B, Machado D: Treatment of refractory pain with botulinum toxins – An evidence-based review. *Pain Med* 2011;12(11):1594-1606.

35. Climent JM, Mondejar-Gomez F, Rodriguez-Ruiz C, Diaz-Llopis I, Gomez-Gallego D, Martin-Medina P: Treatment of Morton neuroma with botulinum toxin A: A pilot study. *Clin Drug Investig* 2013;33(7):497-503.

36. Campbell CM, Diamond E, Schmidt WK, et al: A randomized, double-blind, placebo-controlled trial of injected capsaicin for pain in Morton's neuroma. *Pain* 2016;157(6):1297-1304.

37. Thomson L, Aujla RS, Divall P, Bhatia M: Non-surgical treatments for Morton's neuroma: A systematic review. *Foot Ankle Surg* 2020;26(7):736-743.

This is a systematic review of nonsurgical treatment in Morton neuroma. The review recommended corticosteroid injection although with the caveat that symptoms may recur over time. Although some studies indicate radiofrequency ablation and cryotherapy may be effective, further high-quality studies are needed to evaluate its efficacy. Level of evidence: IV.

38. Chuter GSJ, Chua YP, Connell DA, Blackney MC: Ultrasound-guided radiofrequency ablation in the management of interdigital (Morton's) neuroma. *Skeletal Radiol* 2013;42(1):107-111.

39. Deniz S, Purtuloglu T, Tekindur S, et al: Ultrasound-guided pulsed radio frequency treatment in Morton's neuroma. *J Am Podiatr Med Assoc* 2015;105(4):302-306.

40. Paolo RRA, Mihai BP: Radiofrequency thermo-ablation of Morton's neuroma: A valid minimally invasive treatment procedure in patients resistant to conservative treatment. *Open J Orthop* 2013;13(8):325-330.

41. Caporusso EF, Fallat LM, Savoy-Moore R: Cryogenic neuroablation for the treatment of lower extremity neuromas. *J Foot Ankle Surg* 2002;41(5):286-290.

42. Fridman R, Cain JD, Weil L Jr: Extracorporeal shockwave therapy for interdigital neuroma: A randomized, placebo-controlled, double-blind trial. *J Am Podiatr Med Assoc* 2009;99(3):191-193.

43. Seok H, Kim SH, Lee SY, Park SW: Extracorporeal shockwave therapy in patients with Morton's neuroma A randomized, placebo-controlled trial. *J Am Podiatr Med Assoc* 2016;106(2):93-99.

44. Gimber LH, Melville DM, Bocian DA, Krupinski EA, Guidice MPD, Taljanovic MS: Ultrasound evaluation of Morton neuroma before and after laser therapy. *AJR Am J Roentgenol* 2017;208(2):380-385.

45. Mahadevan D, Salmasi M, Whybra N, Nanda A, Gaba S, Mangwani J: What factors predict the need for further intervention following corticosteroid injection of Morton's neuroma? *Foot Ankle Surg* 2016;22(1):9-11.

46. Coughlin MJ, Pinsonneault T: Operative treatment of interdigital neuroma. A long-term follow-up study. *J Bone Joint Surg Am* 2001;83(9):1321-1328.

47. Womack JW, Richardson DR, Murphy GA, Richardson EG, Ishikawa SN: Long-term evaluation of interdigital neuroma treated by surgical excision. *Foot Ankle Int* 2008;29(6):574-577.

48. Bucknall V, Rutherford D, MacDonald D, Shalaby H, McKinley J, Breusch SJ: Outcomes following excision of Morton's interdigital neuroma: A prospective study. *Bone Joint J* 2016;98-B(10):1376-1381.

49. Kasparek M, Schneider W: Surgical treatment of Morton's neuroma: Clinical results after open excision. *Int Orthop* 2013;37(9):1857-1861.

50. Abdel A, Whitelaw K, Waryasz G, Guss D, Johnson A, DiGiovanni C: Isolated intermetatarsal ligament release as primary surgical management for Morton's neuroma: The carpal tunnel of the foot? *Foot Ankle Orthop* 2018;3(3):2473011418S0013.

51. Koti M, Sharma H, Parikh M, Edwards M, McAllister J: Comparative analysis of dorsal nerve relocation versus dorsal neurectomy in the surgical management of Morton's neuroma. *J Foot Ankle Surg* 2020;59(6):1148-1155.

A retrospective case series evaluated neurectomy vs dorsal nerve relocation. The results indicated similar findings of relocation vs neurectomy although relocation group had better resolution of symptoms, earlier return to footwear, and earlier return to activities. Those undergoing translocation may have less residual neuroma formation although more studies are needed. Level of evidence: IV.

52. Song JH, Kang C, Hwang DS, Kang DH, Kim YH: Dorsal suspension for Morton's neuroma: A comparison with neurectomy. *Foot Ankle Surg* 2019;25(6):748-754.

A retrospective study evaluated the efficacy of neurectomy versus dorsal suspension for Morton neuroma. The results indicated improved healing compared with neurectomy alone, with fewer complications in the dorsal suspension group. Level of evidence: IV.

53. Shapiro SL: Endoscopic decompression of the intermetatarsal nerve for Morton's neuroma. *Foot Ankle Clin* 2004;9(2):297-304.

54. Zelent ME, Kane RM, Neese DJ, Lockner WB: Minimally invasive Morton's intermetatarsal neuroma decompression. *Foot Ankle Int* 2007;28(2):263-265.

55. Iborra-Marcos A, Villanueva-Martinez M, Barrett SL, Sanz-Ruiz P: Ultrasound-guided decompression of the intermetatarsal nerve for Morton's neuroma: A novel closed surgical technique. *J Am Podiatr Med Assoc* 2020;110(6):Article_8.

A two-part study with a cadaver study evaluated the safety of ultrasound-guided decompression and a retrospective case series of the technique. The results indicated that 54 of 56 patients had significant pain relief with releasing the IML by ultrasound. Two patients required open neurectomy. Level of evidence: IV.

56. Archuleta AF, Darbinian J, West T, Weintraub MLR, Pollard JD: Minimally invasive intermetatarsal nerve decompression for Morton's neuroma: A review of 27 cases. *J Foot Ankle Surg* 2020;59(6):1186-1191.

This is a retrospective review of 27 patients who underwent minimally invasive nerve decompression for Morton neuroma. Results indicated poor results in up to 40% of patients with 18.5% of patients requiring neurectomy. Technique may be indicated in patients with a small neuroma with negative Mulder click. Level of evidence: IV.

57. Akermark C, Crone H, Skoog A, Weidenhielm L: A prospective randomized controlled trial of plantar versus dorsal incisions for operative treatment of primary Morton's neuroma. *Foot Ankle Int* 2013;34(9):1198-1204.

58. Benedetti RS, Baxter DE, Davis PF: Clinical results of simultaneous adjacent interdigital neurectomy in the foot. *Foot Ankle Int* 1996;17(5):264-268.

59. Su E, Di Carlo E, O'Malley M, Bohne WHO, Deland JT, Kennedy JG: The frequency of digital artery resection in Morton interdigital neurectomy. *Foot Ankle Int* 2006;27(10):801-803.

60. Rungprai C, Cychosz CC, Phruetthiphat O, Femino JE, Amendola A, Phisitkul P: Simple neurectomy versus neurectomy with intramuscular implantation for interdigital neuroma: A comparative study. *Foot Ankle Int* 2015;36(12):1412-1424.

61. Amis JA, Siverhus SW, Liwnicz BH: An anatomic basis for recurrence after Morton's neuroma excision. *Foot Ankle* 1992;13(3):153-156.

62. Johnson JE, Johnson KA, Unni KK: Persistent pain after excision of an interdigital neuroma. Results of reoperation. *J Bone Joint Surg Am* 1988;70(5):651-657.

63. Stamatis ED, Myerson MS: Treatment of recurrence of symptoms after excision of an interdigital neuroma. A retrospective review. *J Bone Joint Surg Br* 2004;86(1):48-53.

64. Wolfort SF, Dellon AL: Treatment of recurrent neuroma of the interdigital nerve by implantation of the proximal nerve into muscle in the arch of the foot. *J Foot Ankle Surg* 2001;40(6):404-410.

65. Keck C: The tarsal-tunnel syndrome. *J Bone Joint Surg Am* 1962;44(1):180-182.

66. Takakura Y, Sugimoto K, Tanaka Y, Tamai S: Symptomatic talocalcaneal coalition. Its clinical significance and treatment. *Clin Orthop Relat Res* 1991;269:249-256.

67. Lalevee M, Coillard JY, Gauthe R, et al: Tarsal tunnel syndrome: Outcome according to etiology. *J Foot Ankle Surg* 2022;61(3):583-589.

   This retrospective series compared three groups of patients with TTS including space-occupying lesion, venous dilatation, and idiopathic tarsal tunnel. Patients with a permanent space-occupying lesion demonstrated the most improvement. Neuropathy on preoperative ultrasound and idiopathic tarsal tunnel was associated with poor outcomes. In addition, in patients with venous dilatation as a cause of TTS, patients with continuous dilatation had better results versus patients with intermittent dilatation. Level of evidence: IV.

68. Havel PE, Ebraheim NA, Clark SE, Jackson WT, DiDio L: Tibial nerve branching in the tarsal tunnel. *Foot Ankle* 1988;9(3):117-119.

69. Park TA, Del Toro DR: The medial calcaneal nerve: Anatomy and nerve conduction technique. *Muscle Nerve* 1995;18(1):32-38.

70. Trepman E, Kadel NJ, Chisholm K, Razzano L: Effect of foot and ankle position on tarsal tunnel compartment pressure. *Foot Ankle Int* 1999;20(11):721-726.

71. Kinoshita M, Okuda R, Morikawa J, Jotoku T, Abe M: The dorsiflexion-eversion test for diagnosis of tarsal tunnel syndrome. *J Bone Joint Surg Am* 2001;83(12):1835-1839.

72. Frey C, Kerr R: Magnetic resonance imaging and the evaluation of tarsal tunnel syndrome. *Foot Ankle* 1993;14(3):159-164.

73. Bracilovic A, Nihal A, Houston VL, Beattie AC, Rosenberg ZS, Trepman E: Effect of foot and ankle position on tarsal tunnel compartment volume. *Foot Ankle Int* 2006;27(6):431-437.

74. Galardi G, Amadio S, Maderna L, et al: Electrophysiologic studies in tarsal tunnel syndrome. Diagnostic reliability of motor distal latency, mixed nerve and sensory nerve conduction studies. *Am J Phys Med Rehabil* 1994;73(3):193-198.

75. Patel AT, Gaines K, Malamut R, et al: Usefulness of electrodiagnostic techniques in the evaluation of suspected tarsal tunnel syndrome: An evidence-based review. *Muscle Nerve* 2005;32(2):236-240.

76. Lau JT, Daniels TR: Tarsal tunnel syndrome: A review of the literature. *Foot Ankle Int* 1999;20(3):201-209.

77. Gould JS: Tarsal tunnel syndrome. *Foot Ankle Clin* 2011;16(2):275-286.

78. Dellon AL: The four medial ankle tunnels: A critical review of perceptions of tarsal tunnel syndrome and neuropathy. *Neurosurg Clin N Am* 2008;19(4):629-648, vii.

79. Barker AR, Rosson GD, Dellon AL: Pressure changes in the medial and lateral plantar and tarsal tunnels related to ankle position: A cadaver study. *Foot Ankle Int* 2007;28(2):250-254.

80. Rosson GD, Larson AR, Williams EH, Dellon AL: Tibial nerve decompression in patients with tarsal tunnel syndrome: Pressures in the tarsal, medial plantar, and lateral plantar tunnels. *Plast Reconstr Surg* 2009;124(4):1202-1210.

81. Mullick T, Dellon AL: Results of decompression of four medial ankle tunnels in the treatment of tarsal tunnels syndrome. *J Reconstr Microsurg* 2008;24(2):119-126.

82. Krishnan KG, Pinzer T, Schackert G: A novel endoscopic technique in treating single nerve entrapment syndromes with special attention to ulnar nerve transposition and tarsal tunnel release: Clinical application. *Neurosurgery* 2006;59(1 suppl 1):ONS89-ONS100.

83. Fernandez-Gibello A, Moroni S, Camunas G, et al: Ultrasound-guided decompression surgery of the tarsal tunnel: A novel technique for the proximal tarsal tunnel syndrome-Part II. *Surg Radiol Anat* 2019;41(1):43-51.

   A cadaver anatomic study evaluated the technique for ultrasound-guided release of the proximal tarsal tunnel. Level of evidence: V.

84. Moroni S, Gibello AF, Zwierzina M, et al: Ultrasound-guided decompression surgery of the distal tarsal tunnel: A novel technique for the distal tarsal tunnel syndrome-part III. *Surg Radiol Anat* 2019;41(3):313-321.

   A cadaver anatomic study evaluated the technique for ultrasound-guided release of the distal tarsal tunnel. Level of evidence: V.

85. Iborra Marcos A, Villanueva Martinez M, Sanz-Ruiz P, Barrett SL, Zislis G: Ultrasound-guided proximal and distal tarsal decompression: An analysis of pressures in the tarsal, medial plantar, and lateral plantar tunnels. *Foot Ankle Spec* 2021;14(2):133-139.

A study evaluated the intracompartment pressure before and after ultrasound-guided tarsal tunnel decompression. The results indicated that mean pressure values dropped to normal after the procedure. Level of evidence: IV.

86. Iborra A, Villanueva M, Sanz-Ruiz P: Results of ultrasound-guided release of tarsal tunnel syndrome: A review of 81 cases with a minimum follow-up of 18 months. *J Orthop Surg Res* 2020;15(1):30.

This is a retrospective case series of tarsal tunnel release by ultrasonographic guidance. Eighty-one patients were evaluated demonstrating greater than 90% excellent to good improvement after the procedure. Poor results were seen in 9.8% of patients, especially in those who had long-term TTS. Level of evidence: IV.

87. Nagaoka M, Satou K: Tarsal tunnel syndrome caused by ganglia. *J Bone Joint Surg Br* 1999;81(4):607-610.

88. Pfeiffer WH, Cracchiolo A III: Clinical results after tarsal tunnel decompression. *J Bone Joint Surg Am* 1994;76(8):1222-1230.

89. Sung KS, Park SJ: Short-term operative outcome of tarsal tunnel syndrome due to benign space-occupying lesions. *Foot Ankle Int* 2009;30(8):741-745.

90. Doneddu PE, Coraci D, Loreti C, Piccinini G, Padua L: Tarsal tunnel syndrome: Still more opinions than evidence. Status of the art. *Neurol Sci* 2017;38(10):1735-1739.

91. Sammarco GJ, Chang L: Outcome of surgical treatment of tarsal tunnel syndrome. *Foot Ankle Int* 2003;24(2):125-131.

92. Gondring WH, Trepman E, Shields B: Tarsal tunnel syndrome: Assessment of treatment outcome with an anatomic pain intensity scale. *Foot Ankle Surg* 2009;15(3):133-138.

93. Ahmad M, Tsang K, Mackenney PJ, Adedapo AO: Tarsal tunnel syndrome: A literature review. *Foot Ankle Surg* 2012;18(3):149-152.

94. Reichert P, Zimmer K, Wnukiewicz W, Kuliński S, Mazurek P, Gosk J: Results of surgical treatment of tarsal tunnel syndrome. *Foot Ankle Surg* 2015;21(1):26-29.

95. Rungprai C, Phisitkul P, Femino J, Amendola A, Sittapairoj T: Tarsal tunnel release: Medium-term outcomes and complications. *Foot Ankle Orthop* 2016;1(1):2473011416S00287.

96. Gould JD, DiGiovanni BF: Plantar fascia release in combination with proximal and distal tarsal tunnel release, in Wiesel SW, ed: *Operative Techniques in Orthopedic Surgery.* Wolters Kluwer/Lippincott Williams and Wilkins, 2011, pp 3911-3919.

97. Rask MR: Medial plantar neurapraxia (jogger's foot): Report of 3 cases. *Clin Orthop Relat Res* 1978;134:193-195.

98. Baxter DE, Pfeffer GB: Treatment of chronic heel pain by surgical release of the first branch of the lateral plantar nerve. *Clin Orthop Relat Res* 1992;279:229-236.

99. Gould JF, Ford D: Orthoses and insert management of common foot and ankle problems, in Baxter DE, Porter DA, Schon L, eds: *Baxter's the Foot and Ankle in Sport*, ed 2. Mosby Elsevier, 2008, xv, 636 p.

100. Marinacci AA: Neurological syndromes of the tarsal tunnels. *Bull Los Angeles Neurol Soc* 1968;33(2):90-100.

101. Gessini L, Jandolo B, Pietrangeli A: The anterior tarsal syndrome. Report of four cases. *J Bone Joint Surg Am* 1984;66(5):786-787.

102. Roselle N, Stevens A: Unexpected incidence of neurogenic atrophy of the extensor digitorum brevis muscle in young adults, in Desmedt JE, ed: *New Developments in Electromyography and Clinical Neurophysiology.* S. Karger, 1973.

103. Styf J, Morberg P: The superficial peroneal tunnel syndrome. Results of treatment by decompression. *J Bone Joint Surg Br* 1997;79(5):801-803.

104. Barrett SL, Dellon AL, Rosson GD, Walters L: Superficial peroneal nerve (superficial fibularis nerve): The clinical implications of anatomic variability. *J Foot Ankle Surg* 2006;45(3):174-176.

105. Ucerler H, Ikiz 'ZAA: The variations of the sensory branches of the superficial peroneal nerve course and its clinical importance. *Foot Ankle Int* 2005;26(11):942-946.

106. Kennedy JG, Baxter DE: Nerve disorders in dancers. *Clin Sports Med* 2008;27(2):329-334.

107. Young BH, Flanigan RM, DiGiovanni BF: Complications of ankle arthroscopy utilizing a contemporary noninvasive distraction technique. *J Bone Joint Surg Am* 2011;93(10):963-968.

108. Styf J: Entrapment of the superficial peroneal nerve. Diagnosis and results of decompression. *J Bone Joint Surg Br* 1989;71(1):131-135.

109. Stephens MM, Kelly PM: Fourth toe flexion sign: A new clinical sign for identification of the superficial peroneal nerve. *Foot Ankle Int* 2000;21(10):860-863.

110. Yang LJS, Gala VC, McGillicuddy JE: Superficial peroneal nerve syndrome: An unusual nerve entrapment. Case report. *J Neurosurg* 2006;104(5):820-823.

111. Riedl O, Frey M: Anatomy of the sural nerve: Cadaver study and literature review. *Plast Reconstr Surg* 2013;131(4):802-810.

112. Joplin RJ: The proper digital nerve, vitallium stem arthroplasty, and some thoughts about foot surgery in general. *Clin Orthop Relat Res* 1971;76:199-212.

113. Im S, Park JH, Kim HW, Yoo SH, Kim HS, Park GY: New method to perform medial plantar proper digital nerve conduction studies. *Clin Neurophysiol* 2010;121(7):1059-1065.

114. Sandroni P, Benrud-Larson LM, McClelland RL, Low PA: Complex regional pain syndrome type I: Incidence and prevalence in Olmsted county, a population-based study. *Pain* 2003;103(1-2):199-207.

115. Bruehl S, Chung OY: How common is complex regional pain syndrome-Type I? *Pain* 2007;129(1-2):1-2.

116. Jänig W, Baron R: Complex regional pain syndrome is a disease of the central nervous system. *Clin Auton Res* 2002;12(3):150-164.

117. Bruehl S: An update on the pathophysiology of complex regional pain syndrome. *Anesthesiology* 2010;113(3):713-725.

118. Beerthuizen A, Stronks DL, Van't Spijker A, et al: Demographic and medical parameters in the development of complex regional pain syndrome type 1 (CRPS1): Prospective study on 596 patients with a fracture. *Pain* 2012;153(6):1187-1192.

119. Genant HK, Kozin F, Bekerman C, McCarty DJ, Sims J: The reflex sympathetic dystrophy syndrome. A comprehensive analysis using fine-detail radiography, photon absorptiometry, and bone and joint scintigraphy. *Radiology* 1975;117(1):21-32.

120. Hogan CJ, Hurwitz SR: Treatment of complex regional pain syndrome of the lower extremity. *J Am Acad Orthop Surg* 2002;10(4):281-289.

121. Daly AE, Bialocerkowski AE: Does evidence support physiotherapy management of adult complex regional pain syndrome type one? A systematic review. *Eur J Pain* 2009;13(4):339-353.

122. Goebel A, Baranowski A, Maurer K, Ghiai A, McCabe C, Ambler G: Intravenous immunoglobulin treatment of the complex regional pain syndrome: A randomized trial. *Ann Intern Med* 2010;152(3):152-158.

123. Goebel A, Bisla J, Carganillo R, et al: Low-dose intravenous immunoglobulin treatment for long-standing complex regional pain syndrome: A randomized trial. *Ann Intern Med* 2017;167(7):476-483.

124. Soin A, Soin Y, Dann T, et al: Low-dose naltrexone use for patients with chronic regional pain syndrome: A systematic literature review. *Pain Physician* 2021;24(4):E393-E406.

This is a systematic review of literature using naltrexone to treat CRPS. The study indicated some early evidence using naltrexone to treat pain related to CRPS. However, the review indicated that further prospective studies are needed to determine its true effectiveness. Level of evidence: III.

125. Chopra P, Cooper MS: Treatment of Complex Regional Pain Syndrome (CRPS) using low dose naltrexone (LDN). *J Neuroimmune Pharmacol* 2013;8(3):470-476.

126. Sturn KM, Collin M: Low-dose naltrexone: A new therapy option for complex regional pain syndrome type I patients. *Int J Pharm Compd* 2016;20(3):197-201.

127. Weinstock LB, Myers TL, Walters AS, et al: Identification and treatment of new inflammatory triggers for complex regional pain syndrome: Small intestinal bacterial overgrowth and obstructive sleep apnea. *A A Case Rep* 2016;6(9):272-276.

128. Besse JL, Gadeyne S, Galand-Desmé S, Lerat JL, Moyen B: Effect of vitamin C on prevention of complex regional pain syndrome type I in foot and ankle surgery. *Foot Ankle Surg* 2009;15(4):179-182.

129. Hernigou J, Labadens A, Ghistelinck B, et al: Vitamin C prevention of complex regional pain syndrome after foot and ankle surgery: A prospective randomized study of three hundred and twenty nine patients. *Int Orthop* 2021;45(9):2453-2459.

This is a prospective randomized controlled study using vitamin C for prevention of CRPS. The results demonstrated a significant reduction in CRPS with vitamin C with odds ratio of 0.19. Taking 1 g of vitamin C per day for 40 days was found to be effective in reducing the risk of postoperative CRPS. Level of evidence: I.

130. AbuRahma AF, Robinson PA, Powell M, Bastug D, Boland JP: Sympathectomy for reflex sympathetic dystrophy: Factors affecting outcome. *Ann Vasc Surg* 1994;8(4):372-379.

SECTION **3**

Arthritis of the Foot and Ankle

Section Editors:

Robert D. Santrock, MD, FAAOS
Gregory C. Berlet, MD, FRCS(C), FAAOS, FAOA

CHAPTER 8

Ankle Arthritis: Part I. Joint Preservation Techniques and Arthrodesis

ADAM P. SCHIFF, MD, FAAOS • SAMUEL B. ADAMS, MD, FAAOS, FAOA

ABSTRACT

Ankle arthritis can have a substantial effect on patient quality of life. Patients with ankle arthritis present with pain, dysfunction, activity limitations, swelling, and limited ankle motion. Most ankle arthritis is caused by prior trauma. Nonsurgical management of ankle arthritis can include activity modification, shoewear modification, brace use, physical therapy, and corticosteroid injections. For patients who do not experience acceptable improvement with nonsurgical care, surgical options can be considered. Surgical treatment includes a wide variety of procedures and can be subdivided into joint-sparing and joint-sacrificing options based on the amount of arthrosis, deformity present, and patient expectations. Localized arthritis can be managed with anterior débridement or varus-producing or valgus-producing supramalleolar osteotomies. Diffuse mild to moderate arthritis can be managed with distraction arthroplasty, whereas severe arthritis can be managed with bipolar allograft replacement or arthrodesis.

Dr. Schiff or an immediate family member serves as a paid consultant to or is an employee of DJ Orthopaedics, Regeneration Technologies, Inc., Restor3D, and Stryker and has stock or stock options held in Restor3D. Dr. Adams or an immediate family member serves as a paid consultant to or is an employee of Conventus/Flower, DJO, Exactech, Inc., Orthofix, Inc., Regeneration Technologies, Inc., and Stryker; has stock or stock options held in Medshape; and serves as a board member, owner, officer, or committee member of American Orthopaedic Foot and Ankle Society.

Keywords: ankle arthritis; ankle arthrodesis; distraction arthroplasty; failed ankle arthroplasty; supramalleolar osteotomy

INTRODUCTION

Degenerative joint disease within the ankle has a different etiology from most other weight-bearing joints in the human body. Ankle arthritis can have a substantial effect on patient quality of life, function, and pain. The etiology of most ankle arthritis is posttraumatic in nature, although inflammatory arthropathies, neuroarthropathies, primary osteoarthritis (OA), septic arthritis, hemophilia, and hemochromatosis are other etiologies as well. Because of the posttraumatic nature of ankle arthritis, patients with ankle arthritis tend to be younger and more active than those with arthritis of other joints.

Initial management of ankle arthritis begins with nonsurgical care. Anti-inflammatory and analgesic medications, variable levels of immobilization, intra-articular injections (corticosteroids, viscosupplementation, and platelet-rich plasma [PRP]), dietary supplementation, and orthotic/brace devices are the most commonly used nonsurgical treatment options. If nonsurgical management does not yield acceptable results, surgical intervention is indicated. Surgical treatment includes a wide variety of procedures and can be subdivided into joint-sparing and joint-sacrificing options based on the amount of arthrosis, deformity present, and patient expectations. Joint-preserving techniques, allograft arthroplasty, and arthrodesis are explored as treatment options for ankle arthritis.

This chapter is adapted from Ankle arthritis: Part I. Joint preservation techniques and arthrodesis, in Chou LB, ed: Orthopaedic Knowledge Update®: Foot and Ankle 6. American Academy of Orthopaedic Surgeons, 2020, pp 105-128.

ANATOMY AND BIOMECHANICS

The ankle is a constrained joint that gains most of its stability from the bony anatomy of the medial malleolus, the distal fibula, and the configuration of the tibiotalar articulation (tibial plafond and talar dome). Additional stability is gained through static ligamentous structures, including the interosseous membrane, tibiofibular and collateral ligaments, and dynamic musculotendinous units. The medial ligamentous structures (deltoid confluence) are the primary stabilizers of the ankle[1] but are much less commonly injured than the lateral ligaments (anterior talofibular and calcaneofibular ligaments).

The ankle joint is directly perpendicular to the mechanical axis of the lower extremity. Both the anatomic and mechanical axes are the same in the tibia and should pass through the midpoint of the ankle articulation in the coronal and sagittal planes. In the coronal plane, the tibial plafond forms an angle with the mechanical axis, which is referred to as the distal tibial articular surface (TAS) angle. The tibial lateral surface (TLS) angle is the same measurement in the sagittal plane. The normal TAS angle is 88° to 93°, and a normal TLS angle is 80° to 81°[2,3] (**Figure 1**).

The ankle joint is mainly a rolling joint with highly congruent surfaces, particularly during weight bearing.[1,4] It is smaller than the knee or hip in surface area and consequently experiences a much higher force per area.[1,4,5] When the ankle is not bearing weight, the joint is incongruent. However, when bearing weight, the ankle joint becomes more congruent and allows for more joint surface area contact to dissipate the forces during weight bearing.[1] During normal activities, forces in excess of 3.5 times body weight are transmitted across the ankle joint and increase to 9 to 13.3 times body weight during running.[6] The primary motion of the tibiotalar joint is in the sagittal plane and averages a 43° to 63° arc in dorsiflexion and plantar flexion, with only 30° required for steady-state walking. There is an average of 10° of rotational movement of the talus within the mortise.[1]

INCIDENCE AND ETIOLOGY

Ankle arthritis is estimated to occur in 1% of the population.[4] In contrast to other weight-bearing joints of the lower extremity, the ankle joint is much more resistant to the development of primary degenerative OA but is more susceptible to posttraumatic OA.[7] In fact, 76% to 78% of all ankle arthritis cases can be attributed to trauma, whereas primary OA accounts for 7% to 9% of cases.[4,7,8] The remainder of ankle arthritis cases (12% to 13%) are attributable to secondary arthritis as a result of rheumatoid arthritis, neuroarthropathy, hemochromatosis, and postinfectious degeneration.[4,7]

Joint motion, cartilage thickness, incidence of fractures or ligamentous trauma, and metabolic and mechanical factors differ between the knee and ankle and help explain the difference in incidence of primary OA and posttraumatic OA.[4,7-9] Knee OA affects more women than men, whereas ankle OA affects more men than women.[9] This is explained by the posttraumatic nature of ankle OA.

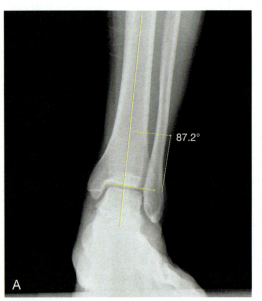 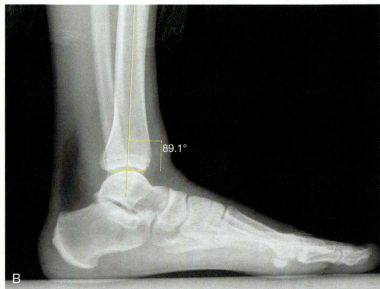

FIGURE 1 **A**, AP radiograph showing the distal tibial articular surface (TAS) angle. **B**, Lateral radiograph showing that the tibial lateral surface (TLS) angle is the same measurement in the sagittal plane. The normal TAS angle is 88° to 93°, and the TLS angle is 80° to 81°.

Although approximately 80% of ankle arthritis is posttraumatic in nature, not all trauma about the ankle results in posttraumatic OA. The overall rate of ankle posttraumatic OA is 14% following all ankle fractures; however, arthritis developed in as many as 33% of patients with Weber C fractures in some studies.[7,10] Large posterior malleolar fractures with displacement are associated with a higher incidence of arthritis.[7,10] Arthritis has been estimated to occur in 13% to 54% of tibial plafond fractures, 40% of bimalleolar fractures, and up to 71% of trimalleolar fractures.[11]

The exact cause of ankle posttraumatic OA is not known. The adequacy of reduction is a strong predictor of outcomes[7,10] (**Figure 2**). However, this mantra is not universally agreed on in the literature, with different conclusions appearing in various studies.[7,10,12] One reason could be the difference in ankle cartilage/chondrocytes. Unlike the knee cartilage, the articular cartilage of the ankle is uniform in thickness, measuring 1 to 1.7 mm, and displays much higher compressive stiffness than hip or knee cartilage.[4,7-9] Although ankle cartilage may develop fissures or fibrillations attributable to aging and wear, these conditions do not progress to OA as they would in the knee or hip.[4,7-9] Ankle cartilage also does not decrease in tensile strength with age.[4,7-9,13]

Additionally, chondrocytes in the ankle respond differently than those in the knee or hip to biochemical and biologic factors and resist degradation. Chondrocytes in cadaver ankle joints have increased proteoglycan and collagen rates in comparison with knee chondrocytes.[14] The increased turnover may allow ankle chondrocytes to respond better to subtle atraumatic wear and tear arthritis than knee chondrocytes. Moreover, ankle chondrocytes are less responsive to inflammatory mediators such as interleukin 1 beta (IL-1β) and synthesize much less of the collagen breakdown molecule, matrix metalloproteinases (MMP) (specifically MMP-8, which is elevated in OA) in response to IL-1 than chondrocytes in the hip or knee.[4,7-9] This decreased sensitivity is likely attributable to a smaller number of differing types of IL-1 receptors on ankle chondrocytes. As a result, the ankle is potentially less susceptible to damage by inflammatory mediators.

However, one potential etiology of ankle posttraumatic OA is related to inflammation. Although inflammation is the initial step in healing of fractures, intra-articular fractures cause an inflammatory burden on the uninjured cartilage throughout the joint. In fact, it has been shown that the intra-articular environment (synovial fluid) after ankle fracture and at end-stage ankle OA (from traumatic causes) is composed of high numbers of inflammatory mediators.[15] In a comparison of 21 patients who sustained intra-articular ankle fractures, several cytokines and MMPs including granulocyte-macrophage colony-stimulating factor, IL-10, IL-1, IL-6, IL-8, tumor necrosis factor, MMP-1, MMP-2, MMP-3, MMP-9, and MMP-10 were identified after intra-articular ankle fractures.[16,17] These inflammatory mediators were found

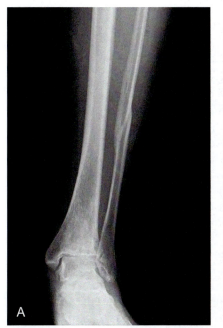
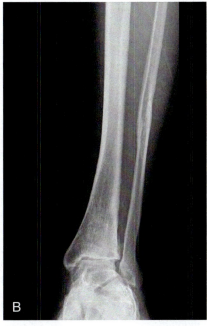
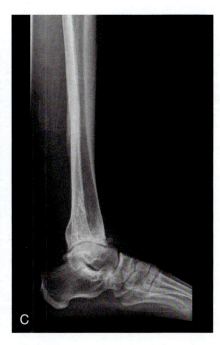

FIGURE 2 **A** through **C**, AP, mortise, and lateral views, respectively, of the ankle of a 43-year-old man with a 10-year history of an ankle fracture managed nonsurgically. Radiographs show evidence of a midfibular shaft fracture with malunion and unstable syndesmosis with substantial joint space narrowing.

Section 3: Arthritis of the Foot and Ankle

to rise acutely after ankle fracture and remained elevated for days to months after injury, providing evidence of a persistent inflammatory environment in synovial fluid after injury.

Primary ankle OA may be secondary to asymmetric cartilage wear. Intra-articular deformities with varus tilting occur as a result of impaction, distal tibial osteonecrosis, or chronic cavovarus. However, flatfoot deformity may develop in patients with chronic ankle instability, hindfoot valgus, and peroneal tendon dysfunction.[2] This could lead to asymmetric wear and/or progression of degeneration (Figure 3). Degeneration in one area can increase the contact pressures and potentially cause degeneration in another area. Although not in end-stage ankle arthritis, this concept has been demonstrated with even subtle mismatch of articular congruency, such as in the setting of osteochondral grafts in the talus. It was demonstrated in a study that with recessed osteochondral grafts, there was transfer of pressure to the opposite side of the talus.[18] Similarly, ankle instability secondary to incompetent ankle ligaments causes incongruity in the ankle joint. A study compared ground reaction forces in patients with chronic ankle instability with those in stable control patients.[19] The chronic ankle instability group had significantly higher impact peak forces and active peak forces compared with the control group. Because this pathology is secondary to an initial traumatic event (ankle sprain), there is debate regarding whether arthritis secondary to chronic ankle instability should be considered posttraumatic OA.

CLINICAL PRESENTATION AND IMAGING

Patients with ankle arthritis present with pain, dysfunction, activity restrictions, swelling, and limited ankle motion. Most patients describe their pain in a transverse line across the anterior ankle. Patients often note pain with any weight-bearing activity, such as prolonged standing, walking, running, and stair climbing. Most patients also have reduced self-perceived function as determined by functional assessments and questionnaires.[13] There is typically a history of ankle trauma or multiple ankle sprains.

Patients often have decreased sagittal plane motion and plantar flexion moment and power.[13] Nonarthritic ankle motion primarily occurs in the sagittal plane, with an arc of 30° required for normal walking.[7] In the setting of end-stage ankle arthritis, motion is limited.[7] As a result, compensation by the hindfoot and forefoot is necessary, which increases the shear forces at the midtarsal joints.[7] Ankle arthritis affects various gait pattern parameters such as walking speed, cadence, and stride length.[7,13] Patients with arthritis also exhibit antalgic gait patterns with abnormal plantar pressures. Those with ankle arthritis also exhibit increased oxygen consumption and decreased gait efficiency.[7] Consequently, sporting activities, prolonged ambulation, fast walking, and running are difficult.[7]

The first step in the management of ankle arthritis is to obtain a thorough history and physical examination. The history should ascertain the etiology of the disease, timing of onset of symptoms, current and prior symptoms, history of traumatic events or recurrent injuries, current level of function, treatment to date, and the desired level of function. Confounding factors, such as systemic diseases, current medications (including current opiate use), prior surgeries, history or suspicion of infections or wound healing problems, and a social history that includes drug abuse and smoking history, should be investigated in depth. A referral to a primary care physician or rheumatologist may help delineate the etiology of arthritis in patients with no history of mechanical causes or trauma. A neurology consultation may be required for patients with atypical pain, numbness, dysesthesias, burning, or non–activity-related pain to rule out spinal or neuropathic etiology. Special attention should be given to rheumatologic causes of ankle arthritis. These systemic arthritides can have an effect on other joints, which affects treatment. For example, rheumatoid arthritis can be associated with cervical spine pathology.

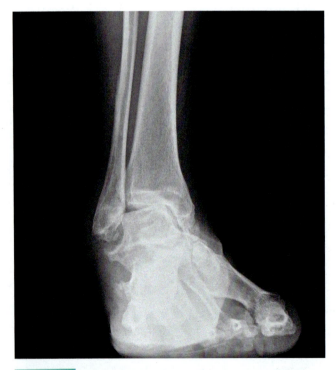

FIGURE 3 AP radiograph of the ankle of a 54-year-old man with a history of chronic ankle instability with multiple ankle inversion injuries reveals substantial varus deformity with medial tibiotalar joint space loss and chronic spurring of the ankle joint.

Cervical spine imaging may be necessary to adequately prepare for anesthesia. Furthermore, there are medication considerations with inflammatory arthritis, where some medications should be stopped preoperatively.

Postoperative complications and adverse outcomes must be mitigated preoperatively. Indolent infections and traumatized soft tissues can pose risks for any surgical intervention, especially when surgical implants are to be placed. Any patient with a history of infection or nonunion should be considered for a staged procedure to obtain deep cultures and inflammatory markers (complete blood count with differential, erythrocyte sedimentation rate, and C-reactive protein level) to rule out any indolent infections. Patients with circulatory dysfunction, diabetes mellitus, smoking history, and a history of osteonecrosis are at much higher risk for wound complications, infections, and nonunions. Smoking is a well-documented cause of postoperative complications in foot and ankle surgery, increasing the risk for nonunion by 16 times versus nonsmokers.[20] Smokers should be encouraged to quit smoking; surgeons have advocated withholding surgical intervention until patients are nicotine free in elective cases. There is no consensus regarding the length of time required for the complications of smoking to dissipate to the level experienced by nonsmokers or if the variance ever completely normalizes. Patients with diabetes or peripheral neuropathy will require more rigid fixation and longer periods of immobilization.[21]

The physical examination should begin with a gait analysis and evaluation of the alignment of the entire extremity to include the hip and knee. It is important to consider proximal deformities before any treatment of the ankle is undertaken. A complete examination of a patient's neurovascular status is essential. A patient with any changes in skin color, weak pulses, differences in vascularity compared with the contralateral side, or lymphedema should have a complete vascular workup or referral to a vascular surgeon. Hair loss on the foot and ankle can be related to vascular disease or neuropathy. The location and condition of all prior incisions and scars should be noted. Range of motion (ROM) of the ankle, subtalar joint, and transverse tarsal joints should be examined and recorded. Care should be taken to isolate motion to the responsible joints because Chopart joint motion (talonavicular and calcaneocuboid joints) often complicates the examination.

The minimum radiographic assessment must include three weight-bearing views of the ankle (AP, mortise, and lateral). These images will reveal the radiographic extent of the ankle arthritis including the intra-articular deformity, joint space narrowing, and ankle osteophytes. One study published a radiographic atlas of ankle arthritis changes and associated Kellgren-Lawrence grades.[22] Another study demonstrated that increasing Kellgren-Lawrence grades significantly correlated with increasing pain and decreasing function as suggested by the American Orthopaedic Foot and Ankle Society ankle-hindfoot scores.[16]

If alignment is questioned at the level of the ankle joint or below, then a hindfoot alignment view should be obtained.[23] Proximal alignment questions or leg-length discrepancies can be assessed on full-length and limb alignment radiographs. The location and degree of deformity are the most important factors in the decision-making process for surgical treatment. The presence of arthritis in the subtalar joint or the transverse tarsal joints may alter treatment algorithms. If radiographs do not correlate with a patient's symptoms or examination, MRI or CT may be indicated. CT may identify adjacent joint arthritis, subchondral cysts, and any specific bony deformities, whereas MRI may be indicated to evaluate for suspected osteonecrosis, bone edema, or associated soft-tissue pathology. These advanced imaging modalities are also important for preoperative planning.

NONSURGICAL TREATMENT

Although the literature is limited regarding the success rate of nonsurgical treatment, all patients with ankle arthritis should undergo a trial of nonsurgical management before proceeding with surgical intervention. However, some authors advocate early surgical intervention for patients with congenital or posttraumatic deformity rather than waiting for symptoms to worsen.[24] This is especially true for severe deformities with impending skin compromise or when the deformity/arthritis causes altered gait that can lead to degeneration of other joints, such as the contralateral hip.

There is no nonsurgical treatment that can restore the degenerative changes that have occurred. Instead, nonsurgical treatment strategies are aimed at symptomatic relief and prolonging the life and function of the native ankle. Rest and activity modification may help relieve the initial inflammation, but these interventions generally are not acceptable long-term solutions for active patients.[24] Walking aids such as canes or walkers are also helpful, but usually are tolerated only by elderly patients. For patients with reports of instability or weakness, a course of physical therapy that includes strength training, proprioceptive training, stretching, and aerobic nonimpact exercise may be beneficial.[24,25]

Oral Therapy

Oral NSAIDs and, on occasion, a short course of oral steroids may be beneficial, especially for patients with inflammatory arthropathies.[25] NSAIDs exert their function by inhibiting cyclooxygenase and reducing prostaglandins, which are inflammatory mediators that protect gastric mucosa.[26] Corticosteroids also function by inhibiting several inflammatory pathways.[26] Care should be taken in long-term use of NSAIDs, and long-term use necessitates monitoring because they can have deleterious effects on liver and kidney function. NSAIDs can also lead to gastric or enteric ulcers and carry an increased risk for bleeding. Analgesic medications, whether topical compounded creams or oral acetaminophen or tramadol, may be useful in controlling pain and increasing function and have a safer adverse effect profile than NSAIDs.[26]

Glucosamine is thought to inhibit the production of IL-1, prostaglandins, and MMPs. It may increase the native production of hyaluronic acid.[27] Chondroitin sulfate inhibits leukocyte elastase and the migration of polymorphonuclear leukocytes, and it may also increase hyaluronic acid production.[27] There is no research on the use of glucosamine or chondroitin sulfate in the ankle. Most of the current literature suggests that glucosamine and chondroitin sulfate may provide symptomatic relief of moderate to severe arthritis of the knee with minimal adverse effects.[27]

Patients with rheumatoid arthritis and other secondary causes of ankle arthrosis would benefit from treatment of the underlying condition. Disease-modifying antirheumatic drugs are medications that halt the progression of the rheumatoid destructive process. These include both biologic (IL-1 and tumor necrosis factor antagonists) and nonbiologic (methotrexate and sulfasalazine) options.[26] However, these drugs typically take months to exert their action and should be managed by a rheumatologist.

Intra-articular Injections

Intra-articular corticosteroid injections may limit pain and inflammation and can be safely used sparingly. Repeated injections carry limited risk for skin discoloration, fat necrosis, and soft-tissue destruction and pose increased risk for infection.[24,25] There has been no evidence to indicate destructive effects to cartilage resulting from these injections. Oral and injectable corticosteroids should be used with caution and monitoring in patients with diabetes because they can lead to alterations in blood glucose levels.

Hyaluronans have been used with success in the knee as well as in other joints. However, limited literature exists to support their use in the ankle. Hyaluronic acid has been shown to inhibit phagocytosis, decrease synovial fluid inflammatory mediators, and stimulate production of hyaluronic acid by chondrocytes.[27] A randomized controlled, double-blind study was performed on 20 patients using sodium hyaluronate over five weekly injections. At 6-month follow-up, there was a decrease in pain and disability and a trend toward better symptomatic relief in the hyaluronate group.[28] It was also found to be as safe as saline.[27,28] This finding was confirmed in other studies that showed a significant decrease in pain and improvement in function with hyaluronate use.[29,30] It is important to consider that hyaluronic acid is not currently FDA approved for use in the ankle.

Although PRP has been used in an expanding number of musculoskeletal disorders, there is minimal evidence to support its use in the ankle. The mechanism of action of PRP is thought to involve platelet degranulation with the subsequent release of various growth factors and the stimulation of stem cell lines involved in the healing and reparative process. In a study of PRP injections in 20 patients with ankle OA,[17] three injections were given at 2-week intervals under ultrasound guidance. Pain was significantly improved even at 24 weeks (study end point) after injection, but maximal pain relief occurred 12 weeks after injection.

Stem (stromal) cell injections have also been tried, but as with other injectables, there are few data to support their use. A meta-analysis of stromal cell injections into various joints, including the ankle, demonstrated a significant decrease in the American Orthopaedic Foot and Ankle Society scores in patients who received an ankle injection but no difference in the American Knee Society Knee Scoring System, the Hospital for Special Surgery Knee Rating Scale, and the International Knee Documentation Committee score for patients receiving knee injections. This may indicate that stem cell injections may be better served for ankle arthritis.[31]

A systematic review of intra-articular injections of steroids, hyaluronic acid, PRP, and stem cells into the ankle was published. Unfortunately, the data were quite limited, and therefore minimal conclusions can be obtained with regard to one therapeutic injection over another.[32]

Brace Treatment

Brace treatment is a valuable option with which to control pain and improve function in ankle arthrosis. Ankle motion occurs mainly in the sagittal plane; however, there is coronal plane motion as well. Therefore, brace options must be able to control both sagittal and frontal plane motion to effectively alleviate symptoms.[33] A custom-made ankle-foot orthosis (AFO) will help decrease symptoms and increase endurance.[24] A leather gauntlet (Arizona type) brace has similar properties as the AFO but is usually much better tolerated.[33] When all weight-bearing activities cause pain, a patellar tendon–bearing AFO may be used to immobilize and offload the

Chapter 8: Ankle Arthritis: Part I. Joint Preservation Techniques and Arthrodesis

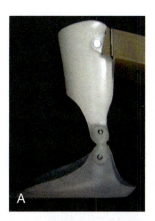
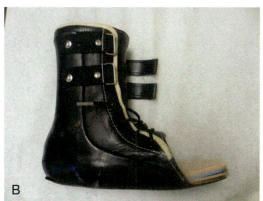
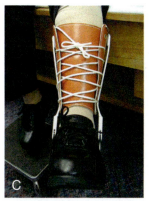
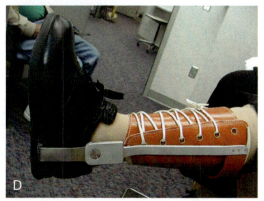
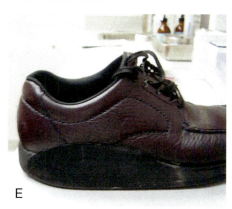

FIGURE 4 Photographs showing examples of braces and shoe modifications typically used in patients with ankle arthritis. **A**, Hinged ankle-foot orthosis, which allows some sagittal plane motion. **B**, Leather ankle gauntlet (Arizona). **C** and **D**, Double upright metal brace with custom-molded calf lacer with built-in shoe and insert (Charcot arthropathy). **E**, Solid ankle cushioned heel with rocker-bottom shoe modifications.

forces across the ankle. Shoe modifications such as a heel lift, solid ankle cushioned heel, and stiff rocker-bottom sole are also useful (**Figure 4**). Heel lifts are used to limit ankle dorsiflexion, reducing the pain from anterior impingement.[24,33] Stiff shank, rocker-bottom shoes/soles can limit ankle motion and normalize gait.[24] They can be effective in the management of ankle arthritis but are more efficacious for midfoot arthritis. A solid ankle cushioned heel dampens heel strike and lessens rapid ankle plantar flexion during heel strike. Additionally, all of these modifications can be combined, such as a heel lift or a solid ankle cushioned heel and an Arizona or AFO brace.[33]

SURGICAL TREATMENT

If nonsurgical care fails to provide adequate pain relief or improve function to a reasonable level, surgical treatment can be considered. Determining the appropriate surgical procedure is an individual decision. Many factors should be considered, including patient demographic information such as age, level of function, desired level of function, and current radiographic studies. The etiology of the arthritis is important as well. For example, joint-preserving options are less effective in osteonecrosis of the talus. There should be an individualized plan that is agreeable to both the patient and surgeon that provides maximal relief and function from a single procedure and does not preclude salvage options. Joint-sparing procedures are listed in **Table 1**. Joint-sacrificing procedures such as allograft transplantation, ankle arthrodesis, or arthroplasty are usually reserved as the last line of treatment.

Joint Preservation Surgery
Synovectomy and Débridement
This surgical option is most effective for patients with predominantly anterior ankle arthritis or symptoms related to anterior impingement. Patients can present with a bony block or limited ankle ROM, or they may have anterior ankle pain with terminal dorsiflexion. There will also be radiographic evidence of a distal anterior tibial

Section 3: Arthritis of the Foot and Ankle

Table 1

Joint-Sparing Procedures

Arthroscopic or open débridement
Subchondral drilling
Osteochondral allografts for defects
Chondrocyte transplantation (autologous, juvenile particulate)
Periarticular osteotomy
Distraction arthroplasty
Interposition arthroplasty

osteophyte. Débridement for mild to moderate arthrosis with osteophytes, synovitis, loose bodies, and mechanical impingement is effective for pain relief and improvements in terminal dorsiflexion ROM[24,25] (**Figure 5**). Patients with rheumatoid arthritis, hemophilia, pigmented villonodular synovitis, and other soft-tissue pathologies may benefit from a simple synovectomy.[34] However, a 5-year survival analysis indicates that débridement is most effective in patients with predominantly anterior ankle impingement and minimal global arthritic changes.[34] In a study of outcomes after anterior débridement, it was found that none of the patients treated for anterior impingement required additional surgery at 5-year follow-up compared with 28% of those with degenerative changes.[34] This finding was independent of patient age.

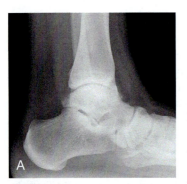
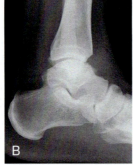
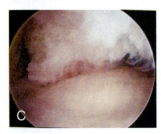
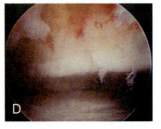

FIGURE 5 **A** and **B**, Preoperative and postoperative lateral radiographs, respectively, of anterior ankle impingement after an ankle arthroscopy and resection of the distal tibial anterior osteophyte. **C** and **D**, Preresection and postresection arthroscopic views, respectively, of the anterior distal tibia.

If there is any anterior talus translation, then this technique should not be used because removal of the anterior tibial lip can cause further anterior talus translation and progression of global arthritis.

Distraction Arthroplasty

Background

Distraction arthroplasty is an alternative to joint replacement procedures, best used in younger patients with arthritis. Ankle distraction arthroplasty was first popularized in 1995.[35] Distraction has been used in other joints with relative success.[36-38] This technique uses an Ilizarov-type external fixator to distract the ankle joint and relies on ligamentotaxis to restore normal joint space, offload the joint, and allow cartilage to recover.[36-38] The exact mechanism of its action is not known. Theories involve mechanical stress relief, continued intermittent intra-articular fluid pressure changes, and increased synovial fluid (thought to enhance chondrocyte reparative activity).[36,38-40] Distraction likely allows for fibrocartilage formation, which may seal cartilage defects and decrease pain from hydrostatic pressure on the subchondral bone.[36,37,41] Maintenance in the fixator for 3 months allows for a reduction of subchondral bone sclerosis, which has been linked to improved clinical outcomes.[36-38]

In vitro and animal studies have supported distraction for the arthritic ankle. It has been shown that chondrocytes have morphologic and biochemical changes when offloaded and when exposed to intermittent hydrostatic pressure changes.[35] Distraction has been shown to increase proteoglycan content in cartilage to near-normal states.[35,38,42] A study evaluating the effects of distraction in a canine model demonstrated a change and normalization of proteoglycan turnover, but failed to demonstrate actual cartilage repair in the short duration of the experiment.[42]

Indications for ankle distraction are a congruent joint, pain, joint mobility, and moderate to severe arthritis.[36,37] Some studies also have included osteonecrosis of the talus as an indication.[37] Ankle distraction is best used for patients who want to avoid an arthrodesis but are too young for arthroplasty. These patients have minimal angular deformity or can undergo concomitant correction. Contraindications for distraction include active infection, coronal plane deformity exceeding 10°, and substantial loss of bone stock.[37,38,43]

Controversy exists regarding the proper amount of distraction and the need for articulation to allow motion.[35,37,44] A study showed early and sustained improvement in patient outcomes with an articulating frame to facilitate ankle motion.[44] Some studies have advocated adjunctive procedures to increase motion, such as elimination of impingement and bony realignment to correct deformity.[37] Others have recommended arthroscopic or open débridement of the joint with synovectomy, loose body removal, and microfracture of exposed bone at the time of external fixator placement.[38,43]

Technique

The original distraction frame was described with the use of two tibial rings. The proximal ring was 5 cm below the knee, and the distal ring was 5 cm above the ankle. Each ring was fixed with two 1.5-mm Kirschner wires (K-wires) through the tibia placed at 90° to each other. The rings were connected with four screw-threaded rods. Two additional pins were then inserted into the calcaneus at 45° to each other. The K-wires were tensioned and fixed to a U-shaped foot ring. Two additional wires were placed into the metatarsals and fixed to a half ring over the forefoot after tensioning. The forefoot and U-shaped rings were then connected to make the foot plate. This foot plate must be dorsal to the equator of the foot to allow for weight bearing. The foot and tibia are then connected with four Ilizarov distraction rods. Distraction started on day 1 at the rate of 0.5 mm twice a day for 5 days, for a total of 5 mm of distraction. Weight bearing was encouraged within a few days of surgery.[39] Between 6 and 12 weeks, previously incorporated hinges were loosened to start motion (**Figure 6**). Later descriptions

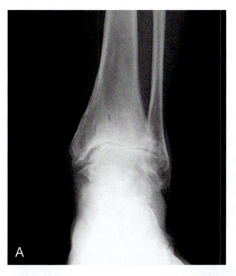
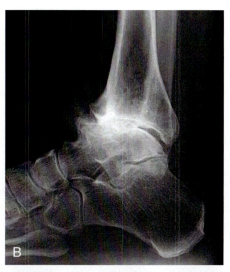
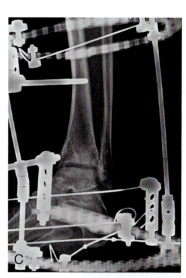
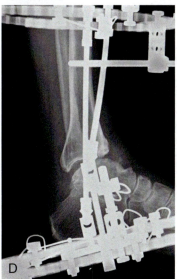
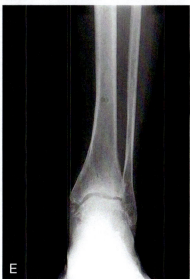
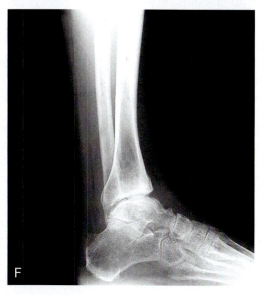

FIGURE 6 Radiographs from a 33-year-old woman with a history of ankle pilon fracture who underwent distraction arthroplasty. **A** and **B**, Preoperative AP and lateral radiographs, respectively. Note the substantial joint space narrowing and osteophyte formation. **C** and **D**, Perioperative radiographs showing the hinged external fixator in place; note the joint space created with maximal distraction. **E** and **F**, One-year postoperative AP and lateral radiographs, respectively, showing preservation of joint space and improvement of the tibial sclerosis.

of the frame added a talar neck pin attached to the foot plate to avoid distraction through the subtalar joint.[37] A study was performed to find the minimum distraction gap needed to ensure that the tibiotalar joint surfaces would not contact each other with full weight bearing while under distraction.[45] The minimum distraction gap was found to be 5.8 mm.

A variation on this technique that used a hinged external fixator that permitted ROM exercise was introduced in 2005.[36,37] The use of concomitant adjunctive procedures was advocated to increase the success rate of the procedure, such as removal of impinging osteophytes, release of joint contractures, correction of equinus deformity, and osseous alignment of the ankle. After application of the two tibial rings, a wire is inserted through the Inman ankle axis of rotation from the tip of the lateral malleolus to the tip of the medial malleolus. Placing this wire across this axis is essential to allow motion in the correct plane. Malposition of the hinges by 10 mm can increase resistance to motion more than fivefold.[46] Threaded rods with hinges are then applied medially and laterally from the distal tibial ring to intersect the axis wire. The medial hinge should be more proximal and anterior to the lateral hinge. The hinge is then connected to the foot ring that is parallel to the sole of the foot. A posterior distraction rod is then added, which can be removed for ROM exercises.

Pin care is performed twice daily with a 50% solution of hydrogen peroxide and saline.[38] Patients should be followed weekly or biweekly until removal of the fixator. The addition of a weight-bearing foot plate or fashioning of accommodative footwear is necessary to ensure compliance with weight bearing.

Results

Results from studies using static ankle distraction showed that 70% of patients experienced significant improvement in their pain with increased function.[35,39,47,48] Although joint motion was maintained, it was still considerably diminished when compared with the unaffected ankle.[35,39,47,48] There was also a progressive increase in joint mobility, widening of the joint, and diminished subchondral sclerosis during the first 5 years after the procedure.[35,38,42,47,49,50]

With the addition of an anatomically located hinge to allow for ROM exercises, it was reported that 78% of a cohort had only occasional mild to moderate pain.[37,41] However, it was noted that after 5 years, the outcome scores significantly decreased; it was concluded that the benefits of distraction treatment decrease after 5 years.[35,37,38,42,47,49,50] A 2019 study examined results after distraction arthroplasty at an average of 4.57 years. Overall, the 5-year survival rate after surgery was 84%. Worse results were seen in patients with osteonecrosis of the talus, leading to the conclusion that caution should be taken in patients with osteonecrosis.[51] Most importantly, the use of distraction arthroplasty does not cause worse results with future surgeries.

The most common complication with distraction arthroplasty is pin tract infections, which can occur in more than 30% of patients. This can often be managed with localized wound care and oral antibiotics.[49]

Periarticular (Supramalleolar) Osteotomies
Background
Any deformity of the ankle joint can lead to abnormal mechanical loads and further degeneration.[11,52-54] Deformity in any plane exceeding 10° should be corrected.[55,56] Recent studies have shown that supramalleolar distal tibial osteotomies are performed to restore anatomic alignment and improve biomechanics by redistributing the joint load onto intact articular cartilage.[55,56]

Patients with minimal ankle OA with substantial varus or valgus deformity may benefit from a periarticular osteotomy.[25] Nonunions and malunions of previous fractures can lead to increased articular loads and pain. These patients may simply benefit from revision of their fixation and realignment if their ankle joint remains salvageable. The osteotomy should be performed at or near the prior fracture line.

With a flexible hindfoot, the ankle is able to tolerate certain amounts of deformity. The subtalar joint is crucial in compensating for any coronal plane deformity. The compensation of these joints can lead to arthritis. Because there is approximately 20° of inversion compared with only 5° of eversion allowed through the subtalar complex, a valgus ankle deformity is much better tolerated than a varus deformity.[57] Consequently, it is critical that any patient being evaluated for a realignment osteotomy be examined for subtalar joint and hindfoot motion, which helps to assess their ability to compensate for the osteotomy. According to a 2020 study, patients with a stiff or misaligned hindfoot should undergo hindfoot realignment concomitantly with the supramalleolar osteotomy.[55]

The goals of periarticular osteotomies are to restore normal TAS and TLS angles. Slight overcorrection is recommended at the time of surgery to allow for some settling.[55] The center of rotation and angulation can be determined by intersecting the mechanical axis of the proximal and distal segments of the tibia. If the osteotomy is performed at the center of rotation and angulation, then the deformity can be corrected without any translation of the distal fragment. However, if the osteotomy needs to be above or below the center of rotation and angulation (as in an intra-articular deformity), the distal fragment must be translated relative to the mechanical axis to avoid a secondary translational deformity.

Multiple osteotomies, fixation methods, and approaches have been described, including opening and closing wedge osteotomies, dome osteotomies, intra-articular osteotomies, and plafondplasty.[2,53,54,58-60] The type and location of the osteotomy are best determined by the surgeon. Varus arthritis/deformity is commonly managed with a medial opening wedge tibial osteotomy. A fibular osteotomy is often required as well, especially if the correction requires more than 10°. Valgus arthritis/deformity is typically managed with a medial closing wedge osteotomy and an oblique fibular lengthening osteotomy. One study recommends a tibial dome osteotomy for varus or valgus deformities greater than 15°.[61] This prevents the excessive translation of the talus in opening wedge osteotomies and shortening of the tibia in closing wedge osteotomies. Although these techniques are described for deformities originating from the ankle joint (eg, varus ankle from lateral ligamentous laxity), the study authors prefer to perform supramalleolar osteotomies when the deformity originates from the tibia.

There are theoretical advantages to each type of osteotomy. For example, a closing wedge osteotomy allows for direct bone contact with the need for an interposition graft. This will allow for earlier bone healing and faster time to initiate weight bearing. An opening wedge osteotomy, on the hand, prevents shortening that can be seen with closing wedge osteotomies.

Both of these osteotomies can be used to correct multiplanar deformities. The wedges, although based medially or laterally, can be directed anteriorly or posteriorly to address sagittal plane deformity. Dome osteotomies, while powerful coronal plane deformity, cannot correct multiplanar or sagittal deformities and cannot be translated. The choice of osteotomy, graft, and fixation should be individualized based on the condition of the soft tissues, history or suspicion of infection, and limb-length discrepancy.

Brief Technique

Patients are positioned supine with an ipsilateral hip bump. If a fibular osteotomy is required, it is performed at the level of the planned tibial osteotomy through a lateral incision. This technique has been described in detail.[52,59] A medial osteotomy is usually performed through a medial longitudinal incision, and a lateral osteotomy is typically performed through the same incision as the fibular osteotomy. Care is taken to avoid excessive stripping and soft-tissue tension.

For opening wedge osteotomies, whether medial or lateral, a K-wire is inserted parallel to the ankle joint as a cutting guide. The osteotomy is performed using a sagittal saw with irrigation to avoid thermal injury to the bone. Alternatively, multiple drill holes can be used. The opposite cortex is left intact. An osteotome is used to greenstick the osteotomy, and a lamina spreader is used to spread the osteotomy until the distal TAS is parallel to the floor or slightly overcorrected. An iliac crest structural autograft or tricortical allograft is then inserted and fixation is obtained (**Figure 7**).

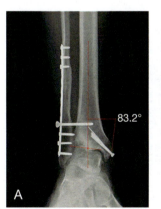 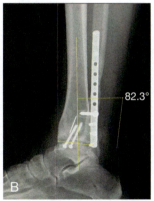 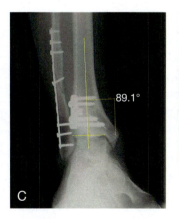 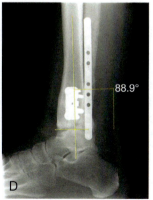

FIGURE 7 Radiographs from a 38-year-old man after sustaining an ankle fracture-dislocation with open reduction and internal fixation. Note that this patient appears to have continued shortening of the fibula and collapse of the lateral aspect of the tibial plafond. **A** and **B**, AP and lateral radiographs, respectively, before revision surgery showing the tibial articular surface (TAS) angle and tibial lateral surface (TLS) angle. **C** and **D**, AP and lateral radiographs, respectively, after fibular osteotomy and lengthening through his existing fibular plate. The same lateral incision was used to approach the lateral aspect of the tibia to perform the opening wedge osteotomy with an opening wedge plate. Note the normalization of the TAS and TLS angles.

A closing wedge osteotomy is performed by inserting two converging K-wires that meet at the opposite cortex, with one parallel to the ankle joint and the other perpendicular to the mechanical axis of the proximal tibia. The osteotomy is then performed along the K-wires. The wedge of bone created is removed and the osteotomy compressed and fixed.

A dome osteotomy is performed through an anterolateral incision. A K-wire is used to mark the plane of the ankle joint. A drill is then used to make multiple holes in the metaphyseal bone in a dome pattern with the dome height at 1 to 1.5 cm. Two 4-mm pins are inserted into each fragment, with the distal pin being parallel to the ankle joint and the proximal pin perpendicular to the proximal mechanical axis. The osteotomy is then completed with a sagittal saw or osteotome, and the pins are made parallel before fixation.

Results

Multiple studies have shown that periarticular osteotomies are a viable option for managing various types of ankle arthritis when various osteotomy techniques are used.[2,11,53,54,60,62] Investigators showed their use in both primary and posttraumatic arthritis with favorable results.[53,58] The study authors attributed their few unsatisfied patients to undercorrection of the deformity and noted stiffness and decreased ROM in the posttraumatic group. One study compared medial opening and closing wedge osteotomies and showed faster time to union with closing wedge osteotomies as well as halted progression of arthritic changes during their 33-month follow-up.[2] Another study reported on the use of external fixation and a percutaneous drilling osteotomy with good results, although the external fixator was used for an average of 5 months.[62] Researchers used a medial opening wedge osteotomy for varus primary ankle arthritis and reported good or excellent results in 20 of 26 ankles at a mean follow-up longer than 8 years.[54] They compared patients with and without involvement of the talar medial dome and found worse outcomes in ankles with talar involvement. Other studies have demonstrated that the results of supramalleolar osteotomies are worse with congruent ankles and when degenerative changes in the medial gutter were present.[54,63]

Osteotomy complications are infrequent, with stiffness being the most commonly reported complication.[2,53] Delayed unions, nonunions, pin site infections, wound breakdown, and superficial or deep infections have also been reported.[2,53,54,58,60,62] Hardware-related complications that necessitated removal were more problematic with the use of medial hardware.[11,54,60]

Joint-Sacrificing Surgery

Allograft Arthroplasty

Background

Allografts have been used successfully in the knee, and there is increasing use of allografts in tibiotalar arthritis. Good outcomes have been reported with osteochondral allografts for small to large talar dome defects.[64-66] The use of bipolar osteochondral joint allografts in the management of end-stage ankle arthritis has been limited. A theoretical advantage of allograft arthroplasty is maintenance of bone, but modern ankle replacement techniques remove much less bone than prior iterations.

The most important concern in allograft transplantation is chondrocyte survival, particularly during the cold storage process.[67,68] It is important to note that frozen grafts should not be used. More than 80% of transplanted chondrocytes can survive in recovered cartilage.[68] The mechanical properties of the matrix are also maintained.[68] Chondrocytes have been shown to survive the transplantation process primarily because cartilage is avascular and predominantly is dependent on synovial fluid for nourishment.[67] Transplanted chondrocytes are not replaced by host chondrocytes. In a long-term retrieval case report in which female donor cartilage was implanted into a male recipient, the retrieved cartilage at 29 years continued to express female chromosomes.[69]

The time from harvest of the donor to implantation has profound effects on the viability of the chondrocytes. In a study of specimens stored fewer than 14 days, there was no decrease in chondrocyte viability or density; when tested beyond 28 days, specimens showed significant loss of chondrocytes.[68] These losses were most notable in the important superficial zone of the cartilage.[67] Cold storage in fetal bovine serum and gradual rewarming in a nitric oxide synthase inhibitor also help to increase chondrocyte viability and proteoglycan synthesis and reverse the metabolic suppression of cold storage.[67] In addition to chondrocyte viability, the potential for bone collapse is present as well. As the allograft bone incorporates, it is replaced by host bone through creeping substitution.[67] During the revascularization period, there is increased risk for graft collapse.

The use of any allograft tissue offers the risk of disease transmission from the donor. There have been no cases of disease transmission from allograft arthroplasty; regardless, this risk should be discussed with patients.

Surgical Technique

The patient is placed supine with an ipsilateral hip bump. An anterior approach to the ankle is performed through a midline incision using the interval between the tibialis anterior and the extensor hallucis longus. The neurovascular bundle is identified and retracted laterally, and synovectomy and anterior osteophyte débridement is performed. A joint distraction device is applied to increase exposure.

A total ankle arthroplasty (TAA) tibial cutting block is applied and fluoroscopically confirmed to ensure appropriate positioning and then fixed to the tibia. The distal tibia and medial malleolus are cut using a sagittal saw. The talar cut is then made with or without the aid of a cutting jig, depending on the thickness of the planned cut. The resection from each side of the joint should be between 4 and 10 mm, depending on the amount of bone loss. Any cystic lesions are filled with autograft from the resected plafond and talar dome.

The donor allograft is cut in the same manner using a guide one size larger than that used for the host. This ensures that the tibial graft is not too thin and does not lead to fracture. The donor talus cut is done freehand. Each graft then undergoes pulsed lavage to remove any marrow elements and debris. The graft is then placed into the host and verified fluoroscopically; the external fixator is removed; and the ankle is ranged to ensure the grafts find their preferred position. The grafts are fixed with two headless or countersunk screws each (**Figure 8**).

Postoperatively, patients are in a non–weight-bearing splint until suture removal at 2 weeks. They are then transitioned to a controlled ankle motion boot and allowed to work on ROM but do not bear weight. At 6 weeks, patients are allowed to begin partial weight bearing until 12 weeks or until the graft is incorporated, at which time they are allowed full weight bearing. High-impact activities should be limited.

Results of Allograft Arthroplasty

A study reported a 42% failure rate at 148 months in seven patients with posttraumatic ankle arthritis who underwent allograft replacement.[70] However, it was noted that radiographic and clinical results may not correlate, attributing failures to graft fragmentation, subluxation, poor graft fit, and nonunions. These procedures were performed with freehand cuts. One study reported on nine patients with bipolar allografts with no failures at 21 months using the Agility (DePuy) total ankle cutting guides.[71] There was one allograft failure in a partial unipolar lateral talar dome. In another study by the same group,[71] only 6 of 11 allografts survived at 33 months. Three failures were revised to a repeat allograft, one to a TAA, and one had not yet been revised. Investigators also showed a correlation between graft thickness and survival, with grafts smaller than 7 mm showing poorer results. Six failures at a 2-year follow-up were reported in a cohort of 32 patients.[72]

One of the largest populations and longest follow-up studies of patients who underwent ankle allograft replacement was conducted, although it is unclear how many of these patients were included in previous studies by the same group.[73] At a mean follow-up of 5.3 years on 86 ankles (82 patients), there was a revision surgery rate of 42% and a failure rate of 29%, with a mean time to failure of 3.7 years. The study authors defined failure as any revision surgery in which the graft was replaced; however, some patients underwent distraction arthrodiastasis for arthritic changes in the grafts, and these patients were not considered part of the failure group. The failure group included 10 patients who underwent revision allografting, 7 who were revised to arthrodesis, 6 who had TAAs, and 2 who underwent transtibial amputations. Survivorship of the allograft was reported as 76% at 5 years and 44% at 10 years. However, 92% of the patients reported satisfaction with the procedure, 85% reported improvement in their pain, and 83% reported improved function.

Although these results reflect a higher failure rate than those of arthrodesis or arthroplasty,[74] allograft arthroplasty remains a viable alternative for the management of end-stage ankle arthritis. This remains an option for patients who are too young for a traditional arthroplasty and seek to avoid ankle arthrodesis because of long-term complications and those with contralateral ankle arthritis or hindfoot arthrosis.

Ankle Arthrodesis

Ankle arthrodesis is considered by many authors as the preferred surgical management of ankle arthritis.[1,24,75,76] Although ankle replacement is increasing in its use and its outcomes, ankle arthrodesis remains a successful surgical procedure. Although it is arguably the most reliable and reproducible form of pain relief in end-stage ankle arthritis, the development of adjacent joint arthritis remains the largest dissatisfier.[7,76,77] The development of arthritis in adjacent joints in the hindfoot was estimated to occur in as many as 50% of patients within 7 to 8 years and 100% of patients within 22 years.[77] The development of adjacent joint arthritis is likely from joint overload. One study demonstrated increased subtalar and talonavicular joint motion in cadavers after simulated ankle arthrodesis.[78] The study postulated that the increased biomechanical burden may lead to degeneration. Another study highlighted the increased ROM that occurs through the talonavicular joint after an ankle arthrodesis.[79]

Functionally, patients who undergo arthrodesis often experience difficulty navigating uneven terrain and inclines, pain with rigorous activities, and increased contact stress at the talonavicular and calcaneocuboid

Section 3: Arthritis of the Foot and Ankle

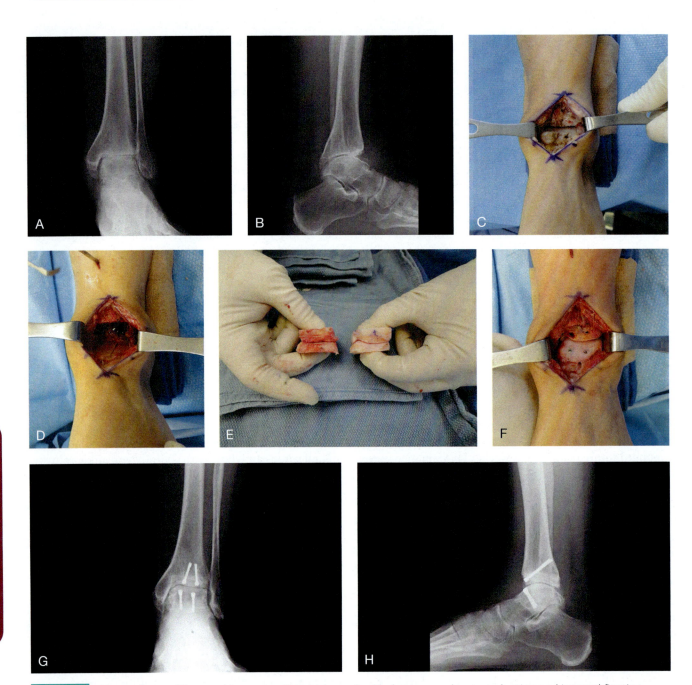

FIGURE 8 Images from a 38-year-old woman with a history of ankle fracture and open reduction and internal fixation. **A** and **B**, AP and lateral radiographs, respectively, showing angular deformity and end-stage arthritis with joint space loss. **C**, Intraoperative anterior approach photograph showing significant degenerative changes. **D**, Photograph of anterior view showing the defect after the resection of the distal tibia and talus. **E**, Intraoperative photograph of the patient's match graft (left) and the donor allograft (right). **F**, Photograph of anterior ankle view showing the allograft in place. **G** and **H**, AP and lateral radiographs, respectively, from the patient 3 years postoperatively. Radiographs show well-incorporated bony interface with some joint space narrowing.

joints.[76,80] Loss of up to 74% of sagittal, 70% of inversion, and 77% of eversion motion has been noted after successful arthrodesis.[81] Additionally, patients with an arthrodesis experience a 16% decrease in gait velocity, a 3% increase in oxygen consumption, and a 10% decrease in gait efficiency. These numbers must be considered in the context of ankle arthritis. In end-stage arthritis, there already is loss of motion at the ankle joint, which leads to loss of function. If deformity is present preoperatively, there is often improvement in gait once that deformity is corrected through the ankle fusion.

The clinical results of ankle arthrodesis have been favorable overall. Symptom relief is highly reliable and more than 90% of patients are satisfied with their outcomes.[74,75,77,81,82] When compared with supramalleolar osteotomy, for example, patients with ankle arthrodesis had better pain relief, superior function, and improved alignment at midterm follow-up according to a 2022 study.[83]

The position of the arthrodesis is vital for good long-term performance. The optimal position for arthrodesis of the ankle is 5° of valgus, 5° to 10° of external rotation, neutral to 5° dorsiflexion, and approximately 5 mm of posterior offset to improve the lever arm of the calcaneus.[24,84]

There are many methods and techniques that can be used for a successful ankle arthrodesis. These can include both open and arthroscopic; different approaches such as anterior, lateral, and posterior; and different methods of fixation.[24]

Internal and external fixation techniques have been described. In the absence of open wounds or infections, internal fixation is typically preferred because of a patient's dissatisfaction with an external fixator. Compression screws and lateral, anterior, or posterior plating are all options for fixation. Crossed screws form a stronger construct than parallel screws but may prevent compression if not performed sequentially.[85,86] Some authors have advocated that the most important screw is one that is placed from the posterior malleolus into the talar neck and head and is referred to as the home run screw.[87] Alternatively, screws can be placed through the medial or lateral malleoli or both.

Complications following arthrodesis involve wound healing, infection, neurovascular injuries, complex regional pain syndrome, venous thromboembolic events, nonunion, or malunion. Most early-onset complications can be avoided with careful patient selection, recognition of high-risk patients, careful dissection, and careful handling and repair of the soft tissues. Aggressive early treatment is necessary for any suspected infection or wound complication.

Overall, union rates for ankle arthrodesis are quite favorable. Although there are historic reports of up to 60% nonunion, most recent studies using modern fixation demonstrate union rates over 87%. Most studies examining the success of ankle arthrodesis include all patient types. Many of these are patients who are considered poor hosts or have significant prior ankle surgeries or deformity, which necessitates arthrodesis over arthroplasty. A large retrospective meta-analysis demonstrated a nonunion rate of 7.9%.[88] Patients with peripheral neuropathy, osteonecrosis of the talus, prior or current deep infections, open injuries, talar dome or pilon fractures, prior subtalar arthrodesis, spasticity, smoking history, and various medical problems are at higher risk for nonunion.[24,89]

Malunions can be quite problematic. Plantar flexion malunions can lead to a vaulting gait pattern and a recurvatum thrust and degeneration at the knee. This may eventually lead to medial collateral ligament failure attributable to an externally rotated gait resulting from attempts to place the foot flat on the ground. Furthermore, stress fractures and metatarsalgia may develop. Dorsiflexion malunions lead to increased pressure on the heel pad and ulcers or a flexed knee gait. Coronal plane deformities usually lead to ligamentous laxity and added stress on the nearby joints and musculotendinous units leading to early degeneration. Valgus malunions are more tolerated than varus malunions because the subtalar joint can compensate for the valgus position of the talus.

Arthroscopic Technique

Arthroscopic ankle arthrodesis is a minimally invasive technique for patients with minimal deformity.[82,90,91] It has been shown to lead to faster fusion rates than open procedures, likely because of decreased tissue stripping and retention of the blood supply.[82,90-92] Fixation is usually obtained with crossing screws, placed percutaneously. During arthroscopic débridement, a noninvasive distractor can be used instead of an external fixator, which has been shown to be associated with more complications.[93] Positioning and fixation are performed under fluoroscopic guidance. With the advent of newer arthroscopic débridement instruments, arthroscopic ankle arthrodesis has become easier and less time consuming (**Figure 9**).

The major advantages of the arthroscopic technique are significantly less morbidity, shorter surgical and tourniquet times, less blood loss, shorter hospital stays, and better improvement in outcome scores for up to 2 years postoperatively.[90-92] The technique produces similar fusion rates compared with open techniques with minimal complications.[87,91-94] A contraindication to this procedure may be substantial preoperative deformity, which may make final positioning extremely difficult and limit the use of this technique; guidelines for the amount of deformity that is tolerated for arthroscopic arthrodesis have not been established.[82] A study that demonstrated the success with ankle arthrodesis elected for open ankle arthrodesis instead of arthroscopic ankle arthrodesis in patients with tibial plafond angles greater than 19°.[95]

A 2022 comparative study examining open and arthroscopic ankle arthrodesis in high-risk patients identified higher union rates, lower complications, and fewer revision surgeries in the arthroscopic arthrodesis group.[96]

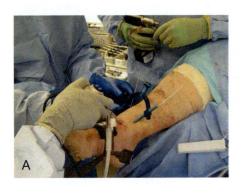 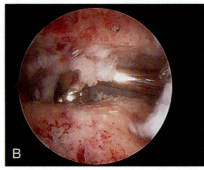 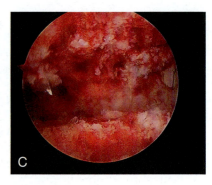

FIGURE 9 **A**, Intraoperative photograph showing noninvasive ankle distraction; also note the intra-articular targeting system with guidewires in place before fixation. **B**, Intra-articular arthroscopic view showing curettage of the joint space. **C**, Intra-articular arthroscopic view after complete preparation; note the guide pin for fixation in the upper left corner.

Open Technique

Various approaches have been described for arthrodesis of the ankle, including anterior, lateral transfibular with or without an accessory medial incision, and posterior approaches. Traditionally, the lateral transfibular approach with partial resection of the fibula was the most popular. The fibula should be maintained if there is a future potential for conversion to ankle arthroplasty. Because most patients who undergo ankle arthrodesis are not candidates for ankle replacement, partial fibula resection is still a viable option. According to recent studies, the anterior approach has gained in popularity.[97,98] This is performed through the interval between the anterior tibialis tendon and extensor hallucis longus. The neurovascular bundle is retracted laterally. The technique allows the use of a single incision to approach both the medial and lateral gutter, preserves the fibula, and makes use of the same incision used for most TAAs for possible later conversion. However, this approach places the neurovascular bundle and the superficial peroneal nerve at risk. Although it is difficult to reach the posterior aspect of the joint for débridement and it also may be difficult to reduce the talus under the tibia, these challenges have not been known to affect the excellent results achieved with this approach (**Figure 10**).

The lateral approach necessitates a fibular osteotomy to access the ankle joint. Traditionally, the fibula was morcellized or used as an onlay graft. Preserving the fibula allows for the potential of a total ankle replacement in the future. A posterior approach may be carried out by splitting the Achilles tendon, performing a long Z-shaped tenotomy of the Achilles tendon, or performing a calcaneal osteotomy of the insertion of the Achilles tendon and reflecting it superiorly. Although used primarily for tibiotalocalcaneal (TTC) arthrodesis, the posterior approach can be used for an isolated ankle arthrodesis if needed.

The mini-open approach was developed to provide the same advantages as an arthroscopic technique, which involves less soft-tissue stripping and quicker time to fusion.[94] It is performed through anteromedial and anterolateral incisions, which are essentially extended arthroscopic portals and are in the same intervals. The superficial peroneal nerve is at risk with an anterolateral incision.

The ankle joint can be prepared in multiple configurations, including simple denuding of the cartilage and subchondral plate while maintaining the congruent curved surfaces, which is the current preferred method. Alternatively, parallel flat cuts can be performed at the apex of the tibia and 5 mm below the apex of the talus.[99] This leads to slight shortening of the limb but is usually well tolerated. Technically, however, this can lead to difficulty determining the exact arthrodesis position rotationally and anterior or posterior translation of the talus relative to the tibia. To avoid this challenge, the use of matching chevron cuts has been described in the tibia and talus.[100] An anterior or posterior sliding tibial, medial, and/or lateral malleoli onlay grafting have also been reported.[24]

Results

Midterm and long-term outcomes of ankle arthrodesis are favorable. One study reported on 72 ankle arthrodeses at a mean follow-up of 4.8 years and found a 99% fusion rate.[101] Another study reported on 60 patients (66 ankles) with a mean follow-up of 9 years. There was a 91% primary arthrodesis rate.[102] The remaining six patients achieved fusion after a second arthrodesis

Chapter 8: Ankle Arthritis: Part I. Joint Preservation Techniques and Arthrodesis

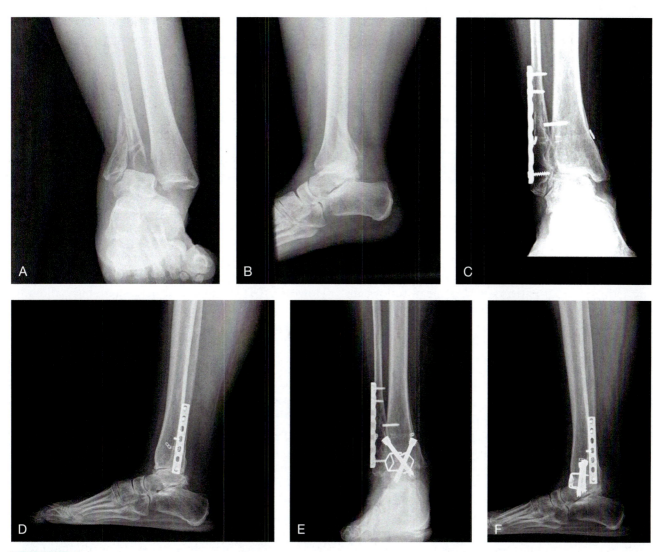

FIGURE 10 Radiographs from a 56-year-old woman with a history of ankle fracture and open reduction and internal fixation with end-stage ankle arthritis. **A** and **B**, AP and lateral radiographs, respectively, at the time of her original fracture-dislocation. **C** and **D**, AP and lateral radiographs, respectively, 3 year after injury showing significant posttraumatic arthritis. **E** and **F**, AP and lateral radiographs, respectively, after an ankle arthrodesis. Crossed headless screws are the preferred vernacular for this treatment.

procedure. Although a downside to ankle arthrodesis is altered gait, a study demonstrated that ankle arthrodesis improves multiple temporal-spatial, kinematic, and kinetic measures, including step length and velocity, over preoperative gait in patients with ankle arthritis.[103]

One study compared the anterior and transfibular approaches and found no differences in the American Orthopaedic Foot and Ankle Society scores.[98] The anterior approach had a longer time to fusion and a slightly higher nonunion rate, but these issues were not significant. There are no data to support one approach over another, and therefore, the approach should be at the discretion of the surgeon based on previous incisions/wounds and any hardware removal needed.

Hardware fixation has been the topic of many reports. Screw fixation alone has achieved a 99% union rate.[101] A cadaver study demonstrated that anterior plate supplementation increased construct rigidity and decreased micromotion at the ankle fusion interface.[104] In one study, compression screws alone versus compression screws supplemented with anterior plate fixation were compared.[105] Expectedly, the nonunion rate in the compression screw–only cohort was 15.4% versus only 7.7% when anterior plate augmentation was used. These rates were not significantly different but were likely based on the numbers in each cohort. Similar to the approach, there is no conclusive evidence to recommend one hardware construct over another.

One of the major problems with arthrodesis is the potential for nonunion. One study identified risk factors affecting union and found that nonunion was significantly more likely to occur with previous ipsilateral subtalar fusion and preoperative varus alignment.[106] Progression of adjacent joint (subtalar and/or talonavicular) disease following ankle arthrodesis is one reason ankle arthroplasty may be more favorable. In a study of 66 ankle fusions, significant radiologic progression of arthritis was reported in all adjacent joints.[102] Additionally, another study reported adjacent joint arthritis in 23 patients with a mean follow-up of 22 years.[77] It was found that moderate to severe arthritis developed in 91% and 57% of subtalar and talonavicular joints, respectively. However, the clinical significance of adjacent joint disease progression is unknown.

Salvage of Failed TAA

With the rising number of TAAs performed, the number of failed arthroplasties will also increase. Ten-year TAA survival ranges between 63% and 91%.[74] Although newer implants and techniques may improve the survival rate, the expanding indications for deformity correction with TAA may lead to an increase in instability and subsidence. Consequently, the need for likely conversion to an arthrodesis will remain.

When a TAA becomes infected, treatment should be staged, with the first stage including removal of all implants, irrigation and débridement, an antibiotic spacer if needed, temporary stabilization, and long-term intravenous antibiotic use based on intraoperative cultures. This is followed by arthrodesis, preferably using external fixation and bone grafting.

In noninfectious failed TAA with minimal bone loss, a single-stage procedure is recommended. With minimal bone loss, a revision arthroplasty may be attempted. However, if unsalvageable, isolated ankle fusion should be attempted. Multiple studies have demonstrated favorable results with high fusion rates for primary conversion arthrodesis after failed TAA with minimal bone loss.[107,108]

When significant bone loss is present after removal of the TAA, a TTC fusion with bulk grafting may be performed. TTC fusion following failed TAA is fraught with complications. The procedure carries a much higher nonunion rate than primary arthrodesis and higher risk for complications. With the use of autograft bone, fusion rates of 20% to 93% have been reported.[108] The use of an intramedullary TTC nail was shown to increase the union rate over compression screws.[108] However, TTC fusions that necessitate bulk allograft such as a femoral head allograft are associated with nonunion rates as high as 50%; nonunions developed in all of the patients with diabetes, and 19% of nonunions eventually resulted in transtibial amputation[109] (**Figures 11** and **12**).

ACUTE ANKLE ARTHRODESIS

According to a 2020 study, intra-articular distal tibia fractures have a high rate of development of ankle arthritis.[110] As discussed in a 2022 study, in elderly patients and patients with diabetes and peripheral neuropathy, these fractures carry a high rate of complications in the acute management, in addition to long-term ankle arthritis.[111] Acute arthrodesis offers the long-term definitive management, avoiding the long-term sequelae of development of ankle arthritis. There is a high union rate with acute arthrodesis. A systematic review reported a 94.5% union rate with acute TTC arthrodesis. Specifically looking at patients with diabetic neuropathy, a 2020 study reported an acceptable union rate in a high-risk population.[112]

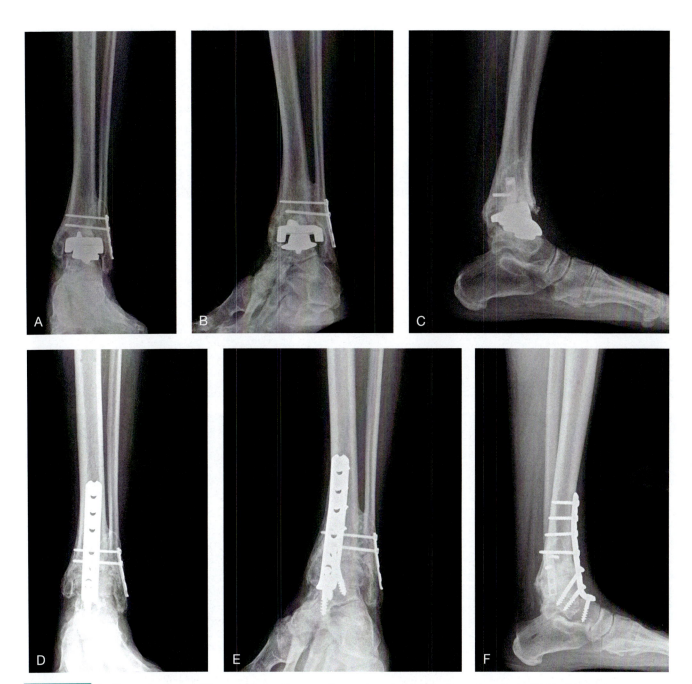

FIGURE 11 Radiographs from a 67-year-old man 2 years after undergoing total ankle arthroplasty (TAA) with previous attempted bone grafting and revision who continues to have pain and significant functional limitations. **A** through **C**, AP, mortise, and lateral radiographs, respectively, showing the substantial subsidence and lucency of both the tibial and talar components. The lateral radiograph shows the substantial anterior distal tibial bone loss and subsidence. **D** through **F**, Mortise, AP, and lateral radiographs, respectively, 18 months after surgery. The patient underwent removal of the TAA with aggressive débridement. The defect was filled with a femoral head allograft and an ankle arthrodesis was performed with an anterior arthrodesis plate. Currently, the patient is ambulating with a rocker-bottom shoe without pain.

Section 3: Arthritis of the Foot and Ankle

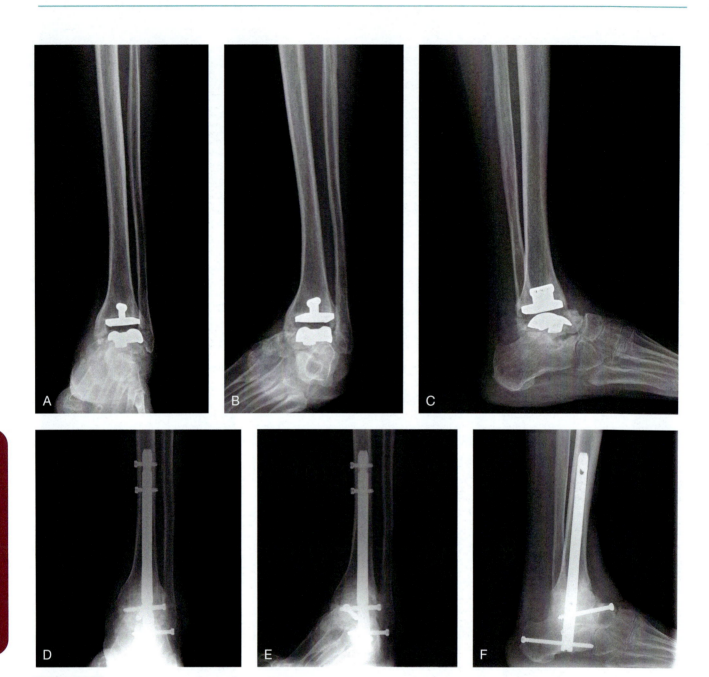

FIGURE 12 Radiographs from a 65-year-old woman after total ankle arthroplasty. Substantial talar component subsidence and pain developed within 1 year. **A** through **C**, AP, mortise, and lateral radiographs, respectively, showing the substantial subsidence (best seen on the lateral) of the talar component. **D** through **F**, AP, mortise, and lateral radiographs, respectively, 30 months after a revision to a pantalar arthrodesis. A femoral head allograft was used to fill the defect and prevent substantial limb shortening. A tibiotalar-calcaneal retrograde rod was used.

SUMMARY

The ankle is a highly congruent joint that experiences large forces through a small surface area. Ankle arthritis can be debilitating. The treatment algorithm should consider all factors including age, activity level, etiology, alignment, history, comorbidities, and physical examination and radiographic findings. Surgical treatment strategies include débridement, distraction arthroplasty, interposition arthroplasty, osteotomies, reconstruction, allograft arthroplasty, arthrodesis, and arthroplasty. Further research is necessary to elucidate the optimal treatment strategies and best candidates and to advance current implant constructs and techniques.

KEY STUDY POINTS

- Posttraumatic OA is the most common form of arthritis affecting the ankle.
- Nonsurgical management of ankle arthritis includes NSAIDs, injections, and brace treatment.
- Surgical management of ankle arthritis is divided into joint-sparing and joint-sacrificing procedures.
- Joint-sparing procedures including débridement, distraction arthroplasty, and supramalleolar osteotomy are mainly reserved for mild or moderate ankle arthritis.
- Joint-sacrificing procedures including allograft resurfacing and ankle arthrodesis are reserved for end-stage arthritis.
- Ankle arthrodesis is a viable treatment option for failed ankle arthroplasty.

ANNOTATED REFERENCES

1. Thomas R, Daniels TR: Ankle arthritis. *J Bone Joint Surg Am* 2003;85(5):923-936.

2. Stamatis ED, Cooper PS, Myerson MS: Supramalleolar osteotomy for the treatment of distal tibial angular deformities and arthritis of the ankle joint. *Foot Ankle Int* 2003;24(10):754-764.

3. Stamatis ED, Myerson MS: Supramalleolar osteotomy: Indications and technique. *Foot Ankle Clin* 2003;8(2):317-333.

4. Valderrabano V, Horisberger M, Russell I, Dougall H, Hintermann B: Etiology of ankle osteoarthritis. *Clin Orthop Relat Res* 2009;467(7):1800-1806.

5. Saltzman CL, Salamon ML, Blanchard GM, et al: Epidemiology of ankle arthritis: Report of a consecutive series of 639 patients from a tertiary orthopaedic center. *Iowa Orthop J* 2005;25:44-46.

6. Buett R: Forces predicted at the ankle during running. *Med Sci Sports Exerc* 1982;14:308.

7. Daniels T, Thomas R: Etiology and biomechanics of ankle arthritis. *Foot Ankle Clin* 2008;13(3):341-352, vii.

8. Thomas AC, Hubbard-Turner T, Wikstrom EA, Palmieri-Smith RM: Epidemiology of posttraumatic osteoarthritis. *J Athl Train* 2017;52(6):491-496.

9. Huch K, Kuettner KE, Dieppe P: Osteoarthritis in ankle and knee joints. *Semin Arthritis Rheum* 1997;26(4):667-674.

10. Lindsjö U: Operative treatment of ankle fracture-dislocations. A follow-up study of 306/321 consecutive cases. *Clin Orthop Relat Res* 1985;199:28-38.

11. Harstall R, Lehmann O, Krause F, Weber M: Supramalleolar lateral closing wedge osteotomy for the treatment of varus ankle arthrosis. *Foot Ankle Int* 2007;28(5):542-548.

12. Marsh JL, Buckwalter J, Gelberman R, et al: Articular fractures: Does an anatomic reduction really change the result? *J Bone Joint Surg Am* 2002;84(7):1259-1271.

13. Segal AD, Shofer J, Hahn ME, Orendurff MS, Ledoux WR, Sangeorzan BJ: Functional limitations associated with end-stage ankle arthritis. *J Bone Joint Surg Am* 2012;94(9):777-783.

14. Hendren L, Beeson P: A review of the differences between normal and osteoarthritis articular cartilage in human knee and ankle joints. *Foot (Edinb)* 2009;19(3):171-176.

15. Adams SB, Setton LA, Bell RD, et al: Inflammatory cytokines and matrix metalloproteinases in the synovial fluid after intra-articular ankle fracture. *Foot Ankle Int* 2015;36(11):1264-1271.

16. Holzer N, Salvo D, Marijnissen AC, et al: Radiographic evaluation of posttraumatic osteoarthritis of the ankle: The Kellgren–Lawrence scale is reliable and correlates with clinical symptoms. *Osteoarthritis Cartilage* 2015;23(3):363-369.

17. Fukawa T, Yamaguchi S, Akatsu Y, Yamamoto Y, Akagi R, Sasho T: Safety and efficacy of intra-articular injection of platelet-rich plasma in patients with ankle osteoarthritis. *Foot Ankle Int* 2017;38(6):596-604.

18. Latt LD, Glisson RR, Montijo HE, Usuelli FG, Easley ME: Effect of graft height mismatch on contact pressures with osteochondral grafting of the talus. *Am J Sports Med* 2011;39(12):2662-2669.

19. Bigouette J, Simon J, Liu K, Docherty CL: Altered vertical ground reaction forces in participants with chronic ankle instability while running. *J Athl Train* 2016;51(9):682-687.

20. Thevendran G, Younger A, Pinney S: Current concepts review: Risk factors for nonunions in foot and ankle arthrodeses. *Foot Ankle Int* 2012;33(11):1031-1040.

21. Stuart MJ, Morrey BF: Arthrodesis of the diabetic neuropathic ankle joint. *Clin Orthop Relat Res* 1990;253:209-211.

22. Kraus VB, Kilfoil TM, Hash TW 2nd, et al: Atlas of radiographic features of osteoarthritis of the ankle and hindfoot. *Osteoarthritis Cartilage* 2015;23(12):2059-2085.

23. Saltzman CL, El-Khoury GY: The hindfoot alignment view. *Foot Ankle Int* 1995;16(9):572-576.

24. Katcherian DA: Treatment of ankle arthrosis. *Clin Orthop Relat Res* 1998;349:48-57.

25. Demetriades L, Strauss E, Gallina J: Osteoarthritis of the ankle. *Clin Orthop Relat Res* 1998;349:28-42.

26. Anain JM, Bojrab AR, Rhinehart FC: Conservative treatments for rheumatoid arthritis in the foot and ankle. *Clin Podiatr Med Surg* 2010;27(2):193-207.

27. Khosla SK, Baumhauer JF: Dietary and viscosupplementation in ankle arthritis. *Foot Ankle Clin* 2008;13(3):353-361, vii.

28. Salk RS, Chang TJ, D'Costa WF, Soomekh DJ, Grogan KA: Sodium hyaluronate in the treatment of osteoarthritis of the ankle: A controlled, randomized, double-blind pilot study. *J Bone Joint Surg Am* 2006;88(2):295-302.

29. Sun S-F, Chou YJ, Hsu CW, et al: Efficacy of intra-articular hyaluronic acid in patients with osteoarthritis of the ankle: A prospective study. *Osteoarthritis Cartilage* 2006;14(9):867-874.

30. Sun S-F, Hsu CW, Sun HP, Chou YJ, Li HJ, Wang JL: The effect of three weekly intra-articular injections of hyaluronate on pain, function, and balance in patients with unilateral ankle arthritis. *J Bone Joint Surg Am* 2011;93(18):1720-1726.

31. Xu S, Liu H, Xie Y, Sang L, Liu J, Chen B: Effect of mesenchymal stromal cells for articular cartilage degeneration treatment: A meta-analysis. *Cytotherapy* 2015;17(10):1342-1352.

32. Vannabouathong C, Del Fabbro G, Sales B, et al: Intra-articular injections in the treatment of symptoms from ankle arthritis: A systematic review. *Foot Ankle Int* 2018;39(10):1141-1150.

33. John S, Bongiovanni F: Brace management for ankle arthritis. *Clin Podiatr Med Surg* 2009;26(2):193-197.

34. Hassouna H, Kumar S, Bendall S: Arthroscopic ankle debridement: 5-year survival analysis. *Acta Orthop Belg* 2007;73(6):737-740.

35. van Valburg AA, van Roermund PM, Lammens J, et al: Can Ilizarov joint distraction delay the need for an arthrodesis of the ankle? A preliminary report. *J Bone Joint Surg Br* 1995;77(5):720-725.

36. Paley D, Lamm BM: Ankle joint distraction. *Foot Ankle Clin* 2005;10(4):685-698, ix.

37. Paley D, Lamm BM, Purohit RM, Specht SC: Distraction arthroplasty of the ankle – How far can you stretch the indications? *Foot Ankle Clin* 2008;13(3):471-484, ix.

38. Morse KR, Flemister AS, Baumhauer JF, DiGiovanni BF: Distraction arthroplasty. *Foot Ankle Clin* 2007;12(1):29-39.

39. van Valburg AA, van Roermund PM, Marijnissen AC, et al: Joint distraction in treatment of osteoarthritis: A two-year follow-up of the ankle. *Osteoarthritis Cartilage* 1999;7(5):474-479.

40. van Roermund PM, Lafeber FP: Joint distraction as treatment for ankle osteoarthritis. *Instr Course Lect* 1999;48:249-254.

41. Tellisi N, Fragomen AT, Kleinman D, O'Malley MJ, Rozbruch SR: Joint preservation of the osteoarthritic ankle using distraction arthroplasty. *Foot Ankle Int* 2009;30(4):318-325.

42. Valburg AAV, van Roermund PM, Marijnissen AC, et al: Joint distraction in treatment of osteoarthritis (II): Effects on cartilage in a canine model. *Osteoarthritis Cartilage* 2000;8:1-8.

43. Chiodo CP, McGarvey W: Joint distraction for the treatment of ankle osteoarthritis. *Foot Ankle Clin* 2004;9(3):541-553, ix.

44. Saltzman CL, Hillis SL, Stolley MP, Anderson DD, Amendola A: Motion versus fixed distraction of the joint in the treatment of ankle osteoarthritis: A prospective randomized controlled trial. *J Bone Joint Surg Am* 2012;94(11):961-970.

45. Fragomen AT, McCoy TH, Meyers KN, Rozbruch SR: Minimum distraction gap: How much ankle joint space is enough in ankle distraction arthroplasty? *Hss J* 2014;10(1):6-12.

46. Bottlang M, Marsh JL, Brown TD: Articulated external fixation of the ankle: Minimizing motion resistance by accurate axis alignment. *J Biomech* 1999;32(1):63-70.

47. Marijnissen AC, van Roermund PM, van Melkebeek J, Lafeber FP: Clinical benefit of joint distraction in the treatment of ankle osteoarthritis. *Foot Ankle Clin* 2003;8(2):335-346.

48. Ploegmakers JJ, van Roermund PM, van Melkebeek J, et al: Prolonged clinical benefit from joint distraction in the treatment of ankle osteoarthritis. *Osteoarthritis Cartilage* 2005;13(7):582-588.

49. Marijnissen AC, Van Roermund PM, Van Melkebeek J, et al: Clinical benefit of joint distraction in the treatment of severe osteoarthritis of the ankle: Proof of concept in an open prospective study and in a randomized controlled study. *Arthritis Rheum* 2002;46(11):2893-2902.

50. van Roermund PM, Marijnissen AC, Lafeber FP: Joint distraction as an alternative for the treatment of osteoarthritis. *Foot Ankle Clin* 2002;7(3):515-527.

51. Greenfield S, Matta KM, McCoy TH, Rozbruch SR, Fragomen A: Ankle distraction arthroplasty for ankle osteoarthritis: A survival analysis. *Strategies Trauma Limb Reconstr* 2019;14(2):65-71.

This study examines intermediate follow-up of 144 patients treated with ankle distraction arthroplasty, with 4.5-year follow-up. Eighty-four percent of patients who underwent a distraction arthroplasty were able to avoid a definitive ankle arthritis procedure, such as replacement or arthrodesis, in this time frame. Female sex and radiographic osteonecrosis were risk factors for more definitive ankle arthritis procedures. Level of evidence: IV.

52. Mann HA, Filippi J, Myerson MS: Intra-articular opening medial tibial wedge osteotomy (plafond-plasty) for the treatment of intra-articular varus ankle arthritis and instability. *Foot Ankle Int* 2012;33(4):255-261.

53. Takakura Y, Takaoka T, Tanaka Y, Yajima H, Tamai S: Results of opening-wedge osteotomy for the treatment of a post-traumatic varus deformity of the ankle. *J Bone Joint Surg Am* 1998;80(2):213-218.

54. Tanaka Y, Takakura Y, Hayashi K, Taniguchi A, Kumai T, Sugimoto K: Low tibial osteotomy for varus-type osteoarthritis of the ankle. *J Bone Joint Surg Br* 2006;88(7):909-913.

55. Lacorda JB, Jung H-G, Im J-M: Supramalleolar distal tibiofibular osteotomy for medial ankle osteoarthritis: Current concepts. *Clin Orthop Surg* 2020;12(3):271-278.

This review article highlights the indications, potential complications, and outcomes following supramalleolar osteotomy for medial ankle osteoarthritis. Surgical techniques for this procedure are also reviewed. Level of evidence: V.

56. Krähenbühl N, Susdorf R, Barg A, Hintermann B: Supramalleolar osteotomy in post-traumatic valgus ankle osteoarthritis. *Int Orthop* 2020;44(3):535-543.

This retrospective study examines 56 patients who underwent an extra-articular medial closing wedge osteotomy for posttraumatic valgus ankle arthritis. Overall, satisfactory clinical and radiographic outcomes are seen with intermediate follow-up. Patients with supramalleolar deformity tend to have better results compared with those with intra-articular deformity. Furthermore, the more advanced preoperative arthritis results in worse radiographic but not clinical outcomes. Level of evidence: III.

57. Heywood AW: Supramalleolar osteotomy in the management of the rheumatoid hindfoot. *Clin Orthop Relat Res* 1983;177:76-81.

58. Takakura Y, Tanaka Y, Kumai T, Tamai S: Low tibial osteotomy for osteoarthritis of the ankle. Results of a new operation in 18 patients. *J Bone Joint Surg Br* 1995;77(1):50-54.

59. Becker AS, Myerson MS: The indications and technique of supramalleolar osteotomy. *Foot Ankle Clin* 2009;14(3):549-561.

60. Pagenstert GI, Hintermann B, Barg A, Leumann A, Valderrabano V: Realignment surgery as alternative treatment of varus and valgus ankle osteoarthritis. *Clin Orthop Relat Res* 2007;462:156-168.

61. Hintermann B, Knupp M, Barg A: Supramalleolar osteotomies for the treatment of ankle arthritis. *J Am Acad Orthop Surg* 2016;24(7):424-432.

62. Sen C, Kocaoglu M, Eralp L, Cinar M: Correction of ankle and hindfoot deformities by supramalleolar osteotomy. *Foot Ankle Int* 2003;24(1):22-28.

63. Knupp M, Stufkens SA, Bolliger L, Barg A, Hintermann B: Classification and treatment of supramalleolar deformities. *Foot Ankle Int* 2011;32(11):1023-1031.

64. Raikin SM: Fresh osteochondral allografts for large-volume cystic osteochondral defects of the talus. *J Bone Joint Surg Am* 2009;91(12):2818-2826.

65. Adams SB, Dekker TJ, Schiff AP, Gross CP, Nunley JA, Easley ME: Prospective evaluation of structural allograft transplantation for osteochondral lesions of the talar shoulder. *Foot Ankle Int* 2018;39(1):28-34.

66. Adams SB, Viens NA, Easley ME, Stinnett SS, Nunley JA: Midterm results of osteochondral lesions of the talar shoulder treated with fresh osteochondral allograft transplantation. *J Bone Joint Surg Am* 2011;93(7):648-654.

67. Jeng CL, Myerson MS: Allograft total ankle replacement – A dead ringer to the natural joint. *Foot Ankle Clin* 2008;13:539-547.

68. Williams SK, Amiel D, Ball ST, et al: Prolonged storage effects on the articular cartilage of fresh human osteochondral allografts. *J Bone Joint Surg Am* 2003;85(11):2111-2120.

69. Jamali AA, Hatcher SL, You Z: Donor cell survival in a fresh osteochondral allograft at twenty-nine years. A case report. *J Bone Joint Surg Am* 2007;89(1):166-169.

70. Kim CW, Jamali A, Tontz W Jr, Convery FR, Brage ME, Bugbee W: Treatment of post-traumatic ankle arthrosis with bipolar tibiotalar osteochondral shell allografts. *Foot Ankle Int* 2002;23(12):1091-1102.

71. Meehan R, McFarlin S, Bugbee W, Brage M: Fresh ankle osteochondral allograft transplantation for tibiotalar joint arthritis. *Foot Ankle Int* 2005;26(10):793-802.

72. Giannini S, Buda R, Grigolo B, et al: Bipolar fresh osteochondral allograft of the ankle. *Foot Ankle Int* 2010;31(1):38-46.

73. Bugbee WD, Khanna G, Cavallo M, McCauley JC, Görtz S, Brage ME: Bipolar fresh osteochondral allografting of the tibiotalar joint. *J Bone Joint Surg Am* 2013;95(5):426-432.

74. Haddad SL, Coetzee JC, Estok R, Fahrbach K, Banel D, Nalysnyk L: Intermediate and long-term outcomes of total ankle arthroplasty and ankle arthrodesis. A systematic review of the literature. *J Bone Joint Surg Am* 2007;89(9):1899-1905.

75. Ahmad J, Raikin SM: Ankle arthrodesis: The simple and the complex. *Foot Ankle Clin* 2008;13(3):381-400.

76. Thomas R, Daniels TR, Parker K: Gait analysis and functional outcomes following ankle arthrodesis for isolated ankle arthritis. *J Bone Joint Surg Am* 2006;88(3):526-535.

77. Coester LM, Saltzman CL, Leupold J, Pontarelli W: Long-term results following ankle arthrodesis for post-traumatic arthritis. *J Bone Joint Surg Am* 2001;83(2):219-228.

78. Sturnick DR, Demetracopoulos CA, Ellis SJ, et al: Adjacent joint kinematics after ankle arthrodesis during cadaveric gait simulation. *Foot Ankle Int* 2017;38(11):1249-1259.

79. Morash J, Walton DM, Glazebrook M: Ankle arthrodesis versus total ankle arthroplasty. *Foot Ankle Clin* 2017;22(2):251-266.

80. Jung H-G, Parks BG, Nguyen A, Schon LC: Effect of tibiotalar joint arthrodesis on adjacent tarsal joint pressure in a cadaver model. *Foot Ankle Int* 2007;28(1):103-108.

81. Mann RA, Rongstad KM: Arthrodesis of the ankle: A critical analysis. *Foot Ankle Int* 1998;19(1):3-9.

82. Myerson MS, Quill G: Ankle arthrodesis. A comparison of an arthroscopic and an open method of treatment. *Clin Orthop Relat Res* 1991;268:84-95.

83. Yang X-Q, Zhang Y, Wang Q, et al: Supramalleolar osteotomy vs arthrodesis for the treatment of Takakura 3B ankle osteoarthritis. *Foot Ankle Int* 2022;43(9):1185-1193.

This retrospective study examined the clinical results after supramalleolar osteotomy and ankle arthrodesis, with more than 4-year follow-up. Although both cohorts had improvement in function, pain, alignment, and quality of life after surgery, the patients who underwent arthrodesis experienced better pain relief and lower reoperation rates. Level of evidence: III.

84. Buck P, Morrey BF, Chao EY: The optimum position of arthrodesis of the ankle. A gait study of the knee and ankle. *J Bone Joint Surg Am* 1987;69(7):1052-1062.

85. Dohm MP, Benjamin JB, Harrison J, Szivek JA: A biomechanical evaluation of three forms of internal fixation used in ankle arthrodesis. *Foot Ankle Int* 1994;15(6):297-300.

86. Ogilvie-Harris DJ, Fitsialos D, Hedman TP: Arthrodesis of the ankle. A comparison of two versus three screw fixation in a crossed configuration. *Clin Orthop Relat Res* 1994;304:195-199.

87. Raikin SM: Arthrodesis of the ankle: Arthroscopic, mini-open, and open techniques. *Foot Ankle Clin* 2003;8(2):347-359.

88. Lawton CD, Butler BA, Dekker RG, Prescott A, Kadakia AR: Total ankle arthroplasty versus ankle arthrodesis – A comparison of outcomes over the last decade. *J Orthop Surg Res* 2017;12(1):76.

89. Raikin SM, Rampuri V: An approach to the failed ankle arthrodesis. *Foot Ankle Clin* 2008;13(3):401-416, viii.

90. Glick JM, Morgan CD, Myerson MS, Sampson TG, Mann JA: Ankle arthrodesis using an arthroscopic method: Long-term follow-up of 34 cases. *Arthroscopy* 1996;12(4):428-434.

91. Townshend D, Di Silvestro M, Krause F, et al: Arthroscopic versus open ankle arthrodesis: A multicenter comparative case series. *J Bone Joint Surg Am* 2013;95(2):98-102.

92. O'Brien TS, Hart TS, Shereff MJ, Stone J, Johnson J: Open versus arthroscopic ankle arthrodesis: A comparative study. *Foot Ankle Int* 1999;20(6):368-374.

93. Crosby LA, Yee TC, Formanek TS, Fitzgibbons TC: Complications following arthroscopic ankle arthrodesis. *Foot Ankle Int* 1996;17(6):340-342.

94. Paremain GD, Miller SD, Myerson MS: Ankle arthrodesis: Results after the miniarthrotomy technique. *Foot Ankle Int* 1996;17(5):247-252.

95. Schmid T, Krause F, Penner MJ, Veljkovic A, Younger ASE, Wing K: Effect of preoperative deformity on arthroscopic and open ankle fusion outcomes. *Foot Ankle Int* 2017;38(12):1301-1310.

96. Martinelli N, Bianchi A, Raggi G, Parrini MM, Cerbone V, Sansone V: Open versus arthroscopic ankle arthrodesis in high-risk patients: A comparative study. *Int Orthop* 2022;46(3):515-521.

    This study retrospectively evaluated two fusion techniques, open and arthroscopic, in patients considered high risk for nonunion. The arthroscopic ankle arthrodesis group had a higher union rate, lower complication rate, and lower reoperation rate compared with the open arthrodesis group. Level of evidence: III.

97. Lindsey BB, Hundal R, Bakshi NK, Holmes JR, Talusan PG, Walton DM: Ankle arthrodesis through an anterior approach. *J Orthop Trauma* 2020;34(suppl 2):S42-S43.

    This article and corresponding video demonstrate the anterior approach and fixation options for an ankle arthrodesis. Level of evidence: V.

98. Kim J-G, Ha DJ, Gwak HC, et al: Ankle arthrodesis: A comparison of anterior approach and transfibular approach. *Clin Orthop Surg* 2018;10(3):368-373.

99. Mann RA, van Manen JW, Wapner K, Martin J: Ankle fusion. *Clin Orthop Relat Res* 1991;268:49-55.

100. Marcus RE, Balourdas GM, Heiple KG: Ankle arthrodesis by chevron fusion with internal fixation and bone-grafting. *J Bone Joint Surg Am* 1983;65(6):833-838.

101. Zwipp H, Rammelt S, Endres T, Heineck J: High union rates and function scores at midterm followup with ankle arthrodesis using a four screw technique. *Clin Orthop Relat Res* 2010;468(4):958-968.

102. Hendrickx RPM, Stufkens SA, de Bruijn EE, Sierevelt IN, van Dijk CN, Kerkhoffs GM: Medium- to long-term outcome of ankle arthrodesis. *Foot Ankle Int* 2011;32(10):940-947.

103. Brodsky JW, Kane JM, Coleman S, Bariteau J, Tenenbaum S: Abnormalities of gait caused by ankle arthritis are improved by ankle arthrodesis. *Bone Joint J* 2016;98-B(10):1369-1375.

104. Tarkin IS, Mormino MA, Clare MP, Haider H, Walling AK, Sanders RW: Anterior plate supplementation increases ankle arthrodesis construct rigidity. *Foot Ankle Int* 2007;28(2):219-223.

105. Mitchell PM, Douleh DG, Thomson AB: Comparison of ankle fusion rates with and without anterior plate augmentation. *Foot Ankle Int* 2017;38(4):419-423.

106. Chalayon O, Wang B, Blankenhorn B, et al: Factors affecting the outcomes of uncomplicated primary open ankle arthrodesis. *Foot Ankle Int* 2015;36(10):1170-1179.

107. Culpan P, Le Strat V, Piriou P, Judet T: Arthrodesis after failed total ankle replacement. *J Bone Joint Surg Br* 2007;89(9):1178-1183.

108. Hopgood P, Kumar R, Wood PL: Ankle arthrodesis for failed total ankle replacement. *J Bone Joint Surg Br* 2006;88(8):1032-1038.

109. Jeng CL, Campbell JT, Tang EY, Cerrato RA, Myerson MS: Tibiotalocalcaneal arthrodesis with bulk femoral head allograft for salvage of large defects in the ankle. *Foot Ankle Int* 2013;34(9):1256-1266.

110. Swords MP, Weatherford B: High-energy pilon fractures: Role of external fixation in acute and definitive treatment. What are the indications and technique for primary ankle arthrodesis? *Foot Ankle Clin* 2020;25(4):523-536.

    This review article highlights the role for external fixation in high-energy pilon fractures. The use of thin wire external fixation and the role for acute arthrodesis with the external fixator are reviewed. Level of evidence: V.

111. Fadhel WB, Taieb L, Villain B, et al: Outcomes after primary ankle arthrodesis in recent fractures of the distal end of the tibia in the elderly: A systematic review. *Int Orthop* 2022;46(6):1405-1412.

    This systematic review evaluates the outcomes of primary ankle and subtalar arthrodesis for the distal tibia fractures in elderly patients. There is an over 94% successful arthrodesis rate in this patient population. About 19% of patients had a complication and 11% required revision arthrodesis. All patients were treated using a retrograde hindfoot fusion nail, with a higher complication rate and revision fusion rate in patients undergoing a short hindfoot nail. Level of evidence: I.

112. Wallace SJ, Liskutin TE, Schiff AP, Pinzur MS: Ankle fusion following failed initial treatment of complex ankle fractures in neuropathic diabetics. *Foot Ankle Surg* 2020;26(2):189-192.

    This study retrospectively evaluated the success of acute ankle arthrodesis for patients sustaining an acute ankle fracture in the setting of neuropathy. Although there is a risk of complications, including a nonunion rate of approximately 47%, primary ankle fusion was determined to be a reasonable option for patients with diabetic neuropathy and acute ankle fractures. Level of evidence: IV.

CHAPTER 9

Ankle Arthritis: Part II. Total Ankle Arthroplasty

STEVEN L. HADDAD, MD, FAAOS • JUSTIN DAIGRE, MD, FAAOS

ABSTRACT

Total joint registries worldwide show a growing trend for ankle arthritis to be managed with total ankle arthroplasty (TAA). Midterm data show increasing survivorship and promising outcomes with TAA. Simplified surgical technique, patient-specific instrumentation, and increased revision options have improved surgeon confidence in TAA procedures. TAA literature is advancing rapidly along with implant innovation and technology; therefore, a thorough understanding of TAA is vital for the foot and ankle surgeon. It is important to review the history of TAA, currently available implants in the United States, implant design and rationale, general surgical technique, deformity and adjacent joint pathologies, and recent outcomes data.

Keywords: ankle fusion; ankle replacement; end-stage ankle arthritis; revision ankle replacement; total ankle arthroplasty

---

Dr. Haddad or an immediate family member has received royalties from Stryker; serves as a paid consultant to or is an employee of Extremity Medical and Wright Medical Technology, Inc.; and serves as a board member, owner, officer, or committee member of American Academy of Orthopaedic Surgeons and American Orthopaedic Foot and Ankle Society. Dr. Daigre or an immediate family member has received royalties from In2Bones/Conmed; serves as a paid consultant to or is an employee of In2Bones and Treace Medical Concepts, Inc.; and has stock or stock options held in Treace Medical.

INTRODUCTION

Much progress and innovation have occurred since the first total ankle arthroplasty (TAA) was performed in 1970. The advent of patient-specific instrumentation (PSI), the ability to address coronal plane deformity of the ankle joint with more consistent results, and more recent data on the safety of single-stage versus multistage procedures with TAA to address adjacent foot deformity and adjacent joint arthritis have provided expanded indications for TAA over ankle arthrodesis. In fact, Medicare data in the United States, along with worldwide joint registries, are revealing trends of end-stage ankle arthritis being managed with joint replacement rather than ankle arthrodesis. The prevalence of total hip and knee arthroplasty research in the literature has greatly outweighed TAA literature, but over the past 10 years, this gap has begun to close. Most important, outcomes data from patients with ankle arthritis are showing promising results with TAA.

BACKGROUND

Historically, short-term studies of first-generation total ankle implants demonstrated promising results, but midterm follow-up revealed evidence of substantial radiographic loosening and high failure rates.[1,2] First-generation total ankle implants required substantial bone resection, placing the components in softer, metaphyseal bone. This becomes an issue in ankle arthroplasty given compressive resistance of the metaphyseal bone is directly correlated with the height of the resection margin.[3] Resistance in the distal tibia subchondral bone can reach levels of 450 MPa. Simply resecting 1 cm of tibial

---

This chapter is adapted from Harnroongroj T, Demetracopoulos CA: Ankle arthritis: Part II. Total ankle arthroplasty, in Chou LB, ed: *Orthopaedic Knowledge Update®: Foot and Ankle 6*. American Academy of Orthopaedic Surgeons, 2020, pp 129-144.

© 2025 American Academy of Orthopaedic Surgeons

Orthopaedic Knowledge Update®: Foot and Ankle 7

bone decreases that resistance by 30% to 50%, increasing the risk of component subsidence. In addition, most early implants were cemented, creating risk of loosening at the bone-cement interface given the poorer quality bone in posttraumatic ankle arthritis.

Early ankle prostheses were designed as either simple, constrained hinge, or completely unconstrained. Motion was allowed only in the sagittal plane in the constrained devices (ie, Mayo implant) or multiaxial in unconstrained devices (ie, Smith implant). The highly constrained early implant designs transmitted significant forces to the bone-implant interface, which led to early loosening, implant subsidence, and failure.[2] Subsequent first-generation designs were much less constrained and relied on the soft-tissue envelope for stability. These designs also proved inefficient and were associated with impingement and early failure.

Second-generation and third-generation implants emphasized limited bone resection, improved fixation to bone with ongrowth and ingrowth surfaces, became semiconstrained, and restored a more anatomic articulation at the ankle joint. Current TAA implants (third and fourth generation) have two common features: (1) all have porous-coated surface (or three-dimensional [3D] printed titanium surfaces) for enhancing bone ingrowth, and (2) all are made of titanium alloy with a cobalt-chromium polyethylene-talar articulation.[4]

As of this writing, there are 12 FDA-approved TAA implants in the US market. These include the INFINITY Total Ankle System (Stryker) (**Figure 1**), INBONE II Total Ankle System (Stryker) (**Figure 2**), and INVISION Total Ankle Revision System (Stryker) (**Figure 3**); the CADENCE Total Ankle System (Smith & Nephew) (**Figure 4**); the Salto Talaris Total Ankle Prosthesis (Smith & Nephew) (**Figure 5**); the QUANTUM Total Ankle System (In2Bones/CONMED); the Scandinavian Total Ankle Replacement (STAR, Enovis) (**Figure 6**); the Trabecular Metal Total Ankle (Zimmer Biomet); the Vantage Total Ankle System (Exactech) (**Figure 7**); the Hintermann Series H3 Total Ankle Replacement System (DT MedTech); and Kinos Axiom Total Ankle System (restor3d). All are fixed-bearing TAAs in the United States that are FDA cleared for cemented use, except the STAR and Hintermann H3, which are mobile-bearing implants approved by the FDA for use without cement.

DESIGN ISSUES AND RATIONALE

The ankle joint consists of three bony interactions: the tibia, fibula, and talus. The morphology of each bone affects the function and relationship of the ankle joint.

Many patients who present with ankle arthritis will also demonstrate radiographic and clinically significant adjacent joint arthritis in the hindfoot, most commonly the subtalar joint. In addition, adjacent joint arthritis is known to progress following ankle arthrodesis. Altered biomechanics after ankle fusion are likely the cause of adjacent joint degeneration although no consensus has been reached in the literature.[5] Kinematic data in patients with posttraumatic ankle osteoarthritis reveal paradoxical opposite motion in the subtalar joint. This abnormal motion likely contributes to adjacent joint degeneration, thus fueling the search for treatment strategies that restore more normal ankle kinematics.[6]

The current generation of implants has sought to address the shortcomings of initial implants. Improved materials and fixation techniques were implemented.

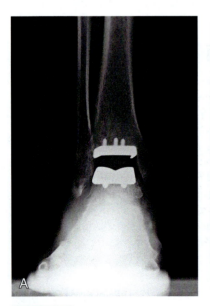
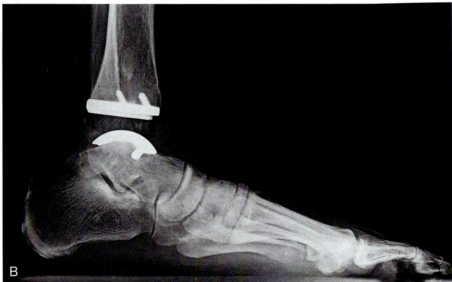

FIGURE 1 The INFINITY Total Ankle System (Stryker). **A**, AP radiograph. **B**, Lateral radiograph.

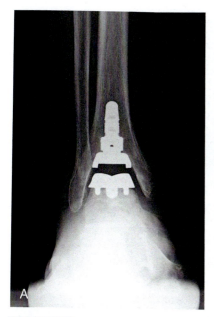
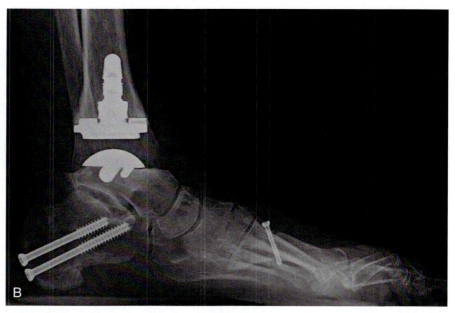

FIGURE 2 The INBONE II Total Ankle System (Stryker). **A**, AP radiograph. **B**, Lateral radiograph.

By minimizing resection, the implants are placed on stronger, subchondral bone. By improving immediate fixation via better ingrowth surfaces, many surgeons use TAA implants off-label without cement. Modern implant designs are semiconstrained, which reduces the stress at the bone-implant interface, and have been successful in improving midterm survivorship.

Because the ankle allows for both gliding and rolling motion, implants are designed to accommodate complex 3D ankle motion. Implant use entails a balance of compromises. Fixed-bearing devices offer inherent stability but sacrifice certain planes of motion, particularly rotational. Mobile-bearing devices not only allow for more rotational motion, thus decreasing stress to the implant, but they also reduce stability; allow for possible bearing impingement, secondary coronal plane deformity, and edge loading of the polyethylene; and create the potential for backside polyethylene wear.

Current ankle prostheses can strike the necessary balance between providing implant stability and decreasing

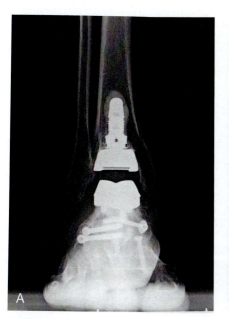
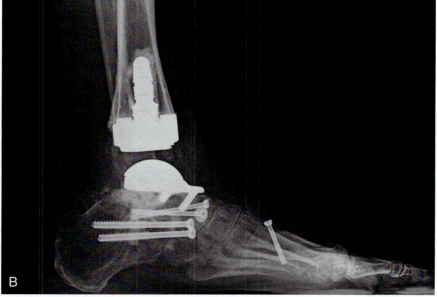

FIGURE 3 The INVISION Total Ankle System (Stryker). **A**, AP radiograph. **B**, Lateral radiograph.

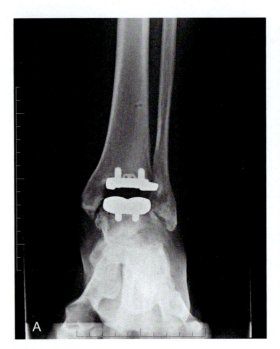
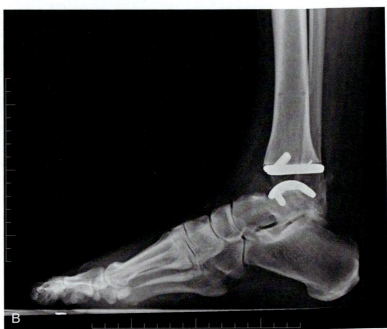

FIGURE 4 The CADENCE Total Ankle System (Smith & Nephew, Inc.). **A**, AP radiograph. **B**, Lateral radiograph.

stress transfer to bone. On the tibial side, most current generation implants emphasize a common approach of minimizing bone resection to allow for stable fixation on the cortical rim of the distal tibia. Additional stability of the tibial component is achieved with either a keel, barrels, pegs, a cage, or a stem. Preserving bone with minimal resection technique potentially allows for the option of revising the failed total ankle prosthesis, though significant subsidence in even low-profile implants can result in challenges for revision.

The complex anatomy of the talus poses challenges to both implant designers and surgeons. Talar anatomy features complex 3D conical wedges. The radii of curvature on each side of the talus (medial, lateral, anterior, and posterior) all differ. Current primary total ankle implants have a resurfacing talar component. Most implant

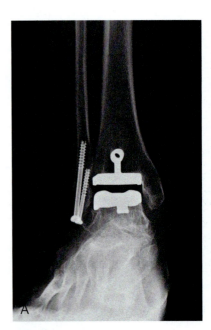
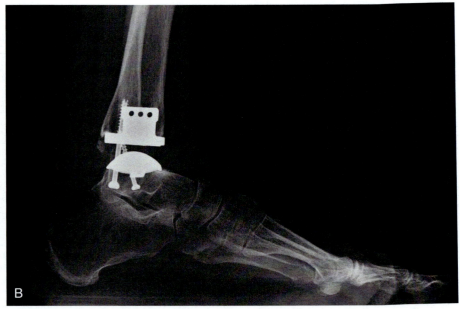

FIGURE 5 The Salto Talaris Total Ankle Prosthesis (Smith & Nephew, Inc.). **A**, AP radiograph. **B**, Lateral radiograph.

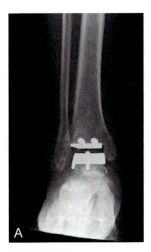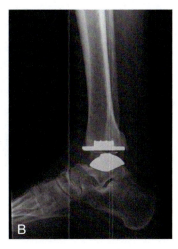

FIGURE 6 The Scandinavian Total Ankle Replacement (DJO Global). **A**, AP radiograph. **B**, Lateral radiograph.

systems do so by making chamfer cuts on which the component sits, although other vendors place the talus on a curved surface with thoughts that it better reproduces the natural talus anatomy. Newer talar designs are attempting to reproduce the complex natural anatomy of the talus, though it remains to be seen if this better mimics talar kinematics. All talar components have one or more pegs or a keel to anchor into the talar body.

The axis of rotation of the talus has been described as having a changing instant center of rotation,[7] with the primary axis of rotation correlated with the transmalleolar axis and externally rotated 23°.[8] To further confound the mechanism, the ankle also rotates approximately 5° in the transverse plane.[9] Current literature shows significant variance between the medial gutter line and the transmalleolar axis.[10] Using the tibial tubercle to set rotation may be unreliable given the wide variability of tibial torsion and foot position in different body types (ie, cavovarus, pes planovalgus). Accessing rotation in TAA is challenging and should consider tibial tubercle position, second metatarsal position, and transmalleolar axis position. Relying on one position may lead to malalignment, gutter impingement, incongruent range of motion, and inadvertent excess malleolar resection. Obtaining proper rotation of the implants may decrease gutter impingement and subsequent surgical débridement.[10]

Previously, resurfacing the medial and lateral facets was thought to help reduce the incidence of gutter impingement. However, current implants, which do not resect the bone of the medial and lateral talus to spare bone, do not have a higher incidence of gutter impingement in the postoperative period. Obtaining correct rotation and resecting impinging osteophytes remains the best method in reducing subsequent gutter débridement surgery.[10,11]

The blood supply of the talus is known to be sensitive to injury, instrumentation, and surgical manipulation. Each technique puts different vascular structures at risk. A cadaver injection study reported that individual implants put unique arterial supply at risk given

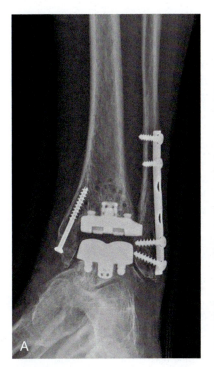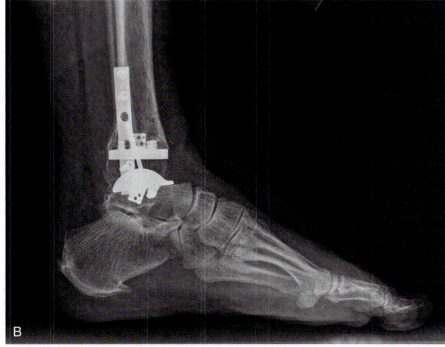

FIGURE 7 The Vantage Total Ankle System (Exactech). **A**, AP radiograph. **B**, Lateral radiograph.

the particular implant's instrumentation.[12] However, follow-up data suggest that this cadaver study is not reproducible in vivo because the anatomy differs under arthritic conditions (especially with deformity). In a 2019 study, follow-up studies using positron emission tomography refuted claims of an insulted blood supply, further confounding the issue.[13] Therefore, the correlation between surgical approach, instrumentation, implant choice, and in vivo blood supply to the talus remains uncertain, and thus, it is unclear how this relationship will affect survivorship of the TAA implants.

INDICATIONS

An unprecedented amount of data on TAA is becoming available. As this information is reviewed, indications and techniques will undoubtedly evolve. TAA is indicated in patients with end-stage ankle arthritis in whom nonsurgical treatment failed. Posttraumatic arthritis is the most common etiology of ankle arthritis, which includes patients with a history of fracture and ankle instability. Other common causes include inflammatory arthropathies, gout, osteonecrosis, and primary ankle osteoarthritis. Patients who have bilateral ankle arthritis and/or those who have significant arthritis in the hindfoot are excellent candidates for TAA.

Patient age is a subjective matter when considering indications for TAA. Initially, it was thought that TAA should be restricted to elderly patients with lower physical demands. Initial research suggested that implant survivorship and functional outcomes are decreased in younger patients undergoing TAA.[14-17] More recent data on outcomes and revision rates have shown equivalency between younger and older patients.[18,19] Because indications for TAA are fluid and somewhat surgeon dependent, reliance on a detailed informed consent allows the patient to make an educated decision in choosing the correct procedure to manage their arthritic condition.

Despite this uncertainty, patients with inflammatory arthropathy such as rheumatoid disease or psoriatic arthritis may have a more functional outcome with TAA over ankle arthrodesis given the potential for progressive arthritic wear in the adjacent joints. Arthrodesis of the hindfoot adjacent to an ankle that has undergone arthrodesis has a detrimental effect on gait. In fact, some literature suggests that patients without neuropathy undergoing a pantalar arthrodesis achieve better gait with a transtibial amputation.[20-22] These patients are best served with hindfoot arthrodesis and TAA.

Postsurgical activity following TAA suggests that low-impact activities are safe and are encouraged.[23,24] Mid-impact to high-impact activities should be addressed individually with patients and should be performed with caution, recognizing they may lead to early implant loosening and

subsidence. A 2020 study suggests that activity level was improved by 10% following TAA and that physical activity outcome scores were better in patients undergoing TAA than those undergoing ankle arthrodesis.[25]

Patients must have sufficient bone stock to support the prosthesis. If the soft-tissue envelope surrounding the implant has the potential for compromise, discussion with a plastic surgeon before the surgery provides necessary guidance in surgical approach and postsurgical management.

Osteonecrosis of the talus was once an absolute contraindication in TAA. Options have improved for patients with osteonecrosis, given the assessment of the magnitude and location of poor-quality bone via CT allows the surgeon to determine if the chosen approach allows good prosthesis coverage after resection of poor-quality bone tissue. As an alternative, total talus arthroplasty is a recognized treatment option for patients with significant osteonecrosis of the talus. Implants were initially constructed with cobalt-chromium alloy. Newer implants are fabricated from titanium alloy, making them much lighter. It is important to note that there are only a few short term studies on total talus arthroplasty,[26-28] and thus this technology must be approached with caution and adequate informed consent. Concerns regarding arthritic pain at the talonavicular joint and subtalar joint without reasonable salvage options should temper overuse of this technology at this time.

CONTRAINDICATIONS

Contraindications to TAA include acute osteomyelitis or unresolvable infection, Charcot or neuropathic joint involvement, complete paralysis of the affected limb, unsalvageable vascular insufficiency, and poor soft-tissue envelope without good reconstructive options.

Relative contraindications include history of infection without resolution, diabetes with neuropathy, morbid obesity, severe osteoporosis, and smoking. This list keeps changing (and decreasing) as technology continues to improve. In addition, patients who have physically demanding employment may have a better long-term outcome with ankle arthrodesis.

SURGICAL TREATMENT

The surgery is traditionally performed under a long-acting spinal, epidural, or general anesthesia with or without a lower extremity nerve block. The patient is positioned supine on a radiolucent surgical table. The surgical hip is elevated and supported to allow for the foot to be positioned neutral. A thigh tourniquet is normally used, and the surgical limb is prepped and draped to thigh level.

Chapter 9: Ankle Arthritis: Part II. Total Ankle Arthroplasty

Most implants require an anterior surgical approach. The incision normally begins approximately 10 cm proximal to the ankle joint and ends at or just distal to the talonavicular joint. An adequate incision should be used to decrease tension on the skin during retraction and allow for good visualization. The interval between the anterior tibialis and extensor hallucis longus is developed. Attention is given to the anterior neurovascular bundle, which should be mobilized, protected, and retracted laterally with the extensor hallucis longus. Minimal handling of the tissue and judicious use of retractors are warranted to limit undue pressure to the soft tissue. Excessive retraction can lead to wound edge necrosis, and wound complications have been reported to be as high as 28%.[29-31]

After the approach has been developed to the level of the ankle joint, the capsule is reflected medial and lateral to expose the entire ankle joint, which includes both the medial and lateral gutters. Anterior osteophytes at the distal tibial plafond can be removed to allow visualization of the joint unless PSI is being used. Ankle deformity should be corrected before making the saw cuts into the tibia and talus (unless using PSI). The ankle should be in neutral dorsiflexion before performing bony resection (unless using PSI). The cuts are completed per the manufacturer-suggested techniques based on the implant being placed.

When performing saw cuts, specific attention is directed to the posterior medial corner because both the posterior neurovascular bundle and posterior tibial tendon are at risk. The flexor hallucis longus is also at risk at the center-posterior aspect of the tibial cut. If these posterior structures are damaged, further exploration is necessary to assess the posterior tibial artery and tibial nerve so that prompt repair is performed.

After the prosthesis has been implanted, a meticulous layered closure is required. In particular, the facial envelope covering the anterior tibial tendon and extensor hallucis longus tendon must be opposed. Postsurgical management is often surgeon dependent, ranging from a well-padded splint with the ankle in a neutral position to a controlled ankle motion boot and compression wraps.[32] Institution of range of motion and time to weight bearing are also surgeon dependent because no published protocols reflect superiority.

ALTERNATIVE SURGICAL APPROACHES

As suggested previously, the anterior approach is most commonly performed and the most studied in the literature. One current implant uses a lateral transfibular approach to access the ankle joint, requiring a fibula osteotomy. In addition, the posterior approach has been considered. Because the posterior soft tissue of the ankle is more often unaffected by traumatic incidents, it has the potential to be an attractive alternative in the patient at risk for poor wound healing anteriorly. A limited number of case reports mention the posterior approach with the current generation of TAA implants.[33]

Concomitant Procedures

Ankle arthritis usually does not exist in isolation. Concomitant pathology typically affects patients with this condition, some of which may be related to underlying arthritis. Retained hardware may need to be addressed in posttraumatic arthritis. Adjacent joint arthritis, deformity of the ankle and foot, equinus contracture, and the quality of bone stock need to be considered in the evaluation of a total ankle procedure.

If there is residual limitation in dorsiflexion following implantation of the ankle prosthesis, a Silfverskiöld test is performed to determine whether a gastrocnemius recession or Achilles tendon lengthening will be effective in restoring adequate dorsiflexion. One study found that TAA with triceps surae lengthening (either gastrocnemius recession or triple hemisection) had significant improvement in both ankle range of motion and peak dorsiflexion angle at 1 year after surgery than TAA alone.[34] There is a risk of plantar flexion weakness following these lengthening procedures that must be considered.[35] Even with such lengthening procedures, the patient should be counseled that restoration of ankle motion to preinjury or prearthritic status is unlikely.[29]

With regard to adjacent joint arthritis, it is useful to ascertain preoperatively (if possible) if the adjacent joints are a significant source of pain. Fluoroscopic-guided injections of local anesthetic can assist this determination. Several studies have shown symptomatic progression in adjacent joint arthritis after TAA.[36,37] However, this rate remains lower (and longer temporally) than what has been reported for those undergoing ankle arthrodesis.[38,39]

Following TAA, a patient with subtalar joint arthritis will often report less hindfoot pain than noted before surgery. Therefore, concomitant subtalar arthrodesis may not be required, even in cases where subtalar joint arthritis is evident radiographically before surgery. Arthrodesis of the subtalar joint may result in additional injury to the blood supply of the talus, which may lead to implant loosening and subsidence. A staged approach is favored with subtalar arthrodesis to limit this risk and to allow the surgeon to alter their implant selection (if necessary) in cases with developing poor-quality talar bone following subtalar arthrodesis.

If concomitant subtalar arthrodesis is performed at the time of TAA, consideration should be given to prepare

Section 3: Arthritis of the Foot and Ankle

the posterior facet in isolation and to not disrupt the vessels within the sinus tarsi.[40] One study observed the outcome of secondary hindfoot arthrodesis after TAA. Although the sample size was small (secondary hindfoot arthrodeses were performed in only 26 of 1,002 patients who underwent TAA [2.6%]), there were 2 patients with delayed union (7.7%) and 2 with nonunion (7.7%). Pain and functional outcome scores improved as well. When comparing the union rate of subtalar arthrodesis with either a TAA or an ankle arthrodesis, subtalar arthrodesis with TAA had a significantly better fusion rate and similar time to fusion.[41]

One study reported the clinical outcomes of 70 patients with hindfoot fusion before, after, or at the time of TAA compared with 334 patients who underwent TAA without hindfoot arthrodesis. Inferior outcomes were found in both pain and functional results in patients undergoing TAA with hindfoot arthrodesis.[42] A 2019 study[43] conducted a prospective database review of the patients who underwent primary TAA with a minimum 5-year follow-up. It was found that ipsilateral hindfoot arthrodesis was one significant factor leading to revision of TAA. Combining the results of both these studies, there is concern that hindfoot arthrodesis may alter the biomechanics of the TAA and affect the long-term clinical outcomes and survivorship of the implant.

Balancing the foot beneath the total ankle prosthesis is critical in improving survival of the implant. Calcaneal osteotomy, procedures on the first ray, tendon transfer, and ligament repair or reconstruction may be necessary. Incision placement is mapped out before surgery to minimize insult and subsequent wound breakdown.

Evaluation of both limb alignment and deformity is important when planning TAA. Radiographic views beyond the standard three radiographs of the ankle are important when deformity is present. Helpful imaging including three radiographic views of the foot, full-limb alignment views (hip-knee-ankle), and a weight-bearing hindfoot alignment view provides great assistance in planning necessary additional procedures.

Weight-bearing CT is becoming more popular in assessing ankle and hindfoot deformity. Preoperative CT imaging software technology found in PSI systems can also assist in determining the correct rotation and axial alignment of the implant, especially in patients with a malunion of the tibia. A 2019 study found that preoperative PSI CT positively affected surgical plan in more than 50% of patients.[10]

Initially, it was thought that coronal plane deformity exceeding 10° to 15° should be managed with ankle arthrodesis instead of TAA given increased failure rates.[44-46] More recent literature has refuted these claims. Numerous studies have shown equivalent outcomes for deformities between 15° and 30°.[9,14,47-49] Specifically, the

literature suggests that if the surgeon corrects the ankle deformity to stable neutral (no matter how large and how unstable the preoperative deformity), results demonstrate a consistent positive outcome.

For management of varus ankle deformity, the most common adjunctive procedures are closing wedge calcaneal osteotomy, deltoid ligament release (fractional or complete), dorsiflexion osteotomy of the first metatarsal (or dorsiflexion arthrodesis of the first tarsometatarsal joint), peroneal tendon transfer, and lateral ligament reconstruction (secondary or with weaved allograft).[9,47-51]

Deformity adjacent to the tibial implant (within the tibial bone) may require staged correction to achieve better bone quality to support the implant. Supramalleolar osteotomy offers the opportunity to correct a variety of deformities that occur proximal to the TAA.

Valgus deformity can occur with or without an associated flatfoot. A medial displacement calcaneal osteotomy, procedures to stabilize the first ray, deltoid ligament secondary repair or reconstruction with allograft, tendon transfer, and even a concomitant talonavicular arthrodesis may be necessary to restore the position of the talus to neutral. Paradoxically, lateral ligament repair/reconstruction may be necessary in cases of valgus ankle arthritis, when the etiology is chronic ankle instability.[52]

Patient-Specific Instrumentation

Some TAA implant systems now offer PSI. A 2021 systematic review of PSI in TAA demonstrates similar implant position and clinical outcome compared with standard instrumentation while shortening both surgical and fluoroscopic imaging time.[53]

COMPLICATIONS

The potential for complications surrounding TAA may lead to reticence in performing the procedure for the uninitiated. Wound dehiscence, acute infection, malleolar fracture, early implant loosening, and hardware complications are the most common early complications (**Figure 8**). The most common intraoperative complication is malleolar fracture. Intraoperative inspection should help to identify medial or lateral malleolar fractures, which require fixation to maintain implant stability. When in doubt, prophylactic fixation may be placed with little additional morbidity (although additional incisions may increase the risk of wound complication). If fractures are diagnosed in early postoperative radiographs, treatment may involve cast immobilization or open reduction and internal fixation depending on the severity, displacement, and potential for implant instability.[54] Again, if there is any doubt, the fracture should be fixed. Ignoring a fracture that can be simply fixed acutely may result in secondary failure that is much more difficult to salvage at a later date.

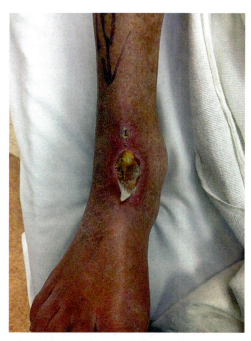

FIGURE 8 Photograph of anterior wound dehiscence during the postoperative period, an unfortunate complication seen with total ankle arthroplasty.

Wound-healing issues should be managed early and aggressively. Patients who smoke, those with diabetes, those who have prior incisions, and those who have inflammatory arthritis may experience increased incision-healing issues.[55] Patients with these associated comorbidities should be counseled accordingly before surgery regarding the potential for additional procedures (occasionally major) to manage this complication.

If a wound shows signs of drainage or persistent erythema, if duskiness is visible, or the wound edges appear necrotic, close monitoring is necessary and early intervention may be needed to avoid deep infection. A surgeon who refers such a patient to a wound care center must still take responsibility for the patient and continue to evaluate the incision for progressive failure. Again, lack of persistent monitoring of the incision may turn a simple irrigation and débridement into explantation of the implant and a free flap. If drainage persists after 3 to 4 weeks, or if the wound begins to break down, the surgeon should consider returning to the operating room for irrigation and débridement. Intravenous antibiotics and negative pressure wound therapy should be considered. In more severe situations, early soft-tissue coverage can salvage the total ankle prosthesis. If wound-healing problems occur during the first 4 to 6 weeks and there is evidence of deep infection or fluid collection, deep tissue cultures and polyethylene exchange are recommended. In the authors' experience, this approach has been successful in managing early infections, though diligence in monitoring for secondary infection is necessary.

Diagnostic methods to detect infection following TAA are evolving. Evaluation may include aspiration of the ankle joint after a minimum 2-week period without antibiotic treatment to enhance accuracy of the results. Serum markers for infection, which include erythrocyte sedimentation rate and C-reactive protein level, are also monitored for abnormal elevation. Tagged white blood cell scan has also been found helpful and certainly better than an isolated technetium bone scan. More recently, single-photon emission CT has been used as a diagnostic measure in infection. In addition, methods to detect human alpha defensins through aspiration of the synovial fluid are under investigation. Alpha defensins are antimicrobial proteins released by activated neutrophils and thus may assist with early detection when other techniques produce a false-negative result.[56]

Subacute and chronic infection involving TAA, especially in the case of component loosening, often requires a two-stage approach involving implant/hardware removal, thorough irrigation and débridement, and antibiotic cement spacer placement at the index procedure. This is followed by reimplantation of components after completion of an appropriate course of antibiotics (often intravenous). Such situations have less favorable outcomes and a lower chance of implant retention. In the elderly or infirm patients, chronic antibiotic suppression is a poor but necessary substitute.

In a study reporting on surgical management of infected TAA, the infected TAA was found in 19 of 613 replacements (3%) and consisted of 15 late chronic, 3 early postoperative, and 1 acute hematogenous infection. Only 3 of 19 patients (16%) underwent successful revision.[57] Another study found a 53.9% long-term failure rate with irrigation, débridement, and polyethylene exchange and component retention in 14 patients who underwent TAA and had an acute hematogenous prosthetic infection.[58] Late infections of a TAA may occur as a result of hematogenous seeding independent of intraoperative causation. Aggressive irrigation and débridement with removal of the prosthesis and placement of an antibiotic spacer is typically necessary. Consultation with an infectious diseases specialist with experience in prosthetic infections is recommended to ensure optimal results.

Medial or lateral (or both) gutter impingement is the most common reason for revision surgery after TAA, with up to 7% of patients who underwent TAA returning to the operating room for gutter débridement.[11,59-61] Inadequate gutter débridement at the index procedure is one likely cause of postoperative gutter impingement (and the simplest to correct by ensuring adequate débridement at the index procedure). A 2019 study demonstrated

Section 3: Arthritis of the Foot and Ankle

with weight-bearing CT data that malrotation can also be a significant cause of gutter impingement.[10] Adequate débridement of bony impingement and correct rotation are essential in lowering TAA reoperation rates.

OUTCOMES

Several studies demonstrate a surgical learning curve associated with TAA. The learning curve seems to be related to surgeon experience and implant familiarity. These studies reveal initial outcome with a new implant and/or surgeon inexperience will likely generate inferior patient outcomes.[29,30,62,63] These data suggest the importance of fellowship training and exposure of foot and ankle surgeons to TAA, if only to appreciate methods of correcting foot and ankle deformity that might not be commonplace with other total joint surgeons. Still, with proper training, monitoring results for success and failure, and using that knowledge to develop refined protocols, low-volume centers can achieve good results and positive patient outcomes.[64]

A 2020 TAA survivorship meta-analysis showed an overall implant survival rate of 93% with at least 5-year follow-up.[65] This level I midterm survivorship study featured second-generation and third-generation implants available in the United States. Patient age and fixed-bearing versus mobile-bearing implants showed no statistically significant difference in survivorship.

The most common reasons for revision of an ankle implant are aseptic loosening and instability and component subsidence.[17,66,67] Because no clear superiority has been established with regard to specific implants, surgeons must evaluate the available literature on the specific implants they are considering and ensure proper training before undertaking their first procedure.

Most studies are published by high-volume centers and surgeon developers of a particular implant. Therefore, their work may not reflect the average surgeon's experience with certain implants, and this makes the interpretation of these results challenging.[68] Registry data can be beneficial in this setting but must be interpreted with caution given the variability in experience of the user. One report based on national registry results reveals the rate of revision surgery was 21.8% at 5 years and 43.5% at 10 years.[69] Several other national registries have shown 5-year survivorship to be between 78% and 86%.[17,66,67] However, most registry studies on TAA include implants that are not available in the United States. In addition, most implants used in registry studies are mobile bearing and may not reflect the outcomes expected with the more commonly used fixed-bearing implants. In addition, because it is not possible to know how a case was coded, less-involved procedures such as

exchange of a polyethylene spacer may be considered the same as complete revision of the entire implant. In the future, failure of TAA implants may be reported more accurately through metrics such as measured component subsidence and/or patient pain/dysfunction rather than the current method of revision of one or more of the metallic components. It is clear that many patients with failed total ankle implants choose to retain their implant rather than undergo often complex revision surgery with unverified results. This is particularly true in elderly patients with poor bone stock.

REVISION TAA

A TAA revision may be the best alternative when the primary TAA has failed. Failure can be characterized by recalcitrant pain, recurrent deformity, bone impingement, progressive bone loss compromising implant stability, subsidence of one or both components, or polyethylene failure by wear or fracture leading to osteolysis.

Revision TAA involves challenges with the soft-tissue envelope, bone loss, and mechanical issues that may have predisposed the previous implant to fail.

Bone defects are variable and are influenced by the implant type. The original levels of bone resection for an implant correlates poorly with the residual preserved bone following implant failure. Compromised malleoli following subsidence or recurrent deformity can present challenges in determining the rotation of the revision implant. Proximal rotational control built into the revision prosthesis is desirable. In addition, more proximal resection on the tibial side may compromise the syndesmosis and place the medial malleolus at risk for fracture as the medial portion of the tibia narrows. Fixation into the tibia itself is challenging because there is little distal bone. This favors vertical fixation with stems on the tibial implant. The joint line can be reestablished by using an augmented tibial baseplate or, less desirably, large polyethylene spacers.

Talar bone defects pose larger challenges during revision TAA. The maximum height of the native talus is 2.4 cm, so subsidence of the primary talar component can easily limit sufficient bone support. In addition, cysts within the body of the talus may compromise implant support. The etiology of cystic disease of the talus remains unclear (its source may be particle-based osteolysis, compromise in blood supply with subsequent osteonecrosis, or progression of preexisting arthritic cysts), and the end result is the common pathway of a loose talar component that subsides. Subsidence typically occurs inferiorly and posteriorly, and ultimately, the implant may violate the subtalar joint. Reconstruction options may include explant of the primary prosthesis followed by a subtalar joint arthrodesis to reestablish a stable base for the prosthesis. In this scenario, the revision procedure is performed in the second stage following union of the arthrodesis. In the event of a contained talar defect (cyst), impaction grafting may be effective, but only with excellent preparation of the native residual talar bone. In some circumstances, that residual talar bone has a blood supply, which is too compromised to allow ingrowth of the impaction graft, and cement becomes a better alternative to provide immediate stability to the revision talar component.[70] Augmented talar components are also available to restore height, but specific metallic augments are currently prohibited in the United States by the FDA.

With respect to cyst formation and detection, radiolucencies that appear in postoperative follow-up radiographs warrant further evaluation. If periprosthetic cyst formation is identified, it should be evaluated using CT. In one study, CT detected cysts twice as often as plain radiographs, and the mean size of the lesion by CT was three times higher than that same lesion detected on plain radiographs.[71] Although the presence of lucency or cyst does not indicate pending failure of an implant, the cyst must be followed for progression, and cyst location should be taken into account when intervention is considered, even in asymptomatic cases.[22,37,46,62,72,73] If cyst formation is progressive and the implant appears stable, bone grafting should be performed to maintain the implant[16,22,37,44,62,72,74] (**Figure 9**).

When performing revision arthroplasty, the surgeon must also evaluate the mechanical alignment and provide periarticular osteotomies to reestablish the mechanical axis if necessary. Published case series on revision arthroplasty with implants currently available in the United States are limited.[75-77] Current literature, however, supports the benefit of revision arthroplasty in terms of maintaining ankle range of motion and preserving the adjacent joints.[78] In addition, given that the high incidence of nonunion and complications was 10.6% and 18.2%, respectively, in cases of salvage arthrodesis, revision TAA is favored when technically achievable.[79]

When a failed TAA is not amenable to revision prosthesis, an arthrodesis procedure is considered. Hindfoot nail systems, plate-and-screw fixation options, or ring-and-wire fixation devices all could be considered as options for salvage procedures. Surgeon experience and preference will likely determine the path for treatment.

Acceptable fusion rates have been demonstrated with both local bone grafting and structural bone grafting techniques.[79-82] A common option is arthrodesis with a femoral head allograft and intramedullary

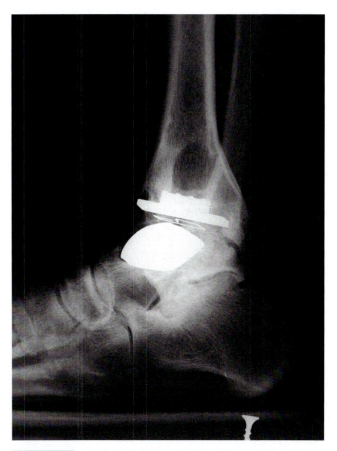

FIGURE 9 Lateral radiograph showing total ankle arthroplasty with cystic lysis and failure of the implant.

fixation with a nail (or plate) in cases of aseptic failure. This allows preservation of appropriate limb length. The malleoli are also preserved by this method. A posterior approach may offer advantages because it allows preparation of both the ankle and subtalar joints through a single incision. This approach also ensures that the graft may be taller posteriorly to prevent the hindfoot from being positioned into equinus. Posterior plate fixation is optimal through this approach, and a variety of robust plates have been designed to accommodate this technique.

In situations where infection was present, tibiocalcaneal arthrodesis is performed with either an external ring fixator or an antibiotic-coated intramedullary nail. Shortening is accepted, and patients will compensate with a lift placed in their shoe. At a later time, these patients may be treated with proximal lengthening of the tibia.

Among patients with underlying inflammatory arthritis, careful evaluation and follow-up is important because there is an increased risk of nonunion in this population.[80,81] The overall complication rate and nonunion rate of arthrodesis after failed TAA have been reported at 18.2% and 10.6%, respectively.[79,82]

Amputation may also be considered in certain situations, such as a recalcitrant infection or when a salvage arthrodesis fails. Amputation rates following attempted salvage of failed total ankle implants have been reported as high as 19%.[83] However, these generally represent complex cases, and most primary ankle replacements have a low risk of eventually requiring amputation because of failure. Diabetes, and the presence of preoperative ulcers, appears to increase risk for amputation after salvage procedures.[83,84]

Counseling is warranted for patients with risk factors placing them at increased risk for amputation. Some patients may elect amputation instead of a salvage procedure, which may be reasonable for that particular patient. Every attempt is made to provide a patient the most acceptable residual limb to allow for prosthesis wear. It is advisable to send a patient for a preoperative consultation with a prosthetist to discuss future needs after surgery.

ARTHRODESIS VERSUS ARTHROPLASTY

Ankle arthritis has been shown to create as much disability—both mentally and physically—as end-stage hip arthrosis.[85] Ankle arthritis can substantially influence the quality of life; as a result, treatment options include both ankle arthrodesis and TAA. Patients with end-stage ankle arthritis are typically younger than their hip and knee counterparts, which plays a significant role in their needs and expectations.[86]

Comparisons between ankle arthrodesis and TAA often involve gait, pain relief, functional outcome, range of motion, and cost-effectiveness. Complications associated with both procedures have also been studied. Both ankle arthrodesis and TAA result in significant pain relief.[62,87,88] Because pain reduction is the primary component of most clinical outcome questionnaires, studies using standard patient-reported outcome scores have not demonstrated a significant difference between patients undergoing TAA or ankle arthrodesis.[62] In contrast, another study evaluating patients on uneven surfaces and stairs showed improved outcome in patients undergoing ankle replacement compared with those undergoing ankle arthrodesis.[89]

Complications such as infection, wound issues, and neurovascular injury can occur with both ankle arthrodesis and TAA. Each procedure involves unique potential complications. Unique to ankle arthrodesis is nonunion. The rate of nonunion is reported to be approximately 10%.[16] Malunion, limb shortening and atrophy, and adjacent joint arthritis also can be seen following ankle arthrodesis.

TAA also presents unique long-term complications. Polyethylene wear, implant loosening, and instability can occur following TAA, conditions not associated with ankle arthrodesis.[17,66,67]

For many patients, the antalgic gait associated with end-stage ankle arthritis, and the loss of function, is the primary motivation for intervention. The inability to participate in desired activities, and the potential to return to these activities after intervention, often carries substantial weight when patients make decisions concerning surgical intervention. Several studies have shown that gait parameters are affected differently by arthrodesis and arthroplasty.[90,91] Studies have been performed comparing patients who have undergone ankle fusion and TAA using age-adjusted norms with respect to gait.[91-93] Patients with ankle arthritis have a shorter stride length, reduced walking speed, and shorter duration of the stance phase in the affected limb during the gait cycle.[91,94,95]

End-stage ankle arthritis substantially influences quality-of-life indicators and overall well-being.[96] Both arthrodesis and TAA have been shown to improve patient quality of life.[96] There are significant differences in postoperative gait for people undergoing both arthrodesis and arthroplasty. Patients undergoing ankle arthrodesis exhibit more asymmetry in gait and increased hip range of motion.[92,93] In contrast, patients undergoing TAA demonstrate increased ankle and knee range of motion, reduced limp, and a more normal gait cycle.[90-93,97] It has been noted, however, that neither arthrodesis nor arthroplasty returns the gait cycle to normal parameters.[90,91] The improvement in gait after TAA is sustainable over several years according to midterm data presented in a 2021 study.[98]

CONVERSION OF ARTHRODESIS TO ARTHROPLASTY

There are limited circumstances in which conversion from ankle arthrodesis to TAA is appropriate. Early conversion of an ankle arthrodesis that did not unite is probably the best example for this procedure. The improved outcome for this conversion is similar to performing a primary TAA. A malunited ankle fusion with symptomatic adjacent joint arthritis also is a good indication for conversion to a TAA to create a mobile ankle segment while the adjacent arthritic joints are fused for pain relief.

Despite conversion of a fused ankle to a mobile ankle, motion itself will remain restricted because of the soft-tissue envelope, which has adapted to the prior ankle arthrodesis. Outcome studies on conversions reveal improvement in pain and clinical function despite the technically challenging nature of the procedure.[99-101] The most frequent complication after conversion is arthrofibrosis.[102] Malleolar fracture is also a concern both at the time of surgery and in the early postoperative period. The malleolar bone becomes osteoporotic over years following ankle arthrodesis given the lack of anatomic loading given the absence of ligament tension and repetitive impact. Loss of subchondral bone in long-standing ankle arthrodesis poses a significant challenge for implant fixation in the setting of a conversion. Conversion of a well-positioned and solidly fused ankle arthrodesis with minimal adjacent joint arthritis is not indicated.

SUMMARY

TAA has evolved into a predictable and sustainable treatment option for end-stage arthritis of the ankle. The contrasts and similarities between ankle arthrodesis and TAA should be objectively discussed as a part of a comprehensive preoperative consultation. The decision algorithm should emphasize the primary goal of pain relief, preservation of motion at the ankle, activity expectation, implant longevity, and adjacent joint arthritis.

KEY STUDY POINTS

- The improvement of the current generation of TAA implants includes limited bony resection and improved fixation providing better initial stability and encouraging bony ingrowth, while seeking to restore the physiologic constraint and articulation of the ankle joint.
- Proper selection of patients undergoing TAA is critical for achieving a satisfactory clinical outcome. The indications and contraindications must be scrutinized.
- The 10° to 15° threshold in coronal plane deformity correction through TAA is no longer valid. Recent literature reveals equivalent outcomes and alignment in patients with either mild or severe coronal plane deformity. The surgeon's ability to correct this deformity to neutral at the time of the surgery plays an important role for achieving these good results.
- Gutter impingement is the most common reason for secondary surgery following primary TAA. Therefore, aggressive resection of both medial and lateral gutter impingement should be performed during the primary procedure.
- Revision TAA systems are readily available. The challenges for revision TAA include a thin soft-tissue envelope, prior incisions, bone defects/bone loss of tibia and talus, and mechanical issues that may have predisposed the original implant to fail.

ANNOTATED REFERENCES

1. Lord G, Marotte JH: Total ankle prosthesis: Technic and 1st results. Apropos of 12 cases [French]. *Rev Chir Orthop Reparatrice Appar Mot* 1973;59(2):139-151.

2. Vickerstaff JA, Miles AW, Cunningham JL: A brief history of total ankle replacement and a review of the current status. *Med Eng Phys* 2007;29(10):1056-1064.

3. Aitken G, Bourne R, Finlay J, Rorabeck CH, Andreae PR: Indentation stiffness of the cancellous bone in the distal human tibia. *Clin Orthop Relat Res* 1985;201:264-270.

4. Cracchiolo A 3rd, DeOrio JK: Design features of current total ankle replacements: Implants and instrumentation. *J Am Acad Orthop Surg* 2008;16(9):530-540.

5. Ling J, Smyth N, Fraser E, et al: Investigating the relationship between ankle arthrodesis and adjacent -joint arthritis in the hindfoot a systematic review. *J Bone Joint Surg Am* 2015;97(9):e43-e519.

6. Kozanek M, Rubash HE, Li G, de Asla RJ: Effect of post-traumatic tibiotalar osteoarthritis on kinematics of the ankle joint complex. *Foot Ankle Int* 2009;30(8):734-740.

7. Chou LB, Coughlin MT, Hansen S Jr, et al: Osteoarthritis of the ankle: The role of arthroplasty. *J Am Acad Orthop Surg* 2008;16(5):249-259.

8. Buechel FF, Pappas MJ, Iorio LJ: New Jersey low contact stress total ankle replacement: Biomechanical rationale and review of 23 cementless cases. *Foot Ankle* 1988;8(6):279-290.

9. Kim BS, Choi WJ, Kim YS, Lee JW: Total ankle replacement in moderate to severe varus deformity of the ankle. *J Bone Joint Surg Br* 2009;91(9):1183-1190.

10. Najefi A, Ghani Y, Goldberg A: Role of rotation in total ankle replacement. *Foot Ankle Int* 2019;40(12):1358-1367.

    Findings show large variation in axial rotation, particularly between the medial gutter line and the transmalleolar axis. Careful clinical assessment and preoperative CT are recommended. Level of evidence: II.

11. Schuberth JM, Babu NS, Richey JM, Christensen JC: Gutter impingement after total ankle arthroplasty. *Foot Ankle Int* 2013;34(3):329-337.

12. Tennant JN, Rungprai C, Pizzimenti MA, et al: Risks to the blood supply of the talus with four methods of total ankle arthroplasty: A cadaveric injection study. *J Bone Joint Surg Am* 2014;96(5):395-402.

13. Dyke J, Garfinkel J, Volpert L, et al: Imaging of bone perfusion and metabolism in subjects undergoing total ankle arthroplasty using 18F-Fluoride positron emission tomography. *Foot Ankle Int* 2019;40(12):1351-1357.

    This study quantified perfusion within the talus beneath the TAA implant, supporting the hypothesis that perfusion of the talus remained intact after surgery. Level of evidence: II.

14. Spirt AA, Assal M, Hansen ST Jr: Complications and failure after total ankle arthroplasty. *J Bone Joint Surg Am* 2004;86(6):1172-1178.

15. Fevang BT, Lie SA, Havelin LI, Brun JG, Skredderstuen A, Furnes O: 257 ankle arthroplasties performed in Norway between 1994 and 2005. *Acta Orthop* 2007;78(5):575-583.

16. Haddad SL, Coetzee JC, Estok R, Fahrbach K, Banel D, Nalysnyk L: Intermediate and long-term outcomes of total ankle arthroplasty and ankle arthrodesis. A systematic review of the literature. *J Bone Joint Surg Am* 2007;89(9): 1899-1905.

17. Henricson A, Skoog A, Carlsson A: The Swedish Ankle Arthroplasty Register: An analysis of 531 arthroplasties between 1993 and 2005. *Acta Orthop* 2007;78(5): 569-574.

18. Demetracopoulos CA, Adams SB Jr, Queen RM, DeOrio JK, Nunley JA 2nd, Easley ME: Effect of age on outcomes in total ankle arthroplasty. *Foot Ankle Int* 2015;36(8):871-880.

19. Gaugler M, Krähenbühl N, Barg A, et al: Effect of age on outcome and revision in total ankle arthroplasty. *Bone Joint J* 2020;102-B(7):925-932.

   Outcomes of TAA in younger patients were similar to those in older patients at early follow-up. Level of evidence: II.

20. Hurowitz EJ, Gould JS, Fleisig GS, Fowler R: Outcome analysis of agility total ankle replacement with prior adjunctive procedures: Two to six year followup. *Foot Ankle Int* 2007;28(3):308-312.

21. van der Heide HJ, Schutte B, Louwerens JW, van den Hoogen FH, Malefijt MC: Total ankle prostheses in rheumatoid arthropathy: Outcome in 52 patients followed for 1-9 years. *Acta Orthop* 2009;80(4):440-444.

22. Mann JA, Mann RA, Horton E: STAR™ ankle: Long-term results. *Foot Ankle Int* 2011;32(5):S473-S484.

23. Bonnin MP, Laurent JR, Casillas M: Ankle function and sports activity after total ankle arthroplasty. *Foot Ankle Int* 2009;30(10):933-944.

24. Naal FD, Impellizzeri FM, Loibl M, Huber M, Rippstein PF: Habitual physical activity and sports participation after total ankle arthroplasty. *Am J Sports Med* 2009;37(1): 95-102.

25. Johns WL, Sowers CB, Walley KC, et al: Return to sports and activity after total ankle arthroplasty and arthrodesis: A systematic review. *Foot Ankle Int* 2020;41(8): 916-929.

   Participation in sports activity was approximately 10% improved after TAA and minimally improved after ankle arthrodesis. Patients who underwent ankle arthrodesis were more active at baseline. High-impact sports were still limited overall. Level of evidence: III.

26. Kadakia RJ, Akoh CC, Chen J, Sharma A, Parekh SG: 3D printed total talus replacement for avascular necrosis of the talus. *Foot Ankle Int* 2020;41(12):1529-1536.

   Patients demonstrated significant improvements in pain scores and patient-reported outcomes with total talus replacement. Total talus replacement is an alternative for patients with talar collapse and osteonecrosis. Level of evidence: IV.

27. Taniguchi A, Takakura Y, Tanaka Y, et al: An alumina ceramic total talar prosthesis for osteonecrosis of the talus. *J Bone Joint Surg Am* 2015;97(16):1348-1353.

28. Morita S, Taniguchi A, Miyamoto T, et al: The long-term clinical results of total talar replacement at 10 years or more after surgery. *J Bone Joint Surg Am* 2022;104(9):790-795.

   Patients who underwent total talus replacement showed favorable clinical results over at least a 10-year follow-up period. Level of evidence: IV.

29. Gougoulias N, Khanna A, Maffulli N: How successful are current ankle replacements? A systematic review of the literature. *Clin Orthop Relat Res* 2010;468(1):199-208.

30. Lee KT, Lee YK, Young KW, Kim JB, Seo YS: Perioperative complications and learning curve of the mobility total ankle system. *Foot Ankle Int* 2013;34(2):210-214.

31. Whalen JL, Spelsberg SC, Murray P: Wound breakdown after total ankle arthroplasty. *Foot Ankle Int* 2010;31(4): 301-305.

32. Hsu A, Franceschina D, Haddad S: A novel method of postoperative wound care following total ankle arthroplasty. *Foot Ankle Int* 2014;35(7):719-724.

33. Bibbo C: Posterior approach for total ankle arthroplasty. *J Foot Ankle Surg* 2013;52(1):132-135.

34. Queen RM, Grier AJ, Butler RJ, et al: The influence of concomitant triceps surae lengthening at the time of total ankle arthroplasty on postoperative outcomes. *Foot Ankle Int* 2014;35(9):863-870.

35. DeOrio JK, Lewis JS Jr: Silfverskiöld's test in total ankle replacement with gastrocnemius recession. *Foot Ankle Int* 2014;35(2):116-122.

36. Knecht SI, Estin M, Callaghan JJ, et al: The agility total ankle arthroplasty: Seven to sixteen-year follow-up. *J Bone Joint Surg Am* 2004;86(6):1161-1171.

37. Wood PL, Prem H, Sutton C: Total ankle replacement: Medium-term results in 200 Scandinavian total ankle replacements. *J Bone Joint Surg Br* 2008;90(5):605-609.

38. SooHoo NF, Zingmond DS, Ko CY: Comparison of reoperation rates following ankle arthrodesis and total ankle arthroplasty. *J Bone Joint Surg Am* 2007;89(10): 2143-2149.

39. Dekker TJ, Walton D, Vinson EN, et al: Hindfoot arthritis progression and arthrodesis risk after total ankle replacement. *Foot Ankle Int* 2017;38(11):1183-1187.

40. DeOrio JK: Total ankle replacement with subtalar arthrodesis: Management of combined ankle and subtalar arthritis. *Tech Foot Ankle Surg* 2010;9(4):182-189.

41. Gross CE, Lewis JS, Adams SB, Easley M, DeOrio JK, Nunley JA 2nd: Secondary arthrodesis after total ankle arthroplasty. *Foot Ankle Int* 2016;37(7):709-714.

42. Lewis JS Jr, Adams SB Jr, Queen RM, DeOrio JK, Nunley JA, Easley ME: Outcomes after total ankle replacement in association with ipsilateral hindfoot arthrodesis. *Foot Ankle Int* 2014;35(6):535-542.

43. Cody EA, Bejarano-Pineda L, Lachman JR, et al: Risk factors for failure of total ankle arthroplasty with a minimum five years of follow up. *Foot Ankle Int* 2019;40(3):249-258.

Retrospective cohort study evaluating independent risk factors for total ankle implant failure at mid- to long-term follow-up. Patients with ipsilateral hindfoot fusion or those who received an INBONE I prosthesis were at significantly higher risk of implant failure. Age, BMI, and amount of deformity were not associated with higher implant failure rates. Level of evidence: III.

44. Wood PL, Deakin S: Total ankle replacement. The results in 200 ankles. *J Bone Joint Surg Br* 2003;85(3):334-341.

45. Nagashima M, Takahashi H, Kakumoto S, Miyamoto Y, Yoshino S: Total ankle arthroplasty for deformity of the foot in patients with rheumatoid arthritis using the TNK ankle system: Clinical results of 21 cases. *Mod Rheumatol* 2004;14(1):48-53.

46. Wood PL, Sutton C, Mishra V, Suneja R: A randomised, controlled trial of two mobile-bearing total ankle replacements. *J Bone Joint Surg Br* 2009;91(1):69-74.

47. Hobson SA, Karantana A, Dhar S: Total ankle replacement in patients with significant pre-operative deformity of the hindfoot. *J Bone Joint Surg Br* 2009;91(4):481-486.

48. Reddy SC, Mann JA, Mann RA, Mangold DR: Correction of moderate to severe coronal plane deformity with the STAR ankle prosthesis. *Foot Ankle Int* 2011;32(7):659-664.

49. Trincat S, Kouyoumdjian P, Asencio G: Total ankle arthroplasty and coronal plane deformities. *Orthop Traumatol Surg Res* 2012;98(1):75-84.

50. Doets HC, van der Plaat LW, Klein JP: Medial malleolar osteotomy for the correction of varus deformity during total ankle arthroplasty: Results in 15 ankles. *Foot Ankle Int* 2008;29(2):171-177.

51. Daniels TR, Cadden AR, Lim K: Correction of varus talar deformities in ankle joint replacement. *Oper Tech Orthop* 2008;18(4):282-286.

52. Demetracopoulos CA, Cody EA, Adams SB Jr, DeOrio JK, Nunley JA 2nd, Easley ME: Outcomes of total ankle arthroplasty in moderate and severe valgus deformity. *Foot Ankle Spec* 2019;12(3):238-245.

Therapeutic study evaluating clinical, radiographic, and patient-reported outcomes of patients with moderate to severe valgus deformity who underwent TAA. Mean preoperative valgus deformity of 15.5° was corrected to a mean of 1.2° of valgus postoperatively. This correction was sustained between 1 year and final follow-up. Outcome scores improved significantly in all patients. Level of evidence: IV.

53. Wang Q, Zhang N, Guo W, Wang W, Zhang Q: Patient-specific instrumentation (PSI) in total ankle arthroplasty: A systematic review. *Int Orthop* 2021;45(9):2445-2452.

PSI showed slightly decreased surgical times and fluoroscopy times. Implant position was similar to that of PSI. Current evidence is lacking to evaluate PSI TAA. Level of evidence: III.

54. Manegold S, Haas NP, Tsitsilonis S, Springer A, Märdian S, Schaser KD: Periprosthetic fractures in total ankle replacement: Classification system and treatment algorithm. *J Bone Joint Surg Am* 2013;95(9):815-820, S1-S3.

55. Raikin SM, Kane J, Ciminiello ME: Risk factors for incision-healing complications following total ankle arthroplasty. *J Bone Joint Surg Am* 2010;92(12):2150-2155.

56. Bonanzinga T, Ferrari M, Tanzi G, Vandenbulcke F, Zahar A, Marcacci M: The role of alpha defensin in prosthetic joint infection (PJI) diagnosis: A literature review. *EFORT Open Rev* 2019;4(1):10-13.

The laboratory-based alpha defensin enzyme-linked immunosorbent assay test demonstrated the highest ever reported accuracy for prosthetic joint infection diagnosis. Alpha defensin synovial biomarkers currently have the highest specificity and sensitivity for diagnosing prosthetic joint infections. Level of evidence: III.

57. Myerson MS, Shariff R, Zonno AJ: The management of infection following total ankle replacement: Demographics and treatment. *Foot Ankle Int* 2014;35(9):855-862.

58. Lachman JR, Ramos JA, DeOrio JK, Easley ME, Nunley JA, Adams SB: Outcomes of acute hematogenous periprosthetic joint infection in total ankle arthroplasty treated with irrigation, debridement, and polyethylene exchange. *Foot Ankle Int* 2018;39(11):1266-1271.

59. Kurup HV, Taylor GR: Medial impingement after ankle replacement. *Int Orthop* 2008;32(2):243-246.

60. Choi WJ, Lee JW: Heterotopic ossification after total ankle arthroplasty. *J Bone Joint Surg Br* 2011;93(11):1508-1512.

61. Lee KB, Cho YJ, Park JK, Song EK, Yoon TR, Seon JK: Heterotopic ossification after primary total ankle arthroplasty. *J Bone Joint Surg Am* 2011;93(8):751-758.

62. Saltzman CL, Mann RA, Ahrens JE, et al: Prospective controlled trial of STAR total ankle replacement versus ankle fusion: Initial results. *Foot Ankle Int* 2009;30(7):579-596.

63. Rippstein PF, Huber M, Naal FD: Management of specific complications related to total ankle arthroplasty. *Foot Ankle Clin* 2012;17(4):707-717.

64. Reuver JM, Dayerizadeh N, Burger B, Elmans L, Hoelen M, Tulp N: Total ankle replacement outcome in low volume centers: Short-term followup. *Foot Ankle Int* 2010;31(12):1064-1068.

65. McKenna B, Cook J, Cook E, et al: Total ankle arthroplasty survivorship: A meta-analysis. *J Foot Ankle Surg* 2020;59(5):1040-1048.

Overall survivorship of this meta-analysis was high at 93.0%. These results are promising although high-quality studies are needed. Level of evidence: I.

66. Hosman AH, Mason RB, Hobbs T, Rothwell AG: A New Zealand national joint registry review of 202 total ankle replacements followed for up to 6 years. *Acta Orthop* 2007;78(5):584-591.

67. Skyttä ET, Koivu H, Eskelinen A, Ikävalko M, Paavolainen P, Remes V: Total ankle replacement: A population-based

study of 515 cases from the Finnish Arthroplasty Register. *Acta Orthop* 2010;81(1):114-118.

68. Labek G, Klaus H, Schlichtherle R, Williams A, Agreiter M: Revision rates after total ankle arthroplasty in sample-based clinical studies and national registries. *Foot Ankle Int* 2011;32(8):740-745.

69. Jastifer JR, Coughlin MJ: Long-term follow-up of mobile bearing total ankle arthroplasty in the United States. *Foot Ankle Int* 2015;36(2):143-150.

70. Prissel MA, Roukis TS: Management of extensive tibial osteolysis with the Agility™ total ankle replacement systems using geometric metal-reinforced polymethylmethacrylate cement augmentation. *J Foot Ankle Surg* 2014;53(1): 101-107.

71. Hanna R, Haddad S, Lazarus M: Evaluation of periprosthetic lucency after total ankle arthroplasty: Helical CT versus conventional radiography. *Foot Ankle Int* 2007;28(8): 921-926.

72. Bonnin M, Gaudot F, Laurent JR, Ellis S, Colombier JA, Judet T: The Salto total ankle arthroplasty: Survivorship and analysis of failures at 7 to 11 years. *Clin Orthop Relat Res* 2011;469(1):225-236.

73. Rippstein PF, Huber M, Coetzee JC, Naal FD: Total ankle replacement with use of a new three-component implant. *J Bone Joint Surg Am* 2011;93(15):1426-1435.

74. Nelissen RG, Doets HC, Valstar ER: Early migration of the tibial component of the buechel-pappas total ankle prosthesis. *Clin Orthop Relat Res* 2006;448(448):146-151.

75. Devries JG, Berlet GC, Lee TH, Hyer CF, Deorio JK: Revision total ankle replacement: An early look at agility to INBONE. *Foot Ankle Spec* 2011;4(4):235-244.

76. Ellington JK, Gupta S, Myerson MS: Management of failures of total ankle replacement with the agility total ankle arthroplasty. *J Bone Joint Surg Am* 2013;95(23): 2112-2118.

77. Horisberger M, Henninger HB, Valderrabano V, Barg A: Bone augmentation for revision total ankle arthroplasty with large bone defects: A technical note in 10 cases. *Acta Orthop* 2015;86(4):412-414.

78. Hordyk PJ, Fuerbringer BA, Roukis TS: Sagittal ankle and midfoot range of motion before and after revision total ankle replacement: A retrospective comparative analysis. *J Foot Ankle Surg* 2018;57(3):521-526.

79. Gross CE, Erickson BJ, Adams SB, Parekh SG: Ankle arthrodesis after failed total ankle replacement: A systematic review of the literature. *Foot Ankle Spec* 2015;8(2):143-151.

80. Culpan P, Le Strat V, Piriou P, Judet T: Arthrodesis after failed total ankle replacement. *J Bone Joint Surg Br* 2007;89(9):1178-1183.

81. Doets HC, Zürcher AW: Salvage arthrodesis for failed total ankle arthroplasty. *Acta Orthop* 2010;81(1):142-147.

82. Berkowitz MJ, Clare MP, Walling AK, Sanders R: Salvage of failed total ankle arthroplasty with fusion using structural allograft and internal fixation. *Foot Ankle Int* 2011;32(5):S49 3-S502.

83. Jeng CL, Campbell JT, Tang EY, Cerrato RA, Myerson MS: Tibiotalocalcaneal arthrodesis with bulk femoral head allograft for salvage of large defects in the ankle. *Foot Ankle Int* 2013;34(9):1256-1266.

84. DeVries JG, Berlet GC, Hyer CF: Predictive risk assessment for major amputation after tibiotalocalcaneal arthrodesis. *Foot Ankle Int* 2013;34(6):846-850.

85. Glazebrook M, Daniels T, Younger A, et al: Comparison of health-related quality of life between patients with end-stage ankle and hip arthrosis. *J Bone Joint Surg Am* 2008;90(3):499-505.

86. Saltzman CL, Salamon ML, Blanchard GM, et al: Epidemiology of ankle arthritis: Report of a consecutive series of 639 patients from a tertiary orthopaedic center. *Iowa Orthop J* 2005;25:44-46.

87. Easley ME, Adams SB Jr, Hembree WC, DeOrio JK: Results of total ankle arthroplasty. *J Bone Joint Surg Am* 2011;93(15):1455-1468.

88. Queen RM, De Biassio JC, Butler RJ, DeOrio JK, Easley ME, Nunley JA: J. Leonard Goldner Award 2011: Changes in pain, function, and gait mechanics two years following total ankle arthroplasty performed with two modern fixed-bearing prostheses. *Foot Ankle Int* 2012;33(7):535-542.

89. Jastifer J, Coughlin MJ, Hirose C: Performance of total ankle arthroplasty and ankle arthrodesis on uneven surfaces, stairs, and inclines: A prospective study. *Foot Ankle Int* 2015;36(1):11-17.

90. Valderrabano V, Nigg BM, von Tscharner V, Stefanyshyn DJ, Goepfert B, Hintermann B: Gait analysis in ankle osteoarthritis and total ankle replacement. *Clin Biomech (Bristol, Avon)* 2007;22(8):894-904.

91. Flavin R, Coleman SC, Tenenbaum S, Brodsky JW: Comparison of gait after total ankle arthroplasty and ankle arthrodesis. *Foot Ankle Int* 2013;34(10):1340-1348.

92. Piriou P, Culpan P, Mullins M, Cardon JN, Pozzi D, Judet T: Ankle replacement versus arthrodesis: A comparative gait analysis study. *Foot Ankle Int* 2008;29(1):3-9.

93. Hahn ME, Wright ES, Segal AD, Orendurff MS, Ledoux WR, Sangeorzan BJ: Comparative gait analysis of ankle arthrodesis and arthroplasty: Initial findings of a prospective study. *Foot Ankle Int* 2012;33(4):282-289.

94. Stauffer RN, Chao EY, Brewster RC: Force and motion analysis of the normal, diseased, and prosthetic ankle joint. *Clin Orthop Relat Res* 1977;127:189-196.

95. Khazzam M, Long JT, Marks RM, Harris GF: Preoperative gait characterization of patients with ankle arthrosis. *Gait Posture* 2006;24(1):85-93.

96. Slobogean GP, Younger A, Apostle KL, et al: Preference-based quality of life of end-stage ankle arthritis treated with arthroplasty or arthrodesis. *Foot Ankle Int* 2010;31(7):563-566.

97. Brodsky JW, Polo FE, Coleman SC, Bruck N: Changes in gait following the Scandinavian total ankle replacement. *J Bone Joint Surg Am* 2011;93(20):1890-1896.

98. Brodsky J, Scott D, Ford S, Coleman S, Daoud Y: Functional outcomes of total ankle arthroplasty at a mean follow-up of 7.6 years: A prospective, 3-dimensional gait analysis. *J Bone Joint Surg Am* 2021;103(6):477-482.

    Patients were shown to have sustained improvement in multiple objective parameters of gait compared with preoperative function. Level of evidence: IV.

99. Greisberg J, Assal M, Flueckiger G, Hansen ST Jr: Take-down of ankle fusion and conversion to total ankle replacement. *Clin Orthop Relat Res* 2004;424:80-88.

100. Hintermann B, Barg A, Knupp M, Valderrabano V: Conversion of painful ankle arthrodesis to total ankle arthroplasty. *J Bone Joint Surg Am* 2009;91(4):850-858.

101. Pellegrini MJ, Schiff AP, Adams SB Jr, et al: Conversion of tibiotalar arthrodesis to total ankle arthroplasty. *J Bone Joint Surg Am* 2015;97(24):2004-2013.

102. Preis M, Bailey T, Marchand LS, Barg A: Can a three-component prosthesis be used for conversion of painful ankle arthrodesis to total ankle replacement? *Clin Orthop Relat Res* 2017;475(9):2283-2294.

CHAPTER 10

Midfoot and Hindfoot Arthrodesis

KSHITIJ MANCHANDA, MD • W. BRET SMITH, DO, FAAOS • TRAPPER LALLI, MD, FAAOS

ABSTRACT

Midfoot and hindfoot arthritis are frequently encountered spectrums of painful and debilitating conditions. Their etiologies may be secondary to trauma, deformity, inflammatory arthritides, neuropathic disease, degenerative arthritis, or idiopathic mechanisms. Joint disease and clinical disability progress in tandem and result in increasing difficulty with shoe wear and ambulation. Nonsurgical measures are the first line of treatment for arthritis and include activity modification, shoe wear modification, orthotics, anti-inflammatory medications, and local joint injections. Many patients can achieve adequate pain relief with nonsurgical management; however, when these fail and patients continue to have progressively worsening pain and deformity, the preferred surgical procedure is arthrodesis and/or deformity correction using osteotomy techniques with or without soft-tissue balancing. Orthobiologics including autograft may augment bony healing in fusion procedures, particularly in high-risk patients.

Keywords: arthrodesis; deformity; hindfoot arthritis; midfoot arthritis; orthobiologics

Dr. Smith or an immediate family member has received royalties from Treace Medical Concepts; serves as a paid consultant to or is an employee of Exactech, Orthofix, Restor3D, and Treace Medical Concepts; and has stock or stock options held in GEO Medical. Dr. Lalli or an immediate family member serves as a paid consultant to or is an employee of Exactech, Inc. Neither Dr. Manchanda nor any immediate family member has received anything of value from or has stock or stock options held in a commercial company or institution related directly or indirectly to the subject of this chapter.

INTRODUCTION

Midfoot and hindfoot arthritis comprise a spectrum of painful and debilitating conditions for which many patients seek the clinical care of a foot and ankle specialist. These conditions are common, but their exact incidence is unknown. Etiologic mechanisms include trauma, deformity, inflammatory arthritides, degenerative arthritis, or idiopathic causes. Because of the different etiologies, arthritis can appear in both younger and older populations. Joint disease and clinical disability progress in tandem and result in increasing difficulty with shoe wear and ambulation. Nonsurgical measures are the first line of treatment; however, when these fail, the preferred surgical procedure is arthrodesis to relieve the progressively worsening pain, deformity, and disability.

ANATOMY

The hindfoot consists of the talus, calcaneus, cuboid, and navicular bones, which articulate through the subtalar, calcaneocuboid, and talonavicular joints. The subtalar joint consists of posterior, middle, and anterior facets. The talonavicular and calcaneocuboid joints are referred to as the transverse tarsal (Chopart) joint. The spring ligament, an important stabilizer of the medial arch, supports the talonavicular joint plantarly.[1] These joints work synchronously and are mainly responsible for inversion and eversion of the hindfoot to accommodate ambulation on uneven ground. Coupled movements of these joints allow the foot to act as a shock absorber at heel strike and to become a rigid lever at push-off.

The midfoot is the junction region connecting the forefoot (metatarsals) to the hindfoot (talus and calcaneus).

Section 3: Arthritis of the Foot and Ankle

This chapter is adapted from O'Donnell SW, Bluman EM: Hindfoot arthritis and Yan AY, Hogan MV: Midfoot arthritis, in Chou LB, ed: *Orthopaedic Knowledge Update®: Foot and Ankle 6*. American Academy of Orthopaedic Surgeons, 2020, pp 145-164.

© 2025 American Academy of Orthopaedic Surgeons

Multiple ligaments, tendons, capsules, interconnected joints, and bony configurations contribute to the construction of this vital junction. The midfoot serves as a stable, load-transferring segment in the unique, bipedal locomotion of human beings.

Articulating between the metatarsals, the three navicular facets, and the cuboid, the midfoot has three distinct longitudinal columns: medial, middle, and lateral (**Figure 1**). The medial column consists of the medial cuneiform–first metatarsal articulation. The middle column includes the middle cuneiform–second metatarsal joint, the lateral cuneiform–third metatarsal joint, and the intercuneiform joints. The lateral column is composed of the cuboid–fourth metatarsal and the cuboid–fifth metatarsal articulations. The keystone and wedged arrangement of the bones of the midfoot joint complex resembles a Roman arch, with the apex at the second metatarsal recessed 4 to 8 mm between the medial and lateral cuneiforms.[2]

In addition to the bony configuration, the midfoot is composed of a strong and complex network of ligamentous connections. Dorsal, plantar, and intercuneiform ligaments provide increased stability to the midfoot. Intermetatarsal ligaments connect the bases of the second through fifth metatarsals to one another. There is no intermetatarsal ligament between the proximal first and second metatarsals. The Lisfranc ligament is the largest ligament of the midfoot ligamentous complex. It links obliquely between the medial cuneiform and the base of the second metatarsal and is composed of three components: dorsal, plantar, and interosseous. The plantar component connects the second and third metatarsals with the medial cuneiform and is the strongest ligament in the Lisfranc complex. Stability of the midfoot is further enhanced by the plantar beam of the peroneus longus as well as contributions from the plantar fascia, anterior tibialis, posterior tibialis, and flexor hallucis brevis.[2]

BIOMECHANICS

The biomechanics of the midfoot and hindfoot are vital to maintaining normal gait. The midfoot is composed of many joints and motion is variable at each joint because of dynamic relationships between the bones. For instance, although the relative motion between the navicular and cuboid bones at the transverse tarsal (Chopart) joint is minor, it plays a significant role in the phases of the gait

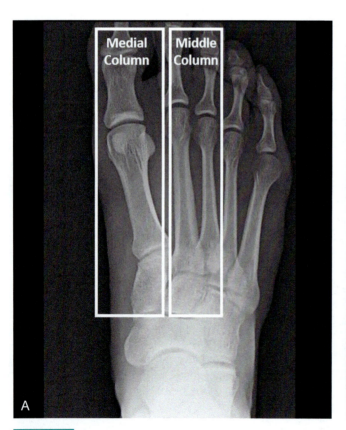 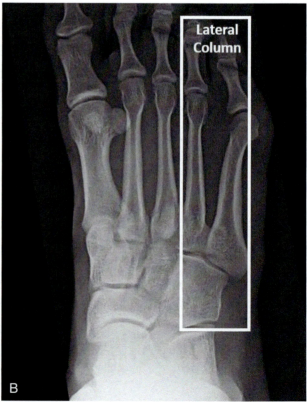

FIGURE 1 **A** AP and **B**, oblique radiographs depicting the columnar anatomy of the midfoot.

cycle. When the subtalar joint everts at heel strike, this aligns the talonavicular and calcaneocuboid joints parallel to each other. This parallelism effectively unlocks the transverse tarsal joint and midfoot, allowing motion and flexibility to absorb impact and balance the foot on the ground during stance. As the foot progresses through the stance phase, the subtalar joint inverts, causing the talonavicular and calcaneocuboid joint axes to diverge and lock the midfoot to create a rigid lever for push-off. The relationship between the Chopart joint and the midfoot complex allows for effective load transfer from the hindfoot and ankle into the midfoot and forefoot.

Considering this complex coupling of multiple joints and facets, it can be difficult to measure their individual motion. Although the entire hindfoot joint complex is involved in inversion and eversion, the transverse tarsal joint is responsible for 26% of foot dorsiflexion and plantar flexion.[3] Cadaver studies of residual joint motion after selective arthrodeses have helped to increase understanding of the complexity of hindfoot motion. Isolated calcaneocuboid arthrodesis has little effect on subtalar motion but decreases talonavicular motion to 67% of its normal value. Subtalar arthrodesis limits calcaneocuboid and talonavicular motion to 56% and 46% of their normal values, respectively. Isolated talonavicular arthrodesis had the most substantial effect, reducing both subtalar and calcaneocuboid motion to less than 8% of normal values.[4,5]

An in vitro study of midfoot motion has shown that the three columns of the midfoot vary at each joint during dorsiflexion–plantar flexion and supination-pronation, with the lateral column having considerably more motion than the medial and middle columns. In the sagittal plane and during supination-pronation, the cuboid-metatarsal joints have approximately 10° of motion, whereas motion at the medial, middle, and lateral cuneiform-metatarsal joints was 3.5°, 0.6°, and 1.6°, respectively. In addition, the second and third tarsometatarsal (TMT) joints have been shown to bear most of the force in the midfoot. As such, the rigid middle column construct may contribute to the more often symptomatic nature of second and third metatarsal-cuneiform arthritis.[6]

PATHOPHYSIOLOGY AND ETIOLOGY

Midfoot and hindfoot arthritis develop in much the same way as arthritis affecting other joints throughout the body. It is the result of direct cartilage or chondrocyte damage from acute macrotrauma, repetitive microtrauma, abnormal weight-bearing stress from articular incongruity, joint malalignment, inflammatory processes adjacent joint arthrodesis, or increased shear stress from ligamentous instability.[1] Any soft-tissue or bony

pathology that causes hindfoot or midfoot deformities can lead to degenerative changes as well. Because of the different etiologies, the age distribution of midfoot arthritis appears to be bimodal: young patients in their 30s with a history of midfoot trauma and patients older than 50 years with primary arthritis.[7] The most common cause of midfoot arthritis is posttraumatic, followed by primary degeneration, and last, inflammatory or neuropathic changes.

The calcaneus is the most commonly fractured tarsal bone, and subtalar posttraumatic arthritis can occur secondary to intra-articular calcaneal fractures. When these injuries are managed nonsurgically, there may be as much as a fivefold increase in the incidence of late subtalar arthrodesis.[8] Damage to the articular surface can occur at the initial injury and over time with the malreduced joint causing uneven loading patterns and progressive cartilage wear. Injury-related cartilage damage can also lead to arthrosis of the midfoot joint complex. Of the various types of midfoot injuries, the incidence rate for midfoot fracture-dislocation is approximately 0.2%. However, there is a 20% rate of missing a fracture-dislocation injury of the midfoot.[9] Thus, it is possible that the incidence of midfoot fracture-dislocation is higher than reported. Furthermore, the literature reports that the development of symptomatic, degenerative arthritis following TMT fracture-dislocation can range from zero to 58%.

Inflammatory arthritis also commonly affects the hindfoot and midfoot. Foot and ankle pain will develop in more than 90% of patients with rheumatoid arthritis. Joint destruction is the result of synovial inflammation leading to cartilage erosion and periarticular bony resorption. This is exacerbated by subsequent ligamentous laxity and possible tendon rupture. Substantial deformity can lead to increased stress on the cartilage and accelerated wear.[10]

Iatrogenic arthritis occurs when foot or ankle surgery leads to increased loads on adjacent joints with subsequent adjacent joint degeneration. One noteworthy example is hindfoot arthritis that develops after ankle arthrodesis. In one study, investigators noted a 90% incidence of adjacent hindfoot arthritis after ankle arthrodesis with a mean follow-up of 22 years.[11] Long-term follow-up of adjacent joint disease following total or partial fusion of the subtalar and midtarsal joints demonstrated high rates of secondary arthritis of the tibiotalar (73%), subtalar (58%), talonavicular (66%), and calcaneocuboid joints (54%); however, the presence of arthritis is not correlated with increased pain at 10-year follow-up.[12]

Development of midfoot arthritis is also related to individual anatomic and biomechanical factors. Long-standing pes planus, first ray instability, short first metatarsal, and long second metatarsal may predispose to deformity and arthritis of the midfoot. The classic deformities of midfoot arthritis include forefoot abduction, collapse of the longitudinal arch, and valgus heel alignment. Collapse of the longitudinal arch results in increased plantar tension and compromises the midfoot lever function during the gait cycle. In addition, sagittal and coronal deformities such as rocker-bottom foot and hallux valgus may be present.[7] Patients with painful midfoot arthritis also demonstrate significantly less first metatarsal plantar flexion excursion during walking and significant calcaneus eversion on step descent when compared with matched control patients.[13] The degenerative process can also result in formation of dorsal and plantar osteophytes, which make shoe wear difficult and may cause callus or ulceration. Injury, inflammation, degeneration, and deformity can cause progressive articular cartilage damage and loss of bony and soft-tissue integrity that result in the painful and debilitating symptoms of midfoot arthritis.

CLINICAL PRESENTATION

Patients with symptomatic midfoot or hindfoot arthritis report pain, swelling, and stiffness. With hindfoot arthritis, the pain is often localized to the sinus tarsi or to areas just distal to the malleoli. Walking on uneven surfaces such as grass, gravel, or sand exacerbates the pain. Pain with loading of the midtarsal region while bearing weight, walking up stairs, or with forced plantar flexion are the most commonly reported symptoms of midfoot arthritis. This can severely restrict a patient's ability to walk and perform daily activities. Patients will often have a deep, aching pain present at rest and may have palpable bony prominences dorsally and/or plantarly, which are associated with swelling and pain that is worse with wearing closed toe shoes. Pain due to irritation of the deep peroneal nerve can also occur because of osteophytes and ganglion cysts developing from capsular rents at the anterior tarsal tunnel. A detailed history of trauma, inflammatory or neuropathic disease, and previous surgeries needs to be assessed during the clinical encounter.

Physical examination with the patient in standing, seated, and dynamic (ie, walking) positions are routinely performed. With the patient standing and undressed from the knees down, overall hindfoot and midfoot alignment should be assessed in the sagittal and coronal planes and any deformities noted and determined to be flexible or rigid.

Palpation of the region occurs during the seated examination and the joints should be assessed for motion as well as point tenderness. Arthritis-associated midfoot pain can be reproduced with the piano key sign or an abduction-pronation stress test of the midtarsal joint.[14] Any limited or painful motion may indicate joint

degeneration and should be compared with the contralateral side. The Coleman block test and the Silfverskiöld test should be performed when there is any malalignment observed and can assist in future surgical decision making. A Silfverskiöld test can help to determine whether the contracture is in the gastrocnemius or the triceps surae. Similarly, the flexibility of the hindfoot in longstanding planovalgus deformity is also critical in guiding treatment. Routine neurovascular examination should always be performed, especially when a neuroarthropathic etiology is suspected. Any motor weakness or sensory loss should be noted because this may indicate a neuromuscular or neuropathic disorder. Patients without palpable pulses should be further evaluated with vascular studies, especially if surgery is being considered.

Diagnostic injections of local anesthetic may aid in identifying specific joint involvement. The subtalar joint can typically be injected in the office setting, whereas injections of the talonavicular, calcaneocuboid, or midfoot joints often necessitate image guidance. Fluoroscopy remains the preferred method for intra-articular injections in the foot and ankle; however, there has been recent interest in the use of ultrasound guidance for diagnostic injections to improve accuracy without ionizing radiation exposure. Although these injections may help to localize pathology, communications can exist between these joints and should be considered when using these diagnostic tests to guide treatment.[15]

IMAGING

AP, lateral, and oblique standing radiographs of the foot are used routinely as part of the initial evaluation to identify the location and extent of the disease as well as to detect any deformity. Weight-bearing radiographs accurately assess alignment and the degree of degenerative joint changes. The AP view will reveal arthritic change as well as forefoot adduction or abduction through the talonavicular joint. Talar head uncovering is frequently used to indicate the amount of abduction present and guide surgical treatment of flatfoot disorder. Arthritis of the calcaneocuboid joint is best seen on an oblique radiograph. The subtalar and talonavicular joints are well visualized on lateral radiographs, as are pes planus or cavus deformities. A radiograph showing primary midfoot arthritis may reveal a lower medial cuneiform height and a negative talar–first metatarsal angle (Meary angle) compared with those of traumatic midfoot arthritis. Recognition of the apex of any collapse of the midfoot in the coronal and sagittal planes helps surgical decision making and planning for future reconstruction.[7] Hindfoot alignment and axillary views are also useful to assess varus or valgus hindfoot deformity[16] (**Figure 2**).

Chapter 10: Midfoot and Hindfoot Arthrodesis

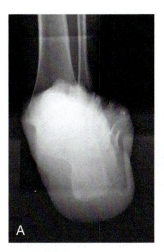 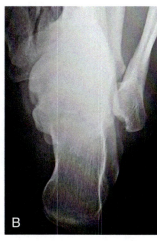

FIGURE 2 Radiographic views showing hindfoot alignment (**A**) and axillary heel (**B**) demonstrating valgus and varus malalignment, respectively.

CT may be useful when there is symptomatic disease that is not easily revealed by plain radiographs. CT also provides the most accurate assessment of the hindfoot joints and may be useful in surgical planning. CT is usually done non–weight bearing and provides a three-dimensional reconstruction to show the extent of arthritis and deformities in the specific, symptomatic joints. With recent advances, cone beam CT technology has made weight-bearing CT more readily available in the foot and ankle clinical setting.[17] This allows radiographic analysis of the foot under physiologic loads. This may be a useful adjunct in measuring hindfoot/midfoot alignment and aid in surgical decision making and therapeutic planning.[18] However, standardization and validation of measurement are still needed for future adoption of cone beam CT as a standard diagnostic approach.

Ultrasonography can effectively identify cortical erosions and synovitis in inflammatory arthritides at low cost and without ionizing radiation exposure. However, ultrasonography's efficacy is operator dependent and is not routinely used in the workup for arthritis. MRI has high sensitivity for detecting arthritic changes in joints but may not be routine imaging for arthritides. Nuclear medicine studies and magnetic resonance arthrography may not be as clinically useful as CT studies. Both modalities have good sensitivity for disease detection but often do not provide the bony resolution of radiograph-based imaging.[19]

When physical examination and imaging studies provide inconclusive information, selective joint injection of local anesthetics under ultrasonographic or fluoroscopic guidance can be done. Selective local anesthetic injection can be very helpful when coupled with use of a pain diary to assist in identifying the diseased joints and ultimately allows for prediction of a future response to arthrodesis.

NONSURGICAL TREATMENT

Nonsurgical management is the initial treatment for midfoot and hindfoot arthritis. The purpose and rationale of nonsurgical management is based on offloading and stabilization. As such, nonsurgical treatment includes activity and shoe modification, anti-inflammatory medications, foot orthoses, and local corticosteroid and anesthetic injections. NSAIDs are often used as a pharmaceutical treatment; however, they are only recommended for short-term use because of their systemic side effects. High-impact activity such as running should be avoided. Low-impact activities involving elliptical trainers, stationary bicycles, or swimming may provide good substitutes. Avoiding uneven terrain and wearing appropriate shoes may also provide substantial relief of symptoms. The next step in management includes the use of orthotic devices. A variety of orthotic devices, braces, and shoe modifications exist for the treatment of foot arthritis. These orthotic devices may provide temporary pain relief for patients who want to delay or avoid surgical procedures or are poor surgical candidates. Although these devices cannot correct deformities or heal existing degenerative joints, they may provide pain relief through soft-tissue rest. Their use can be considered successful if they eliminate the need for surgical intervention by reducing pain, preventing deformity progression, or slowing the development of arthritis.[20]

The extent of joint disease and the presence of deformity will determine the appropriate orthotic device. A simple shoe modification such as a rocker-bottom sole may be sufficient to offload the foot and decrease pain. When degenerative disease or deformity is more advanced, a stabilizing or position correcting device can be added to relieve pressure, reduce flexible deformities, limit motion, and/or accommodate fixed deformities. Flexible deformities may be stabilized or corrected by adding a post to an orthotic device; fixed deformities may be accommodated using soft, moldable contours to protect against skin breakdown and ulceration.[20] The University of California Biomechanics Laboratory orthotic device can be used to limit painful hindfoot motion and correct flexible hindfoot deformity. An advantage of this device is that it will fit inside of a regular shoe; however, it is rigid and may be poorly tolerated by some patients. More severe deformity or advanced arthrosis cannot be managed with a foot orthotic device alone, and an orthotic device that incorporates the ankle joint (ankle-foot orthosis) to more effectively offload arthritic joints and correct or accommodate deformity

Section 3: Arthritis of the Foot and Ankle

is necessary. One common ankle-foot orthosis is the Arizona Brace, which is a custom-molded leather brace that limits ankle and hindfoot motion and decreases pain at these arthritic joints. Stiff carbon fiber shoe inserts for arch support, soft or hard braces, and cupped heels are also commonly recommended to minimize motion and modify the load of the midfoot to help maintain functional biomechanics and reduce symptoms of pain.

Corticosteroid injections have been used to reduce inflammation and provide temporary pain relief for foot arthritis. A study reported on 63 patients who underwent steroid injection for midfoot arthritis.[21] Approximately 60% of patients experienced relief that persisted for up to 3 months after injection; however, fewer than 15% of patients experienced relief beyond 3 months. A retrospective review of image-guided injections of the foot and ankle reported that 86% of patients provided significant improvement with an average recurrence of pain at 3 months and a complication rate of 1.3%. Almost one-fourth of patients underwent surgical intervention within the 2-year follow-up period.[22] Complications of steroid injections should be discussed with patients and include skin hypopigmentation, subcutaneous fat atrophy, and tendon rupture.

SURGICAL TREATMENT

For patients failing to respond to aggressive nonsurgical management, surgical management is indicated. Arthrodesis of the involved joints remains the gold standard after failed nonsurgical treatment.

Active infection is the only absolute contraindication to fusion. Caution should be exercised when treating patients with peripheral vascular disease. These patients should undergo the appropriate vascular studies and, possibly, a vascular surgery consultation before arthrodesis. As discussed in a 2021 study, nicotine use is another relative contraindication to any foot or ankle arthrodesis, with these patients experiencing a higher rate of infection, increased need for bone stimulator use, and trend toward nonunion or delayed union (5.81 relative risk) in both hindfoot and midfoot arthrodesis.[23]

Medial and Middle Column

The mainstay treatment of medial and middle column midfoot arthritis is arthrodesis of the symptomatic joints: TMT, intercuneiform, and naviculocuneiform joints. The pattern of instability, deformity, and symptoms dictates the extent of the surgical treatment. In situ arthrodesis is only indicated for those with less than 2 mm of displacement and no more than 15° of deformity angulation. Otherwise, realignment procedures are needed in addition to fusion of the joints.[24] Arthrodesis most often involves the medial and middle columns (first, second,

and third TMT joints). If there is noticeable instability and extending the fusion will prevent further load shifting, the intercuneiform and the naviculocuneiform joints can also be included. Fusion of the lateral column is rarely performed.

Thorough joint preparation and absolute rigid fixation are the keys for a successful fusion. The most common approach involves one or two dorsal longitudinal incisions of the foot with provision of adequate skin bridges. Choices for internal fixation include both cannulated and noncannulated screws ranging in size from 2.7 to 4.5 mm. The screws can be headless, fully (lag by technique) or partially threaded (lag by design). In addition, intramedullary screws have been used for fixation in patients with Charcot arthropathy. Often in combination with transarticular screws, dorsal, medial, and/or plantar plating can be used to provide rigid internal fixation. There are many plate configurations, from single plates on each joint of interest to one plate covering multiple articulations, to facilitate fusion across multiple joints (**Figure 3**).

A 2020 retrospective study found that the use of compression staples had similar fusion rates and patient satisfaction scores when compared with other methods.[25] Similarly, a retrospective case series in 2021 reported on the use of plantar-positioned implants and found few complications with maintenance of correction.[26] Comparisons of screws only, staples only, plates only, and plate with lag-screw constructs in midfoot arthrodesis concluded that all methods of fusion provide improved function and pain. However, according to a 2021 study, using screws only might produce lower rates of bony healing.[27] In a review of 16 patients who underwent arthrodesis following failed fixation of a TMT fracture-dislocation, it was concluded that reduction was the key to good outcomes.[28]

Surgical realignment is needed for patients with increased angulation or residual deformity in the sagittal, coronal, and/or transverse planes at the time of fusion. Realignment procedures are mostly a combination of corrective osteotomies with soft-tissue balancing. Soft-tissue balancing may include peroneus brevis release or lengthening, peroneus longus to brevis transfer, and Achilles or gastrocnemius lengthening. A study reported a significant improvement of American Orthopaedic Foot and Ankle Society (AOFAS) score in patients with midfoot arthritis who underwent correction of residual malalignment in addition to arthrodesis. These patients had at least 3 mm of displacement and 15° of malalignment.[24]

Lateral Column

Surgical management of the lateral column of the midfoot remains controversial. As shown in an in vitro study, the sagittal mobility of the lateral column is approximately

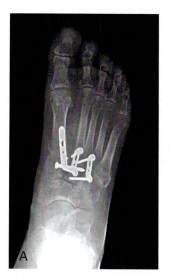
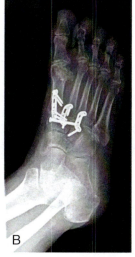
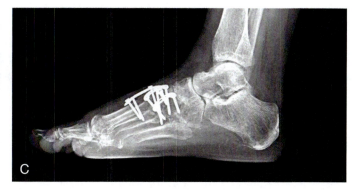

FIGURE 3 **A**, AP, **B**, oblique, and **C**, lateral radiographs following midfoot arthrodesis using a combination, plate-and-screw construct.

10°.[6] Many surgeons leave the lateral column free of fusion based on concern that arthrodesis of the more mobile, lateral column could cause stress fractures, nonunion, and formation of a rigid prominence, and ultimately cause further pain.[24] However, a study showed a significant reduction of functional incapacity as well as improvement in AOFAS scores and pain scores at 2-year follow-up in 23 patients who underwent lateral column arthrodesis. In particular, the study recommended lateral column arthrodesis in patients with uncorrectable lateral column collapse and rocker-bottom foot deformity.[29]

In an effort to maintain motion across the fourth and fifth TMT joints, resection arthroplasty and interpositional arthroplasty with soft-tissue or ceramic spheres are appropriate surgical alternatives to arthrodesis. A study showed a 35% decrease in both pain and subjective maintenance of lateral column motion in 12 patients who underwent soft-tissue interposition of the lateral TMT joints using the peroneus tertius tendon.[30] Ceramic spherical interpositional arthroplasty has been another alternative procedure for treatment of lateral column arthritis, with little support in the literature to date. One study reported an average AOFAS score improvement of 87% and pain improvement of 42% at 34 months' follow-up in 11 patients who underwent placement of a ceramic spherical implant into the resected fourth and/or fifth TMT joint.[31]

Subtalar Arthrodesis

Isolated subtalar arthritis commonly occurs after intra-articular calcaneal fractures are sustained, but also can be the result of rheumatoid arthritis, subtalar coalition, or a long-standing hindfoot deformity.[8] Subtalar arthrodesis is typically performed through a lateral approach. The hindfoot should be positioned in approximately 5° of valgus (**Figure 4**).

With the advancements in arthroscopy, arthroscopic subtalar arthrodesis has been advocated when distraction or large deformity correction is not required. One potential advantage of arthroscopic arthrodesis is preservation of the talar and calcaneal blood supply because the interosseous ligament and its associated vasculature are

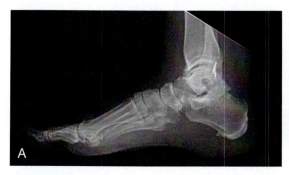
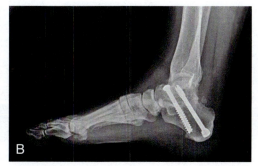
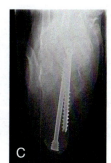

FIGURE 4 Radiographs showing subtalar arthritis. **A**, Preoperative lateral view. **B**, Postoperative lateral view. **C**, Axillary view.

preserved. This technique can be performed in the supine, lateral, or prone positions with no appreciable difference in outcomes. Fusion rates are reported to be approximately 95.8%, and time to union is approximately 11.9 weeks. Advantages of the arthroscopic technique include shorter hospitalization and decreased wound complications and sural nerve injuries. Clinical outcomes tend to be similar to those of open arthrodesis and therefore it is a safe and effective alternative option with high patient satisfaction rate and low complication rates.[32,33]

Talonavicular Arthrodesis

Talonavicular arthritis can develop after traumatic injury, rheumatoid arthritis, or osteoarthritis (**Figure 5**). Arthrodesis is used to treat all of these conditions, as well as flatfoot deformity with an unstable talonavicular joint.[34] Osteonecrosis of the navicular can lead to joint degeneration. Navicular osteonecrosis occurs most commonly after fracture but may be idiopathic in nature. Müller-Weiss disease is an adult-onset navicular osteonecrosis characterized by sclerosis, lateral collapse, and fragmentation of the navicular. Definitive treatment depends largely on the extent of arthrosis and collapse at presentation. Patients with disease isolated to the talonavicular joint can appropriately undergo talonavicular arthrodesis, but if substantial fragmentation and collapse are present, a bone block graft may be necessary to restore length. If there is substantial adjacent joint breakdown, additional fusion procedures may be necessary.[35]

Although the most common nonunion site in triple arthrodesis is at the talonavicular joint, likely because of the shear and torsional stresses present, fusion rates for isolated talonavicular arthrodesis are high, ranging between 90% and 97%.[4,36] Adjacent joint degeneration is still seen with isolated talonavicular arthrodesis, particularly in the subtalar and naviculocuneiform joints. However, peak pressure load in the ankle joint is lower and more evenly distributed after talonavicular arthrodesis compared with triple arthrodesis.[4]

Calcaneocuboid Arthrodesis

The calcaneocuboid joint, which is rarely fused in isolation, is more typically fused in double or triple arthrodesis or to correct planovalgus deformity.[37] Lateral column lengthening is a common procedure performed in flatfoot corrective surgery when there is substantial forefoot abduction. It is performed as either an osteotomy 10 to 15 mm posterior to the joint or as a distraction arthrodesis through the calcaneocuboid joint (**Figure 6**). Proponents of distraction arthrodesis argue that lengthening the lateral column increases contact pressure at the calcaneocuboid joint, predisposing it to accelerated degeneration. Although multiple studies suggest increased contact pressure at the calcaneocuboid joint following a lengthening procedure, there is no clear correlation between increased pressure and accelerated calcaneocuboid arthrosis. Those in favor of osteotomy point to the increased

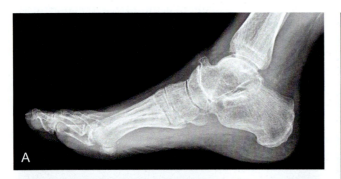
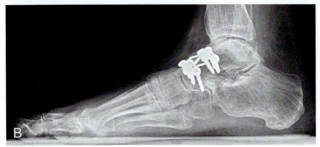
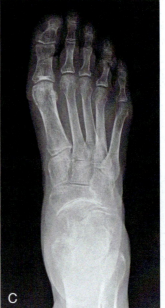
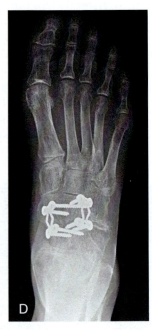

FIGURE 5 Radiographs showing isolated talonavicular arthrodesis. **A**, Preoperative lateral view. **B**, Postoperative lateral view. **C**, Preoperative AP view. **D**, Postoperative AP view.

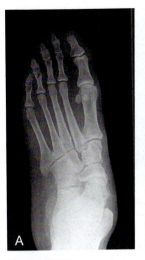
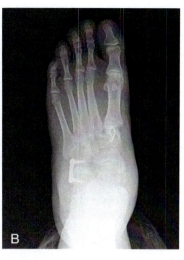

FIGURE 6 Radiographs showing distraction arthrodesis through the calcaneocuboid joint for pes planus. **A**, Preoperative AP view. **B**, Postoperative AP view.

complications associated with distraction arthrodesis and the equivalent outcomes between the two procedures.[38]

Triple Arthrodesis

Standard triple arthrodesis consists of fusion of the talonavicular joint through a medial approach and the calcaneocuboid and subtalar joints through a lateral approach (**Figure 7**). Recent fusion rates are reported at approximately 95%. Adjacent joint degeneration is the major concern, with ankle arthrosis reportedly ranging between 40% and 100% and midfoot arthrosis near 50% at follow-up. Long-term follow-up at 15 years has shown increased ankle arthritis in 47.5% of patients.[39] Nevertheless, clinical outcomes and patient satisfaction remain high after triple arthrodesis, with reports that 95% would undergo the same procedure.[39] Some concern over lateral wound dehiscence in the presence of valgus deformity and contracted lateral soft tissues has led to the development of a single medial approach to triple arthrodesis. In one study, the authors demonstrated that the degree of radiographic correction in medial triple arthrodesis was similar to results achieved with standard two-incision triple arthrodesis.[40] In a 2021 cadaver study,[41] the authors showed that there is a risk of subtotal débridement of the subtalar joint and talar head with a single medial incision approach and therefore greater soft-tissue dissection may be necessary. Although a medial-only approach precludes lateral wound complications, there is also an increased risk for disruption of talar blood supply and a risk to the deltoid ligament (especially with the greater soft-tissue dissection), which can lead to medial instability and valgus tibiotalar tilt.[41]

Double Arthrodesis

Historically, treatment entailed a triple arthrodesis and involved fusion of the subtalar, talonavicular, and calcaneocuboid joints.[42] More recently, there has been a trend toward selective one-joint or two-joint arthrodesis in an attempt to preserve motion and possibly limit adjacent joint degeneration while decreasing surgical time and complications.[43]

The term double arthrodesis refers to selective fusion of two of the three hindfoot joints (**Figure 8**). This concept arose from the idea of fusing only the arthritic joints and preserving the remaining joint in hopes of reducing loads on adjacent joints to prevent or delay adjacent joint breakdown.[4,43] There are potential advantages to double arthrodesis. There is one less surgical site at which potential complications can develop. After double arthrodesis, there is only approximately 2° of residual motion at the calcaneocuboid joint, but this may be enough to reduce the forces across the adjacent joints. A 2022 systematic review has shown nearly equivalent fusion rates and time to fusion, showing that double arthrodesis is an effective alternative.[43]

PRIMARY ARTHRODESIS FOR ACUTE OR SUBACUTE TRAUMA

Posttraumatic subtalar arthritis after calcaneal fracture can pose several additional challenges. A lateral calcaneal wall exostectomy may be required to relieve subfibular impingement. There also may be anterior ankle joint impingement because of loss of calcaneal height, which necessitates distraction arthrodesis. This will restore hindfoot height and talar declination, thereby relieving anterior impingement[44,45] (**Figure 9**). As described in recent studies, a posterior approach for subtalar distraction arthrodesis offers the advantages of avoiding previous surgical incisions, provides excellent subtalar joint exposure, and is optimal for correcting large varus or valgus deformities in addition to joint distraction.[45,46]

Union rates for open subtalar arthrodesis range between 84% and 100%. Controversy exists regarding the optimal time at which to perform an in situ or distraction subtalar arthrodesis. The only clear indication for distraction arthrodesis remains anterior ankle impingement. Even though a distraction arthrodesis necessitates fusion across two surfaces, union rates have been comparable between the two procedures. Clinical outcomes also have been similar for both techniques, although the complications associated with distraction tend to be more numerous and include wound healing problems, neuralgia, and varus malunion.[44] Despite preservation of the transverse tarsal joints, adjacent joint degeneration still occurs, with one study noting a 10% incidence of adjacent joint arthrosis at 4 years after subtalar arthrodesis.[32]

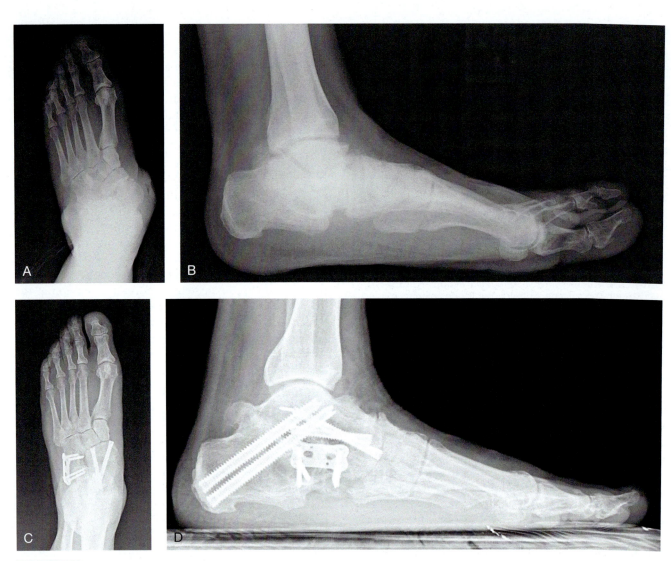

FIGURE 7 Radiographs showing triple arthrodesis. **A** and **B**, Preoperative and lateral images, respectively, of fixed planovalgus deformity. **C** and **D**, Postoperative AP and lateral images, respectively, after triple arthrodesis.

In the midfoot, ongoing debate regarding primary arthrodesis versus open reduction and internal fixation (ORIF) for treatment of fracture-dislocation of the TMT joint has not reached any convincing conclusions. In fact, despite anatomic reduction and fixation of the midtarsal joints, there is a high rate of posttraumatic arthritis following a midtarsal fracture-dislocation injury. One study found that in 25% of patients following ORIF of the TMT joint, posttraumatic arthritis developed at 52 months' follow-up. In addition, posttraumatic arthritis developed in 40% of the pure ligamentous injury cases regardless of anatomic reduction.[47]

A prospective randomized controlled study compared primary arthrodesis with ORIF for initial treatment of primary ligamentous Lisfranc joint injuries. At an average follow-up of 42 months, the arthrodesis group showed significantly higher AOFAS scores, higher returns to preinjury activity level, less pain, and a lower rate of revision surgical treatment.[48] In a 2022 systematic literature review, multiple meta-analyses were compared to determine the outcomes of ORIF versus arthrodesis of Lisfranc injuries. In addition to the increased rate of hardware removal for ORIF, the other factors were similar, including patient satisfaction and return to work.[49]

One study[7] showed a similarly high satisfaction rate, 86.6%, as well as improved functional scores in 59 patients with atraumatic TMT arthritis who were treated with fusion and concomitant deformity correction. Significant improvement following arthrodesis was

Chapter 10: Midfoot and Hindfoot Arthrodesis

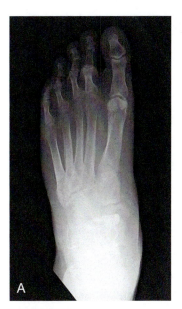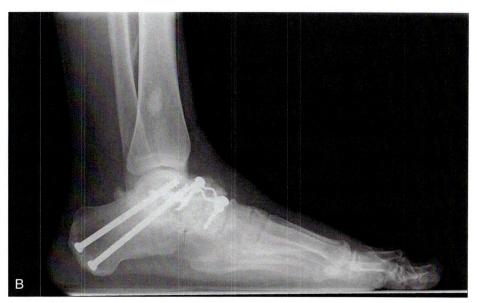

FIGURE 8 Radiographs showing double arthrodesis following selective fusion of the subtalar and talonavicular joints, preserving the calcaneocuboid articulation. **A**, AP view. **B**, Lateral view.

also observed regarding pain, disability, and activity limitation.

Although arthrodesis is commonly used as secondary salvage procedure following failed ORIF, it may be a sensible, primary treatment option for TMT joint fracture-dislocation, particularly within the pure ligamentous injury population.[47] Although these studies serve as a reference for surgical decision making and the treatment of traumatic midfoot injury, no studies have shown definitive superiority of primary arthrodesis over ORIF.

ADJUVANT TREATMENT IN HINDFOOT AND MIDFOOT ARTHRODESIS

There are three basic requirements for bone healing. An osteoconductive matrix must provide the scaffold upon which new bone can grow. Also needed is a local population of osteogenic cells including osteoblasts or their progenitors to populate this matrix. Osteoinductive growth factors to recruit, differentiate cells, and help drive bone formation is the last requirement.[50]

Iliac crest autograft is considered the benchmark bone graft because it meets all three requirements without risk for disease transmission. However, several complications are associated with autograft harvest, including nerve injury, hematoma, and donor site pain. These complications occur in 2.4% to 9.5% of foot and ankle cases. A systematic review of more than 150 studies in the foot and ankle literature favored the use of autograft over no graft material during surgery and reported an average fusion rate of 90% regardless of if autograft or allograft

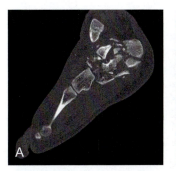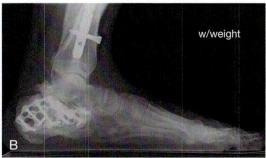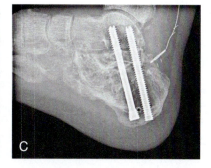

FIGURE 9 **A**, Preoperative CT scan of a comminuted calcaneal fracture. **B**, Lateral radiograph showing initial treatment with open reduction and internal fixation. **C**, Radiograph shows loss of calcaneal height and subtalar arthritis that was then treated with distraction arthrodesis.

material was used.[51] It is often unnecessary to procure the large quantity of bone graft available in the iliac crest for routine foot procedures. The tibia is another common autograft harvest site and has the advantage of proximity to the primary surgical site.[52]

Allograft bone products provide osteoconductive properties with limited osteoinduction in large volumes. Although donor site morbidity is avoided, there is a very small risk of disease transmission. Primary fusion rates and clinical outcomes have been comparable with those of autograft in foot and ankle surgery.[52]

Multiple synthetic bone graft substitute products are available. These materials have a structure and porosity that resembles cancellous bone. Calcium-based ceramics, calcium sulfate, calcium phosphate, and tricalcium phosphate are most commonly used. All are osteoconductive, but they vary in their strength and rate of resorption. These grafts commonly are used in combination with osteoinductive agents to enhance their efficacy.[53]

Osteobiologic agents refer to the osteoinductive proteins and osteogenic cells that are used to promote bone healing. The common agents include demineralized bone matrix, bone morphogenetic protein, bone marrow, and platelet-rich plasma. Demineralized bone matrix is allograft that has been processed to remove the mineral phase and leave the proteinaceous growth factors and as a result its osteoinductive capacity. Studies have demonstrated experimental increases in growth factors, cellular proliferation, and bone healing using osteobiologic agents.[54] However, the content and activity of these osteoinductive agents varies widely between products and the way in which they are processed, making it difficult to standardize their efficacy. A multicenter prospective randomized noninferiority trial of more than 400 patients undergoing ankle or hindfoot arthrodesis demonstrated comparable fusion rates with less pain and fewer side effects when compared with autograft treatment.[55] Retrospective studies have reported orthobiologics to be useful adjuncts in high-risk patients (eg, those with nicotine use, peripheral vascular disease and/or diabetes, a need for revision surgery, and/or a history of nonunion). This is particularly true when orthobiologics are combined with bone autograft or allograft.[56]

Osteobiologic devices can be used as adjuvants to promote bone healing and arthrodesis. These include bone stimulators and high-energy extracorporeal shockwave therapy. Although current literature does not support a specific role for extracorporeal shock wave therapy in primary hindfoot arthrodesis, internal bone stimulators have been reported as adjuncts to successful hindfoot arthrodesis in high-risk patients.[57]

COMPLICATIONS OF ARTHRODESIS

There are several complications related to the treatment of midfoot and hindfoot arthritis. Superficial wound complications reportedly affect between 3% and 30% of patients undergoing foot arthrodesis. Other examples of potential complications include infection, nerve injury, nonunion, implant complications, fracture, and complex regional pain syndrome (CRPS).

For the midfoot, reported complications of arthrodesis include infection (3%), peripheral nerve injury (9%), painful neuroma formation (7%), nonunion (3% to 7%), implant complications (9%), stress fracture (7%), metatarsalgia (6%), sesamoid pain (38.8%), and sural nerve neuralgia (7.5%). There is a higher likelihood of nonunion in elderly patients.[7,24] Long-term complications include development of secondary arthritis in adjacent joints (4.5%), and an additional rare complication is CRPS.[58,59] For instance, in one study to assess pain, AOFAS score, and patient satisfaction in patients with primary midfoot arthritis who underwent arthrodesis and deformity correction with or without gastrocnemius recession, 4% of major complications were due to deep infections and CRPS. In addition, of the 68 patients available for follow-up analysis, there was one instance of delayed union and eight instances of nonunion.[59]

For healthy patients undergoing elective hindfoot fusion, the wound complication rate is approximately 3%. Complication rates increase slightly in the case of revision hindfoot surgical treatment. Patients with diabetes have an overall wound complication rate of approximately 14%, which may increase to as high as 50% for revision or salvage surgeries. Problems involving prominent hardware can occur 20% of the time, and symptoms may necessitate removal in 50% of patients with prominent hardware.[58]

Superficial infections occur in 3% of patients who undergo hindfoot fusion and among elderly patients, the infection rate has been reported as high as 11%.[58] Deep infection and osteomyelitis occurs in approximately 2% of cases.[4,58] Nerve injury can present as a neuroma, neuritis, or CRPS. Direct nerve injury is most common with calcaneocuboid arthrodesis, with the incidence of sural nerve injury as high as 32%. CRPS has been reported in as many as 18% of cases in some studies; however, most literature quotes rates at 2% to 3%.[4,58] This can be particularly difficult to treat and often necessitates a multimodal approach including physical therapy and pain management.

Nonunion is a potentially devastating complication, and unless a patient is stable and asymptomatic, they

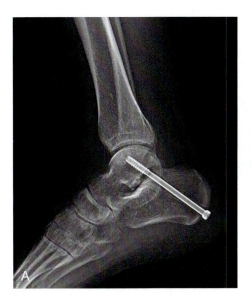 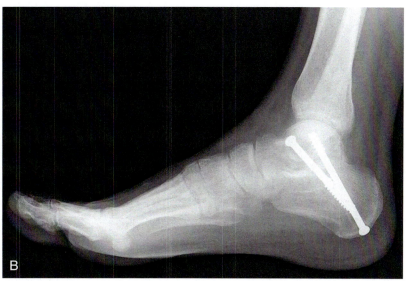

FIGURE 10 Radiographs showing subtalar nonunion (**A**) that was treated with revision arthrodesis (**B**).

will almost always need revision surgical treatment (**Figure 10**). Rates of nonunion after triple arthrodesis range between 3% and 17%. The fusion rates of double (subtalar/talonavicular) arthrodesis are higher, with a nonunion rate of approximately 6%.[58]

A 6% malunion rate is associated with midfoot and hindfoot fusion procedures. The malunion rate after triple arthrodesis is 3%, but this rate doubles in revision cases. The most common deformity is equinovarus, followed by hindfoot varus and hindfoot valgus.[58]

SUMMARY

Midfoot and hindfoot arthritis are painful and debilitating conditions that may occur both in younger and older patients. They can be due to traumatic, inflammatory, or degenerative processes. After exhaustion of nonsurgical management methods including shoe modification, orthoses, anti-inflammatory agents, and anesthetic joint injection, surgical treatment of the symptomatic joints by means of arthrodesis and correction of any underlying anatomic deformity can achieve good clinical results. Trauma is the most common etiology for midfoot arthritis, and primary arthrodesis is a sensible option for initial treatment of traumatic midfoot injury. Techniques continue to evolve to promote improved wound healing and alignment, increase fusion rates while decreasing time to union, reduce postoperative disability, and contribute to optimal patient outcomes. The role of synthetic and biologic adjuvants in arthrodesis continues to expand and will benefit from high-quality trials investigating their efficacy.

KEY STUDY POINTS

- Midfoot and hindfoot arthritis have a variety of etiologies including primary arthritis, traumatic injury, inflammatory degeneration, and neuropathic disease.
- The first step in managing midfoot and hindfoot arthritis is nonsurgical management including activity modification, shoe modification, orthoses, a trial of NSAIDs, and potentially anesthetic joint injections. High-impact activity such as running should be avoided. Bracing may also provide many patients symptomatic relief.
- Surgical management is indicated for progressively painful and debilitating disease and/or deformity that has failed to respond to nonsurgical management. This usually involves arthrodesis and deformity correction using osteotomy techniques with or without soft-tissue balancing.
- Primary arthrodesis may be a sensible initial treatment for displaced and unstable traumatic injuries.
- Adjuvant therapies including bone autograft and allograft, synthetic bone graft substitutes, and osteobiologics are commonly used in fusion procedures without level I and level II evidence in the literature to support this.

ANNOTATED REFERENCES

1. Kelikian AS, Sarrafian SK: *Sarrafian's Anatomy of the Foot and Ankle: Descriptive, Topographic, Functional.* LWW, 2011.

2. Peicha G, Labovitz J, Seibert FJ, et al: The anatomy of the joint as a risk factor for Lisfranc dislocation and fracture-dislocation. An anatomical and radiological case control study. *J Bone Joint Surg Br* 2002;84(7):981-985.

3. Thordarson DB: Fusion in posttraumatic foot and ankle reconstruction. *J Am Acad Orthop Surg* 2004;12:322-333.

4. Crevoisier X: The isolated talonavicular arthrodesis. *Foot Ankle Clin* 2011;16:49-59.

5. Wülker N, Stukenborg C, Savory KM, Alfke D: Hindfoot motion after isolated and combined arthrodeses: Measurements in anatomic specimens. *Foot Ankle Int* 2000;21:921-927.

6. Ouzounian TJ, Shereff MJ: In vitro determination of midfoot motion. *Foot Ankle* 1989;10(3):140-146.

7. Jung HG, Myerson MS, Schon LC: Spectrum of operative treatments and clinical outcomes for atraumatic osteoarthritis of the TMT joints. *Foot Ankle Int* 2007;28(4):482-489.

8. Radnay CS, Clare MP, Sanders RW: Subtalar fusion after displaced intra-articular calcaneal fractures: Does initial operative treatment matter? *J Bone Joint Surg Am* 2009;91:541-546.

9. Richter M, Wipermann B, Krettek C, Schratt HE, Hufner T, Therman H: Fractures and fracture dislocations of the midfoot: Occurrence, causes and long term results. *Foot Ankle Int* 2001;22(5):392-398.

10. Jeng C, Campbell J: Current concepts review: The rheumatoid forefoot. *Foot Ankle Int* 2008;29:959-968.

11. Coester LM, Saltzman CL, Leupold J, Pontarelli W: Long-term results following ankle arthrodesis for post-traumatic arthritis. *J Bone Joint Surg Am* 2001;83-A:219-228.

12. Ebalard M, Le Henaff G, Sigonney G, et al: Risk of osteoarthritis secondary to partial or total arthrodesis of the subtalar and midtarsal joints after a minimum follow-up of 10 years. *Orthop Traumatol Surg Res* 2014;100:S231-S237.

13. Rao S, Baumhauer JF, Tome J, Nawoczenski DA: Comparison of in vivo segmental foot motion during walking and step descent in patients with midfoot arthritis and matched asymptomatic control subjects. *J Biomech* 2009;42(8):1054-1060.

14. Keiserman LS, Cassandra J, Amis JA: The piano key test: A clinical sign for the identification of subtle TMT pathology. *Foot Ankle Int* 2003;24:437-438.

15. Carmont MR, Tomlinson JE, Blundell C, Davies MB, Moore DJ: Variability of joint communications in the foot and ankle demonstrated by contrast-enhanced diagnostic injections. *Foot Ankle Int* 2009;30:439-442.

16. Saltzman CL, el-Khoury GY: The hindfoot alignment view. *Foot Ankle Int* 1995;16:572-576.

17. Barg A, Bailey T, Richter M, et al: Weightbearing computed tomography of the foot and ankle: Emerging technology topical review. *Foot Ankle Int* 2018;39(3):376-386.

18. Godoy-Santos AL, Cesar CD, Weight Bearing CT International Study Group: Weight-bearing computer tomography of the foot and ankle: An update and future directions. *Acta Ortop Bras* 2018;26:135-139.

19. Guermazi A, Hayashi D, Eckstein F, Hunter DJ, Duryea J, Roemer FW: Imaging of osteoarthritis. *Rheum Dis Clin North Am* 2013;39:67-105.

20. Janisse DJ, Janisse E: Shoe modification and the use of orthoses in the treatment of foot and ankle pathology. *J Am Acad Orthop Surg* 2008;16:152-158.

21. Drakonaki EE, Kho JSB, Sharp RJ, Ostlere SJ: Efficacy of ultrasound-guided steroid injections for pain management of midfoot joint degenerative disease. *Skeletal Radiol* 2011;40:1001-1006.

22. Grice J, Marsland D, Smith G, Calder J: Efficacy of foot and ankle corticosteroid injections. *Foot Ankle Int* 2017;38:8-13.

23. Allport J, Ramaskandhan J, Siddique MS: Nonunion rates in hind- and midfoot arthrodesis in current, ex-, and nonsmokers. *Foot Ankle Int* 2021;42(5):582-588.

A retrospective cohort study was done to examine the effect of smoking status on union rates. Among smokers, higher rate of infection, bone stimulator use, and trend toward nonunion (5.81 relative risk) were found. Heavier smokers also had a trend toward slower union. Level of evidence: III.

24. Komenda GA, Myerson MS, Biddinger KR: Results of arthrodesis of the TMT joints after traumatic injury. *J Bone Joint Surg Am* 1996;78:1665-1676.

25. Dock CC, Freeman KL, Coetzee JC, McGaver RS, Giveans MR: Outcomes of Nitinol compression staples in tarsometatarsal fusion. *Foot Ankle Orthop* 2020;5(3):2473011420944904.

A retrospective case series was done to identify outcomes of patients undergoing TMT fusion with compression staples. All patients improved from preoperatively to their latest follow-up with no wound complications. Fusion rate and patient satisfaction score is similar to other methods. Level of evidence: IV.

26. Fraser TW, Miles DT, Huang N, Davis FB, Dunlap BD, Doty JF: Radiographic outcomes, union rates, and complications associated with plantar implant positioning for midfoot arthrodesis. *Foot Ankle Orthop* 2021;6(3):24730114211027115.

A retrospective case series was done to identify outcomes of patients undergoing TMT fusion with plantar-positioned implants. Implants maintained deformity correction with rare instance of symptomatic hardware. Union rate is similar to that of other implants. Level of evidence: IV.

27. Lee W, Prat D, Wapner KL, Farber DC, Chao W: Comparison of 4 different fixation strategies for midfoot arthrodesis: A retrospective comparative study. *Foot Ankle Spec* 2021; August 2 [Epub ahead of print].

A retrospective chart review was done to examine and compare four different fixation constructs (staples, compression plate, compression plate with lag screws, and compression screws). Compression screw alone was found to have significantly higher nonunion rate than other fixation constructs. Lack of adjuvant bone graft, diabetes, and postoperative nonanatomic alignment also increased the risk of nonunion. Level of evidence: III.

28. Sangeorzan BJ, Veith RG, Hansen ST Jr: Salvage of Lisfranc's TMT joint by arthrodesis. *Foot Ankle Int* 1990;10(4):193-200.

29. Raikin SM, Schon LC: Arthrodesis of the fourth and fifth TMT joints of the midfoot. *Foot Ankle Int* 2003;24(8):584-590.

30. Berlet GC, Hodges Davis W, Anderson RB: Tendon arthroplasty for basal fourth and fifth metatarsal arthritis. *Foot Ankle Int* 2002;23(5):440-446.

31. Shawen SB, Anderson RB, Cohen BE, Hammit MD, Davis WH: Spherical ceramic interpositional arthroplasty for basal fourth and fifth metatarsal arthritis. *Foot Ankle Int* 2007;28(8):896-901.

32. Easley ME, Trnka HJ, Schon LC, Myerson MS: Isolated subtalar arthrodesis. *J Bone Joint Surg Am* 2000;82:613-624.

33. Loewen A, Ge SM, Marwan Y, Berry GK: Isolated arthroscopic-assisted subtalar fusion: A systematic review. *JBJS Rev* 2021;9(8).

    A systematic review was done to determine the outcomes of arthroscopic arthrodesis. Results showed that it is a safe and effective alternative to open approaches with high satisfaction rates and union rates of 95.8%. Level of evidence: V.

34. Lechler P, Graf S, Köck FX, Schaumburger J, Grifka J, Handel M: Arthrodesis of the talonavicular joint using angle-stable mini-plates: A prospective study. *Int Orthop* 2012;36:2491-2494.

35. Doyle T, Napier RJ, Wong-Chung J: Recognition and management of Müller-Weiss disease. *Foot Ankle Int* 2012;33:275-281.

36. Jarrell SE, Owen JR, Wayne JS, Adelaar RS: Biomechanical comparison of screw versus plate/screw construct for talonavicular fusion. *Foot Ankle Int* 2009;30:150-156.

37. Barmada M, Shapiro HS, Boc SF: Calcaneocuboid arthrodesis. *Clin Podiatr Med Surg* 2012;29:77-89.

38. Grunander TR, Thordarson DB: Results of calcaneocuboid distraction arthrodesis. *Foot Ankle Surg* 2012;18:15-18.

39. Klerken T, Kosse NM, Aarts CAM, Louwerens JWK: Long-term results after triple arthrodesis: Influence of alignment on ankle osteoarthritis and clinical outcome. *Foot Ankle Surg* 2017;25(2):247-250.

40. Jeng CL, Vora AM, Myerson MS: The medial approach to triple arthrodesis. Indications and technique for management of rigid valgus deformities in high-risk patients. *Foot Ankle Clin* 2005;10:515-521, vi-vii.

41. MacDonald A, Anderson M, Soin S, Brodell JD Jr. Flemister AS, Ketz JP: Single medial vs 2-incision approach for double hindfoot arthrodesis: Is there a difference in joint preparation? *Foot Ankle Int* 2021;42(8):1068-1073.

    A retrospective cohort study was done in cadavers to determine whether there was a difference in approaches. Single medial incision approach demonstrated increased valgus tibiotalar tilt with risk of subtotal débridement of subtalar joint and talar head. To achieve the débridement, greater soft-tissue dissection may be necessary. Level of evidence: III.

42. Knupp M, Stufkens SAS, Hintermann B: Triple arthrodesis. *Foot Ankle Clin* 2011;16:61-67.

43. Cates NK, Mayer A, Tenley J, et al: Double versus triple arthrodesis fusion rates: A systematic review. *J Foot Ankle Surg* 2022;61(4):907-913.

A systematic review done to review the fusion rates and mean time to fusion in double and triple arthrodesis. There were nearly equivalent fusion rates and time to fusion, showing that double arthrodesis is an effective alternative. Level of evidence: III.

44. Trnka HJ, Easley ME, Lam PW, Anderson CD, Schon LC, Myerson MS: Subtalar distraction bone block arthrodesis. *J Bone Joint Surg Br* 2001;83:849-854.

45. Scott RT, Dujela MD, DeVries JG, et al: Deformity correction of the midfoot/hindfoot/ankle. *Clin Podiatr Med Surg* 2022;39(2):233-272.

    This is a review article discussing the more contemporary solutions for complex corrections needed to correct deformities in the midfoot, hindfoot, or ankle. Modern approaches/techniques to TMT, naviculocuneiform fusions in the midfoot, and the medial double approach are discussed. Not only are the surgical approaches described in detail, but tips are given to have more successful outcomes. Level of evidence: V.

46. Stephens AR, Grujic L: Post-traumatic hindfoot arthritis. *J Orthop Trauma* 2020;34:S32-S37.

    This review article discusses the principles of treatment of hindfoot arthritis in all types of cases including posttraumatic. Emphasis is provided on the importance of proper alignment and approaches are discussed in how to achieve this. New approaches and techniques including arthroscopic/minimally invasive ways are discussed. Level of evidence: IV.

47. Kuo RS, Tejwani NC, Digiovanni CW, et al: Outcome after open reduction and internal fixation of Lisfranc joint injuries. *J Bone Joint Surg Am* 2000;82(11):1609-1618.

48. Ly TV, Coetzee JC: Treatment of primarily ligamentous Lisfranc joint injuries: Primary arthrodesis compared with open reduction and internal fixation. A prospective, randomized study. *J Bone Joint Surg Am* 2006;88(3):514-520.

49. Peters W, Panchbhavi V: Primary arthrodesis versus open reduction and internal fixation outcomes for Lisfranc injuries: An analysis of conflicting meta-analyses results. *Foot Ankle Spec* 2022;15(2):171-178.

    A systematic literature review of meta-analyses was performed to identify outcomes of patients undergoing ORIF or arthrodesis of Lisfranc injuries. The main difference is the rate of hardware removal in arthrodesis; however, other factors were similar including patient satisfaction and return to work. Level of evidence: II.

50. Guyton GP, Miller SD: Stem cells in bone grafting: Trinity allograft with stem cells and collagen/beta-tricalcium phosphate with concentrated bone marrow aspirate. *Foot Ankle Clin* 2010;15:611-619.

51. Lareau CR, Deren ME, Fantry A, Donahue RMJ, DiGiovanni CW: Does autogenous bone graft work? A logistic regression analysis of data from 159 papers in the foot and ankle literature. *Foot Ankle Surg* 2015;21:150-159.

52. Winson IG, Higgs A: The use of proximal and distal tibial bone graft in foot and ankle procedures. *Foot Ankle Clin* 2010;15:553-558.

53. Panchbhavi VK: Synthetic bone grafting in foot and ankle surgery. *Foot Ankle Clin* 2010;15:559-576.

54. Lin SS, Yeranosian MG: The role of orthobiologics in fracture healing and arthrodesis. *Foot Ankle Clin* 2016;21:727-737.

55. DiGiovanni CW, Lin SS, Baumhauer JF, et al: Recombinant human platelet-derived growth factor-BB and beta-tricalcium phosphate (rhPDGF-BB/β-TCP): An alternative to autogenous bone graft. *J Bone Joint Surg Am* 2013;95:1184-1192.

56. El-Amin SF, Hogan MV, Allen AA, Hinds J, Laurencin CT: The indications and use of bone morphogenetic proteins in foot, ankle, and tibia surgery. *Foot Ankle Clin* 2010;15:543-551.

57. Saxena A, DiDomenico LA, Widtfeldt A, Adams T, Kim W: Implantable electrical bone stimulation for arthrodeses of the foot and ankle in high-risk patients: A multicenter study. *J Foot Ankle Surg* 2005;44:450-454.

58. Bibbo C, Anderson RB, Davis WH: Complications of midfoot and hindfoot arthrodesis. *Clin Orthop Relat Res* 2001;391:45-58.

59. Nemec SA, Habbu RA, Anderson JG, Bohay DR: Outcomes following midfoot arthrodesis for primary arthritis. *Foot Ankle Int* 2011;32(4):355-361.

CHAPTER 11

Adult-Acquired Flatfoot Deformity

MATTHEW M. BUCHANAN, MD, FAAOS • FREDERICK R. LEMLEY, MD, FAAOS

ABSTRACT

Adult-acquired flatfoot deformity is a common diagnosis in the fifth and sixth decades of life, arising primarily in individuals with an anatomic predisposition. The deformity involves varying degrees of hindfoot valgus and longitudinal arch collapse, with forefoot abduction and valgus tibiotalar deformity seen in more severe cases. Affected soft-tissue structures can include the posterior tibial tendon, the calcaneonavicular (spring) ligament, and the deltoid ligament of the ankle. Achilles tendon contractures are almost always present. Nonsurgical treatments include a variety of orthotics and braces as well as physical therapy. Surgical treatment is individualized to the deformity and the patient. Typically, joint-sparing procedures (osteotomies and tendon transfers) are performed for flexible deformities without arthritis, whereas hindfoot arthrodesis is performed for rigid deformities and/or arthritis.

Keywords: adult-acquired flatfoot deformity; pes planovalgus; pes planus; posterior tibial tendon dysfunction; progressive collapsing foot deformity

INTRODUCTION

Adult-acquired flatfoot deformity (AAFD) is a common problem. It encompasses a wide range of pathology

Dr. Buchanan or an immediate family member has received royalties from Merete Medical. Neither Dr. Lemley nor any immediate family member has received anything of value from or has stock or stock options held in a commercial company or institution related directly or indirectly to the subject of this chapter.

involving the ankle, hindfoot, and midfoot, including progressive posterior tibial tendon (PTT) dysfunction, failure of the supporting ligamentous structures, and malalignment of the bony architecture. Pes planovalgus deformities can also develop in adults following untreated Lisfranc injuries and inflammatory arthropathies, but like congenital pes planovalgus deformities, these are distinct entities apart from AAFD. Symptoms of AAFD usually begin in the fifth and sixth decades of life and treatment is based on the severity of pain and deformity.

ANATOMY AND PATHOPHYSIOLOGY

The PTT is the primary dynamic stabilizer of the medial longitudinal arch. The tibialis posterior muscle originates from the posterior tibia and fibula and the interosseous membrane. The PTT courses behind and around the medial malleolus and inserts mainly on the navicular but also has attachments to the cuneiforms and metatarsal bases. The PTT adducts and inverts the foot and plantarflexes the ankle. Adduction of the midfoot provides a rigid lever for progression through the gait cycle during midstance and push-off.

Posterior tibial tendon dysfunction (PTTD) is caused by an elongated and/or degenerative tendon over the course of its watershed area, which extends from the tip of the medial malleolus to 2 cm distal.[1] Slow degeneration of the tendon decreases its elastic properties and ability to support the foot's medial column. Inspection of the PTT during surgery usually reveals longitudinal tearing, disorganized collagen, tendinosis, and decreased excursion. Histologically, myxoid and mucinous degeneration is seen.[2] This degenerative process may be painful, and resection of the diseased tendon is considered a useful

Section 3: Arthritis of the Foot and Ankle

This chapter is adapted from Cody EA, Ellis SJ: Adult-acquired flatfoot deformity, in Chou LB, ed: *Orthopaedic Knowledge Update®: Foot and Ankle 6*. American Academy of Orthopaedic Surgeons, 2020, pp 165-177.

© 2025 American Academy of Orthopaedic Surgeons

adjunct during reconstruction to alleviate pain, although this is controversial.

As the ligaments that support the arch of the foot weaken, the PTT may ultimately lose function, leading to plantar flexion of the talus and eversion of the calcaneus. In addition to tendon dysfunction, other plantar structures can attenuate and degenerate as the deformity progresses. The calcaneonavicular (spring) ligament, naviculocuneiform ligament, talonavicular capsule, and deltoid ligament all may become compromised as the stages of flatfoot progress. The calcaneonavicular ligament has two components, superomedial and inferior, which are collectively referred to as the spring ligament complex. The spring ligament creates a sling that supports the talar head between the calcaneus and the navicular. In patients with AAFD, the spring ligament is frequently attenuated or fully ruptured.

With attenuation of the PTT and spring ligament, the talus plantarflexes further and the forefoot abducts, resulting in talonavicular uncoverage. In addition, the forefoot supinates to compensate for the valgus hindfoot deformity and maintain a plantigrade foot. The pull of the Achilles tendon on the everted calcaneus works to exacerbate the hindfoot valgus deformity, and a gastrocnemius-soleus contracture typically develops. With advanced disease, flexible deformities can become rigid, limiting treatment options. And finally, with increasing hindfoot valgus, the deltoid ligament can fail, resulting in valgus talar tilt at the ankle.

New research using weight-bearing CT (WBCT) has shown that patients with AAFD may have an anatomic predisposition for the development of valgus hindfoot collapse and ligament/tendon failure. One study compared patients scheduled for surgical reconstruction of AAFD with control patients and found that the patients with AAFD had significantly more innate talar valgus and more valgus subtalar joint alignment than the control patients.[3] Another study found that patients with peritalar subluxation, as seen in severe AAFD, had greater valgus orientation of the subtalar joint compared with control patients.[4] These patients' tendency toward hindfoot valgus likely puts more stress on the PTT, contributing to development of PTTD. It is possible that in the future, evaluation of bony anatomy will allow surgeons to predict which patients are likely to have progression of deformity and which might benefit from earlier intervention.

CLASSIFICATION

PTTD staging was first described in 1989,[5] was later modified in 1996, and refined in 2007[6,7] (**Tables 1** and **2**). Other classification systems have been described.[8,9] It is important to note that the classification system was created to describe the pathology of the PTT but is commonly used to describe progression of AAFD. The flatfoot deformity itself, as noted earlier, occurs with certain anatomic predispositions as well as ligament failure, involving far more than just the PTT.

Stage I PTTD is defined as tenosynovitis with retained strength (eg, the patient can still perform a single-limb heel rise). No alteration of foot alignment is noted clinically or radiographically. Stage II PTTD is characterized by progressive pes planovalgus deformity, which remains flexible, and decreased strength, demonstrated by the inability to perform a single-limb heel rise. Stage III PTTD is defined by a rigid planovalgus deformity, and stage IV involves changes to the ankle joint with deltoid laxity, resulting in ankle valgus deformity.

Patients presenting with stage I PTTD usually report medial ankle and hindfoot pain. Their foot remains flexible and they are able to perform a single-limb heel rise; however, a patient may have pain with repetitive rising. The tendon has normal function and length. Stage I PTTD typically involves overuse and training errors in active patients participating in high-impact running and jumping sports.

Most patients with AAFD who seek evaluation have stage II PTTD. Patients report progressive pain and deformity in most cases, and they are unable to perform a single-limb heel rise on the affected extremity. However, the deformity remains flexible and they usually can perform a double-limb heel rise. The hindfoot typically does not invert during heel rise in cases of PTTD. Patients may also report lateral hindfoot pain, which is usually attributable to development of subtalar arthritis, sinus tarsi impingement, or calcaneofibular (subfibular) impingement[10] (**Figure 1**). Fibular stress fractures also can

Table 1	
Clinical Staging of Posterior Tibial Tendon Dysfunction	
Stage I	Pain over the posterior tibialis with no deformity
Stage II	Deformity is flexible 1. Medial pain only 2. Lateral pain
Stage III	Deformity is not flexible
Stage IV	Deformity is not flexible and changes at the ankle

Reproduced from Alvarez RG, Price J, Marini A, Turner NS, Kitaoka HB: Adult acquired flatfoot deformity and posterior tibial tendon dysfunction, in Pinzur MS, ed: *Orthopaedic Knowledge Update® Foot and Ankle 4.* American Academy of Orthopaedic Surgeons, 2008, pp 215-229.

Chapter 11: Adult-Acquired Flatfoot Deformity

Table 2

Clinical Classification System for Posterior Tibial Tendon Dysfunction

Stage	Substage	Characteristic Clinical Findings	Radiographic Findings	Treatment
I	A: Inflammatory disease	Normal anatomy, tender PTT	Normal	NSAIDs, immobilization, ice, orthoses, tenosynovectomy, treat specific systemic disease
	B: Partial tear	Normal anatomy, tender PTT	Normal	Same as for substage A
	C: Partial tear with mild HF valgus	Slight HF valgus, tender PTT	Slight HF valgus	Same as for substage A
II	A1: HF valgus with flexible FF varus	Flexible HF valgus, flexible FF varus ± tender PTT	HF valgus, Meary angle disrupted, calcaneal pitch lost	Orthoses, medial slide calcaneal osteotomy, Strayer or Achilles tendon lengthening, FDL transfer (if deformity corrects only with ankle PF)
	A2: HF valgus with rigid FF varus	Flexible HF valgus, rigid FF varus ± tender PTT	Same as A1	Same as for substage A1, Cotton osteotomy
	B: FF abduction	Same as for substages A1 and A2 with FF abduction	HF valgus, talonavicular uncovering, FF abduction	Medial slide calcaneal osteotomy, lateral column lengthening, Strayer or Achilles tendon lengthening, FDL transfer
	C: Medial ray instability	Flexible HF valgus, fixed FF varus, medial column instability, first ray dorsiflexion with HF correction, sinus tarsi pain	HF valgus, first TMT joint plantar gaping	Medial slide calcaneal osteotomy, FDL transfer, Cotton osteotomy, or first TMT joint fusion
III	A: Rigid HF valgus	Rigid HF valgus, sinus tarsi pain	Decreased subtalar joint space, angle of Gissane sclerosis	Triple arthrodesis, custom AFO if not a surgical candidate
	B: FF abduction	Same as for substage IIIA, FF abduction	Same as for substage IIIA, FF abduction	Triple arthrodesis with lateral column lengthening, custom AFO if not a surgical candidate
IV	A: Rigid HF valgus, flexible ankle valgus, deltoid ligament insufficiency, minimal ankle arthritis	Flexible tibiotalar valgus	Tibiotalar valgus, HF valgus	Correct HF valgus, reconstruct deltoid ligament
	B: Significant ankle arthritis, with or without rigid ankle valgus	Rigid tibiotalar valgus	Tibiotalar valgus, HF valgus	Pantalar fusion, TTC fusion, or triple arthrodesis and TAA

AFO = ankle-foot orthosis, FDL = flexor digitorum longus, FF = forefoot, HF = hindfoot, PF = plantar flexion, PTT = posterior tibial tendon, TAA = total ankle arthroplasty, TMT = tarsometatarsal, TTC = tibiotalocalcaneal

Adapted from Bluman EM, Title CI, Myerson MS: Posterior tibial tendon rupture: A refined classification system. *Foot Ankle Clin* 2007;12(2):233-249. Copyright 2007, with permission from Elsevier.

Section 3: Arthritis of the Foot and Ankle

Section 3: Arthritis of the Foot and Ankle

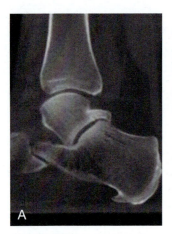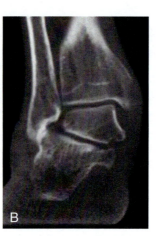

FIGURE 1 **A**, Sinus tarsi and **B**, subfibular impingement seen on weight-bearing CT. (Reproduced with permission from Jeng CL, Rutherford T, Hull MG, Cerrato RA, Campbell JT: Assessment of bony subfibular impingement in flatfoot patients using weight-bearing CT scans. *Foot Ankle Int* 2019:40[2];152-158.)

occur with severe deformity because of calcaneofibular abutment. A 2021 study suggested that prolonged lateral overload due to hindfoot valgus can lead to syndesmotic widening.[11]

Stage III PPTD is characterized by a rigid deformity. The hindfoot is fixed in valgus and patients cannot perform a single-limb heel rise. Often, the subtalar joint is arthritic. Varying degrees of talonavicular and calcaneocuboid arthrosis and deformity may also be present. With advanced disease, deformity may develop further down the medial column, extending to the naviculocuneiform joints and the first tarsometatarsal (TMT) joint. This can be observed on a lateral radiograph or WBCT with collapse at the naviculocuneiform joint and plantar gapping at the first TMT joint (**Figure 2**).

Stage IV PTTD is defined by involvement of the deltoid ligament (**Figure 3**). With prolonged AAFD, the deltoid becomes attenuated and valgus talar tilt develops. The

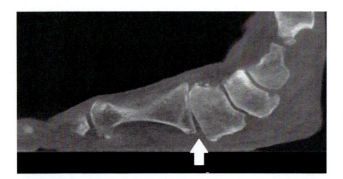

FIGURE 2 Weight-bearing CT sagittal image demonstrating first tarsometatarsal plantar gapping (arrow), representing instability as well as degenerative arthritis.

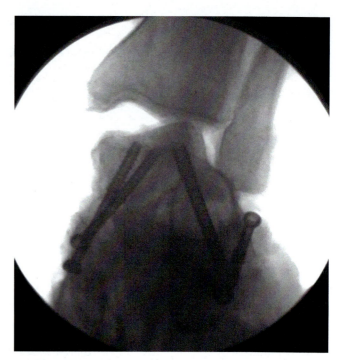

FIGURE 3 Stress radiograph demonstrating significant deltoid laxity. (Reproduced from Ellington JK, Myerson MS: The use of arthrodesis to correct rigid flatfoot deformity. *Instr Course Lect* 2011;60:311-320.)

foot deformity may be flexible or rigid. Once AAFD has progressed to this stage, treatment becomes much more difficult. For this reason, weight-bearing AP ankle radiographs should always be obtained in patients with AAFD to ensure ankle congruity and to assess for arthritis. Patients with ankle involvement may present with either isolated deltoid stretching or tearing, or frank arthritis in the ankle joint itself with lateral cartilage loss contributing to valgus talar tilt. The distinction between these two scenarios has important implications for surgical management.

In 2020, an expert consensus group proposed a new nomenclature and developed an entirely new classification system for AAFD. The name, progressive collapsing foot deformity, acknowledges that a flatfoot deformity does not always involve pathology of the PTT and does not follow a linear progression of deformity. This new classification system (**Table 3**) seeks to improve the reproducibility, reliability, and usefulness of treatment decisions for these complex foot deformities.[12]

CLINICAL PRESENTATION

Patients with AAFD typically present with medial hindfoot pain. However, in some patients, lateral foot pain predominates, and more rarely, patients will present with only ankle pain. Typically, prolonged ambulation and uneven terrain aggravate symptoms. Patients may report

Chapter 11: Adult-Acquired Flatfoot Deformity

Table 3

Consensus Group Classification of Progressive Collapsing Foot Deformity

Stage of the Deformity

Stage I (Flexible) — **Stage II (Rigid)**

Type of deformity (classes—isolated or combined)

	Deformity Type/Location	Consistent Clinical/Radiographic Findings
Class A	Hindfoot valgus deformity	Hindfoot valgus alignment Increased hindfoot moment arm, hindfoot alignment angle, foot and ankle offset
Class B	Midfoot/forefoot abduction deformity	Decreased talar head coverage Increased talonavicular coverage angle Presence of sinus tarsi impingement
Class C	Forefoot varus deformity/medial column instability	Increased talus–first metatarsal angle Plantar gapping first TMT joint/NC joints Clinical forefoot varus
Class D	Peritalar subluxation/dislocation	Significant subtalar joint subluxation/subfibular impingement
Class E	Ankle instability	Valgus tilting of the ankle joint

NC = naviculocuneiform, TMT = tarsometatarsal

Reproduced with permission from Myerson MS, Thordarson DB, Johnson JE, et al: Classification and nomenclature: Progressive collapsing foot deformity. *Foot Ankle Int* 2020;41(10):1271-1276.

uneven shoe wear, with the medial aspect of the heel wearing out faster, or difficulty finding shoes that fit. Some patients report a prior injury, sometimes having heard or felt a pop, and many have been treated by their primary physicians for an ankle sprain. Some patients state that they have had flatfoot their entire life, which has worsened. Comorbidities, particularly inflammatory conditions and diabetes mellitus, should be documented.

PHYSICAL EXAMINATION

Patients should be evaluated in both the standing and seated positions. In the standing position, a patient with AAFD will have a decreased arch, increased hindfoot valgus (**Figure 4**), and the "too many toes sign" (attributable to forefoot abduction) when viewed from behind. In the seated position, the flexibility of the hindfoot and that of the gastrocnemius-soleus complex are assessed. Findings should be compared with those of the opposite foot/ankle. A flexible deformity allows for osteotomies and tendon transfers, whereas rigid deformities require arthrodesis procedures.

The Silfverskiöld test is performed to distinguish between contracture of the Achilles tendon and isolated gastrocnemius contracture. It is important to assess ankle dorsiflexion with the hindfoot held reduced in a neutral position; if this is not done, dorsiflexion will be overestimated. The test is performed by first assessing ankle dorsiflexion with the knee in full extension. The knee is then flexed. If ankle dorsiflexion increases when the knee is flexed, this indicates an isolated gastrocnemius contracture (because of the gastrocnemius origin being above the knee joint). If ankle dorsiflexion does not increase with knee flexion, then the entire gastrocnemius-soleus complex/Achilles tendon is contracted. This detail is important for surgical planning. If the gastrocnemius is contracted, then it is lengthened as part of the surgical procedure. Several gastrocnemius fascia lengthening procedures have been described, including the Strayer recession.[13] If the entire complex is contracted, then Achilles tendon lengthening is performed. This procedure often involves a percutaneous triple-cut hemisection of the Achilles tendon.[14]

Swelling and pain with palpation over the course of the PTT and its insertion on the navicular are also documented. An accessory navicular may become obvious when a painful prominence is present at the PTT insertion. Localized edema over the PTT is common in AAFD and has been shown to be an excellent predictor of PTTD confirmed with MRI. In a study of 49 patients, pitting edema in the distal PTT area had a sensitivity of 86% and specificity of 100% for PTT degeneration.[15] Additional examination findings associated with AAFD include a callus that may develop under the medial column and a medial rocker-bottom deformity. Tenderness may be noted in the sinus tarsi, in the subfibular area, and over the peroneal tendons.

© 2025 American Academy of Orthopaedic Surgeons

Section 3: Arthritis of the Foot and Ankle

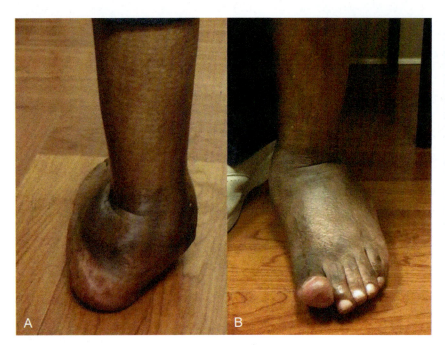
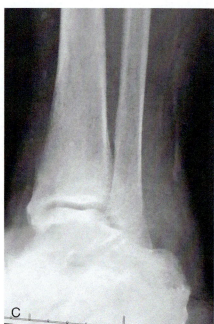

FIGURE 4 **A**, Anterior and **B**, posterior photographs demonstrating substantial adult-acquired flatfoot deformity. **C**, Corresponding radiograph showing subfibular impingement.

Finally, forefoot deformity is assessed in the seated position. With the hindfoot corrected to neutral, compensatory forefoot supination may be apparent (**Figure 5**). It is important to ascertain if the forefoot supination is flexible (ie, the physician can manipulate the medial column back to a plantigrade position) because this will affect surgical planning.

One of the most sensitive tests for PTTD is the single-limb heel rise. The patient must elevate the unaffected limb from the floor. The physician views the patient from behind and asks them to rise up on the toes. PTT insufficiency is demonstrated by either the inability to perform the rise because of weakness or pain or a partial heel rise without evidence of hindfoot inversion as the patient rises onto the ball of the foot.

IMAGING

Weight-bearing foot and ankle radiographs are necessary when evaluating patients with AAFD and should include hindfoot alignment, AP and oblique foot, lateral foot, and AP and mortise ankle views. The hindfoot alignment view is performed in the following manner: the patient stands on an elevated platform and the x-ray beam is positioned behind the patient, raised 20° from the floor. The radiograph cassette is placed in front of the patient and positioned perpendicular to the x-ray beam. This view, performed properly, is important to assess the severity of hindfoot valgus. An AP foot radiograph shows the extent of talonavicular uncoverage.

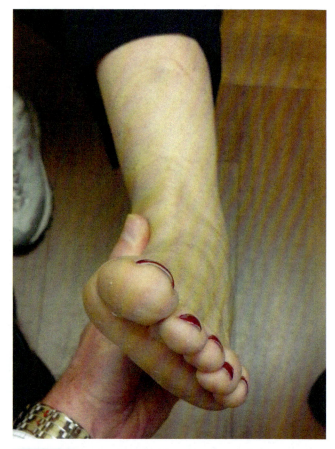

FIGURE 5 Photograph demonstrating residual forefoot varus after the hindfoot has been corrected to neutral.

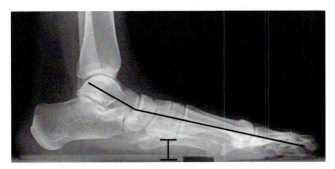

FIGURE 6 Lateral radiograph showing the Meary angle (the line down the axis of the talus and first metatarsal); normal is 0 (±10°). Medial cuneiform height is measured from the floor to the plantar aspect of the medial cuneiform (normal 15 to 25 mm).

A lateral foot radiograph is used to assess for arch collapse and first TMT plantar gapping. Meary angle and medial cuneiform height relative to the base of the fifth metatarsal may be measured, among other parameters (Figure 6). A weight-bearing AP radiograph of the ankle evaluates for talar tilt and subfibular impingement (Figure 4).

Ultrasonography can be used to evaluate the PTT, but its usefulness is user-dependent and no studies have provided prognostic information based on ultrasonographic studies.

After weight-bearing radiographs, MRI is the next most common imaging modality used to assess AAFD. MRI is important to confirm pathology and to assess the spring ligament, deltoid ligament, sinus tarsi impingement, and any arthritic changes. This additional information can be used to develop an individualized treatment plan. Because MRI is a non–weight-bearing study, it does not show the pathology that can be gained from weight-bearing studies, either traditional radiographs or WBCT scans. An example of MRI in a patient with clinical stage I PTTD is shown in Figure 7, with substantial tenosynovitis without tendinopathy.

Traditional CT is not commonly used for the diagnosis because MRI is much more sensitive and accurate. However, WBCT is particularly useful in the evaluation of AAFD because it allows assessment of deformity and joint spaces in the weight-bearing position in which symptoms usually occur. Subtalar subluxation, including middle facet subluxation, which might not be apparent on standard CT, can be readily identified with WBCT.[16] Additional valuable information provided includes assessment of sinus tarsi and subfibular impingement, arthritic changes, and presence of ankle, hindfoot, and midfoot malalignment. Specifically, WBCT helps quantify the degree of peritalar instability, or alignment of the subtalar joint.[17] WBCT has been shown to demonstrate more severe deformity than traditional CT, making it

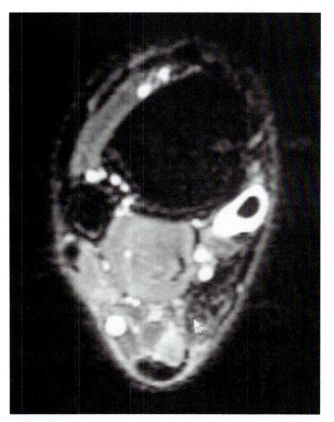

FIGURE 7 Axial T2 magnetic resonance image demonstrating substantial tenosynovitis around the posterior tibial tendon. This patient could perform a single-limb heel rise, signifying stage I posterior tibial tendon dysfunction.

more useful for surgical planning.[18,19] The presence of arthritis and/or subtalar subluxation seen on WBCT may lead a surgeon to consider an arthrodesis procedure instead of a joint-sparing reconstruction. WBCT recently allowed surgeons to quantify complex three-dimensional anatomy into a single measurement called the foot-ankle offset. The foot-ankle offset is an optimized biomechanical assessment of foot alignment and further study will be necessary to determine its role in quantifying foot alignment abnormalities.[20,21] In a 2020 study, an expert consensus panel recommended the use of WBCT (if available) for surgical planning of flatfoot reconstructions.[22]

NONSURGICAL TREATMENT

The goal of nonsurgical treatment is to decrease pain, improve function, protect the PTT, and prevent further deformity. A variety of modalities is available, ranging from custom braces or orthotics to off-the-shelf devices. Flexible deformities are treated with supportive devices and rigid deformities are treated with accommodative devices. Corticosteroid injections should never be administered around the PTT because of risk for tendon rupture but may be useful if administered intra-articularly in the setting of arthritis.

Off-the-shelf options include orthotic devices with a longitudinal arch support and medial heel posting, a variety of lace-up ankle braces (specifically, the Aircast Airlift PTTD brace), and walker boots. Removable boots are an effective means with which to immobilize an inflamed foot. These devices are great options in the clinic setting for patients who are limping and/or experiencing pain or swelling. After the acute inflammatory symptoms resolve with immobilization, physical therapy can be initiated. Home exercises or supervised therapy has been shown to be equally effective in relieving pain and improving functional outcome in patients with stage I to III PTTD.[23]

Customized options include custom-molded orthotic devices and articulated and nonarticulated ankle-foot orthoses (AFOs). In addition to traditional custom-molded orthotic device, the UCBL (University of California Biomechanics Laboratory) is a maximally supportive shoe orthosis with reported success.[24] The brace options include a wide variety of options such as solid molded polypropylene AFOs and customized leather gauntlet (Arizona) braces. Success has also been reported with a shell brace that conserves hindfoot motion[25] and with a short customized articulated AFO combined with a physical therapy–directed exercise program.[26] In a study on use of the AFO-physical therapy combination, patients completed high-repetition exercises, aggressive plantar flexion activities, and an aggressive high-repetition home exercise program that included gastrocnemius-soleus complex tendon stretching. Only 11% of patients progressed to surgery, and 89% were satisfied and demonstrated improved strength.[26] A short customized articulated AFO preserves ankle motion and may have less of a deleterious effect on the gait cycle compared with a nonarticulated AFO.[27]

SURGICAL TREATMENT

Surgical treatment is offered to patients in whom nonsurgical treatment strategies fail to provide adequate relief of symptoms. There are a variety of surgical procedures to consider, usually in combination, each chosen to meet individual needs and components of the deformity. The surgical decision-making process takes into account the extent of deformity, patient age, and activity level/demands. The goal is to reduce pain and improve function by recreating a stable, plantigrade foot. Contraindications include vascular disease or open wounds; these conditions should be treated appropriately before reconstruction.

Surgical procedures for AAFD are typically considered in terms of joint-sparing versus joint-sacrificing (fusion) procedures. Flexible deformities can usually be managed with joint-sparing procedures, including tendon transfers and osteotomies, whereas rigid deformities or those involving substantial arthrosis require hindfoot fusion, consisting of subtalar fusion with or without talonavicular and/or calcaneocuboid fusion. Traditionally, some surgeons have favored fusions in older patients and patients who are overweight because of a perceived higher failure of joint-sparing reconstruction in these patient populations. However, a study has shown that patients older than 65 years have improvement with joint-sparing procedures similar to that of their younger counterparts, without a higher risk of revision surgery.[28] Another study also showed that outcomes of joint-sparing procedures did not vary relative to weight, with similar improvements among patients with normal weight, overweight, and obesity.[29]

Regardless of the procedures undertaken, surgical correction of AAFD should not be underestimated in difficulty by the surgeon or the patient. From the surgeon's perspective, care must be taken to tailor treatment to each patient's individual needs. Caution should be exercised in patients who smoke, those with diabetes, and others at higher risk for healing problems because the success of any surgery is dependent on healing of osteotomy sites or fusion sites and multiple incisions. From the patient's perspective, a prolonged non–weight-bearing period is required. Even after weight bearing is allowed, progress is slow and maximal improvement in symptoms may take 1 to 2 years.

POSTERIOR TIBIAL TENOSYNOVITIS

Surgical treatment is rarely indicated for stage I PTTD. Most patients respond well to immobilization. After symptoms improve, patients benefit from a rehabilitation program and supportive orthotic devices. For patients without deformity, open tenosynovectomy with repair of the PTT can improve symptoms. PTT tendoscopic synovectomy has been described as a minimally invasive and effective surgical procedure to treat patients with stage I PTTD.[30] It offers the advantages of less wound pain and fewer scar and wound complications. The authors advocated that if a tendon tear is observed during tendoscopy, it must be repaired with nonabsorbable sutures using a 3- or 4-cm incision.[30] However, tendoscopic procedures are not the standard in treatment of stage I PTTD. This technique can be technically difficult, visualization may be challenging, and there is a significant learning curve.

FLEXIBLE DEFORMITIES

Surgical treatment of stage II deformities usually entails joint-sparing reconstruction with osteotomies and tendon transfers. Correction of underlying bony deformity is essential to success, and soft-tissue repairs are rarely indicated in isolation. The mainstays of treatment of stage II deformities are medial displacement calcaneal osteotomy (MDCO), débridement of the degenerative PTT, flexor digitorum longus (FDL) tendon transfer to the navicular, and gastrocnemius lengthening. The purpose of these procedures is to improve pain and alignment and to avoid arthrodesis. Although clinical and radiographic parameters improve with these treatments, restoration of normal alignment is not necessarily the goal and is usually not achievable.

Soft-Tissue Procedures

FDL tendon transfer is performed to replace the function of a degenerated or ruptured PTT. The flexor hallucis longus is preferred by some surgeons because it is a stronger tendon.[31] Direct repair of the PTT is controversial because the tendon is degenerated, does not heal well, and is a likely pain generator in the process. To perform the tendon transfer, the FDL is traced into the arch of the foot and tenotomy is performed with care to avoid injury to the nearby neurovascular bundle. The FDL is then transferred to the PTT stump or, more commonly, to the navicular through a drill hole and secured with a biotenodesis screw or suture. The tendon transfer is tensioned with the ankle in mild plantar flexion and inversion of the foot. The peroneus brevis has been described as another option to be used in the revision setting or to augment a weak FDL tendon.[32]

Other soft-tissue procedures include lengthening the Achilles tendon and repairing the spring ligament. Addressing Achilles tendon or gastrocnemius contracture is almost always necessary in the surgical correction of flatfoot deformity. In cases of isolated gastrocnemius contracture, gastrocnemius recession is performed, which entails isolated release of the gastrocnemius fascia in the leg. This can be performed open through a posteromedial incision or endoscopically. The release is commonly done at the musculotendinous junction with care taken to avoid injury to the sural nerve. The fascia is identified and horizontally incised until approximately 10° above neutral ankle dorsiflexion is achieved. In cases of more severe contracture or generalized Achilles tendon contracture, the entire complex can be lengthened by a triple-cut hemisection of the Achilles tendon. This is commonly done percutaneously with three stab incisions, alternating medial and lateral, spaced about 2 cm apart.

Regarding the spring ligament, multiple different repair and reconstruction techniques have been described, with no clear consensus on the optimal method or indication. In 2020, an expert panel recommended a medial soft-tissue reconstruction when a lateral column lengthening (LCL) fails to fully correct the abduction deformity.[33] Techniques to repair the spring ligament vary and include direct end-to-end repair with or without augmentation. One method to reconstruct the ligament using the PTT remnant was described.[34] Another technique using the peroneus longus has also been described.[35] However, there are no data differentiating between methods or even demonstrating the necessity of spring ligament reconstruction.

Periarticular Osteotomies

The MDCO is the single most important procedure for correcting valgus hindfoot alignment, with more medial translation conferring more correction.[36] The standard MDCO is an oblique osteotomy made through a lateral incision. The MDCO has been performed using minimally invasive techniques, which may decrease postoperative pain as well as the incidence of nerve injury[37] The posterior tuberosity is translated medially generally between 7 and 15 mm depending on the amount of deformity.[38] The aim is to correct hindfoot valgus and protect the FDL tendon transfer by restoring neutral hindfoot alignment. This osteotomy can be fixed with headed or headless screws or with lateral step plates or staples (**Figure 8**). When assessing the correction, the surgeon should aim for a clinically straight heel (neutral alignment) confirmed by an intraoperative axial and/or hindfoot alignment view. A study of 55 patients undergoing reconstruction of stage II deformity showed that patients had significantly greater improvement when they were

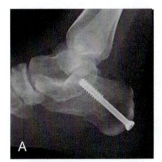
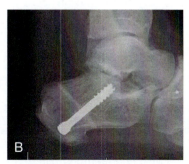
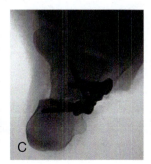
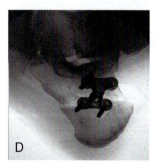

FIGURE 8 Radiographs showing multiple options for medial displacement calcaneal osteotomy fixation. **A**, A headed screw is used. **B**, A headless screw is used. **C** and **D**, Plate fixation is used.

corrected to neutral or mild radiographic varus alignment (0° to 5°) versus valgus or moderate radiographic varus alignment.[39] Clinically, these patients were shown to be in neutral hindfoot alignment.

If preoperative weight-bearing radiographs show talonavicular joint uncoverage above 40%, indicating forefoot abduction, an LCL osteotomy also may be performed (**Figure 9**). This is typically done through a second incision anterior and distal to the MDCO incision. The osteotomy is made at least 1 cm proximal to the calcaneocuboid joint and distracted until satisfactory correction of foot abduction is achieved. The amount of distraction varies but is generally between 5 and 10 mm to reduce the talonavicular joint into anatomic alignment.[40] An appropriately sized cortical autograft, allograft, or porous metal wedge is then placed in the osteotomy site. When performing LCL, care must be taken to avoid overdistraction leading to lateral foot overload or subluxating the calcaneocuboid joint.[41] Overdistraction can be avoided by checking for proper alignment of the talonavicular joint on simulated weight-bearing fluoroscopic imaging. It is also important to maintain the ability of the hindfoot to evert by assessing residual passive eversion range of motion.[40] A comparative study of 72 feet using different corrective options demonstrated that patients who had both LCL and MDCO experienced more improvement in all radiographic parameters (versus MDCO alone).[42] LCL can also be performed using a Z-cut or step-cut calcaneal osteotomy. Compared with a traditional LCL, this procedure has been shown to lead to equivalent deformity correction, similar outcome scores, faster healing times, and fewer nonunions[43] (**Figure 10**).

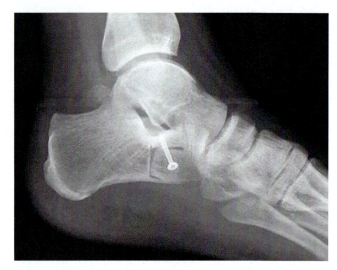

FIGURE 10 Radiograph demonstrating the Z-cut calcaneal osteotomy.

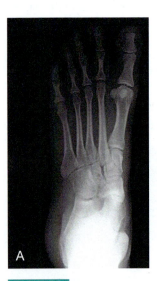 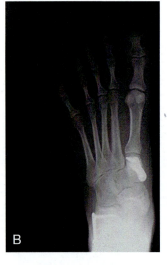

FIGURE 9 **A**, Preoperative and **B**, postoperative AP radiographs demonstrating significant uncoverage and the need for a lateral column lengthening.

A possible alternative to LCL is calcaneocuboid distraction arthrodesis. However, this technique has fallen out of favor and must be used with caution because high nonunion rates (nearly 50%) have been reported.[44]

After MDCO and/or LCL, the forefoot is reassessed. If there is residual forefoot supination, a dorsal opening wedge osteotomy of the medial cuneiform can be added (also known as a Cotton osteotomy) (**Figure 11**). This plantarflexes the medial column to restore the plantigrade foot and weight-bearing tripod. The Cotton osteotomy has been shown to lead to significant correction of longitudinal arch collapse when combined with other flatfoot procedures. In 2020, an expert consensus group reported a typical range of 5 to 11 mm of correction (average size 5 to 6 mm) for Cotton osteotomies.[45] In another study, each additional 2 mm of Cotton osteotomy graft size led to 2.1° improvement in arch collapse measured radiographically.[46]

Some patients with residual forefoot supination may require a midfoot arthrodesis procedure. Indications for first TMT arthrodesis include first TMT hypermobility, first TMT plantar joint gapping, first TMT arthritis, and/or a significant hallux valgus deformity. In these patients, additional plantar flexion of the medial column can be achieved through the arthrodesis site. First TMT fusion in this setting leads to acceptable clinical and radiographic outcomes.[47] Occasionally, medial column instability exists at the naviculocuneiform joint. In such cases, the apex of deformity is seen at the naviculocuneiform joint on a lateral radiograph. This is addressed with either a Cotton osteotomy, a first TMT arthrodesis or naviculocuneiform arthrodesis, or a combination of these procedures (**Figure 12**).

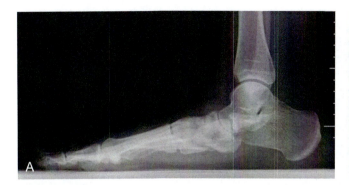 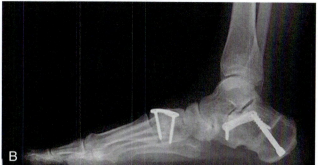

FIGURE 11 **A**, Preoperative and **B**, postoperative lateral radiographs. This patient required a Cotton osteotomy.

Finally, subtalar arthroereisis can be performed as an adjunct to other procedures to help correct hindfoot valgus. There are metallic and bioabsorbable options and removal is debated. Use of this technique is controversial and has decreased over the years. Arthroereisis implants frequently require removal and there are no high-quality clinical data supporting their use for AAFD.

RIGID DEFORMITIES

Arthrodesis procedures are performed for rigid deformities, severe flexible deformities, patients with underlying inflammatory arthropathy, and revision of failed procedures. Triple arthrodesis is the standard procedure; however, future adjacent joint arthrosis is a concern. A triple arthrodesis is appropriate for patients with substantial deformity and underlying arthritis of the three joints (**Figure 13**). Selective arthrodesis is another popular option. This can entail a single joint arthrodesis (talonavicular or subtalar) or a double arthrodesis (ie, fusion of both). A 2019 article described successful results after fusing both the naviculocuneiform and subtalar joints.[48] Isolated talonavicular arthrodesis is a useful and effective alternative to double arthrodesis. It is worth noting that isolated talonavicular arthrodesis is equivalent to double arthrodesis in terms of motion loss: both lead to an approximate 80% reduction in tarsal motion.[49]

A double arthrodesis of the subtalar/talonavicular joints can be performed through an all-medial or combined lateral/medial or lateral/dorsal approach depending on surgeon preference. For the all-medial approach, the incision extends from the tip of the medial malleolus down the midline of the foot. The PTT can be preserved or removed. The surgeon must be careful not to violate the deltoid ligament; this could lead to iatrogenic ankle valgus. The medial approach allows access to both the subtalar and talonavicular joints and has wound healing advantages.[50] When addressing long-standing deformity and contracted lateral skin, the medial approach avoids the lateral foot, which lowers the wound complication rate (specifically, closure difficulty at the time of surgery and wound dehiscence postoperatively). Following correction, redundant medial skin allows closure without tension. The largest published series reported on 96 feet. In this study, 91% of feet had correction maintained at a mean 4.7 years; 15% of the feet required secondary surgery, most commonly for nonunion (6 patients) and progression of deformity with tibiotalar arthritis (5 patients). Regarding clinical outcomes, the mean American Orthopaedic Foot and Ankle Society ankle-hindfoot score was 67 and the mean visual analog scale score for pain was 2.4.[51]

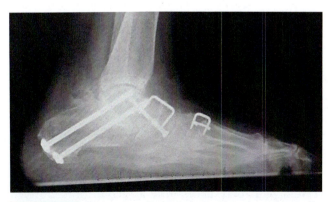

FIGURE 12 Lateral radiograph of the foot of a patient with substantial first tarsometatarsal instability. A tarsometatarsal arthrodesis was needed in addition to the hindfoot double arthrodesis and Achilles tendon lengthening.

DEFORMITIES WITH ANKLE INVOLVEMENT

Stage IV deformity is associated with ankle valgus attributable to prolonged hindfoot valgus and resultant deltoid incompetence. The underlying flatfoot can be rigid or flexible and should be corrected according to the principles described earlier. Often, a triple or double arthrodesis is required.

In cases in which the ankle joint is not yet arthritic, ankle valgus may be corrected with deltoid ligament

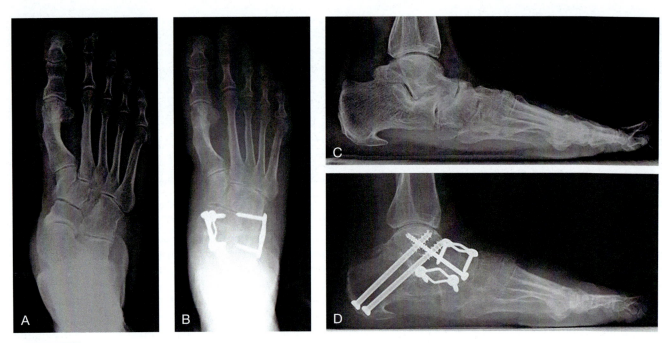

FIGURE 13 AP and lateral radiographs following a triple arthrodesis. **A**, Preoperative AP view. **B**, Postoperative AP view. **C**, Preoperative lateral view. **D**, Postoperative lateral view.

reconstruction in an effort to preserve the ankle joint. These techniques vary from tendon allograft weaved through the medial tibia and into the navicular to use of ACL guides to direct tunnel placement and use of synthetic material to augment the repair. These techniques are challenging and very few outcome reports have been published. One study reported on five patients who had deltoid reconstructions using peroneus longus autograft. None required additional surgery on the ankle by a mean 9 years of follow-up.[52] Another study examined combined allograft reconstruction of both the spring and deltoid ligament complexes. This study concluded that this combined approach was a viable surgical option in advanced AAFD with medial peritalar instability.[53] The spring and deltoid ligament complexes can also be reconstructed at the same time with supplemental internal brace augmentation.[54]

When the ankle shows advanced arthritic changes, arthrodesis or ankle replacement is often required to achieve pain relief and a stable plantigrade extremity. Patients who require tibiotalocalcaneal or pantalar arthrodesis should be counseled on risks and limitations following an extensive arthrodesis. The alternative to ankle fusion is total ankle arthroplasty (TAR), performed with or without deltoid repair. TAR can be performed simultaneously with foot correction or in a staged fashion. Although good outcomes have been reported on TAR for valgus deformities, there are no outcome reports specifically pertaining to TAR performed in the setting of flatfoot deformities. These deformities are complex and necessitate detailed preoperative planning to obtain a satisfactory result.

COMPLICATIONS

Complications are common in patients undergoing reconstruction for AAFD. These include, but are not limited to, infection, nerve (most commonly sural) and vessel injury, wound complications, malunion, nonunion, failure of tendon transfer incorporation, undercorrection, overcorrection (most commonly lateral column overload), progression of deformity, pain or arthritis, and medical complications such as deep vein thrombosis. Risks are directly associated with the deformity and complexity of each case and can be minimized with careful planning. Patients with diabetes should be advised to closely monitor their serum glucose levels, and surgery should be performed with caution in patients with a hemoglobin A1c level above 7.5 mg/dL. Those who smoke should be strongly encouraged to discontinue tobacco use. Patients taking corticosteroids and those with preexisting ulcers caused by chronic deformity are at an increased risk for complications. Also, in patients with long-standing severe deformity, lateral incisions may pose difficulty with closure and healing after hindfoot valgus has been corrected. Hardware-related pain may necessitate a second procedure to remove the implant. Failures following reconstructions with osteotomies and tendon transfers are salvaged with arthrodesis procedures.

Chapter 11: Adult-Acquired Flatfoot Deformity

SUMMARY

AAFD is a common problem and should be considered in patients presenting with medial or lateral hindfoot and ankle pain. A thorough history and physical examination is required for diagnosis and to effectively treat these patients. Treatment is individualized to a patient's age, weight, stage of deformity, activity level, and expectations. Many nonsurgical options are available when treating these patients initially. When nonsurgical management is unsuccessful, a surgical procedure can improve pain, alignment, and function. Recovery may take up to 1 to 2 years.

KEY STUDY POINTS

- AAFD is caused by PTTD and ligamentous failure of the foot that usually develops later in life in individuals with underlying anatomic predisposition. It is a distinct entity from congenital flatfoot and other causes of flatfoot deformities, such as trauma and inflammatory disorders.
- Patients present with hindfoot valgus, a collapsed medial arch, and medial pain over the PTT and/or lateral pain from subfibular impingement. Performing a single-limb heel rise is difficult or impossible because of PTT weakness.
- Treatment is individualized to the patient and the flexibility of the deformity. Flexible deformities may usually be treated with joint-sparing procedures, including tendon transfers and osteotomies, whereas rigid deformities require arthrodesis procedures.

ANNOTATED REFERENCES

1. Frey C, Shereff M, Greenidge N: Vascularity of the posterior tibial tendon. *J Bone Joint Surg Am* 1990;72(6):884-888.

2. Mosier SM, Lucas DR, Pomeroy G, Manoli A II: Pathology of the posterior tibial tendon in posterior tibial tendon insufficiency. *Foot Ankle Int* 1998;19(8):520-524.

3. Cody EA, Williamson ER, Burket JC, Deland JT, Ellis SJ: Correlation of talar anatomy and subtalar joint alignment on weightbearing computed tomography with radiographic flatfoot parameters. *Foot Ankle Int* 2016;37(8):874-881.

4. Apostle KL, Coleman NW, Sangeorzan BJ: Subtalar joint axis in patients with symptomatic peritalar subluxation compared to normal controls. *Foot Ankle Int* 2014;35(11):1153-1158.

5. Johnson KA, Strom DE: Tibialis posterior tendon dysfunction. *Clin Orthop Relat Res* 1989;239:196-206.

6. Myerson MS: Adult-acquired flatfoot deformity: Treatment of dysfunction of the posterior tibial tendon. *Instr Course Lect* 1997;46:393-405.

7. Bluman EM, Title CI, Myerson MS: Posterior tibial tendon rupture: A refined classification system. *Foot Ankle Clin* 2007;12(2):233-249, v.

8. Raikin SM, Winters BS, Daniel JN: The RAM classification: A novel, systematic approach to the adult-acquired flatfoot. *Foot Ankle Clin* 2012;17(2):169-181.

9. Conti S, Michelson J, Jahss M: Clinical significance of magnetic resonance imaging in preoperative planning for reconstruction of posterior tibial tendon ruptures. *Foot Ankle* 1992;13(4):208-214.

10. Ellis SJ, Deyer T, Williams BR, et al: Assessment of lateral hindfoot pain in acquired flatfoot deformity using weight-bearing multiplanar imaging. *Foot Ankle Int* 2010;31(5):361-371.

11. Auch E, Barbachan Mansur NS, Alexandre Alves T, et al: Distal tibiofibular syndesmotic widening in progressive collapsing foot deformity. *Foot Ankle Int* 2021;42(6):768-775.

    Sixty-two symptomatic patients and 29 control patients underwent WBCT. Patients with progressive collapsing foot deformity had significantly increased foot-ankle offset and distal tibiofibular syndesmosis measurements in comparison with control patients. Level of evidence: III.

12. Myerson MS, Thordarson DB, Johnson JE, et al: Classification and nomenclature: Progressive collapsing foot deformity. *Foot Ankle Int* 2020;41(10):1271-1276.

    Expert consensus group recommends renaming PTTD and AAFD to progressive collapsing foot deformity. Level of evidence: V.

13. Strayer LM: Gastrocnemius recession: Five-year report of cases. *J Bone Joint Surg Am* 1958;40-A(5):1019-1030.

14. Hatt RN, Lamphier TA: Triple hemisection: A simplified procedure for lengthening the Achilles tendon. *N Engl J Med* 1947;236(5):166-169.

15. DeOrio JK, Shapiro SA, McNeil RB, Stansel J: Validity of the posterior tibial edema sign in posterior tibial tendon dysfunction. *Foot Ankle Int* 2011;32(2):189-192.

16. de Cesar Netto C, Godoy-Santos AL, Saito GH, et al: Subluxation of the middle facet of the subtalar joint as a marker of peritalar subluxation in adult acquired flatfoot deformity: A case-control study. *J Bone Joint Surg Am* 2019;101(20):1838-1844.

    Thirty patients with stage II AAFD and 30 control patients underwent WBCT scans. The WBCT scans allowed accurate measurements, and significant differences were found in the percentage of joint uncoverage and the incongruence angle compared with control patients. Level of evidence: III.

17. de Cesar Netto C, Silva T, Li S, et al: Assessment of posterior and middle facet subluxation of the subtalar joint in progressive flatfoot deformity. *Foot Ankle Int* 2020;41(10):1190-1197.

Section 3: Arthritis of the Foot and Ankle

© 2025 American Academy of Orthopaedic Surgeons

Orthopaedic Knowledge Update®: Foot and Ankle 7

179

Seventy-six patients with AAFD underwent WBCT with the goal of comparing the amount of subluxation between the medial and posterior facets. Their results indicated that middle facet subluxation may provide an earlier and more pronounced marker of progressive peritalar subluxation in AAFD. Level of evidence: III.

18. De Cesar Netto C, Schon LC, Thawait GK, et al: Flexible adult-acquired flatfoot deformity: Comparison between weight-bearing and non-weight-bearing measurements using cone-beam computed tomography. *J Bone Joint Surg Am* 2017;99(18):e98.

19. Kunas GC, Probasco W, Haleem AM, Burket JC, Williamson ERC, Ellis SJ: Evaluation of peritalar subluxation in adult-acquired flatfoot deformity using computed tomography and weightbearing multiplanar imaging. *Foot Ankle Surg* 2018;24(6):495-500.

20. de Cesar Netto C, Bang K, Mansur NS, et al: Multiplanar semiautomatic assessment of foot and ankle offset in adult acquired flatfoot deformity. *Foot Ankle Int* 2020;41(7):839-848.

    One hundred thirteen patients with stage II AAFD underwent semiautomatic three-dimensional WBCT to measure the foot-ankle offset. The foot-ankle offset significantly correlated with traditional markers of pronounced AAFD and offered a simple and more complete single measurement of the three-dimensional components of AAFD. Level of evidence: III.

21. Day J, de Cesar Netto C, Nishikawa DRC, et al: Three-dimensional biometric weightbearing CT evaluation of the operative treatment of adult-acquired flatfoot deformity. *Foot Ankle Int* 2020;41(8):930-936.

    Nineteen adult patients with stage II AAFD underwent preoperative and postoperative WBCT at mean 19 months after surgery. The foot-ankle offset measurement was calculated and determined to be a reliable and sensitive tool to evaluate preoperative deformity as well as postoperative correction. Level of evidence: II.

22. de Cesar Netto C, Myerson MS, Day J, et al: Consensus for the use of weightbearing CT in the assessment of progressive collapsing foot deformity. *Foot Ankle Int* 2020;41(10):1277-1282.

    Expert consensus group unanimously recommends weight-bearing radiographs (including hindfoot alignment view) and WBCT scans (when available) for preoperative planning in patients with progressive collapsing foot deformity. CT findings to be assessed included sinus tarsi impingement, subfibular impingement, increased valgus inclination of the posterior facet of the subtalar joint, and subluxation of the subtalar joint at the posterior and/or middle facet. Level of evidence: V.

23. Bek N, Simşek IE, Erel S, Yakut Y, Uygur F: Home-based general versus center-based selective rehabilitation in patients with posterior tibial tendon dysfunction. *Acta Orthop Traumatol Turc* 2012;46(4):286-292.

24. Chao W, Wapner KL, Lee TH, Adams J, Hecht PJ: Non-operative management of posterior tibial tendon dysfunction. *Foot Ankle Int* 1996;17(12):736-741.

25. Krause F, Bosshard A, Lehmann O, Weber M: Shell brace for stage II posterior tibial tendon insufficiency. *Foot Ankle Int* 2008;29(11):1095-1100.

26. Alvarez RG, Marini A, Schmitt C, Saltzman CL: Stage I and II posterior tibial tendon dysfunction treated by a structured nonoperative management protocol: An orthosis and exercise program. *Foot Ankle Int* 2006;27(1):2-8.

27. Neville CG, Houck JR: Choosing among 3 ankle-foot orthoses for a patient with stage II posterior tibial tendon dysfunction. *J Orthop Sports Phys Ther* 2009;39(11):816-824.

28. Conti MS, Jones MT, Savenkov O, Deland JT, Ellis SJ: Outcomes of reconstruction of the stage II adult-acquired flatfoot deformity in older patients. *Foot Ankle Int* 2018;39(9):1019-1027.

29. Soukup DS, MacMahon A, Burket JC, Yu JM, Ellis SJ, Deland JT: Effect of obesity on clinical and radiographic outcomes following reconstruction of stage II adult-acquired flatfoot deformity. *Foot Ankle Int* 2016;37(3):245-254.

30. Khazen G, Khazen C: Tendoscopy in stage I posterior tibial tendon dysfunction. *Foot Ankle Clin* 2012;17(3):399-406.

31. Sammarco GJ, Hockenbury RT: Treatment of stage II posterior tibial tendon dysfunction with flexor hallucis longus transfer and medial displacement calcaneal osteotomy. *Foot Ankle Int* 2001;22(4):305-312.

32. Song SJ, Deland JT: Outcome following addition of peroneus brevis tendon transfer to treatment of acquired posterior tibial tendon insufficiency. *Foot Ankle Int* 2001;22(4):301-304.

33. Deland JT, Ellis SJ, Day J, et al: Indications for deltoid and spring ligament reconstruction in progressive collapsing foot deformity. *Foot Ankle Int* 2020;41(10):1302-1306.

    Expert consensus group acknowledges uncertainty but unanimously recommends medial soft-tissue procedures if lateral column lengthening does not fully correct the abduction deformity. Level of evidence: V.

34. Ryssman DB, Jeng CL: Reconstruction of the spring ligament with a posterior tibial tendon autograft: Technique tip. *Foot Ankle Int* 2017;38(4):452-456.

35. Williams BR, Ellis SJ, Deyer TW, Pavlov H, Deland JT: Reconstruction of the spring ligament using a peroneus longus autograft tendon transfer. *Foot Ankle Int* 2010;31(7):567-577.

36. Chan JY, Williams BR, Nair P, et al: The contribution of medializing calcaneal osteotomy on hindfoot alignment in the reconstruction of the stage II adult-acquired flatfoot deformity. *Foot Ankle Int* 2013;34(2):159-166.

37. Sherman TI, Guyton GP: Minimal incision/minimally invasive medializing displacement calcaneal osteotomy. *Foot Ankle Int* 2018;39(1):119-128.

38. Schon LC, Netto CD, Day J, et al: Consensus for the indication of a medializing displacement calcaneal osteotomy in the treatment of progressive collapsing foot deformity. *Foot Ankle Int* 2020;41(10):1282-1285.

    Expert consensus group unanimously recommends an MDCO (with the goal of achieving a neutral heel) as an isolated bony procedure when there is an isolated hindfoot valgus with adequate talonavicular coverage and lack of significant forefoot supination, varus, or abduction. Level of evidence: V.

39. Conti MS, Ellis SJ, Chan JY, Do HT, Deland JT: Optimal position of the heel following reconstruction of the stage II adult-acquired flatfoot deformity. *Foot Ankle Int* 2015;36(8):919-927.

40. Thordarson DB, Schon LC, de Cesar Netto C, et al: Consensus for the indication of lateral column lengthening in the treatment of progressive collapsing foot deformity. *Foot Ankle Int* 2020;41(10):1286-1288.

   Expert consensus group made a strong consensus for LCL when talonavicular uncoverage is greater than 40% and the strongest consensus for evaluating the talonavicular joint on simulated weight-bearing radiographs to avoid overcorrection. They also had unanimous agreement that the range of a typical LCL is between 5 and 10 mm. Level of evidence: V.

41. Oh I, Imhauser C, Choi D, Williams B, Ellis S, Deland J: Sensitivity of plantar pressure and talonavicular alignment to lateral column lengthening in flatfoot reconstruction. *J Bone Joint Surg Am* 2013;95(12):1094-1100.

42. Iossi M, Johnson JE, McCormick JJ, Klein SE: Short-term radiographic analysis of operative correction of adult-acquired flatfoot deformity. *Foot Ankle Int* 2013;34(6):781-791.

43. Saunders SM, Ellis SJ, Demetracopoulos CA, Marinescu A, Burkett J, Deland JT: Comparative outcomes between step-cut lengthening calcaneal osteotomy vs traditional Evans osteotomy for stage IIB adult-acquired flatfoot deformity. *Foot Ankle Int* 2018;39(1):18-27.

44. Grunander TR, Thordarson DB: Results of calcaneocuboid distraction arthrodesis. *Foot Ankle Surg* 2012;18(1):15-18.

45. Ellis SJ, Johnson JE, Day J, et al: Titrating the amount of bony correction in progressive collapsing foot deformity. *Foot Ankle Int* 2020;41(10):1292-1295.

   Expert consensus group met to define the amount of bony correction performed in the setting of progressive collapsing foot deformity. The recommendations included MDCO, LCL, and Cotton osteotomy. Level of evidence: V.

46. Kunas GC, Do HT, Aiyer A, Deland JT, Ellis SJ: Contribution of medial cuneiform osteotomy to correction of longitudinal arch collapse in stage IIb adult-acquired flatfoot deformity. *Foot Ankle Int* 2018;39(8):885-893.

47. Day J, Conti MS, Williams N, Ellis SJ, Deland JT, Cody EA: Contribution of first-tarsometatarsal joint fusion to deformity correction in the treatment of adult-acquired flatfoot deformity. *Foot Ankle Orthop* 2020;5(3):2473011420927321.

   Forty patients were retrospectively analyzed after undergoing first TMT and subtalar fusion as part of a flatfoot reconstructive procedure. Fusion of the TMT joint, in combination with other procedures, led to acceptable clinical and radiographic outcomes. Level of evidence: III.

48. Steiner CS, Gilgen A, Zwicky L, Schweizer C, Ruiz R, Hintermann B: Combined subtalar and naviculocuneiform fusion for treating adult acquired flatfoot deformity with medial arch collapse at the level of the naviculocuneiform joint. *Foot Ankle Int* 2019;40(1):42-47.

   Thirty-one patients were treated with subtalar and naviculocuneiform fusion, which was an effective and safe surgical solution for AAFD. Level of evidence: IV.

49. Thelen S, Rütt J, Wild M, Lögters T, Windolf J, Koebke J: The influence of talonavicular versus double arthrodesis on load dependent motion of the midtarsal joint. *Arch Orthop Trauma Surg* 2010;130(1):47-53.

50. Jeng CL, Vora AM, Myerson MS: The medial approach to triple arthrodesis. Indications and technique for management of rigid valgus deformities in high-risk patients. *Foot Ankle Clin* 2005;10(3):515-521, vi-vii.

51. Röhm J, Zwicky L, Horn Lang T, Salentiny Y, Hintermann B, Knupp M: Mid- to long-term outcome of 96 corrective hindfoot fusions in 84 patients with rigid flatfoot deformity. *Bone Joint J* 2015;97-B(5):668-674.

52. Ellis SJ, Williams BR, Wagshul AD, Pavlov H, Deland JT: Deltoid ligament reconstruction with peroneus longus autograft in flatfoot deformity. *Foot Ankle Int* 2010;31(9):781-789.

53. Brodell JD, MacDonald AM, Perkins JA, Deland JT, Oh I: Deltoid-spring ligament reconstruction in adult acquired flatfoot deformity with medial peritalar instability. *Foot Ankle Int* 2019;40(7):753-761.

   Twelve patients who underwent osseous and deltoid-spring ligament reconstruction for advanced AAFD were evaluated at mean postoperative follow-up of 24 months. The authors concluded the procedure was a viable surgical option for advanced AAFD with medial peritalar instability. Level of evidence: IV.

54. Nery C, Lemos AVKC, Raduan F, Mansur NSB, Baumfeld D: Combined spring and deltoid ligament repair in adult-acquired flatfoot. *Foot Ankle Int* 2018;39(8):903-907.

SECTION 4

The Forefoot

Section Editor:

Elizabeth A. Martin, MD, MSc, FAAOS

CHAPTER 12

Disorders of the Hallux

SARA LYN MINIACI-COXHEAD, MD, MEd, FAAOS

ABSTRACT

The most common disorders of the hallux include hallux valgus, hallux varus, and hallux rigidus. These disorders can be managed nonsurgically; however, if pain persists, then surgical treatment may be necessary. For each disorder, there are considerations regarding patient factors, radiographic findings, and the extent of the deformity that help surgeons determine the most appropriate surgical treatment.

Keywords: arthrodesis; arthroplasty; hallux rigidus; hallux valgus; hallux varus

INTRODUCTION

There are many disorders of the great toe that are evaluated by an orthopaedic surgeon, the most common being hallux valgus, hallux rigidus, and hallux varus. Each of these disorders presents in a characteristic manner, usually with pain and deformity. It is important to discuss the anatomy, pathophysiology, history and physical examination, and treatment options for each of these disorders.

Dr. Miniaci-Coxhead or an immediate family member serves as a paid consultant to or is an employee of Avitus and Exactech, Inc. and serves as a board member, owner, officer, or committee member of American Orthopaedic Foot and Ankle Society.

HALLUX VALGUS

Hallux valgus is a common forefoot deformity in which the first metatarsal deviates medially and the hallux deviates both laterally and into pronation, leaving a prominence on the medial side of the forefoot at the first metatarsal head. The causes of hallux valgus in most patients are thought to be multifactorial, including an intrinsic predisposition to develop a bunion along with a history of extrinsic deforming factors.

Anatomy and Pathogenesis

The stability of the first ray depends on a balance of static and dynamic structures. Loss of stability anywhere along the length of the first ray can contribute to hallux valgus. In addition to the bony architecture of the first tarsometatarsal (TMT) and first metatarsophalangeal (MTP) joints, several soft-tissue structures contribute to joint stability (**Table 1**). The four requirements for stability of the first ray are a congruent and stable MTP joint, a distal metatarsal articular angle (DMAA) that encourages stability, balanced static and dynamic constraints, and a stable TMT joint.[1]

Hallux valgus typically progresses in a stepwise manner. The process is thought to begin with attenuation of the medial soft-tissue supporting structures of the MTP joint (abductor hallucis and the medial joint capsule). As a result, the first metatarsal drifts into varus and the first MTP joint subluxates laterally. Progressive deformity often occurs as the medial supporting structures attenuate further and the lateral structures begin to contract. As the first metatarsal drifts into varus, the sesamoid bones, which are tethered by the transverse metatarsal ligament, displace into the first intermetatarsal space. This causes pronation of the hallux. Moderate to severe

---

This chapter is adapted from Smith JT, Bluman EM: Hallux valgus and hallux varus; Telleria JJM, Kwon JY: Hallux rigidus, in Chou LB, ed: *Orthopaedic Knowledge Update®: Foot and Ankle 6.* American Academy of Orthopaedic Surgeons, 2020, pp 179-204.

© 2025 American Academy of Orthopaedic Surgeons

Section 4: The Forefoot

Table 1

Soft-Tissue Stabilizers of the First Tarsometatarsal and First Metatarsophalangeal Joints

First Tarsometatarsal Joint	First Metatarsophalangeal Joint
Flexor hallucis longus	Abductor hallucis
Tibialis anterior	Adductor hallucis
Intrinsic muscles of the foot	Extensor hallucis brevis
Joint capsule	Extensor hallucis longus and extensor hood
Peroneus longus	Flexor hallucis brevis and sesamoid complex
Plantar fascia	Joint capsule
	Medial and lateral collateral ligaments
	Sesamoid ligaments
	Transverse metatarsal ligament

hallux valgus deformity can significantly compromise the weight-bearing capacity of the first ray, resulting in transfer of weight from the first MTP joint to the adjacent lesser MTP joints.

Numerous factors are thought to contribute to the development of hallux valgus. The possible intrinsic etiologies include metatarsal head morphology, metatarsus primus varus, hypermobility of the first TMT joint, pes planus, generalized ligamentous laxity, tight Achilles tendon, inflammatory arthropathies, and neuromuscular disorders. Heritable anatomic factors such as DMAA, hypermobility, and arch height are thought to have an important role in the development of hallux valgus. Juvenile hallux valgus is more linked to heritable factors than adult hallux valgus. The extrinsic factors that contribute to hallux valgus include poorly fitting shoes that force the toe into an abnormal posture and acute trauma that disrupts the medial capsule, abductor hallucis, or sesamoid complex or fractures of the medial base of the proximal phalanx.

Historically, a much higher prevalence of hallux valgus has been observed in females than in males. There are fundamental anatomic differences between females and males that may predispose females to the development of hallux valgus. In general, females have a smaller and rounder metatarsal head, an adducted first metatarsal, and higher rates of ligamentous laxity than men. Studies report a ratio as high as 15 females to every 1

male treated surgically for this problem.[2] Compared with females, males who undergo surgical treatment for hallux valgus are typically younger and more likely to have a family history of hallux valgus. Radiographic measurements have shown a larger deformity in males having surgical treatment for hallux valgus than in females, as well as a higher rate of first MTP joint congruence.

Diagnostic Evaluation

Patients with hallux valgus typically present with pain over the medial eminence. The patient also may have generalized pain at the first MTP joint, pain from associated lesser toe abnormalities such as hammer toes, or pain at the lesser metatarsal heads caused by abnormal physiologic loading (transfer metatarsalgia). Skin lesions caused by chafing from shoes are common. Guidance and care should be tailored to the patient's symptoms, limitations, goals, and expectations.

The physical examination should include a standing assessment of alignment and a careful inspection for skin lesions including callosities. Neurologic and vascular status should be evaluated for all patients. The specific location of pain should be determined based on direct palpation as well as history. Joint motion and passive correction of the deformity are assessed. To evaluate for contractures, it is important to determine the dorsiflexion and plantar flexion of the first MTP joint in a reduced position. Intrinsic causes of hallux valgus should be assessed by examining for hypermobility of the first TMT joint, pes planus, generalized ligamentous laxity, and a tight Achilles tendon. Patients should also be evaluated for a history of inflammatory arthropathy or neuromuscular disorders.

Weight-bearing AP, lateral, and oblique radiographs of the foot should be obtained. The AP view is used to measure the intermetatarsal angle, hallux valgus angle, DMAA, and hallux valgus interphalangeus angle (**Figure 1**). The deformity is classified as mild, moderate, or severe (**Table 2**). The alignment of the sesamoid bones under the first metatarsal head is assessed. Evaluation of sesamoid position has been described on both plain radiographs and weight-bearing CT.[3] It is important to determine whether the first MTP joint is congruent or incongruent (**Figure 2**). In a congruent deformity, there is a concentric relationship between the first metatarsal head and the base of the proximal phalanx. An incongruent deformity occurs when the hallux is laterally subluxated on the metatarsal head. Finally, the first MTP joint should be evaluated radiographically for arthritic changes.

Instability of the first TMT joint is diagnosed primarily by clinical assessment, although efforts continue to develop an objective way to measure this.[4] Several different devices can be used to measure sagittal plane motion.[5] A study of a mobile fluoroscopic device used

Chapter 12: Disorders of the Hallux

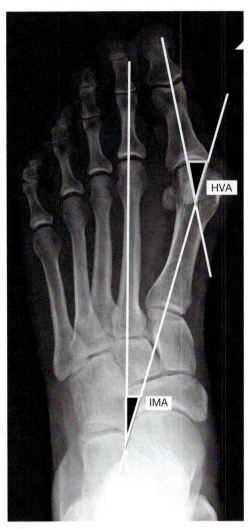

FIGURE 1 Weight-bearing AP radiograph shows the angles measured in hallux valgus. HVA = hallux valgus angle, IMA = intermetatarsal angle

Table 2

Radiographic Angles Used to Measure the Severity of Deformity in Hallux Valgus

Severity of Deformity	Hallux Valgus Angle	First-Second Intermetatarsal Angle	Distal Metatarsal Articular Angle
None (normal)	<15°	<9°	<10°
Mild	<20°	<11°	
Moderate	20°-40°	11°-16°	
Severe	>40°	>16°	

to analyze first ray motion in the sagittal plane during gait found that patients with hallux valgus had increased maximal dorsiflexion of the first TMT.[6] Weight-bearing CT has identified increased motion in multiple joints along the first ray, including the first TMT joint, in patients with hallux valgus compared with a control group.[7,8] As suggested in a 2020 study, inclusion of weight-bearing CT will become the standard of care in the near future, with the ability to define hallux valgus in a three-dimensional way.[9]

Rotational deformity of the first metatarsal has become a topic of interest in recent years. The presence of a rotational deformity associated with hallux valgus was included in early descriptions, but because of the biplanar nature of radiographs, measurements and descriptions have focused solely on two-dimensional angles. A 2021 systematic review addressed the issue of first metatarsal rotation as it relates to hallux valgus deformities. It was concluded that rotational deformity of the metatarsal is consistently present in hallux valgus; however, a standardized way to measure rotation was not provided. Furthermore, no conclusion was made regarding the most appropriate surgical method to address rotational deformities.[10]

Nonsurgical Treatment

Patient education and shoe modification are the mainstays of nonsurgical management of hallux valgus. The patient should understand the importance of shoe modification as a means of minimizing symptoms. Shoes with a wide toe box should be worn to accommodate the widened forefoot, and elevated heels should be avoided to minimize forefoot pressure during gait. Bunion splints, toe spacers, and pads can be used to improve alignment and avoid rubbing on the medial eminence in shoes. In-shoe orthotic devices may be useful to manage transfer metatarsalgia but are unlikely to relieve symptoms directly related to the hallux valgus deformity.

Surgical Treatment

Surgical reconstruction can be considered if the patient has persistent pain that limits their ability to function, despite nonsurgical management. Cosmesis alone is not an appropriate indication for surgical treatment to manage hallux valgus. More than 100 procedures have been described for treating a hallux valgus deformity.

Several basic principles of hallux valgus correction should be considered when selecting the appropriate reconstructive procedure. The first principle is that the choice of procedure depends on whether the deformity is congruent or incongruent. With congruent deformities, surgical treatment should be directed at correcting the intermetatarsal angle and DMAA using osteotomies without altering the normal MTP joint relationship.

A surgical procedure such as an Akin osteotomy, which is a medial closing wedge osteotomy of the great toe proximal phalanx, will help to correct alignment of the toe without altering the alignment of the first MTP joint. Patients with incongruent deformities, in contrast, should undergo soft-tissue balancing of the subluxated MTP joint along with any necessary corrective osteotomies.

The second general principle of hallux valgus correction is that as the severity of the deformity increases, the more proximal the correction needs to be (**Table 2**). For a mild deformity, a procedure that includes a distal osteotomy and soft-tissue balancing is often sufficient. The distal first metatarsal chevron osteotomy is commonly performed for mild deformities. For a moderate deformity, the correction often involves a first metatarsal shaft osteotomy accompanied by a distal soft-tissue procedure. A severe deformity requires a more proximal osteotomy or a first TMT fusion to correct a wide intermetatarsal angle.

The third principle is that in the presence of arthritis or if there is a significant loss of motion when examining the hallux in a reduced position, a first MTP joint arthrodesis should be considered. First MTP joint fusion can be a powerful tool to correct severe deformity.

Regardless of the technique chosen, several details are paramount to durable surgical success. The first of these is that sesamoid reduction under the first metatarsal head is correlated with maintenance of deformity correction. The quality of reduction can be graded using the Hardy-Clapham scale for determining the position of the medial sesamoid with respect to the longitudinal axis of the first metatarsal[11] (**Figure 3**). A significant correlation has been found between the magnitude of sesamoid displacement

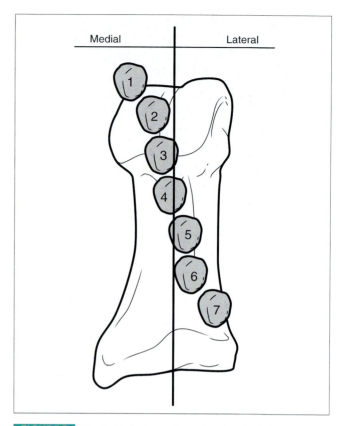

FIGURE 3 Illustration shows how the severity of sesamoid subluxation or dislocation can be graded using a system created by Hardy and Clapham. The medial-to-lateral position of the medial sesamoid (numbered circles) is determined in relation to the longitudinal axis of the first metatarsal (vertical line).

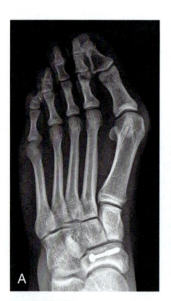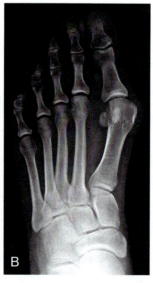

FIGURE 2 Weight-bearing AP radiographs show a congruent (**A**) and an incongruent (**B**) hallux valgus deformity.

at early follow-up and the risk of hallux valgus recurrence. Patients with an abnormal sesamoid position (5, 6, or 7) at the time of early follow-up were found to have a tenfold greater risk of recurrence than those with a normal position (1 to 4).[12] Not surprisingly, the quality of reduction of the subluxated first MTP joint is also critical to avoid recurrence of the deformity. The risk of hallux valgus recurrence was shown in a study to be correlated with both hallux valgus angle and sesamoid position on early postoperative weight-bearing radiographs.[13]

Release of the contracted soft tissues in the distal first-second intermetatarsal space is necessary for complete and durable correction of many hallux valgus deformities. The adductor hallucis tendon, the sesamoid suspensory ligament, and the lateral first MTP capsule should be sequentially released to facilitate the reduction of the proximal phalanx on the metatarsal head as well as of the sesamoids relative to the crista under the metatarsal head. Dorsal, distal, transarticular, and endoscopic approaches have been described to obtain this correction.[14]

Procedures that maintain the length of the first ray theoretically minimize the development of transfer lesions in the lesser metatarsal heads. Surgical procedures using a suture suspension technique or an opening wedge proximal metatarsal osteotomy can maintain first metatarsal length while correcting the intermetatarsal angle. Suture suspensory techniques have been introduced as an alternative to metatarsal osteotomy for mild to moderate deformity.[15] The procedure consists of a distal soft-tissue release, followed by suture suspension to reduce and hold the first-second intermetatarsal angle (**Figure 4**). Several studies have reported success when a suture suspensory device is used to correct a hallux valgus deformity.[16] Although some of the earliest studies reported second metatarsal fractures in patients treated with this technique, an updated smaller device appears to minimize this complication.[17]

A proximal opening wedge osteotomy can also be used to obtain hallux valgus correction without shortening. This medially based osteotomy is made at the proximal metaphysis of the first metatarsal and fixed with a dedicated plate that has a built-in spacer. The gap that is created is typically filled with bone graft. This is combined with a lateral release and medial capsular imbrication to obtain correction at the first MTP joint. The available studies found this technique to modestly lengthen the first metatarsal,[18] with good correction of the hallux valgus deformity achieved. Greater lengthening is claimed to be an advantage of the scarf osteotomy for correcting hallux valgus. Although few studies report on this parameter, lengthening as great as 10 mm was found to be possible.[19] A 10-year follow-up study of patients who underwent scarf osteotomy for hallux valgus correction showed that despite a radiographic recurrence rate of 30%, patients were still found to have substantial improvements in functional outcome scores.[20]

For patients with first TMT joint instability, an arthrodesis of the TMT joint is the preferred treatment for hallux valgus correction. Many surgeons have used two or three crossed screws as the standard fixation for a first TMT joint fusion, also known as a Lapidus procedure. Several cadaver studies examined the relative benefit (in terms of rigidity) of using a locking plate construct or crossed screws. In general, superior rigidity was found when a locking plate was used rather than crossed screws. A retrospective study found better union and earlier return to full weight bearing when a locking plate was used, compared with crossed screws.[21]

For patients with arthritis of the first MTP joint or rigidity of the joint when the hallux is reduced into neutral alignment, a first MTP joint arthrodesis is indicated. A cadaver study of fixation at the first MTP joint demonstrated greater stiffness when a locking plate-and-screw construct was used compared with a nonlocking plate-and-screw construct.[22] Studies have examined whether a proximal corrective procedure should accompany first MTP joint fusion for hallux valgus correction in cases with a wide intermetatarsal angle. Satisfactory correction of the intermetatarsal angle was reported after the first MTP fusion alone in patients with a mean preoperative 33° hallux valgus angle and 13° intermetatarsal angle.[23] The intermetatarsal angle is corrected by the pull of the adductor hallucis tendon on the lateral base of the proximal phalanx. When fused to the first metatarsal, this pulls the first-second intermetatarsal angle into a more reduced position. A similar study of patients with severe hallux valgus deformity treated with first MTP fusion alone found acceptable correction of the intermetatarsal angle.[24]

The outcomes of the surgical treatment of hallux valgus should be assessed using validated functional outcome tools. The Foot and Ankle Outcome Score was validated in patients with hallux valgus.[25] Research examining pain relief after hallux valgus surgery suggests that pain continues to diminish for up to 18 months, with most patients being pain free by 2 years after surgery.[26]

HALLUX VARUS

Hallux varus occurs when the great toe is aligned in varus relative to the first metatarsal (**Figure 5**). Mild hallux varus is usually well tolerated and can be managed nonsurgically. More severe deformities may require surgical intervention with soft-tissue procedures and occasionally bony correction.

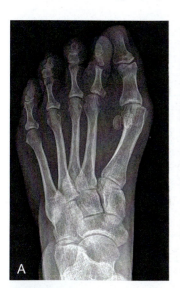
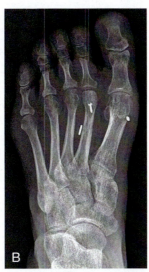

FIGURE 4 Preoperative (**A**) and postoperative (**B**) weight-bearing AP radiographs show hallux valgus deformity corrected with a suture suspensory device and second metatarsal shortening osteotomy.

Section 4: The Forefoot

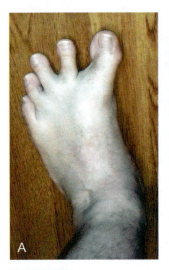
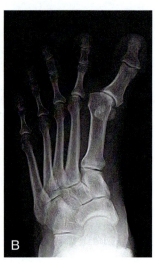

FIGURE 5 Clinical photograph (**A**) and weight-bearing AP radiograph (**B**) show a posttraumatic hallux varus deformity.

Anatomy and Pathogenesis

The first MTP joint is stabilized by its bony architecture and the surrounding soft-tissue restraints (**Table 1**). The lateral capsule, the lateral ligaments, the adductor hallucis, the lateral aspect of the flexor hallucis brevis, and the fibular sesamoid are important restraints to varus deformity. Relative laxity of the lateral soft-tissue structures at the first MTP joint, compared with the medial structures, contributes to hallux varus deformity.

The most common cause of hallux varus is iatrogenic overcorrection during hallux valgus surgery. The reported incidence of hallux varus following bunion surgery is 2% to 15%.[27] Hallux varus can result from excessive release of the lateral soft-tissue structures, excision of the fibular sesamoid, excessive resection of the medial aspect of the first metatarsal head, excessive tightening of the medial capsular structures, overcorrection of the intermetatarsal angle with a metatarsal osteotomy, or malpositioning of a first MTP arthrodesis. Other etiologies for hallux varus include congenital, neurologic, posttraumatic, or idiopathic.

Diagnostic Evaluation

The evaluation of a patient with hallux varus should begin with an assessment of their symptoms. Patients often report pain with shoe wear when the medial tip of the hallux rubs against the inside of the toe box. As with hallux valgus, the clinical examination should include a standing assessment of alignment, an inspection for callosities, and a determination of the specific site of pain. The motion of the MTP and interphalangeal (IP) joints should be measured, and the flexibility of the varus deformity should be assessed.

The radiographic evaluation of the foot should include weight-bearing AP, lateral, and oblique views. These images should be studied to determine the hallux varus angle, the intermetatarsal angle, the location of the sesamoids relative to the first metatarsal head, and the extent of arthrosis at the first MTP joint (**Figure 6**).

An attempt should be made to understand the cause of the deformity. A review of specific features of any earlier procedures may clarify the underlying cause of the deformity. Scars from any previous hallux valgus surgery should be taken into consideration if surgical reconstruction is necessary.

Nonsurgical Treatment

Nonsurgical management of a hallux varus deformity consists of patient education and shoe modifications. A shoe with a wide toe box can best accommodate the foot. The hallux sometimes can be taped or splinted to correct a supple deformity and improve symptoms. Silicone or foam toe caps can protect the hallux from rubbing inside shoes.

Surgical Treatment

Several surgical techniques have been described for management of hallux varus deformity. It is important to assess the extent of arthrosis of the first MTP joint before surgical treatment. If significant degenerative changes are

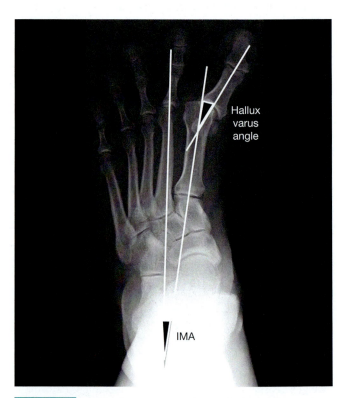

FIGURE 6 Weight-bearing AP radiograph shows the angles measured in hallux varus. IMA = intermetatarsal angle

present, the best treatment option may be arthrodesis of the first MTP joint.[28] In the absence of degenerative changes, joint-sparing realignment procedures may be considered; these include bony as well as soft-tissue procedures such as releases and tendon transfers.

Extensor hallucis longus (EHL) tendon transfer is a reliable method of correcting a flexible, nonarthritic hallux varus deformity. This technique was initially described using the entire EHL tendon. The tendon is transected distally off the dorsum of the distal phalanx, passed deep to the transverse metatarsal ligament in the first web space, and then fixed to the lateral aspect of the proximal phalanx under tension. A complete EHL tendon transfer typically is coupled with an IP joint arthrodesis,[29] which may become problematic if an MTP arthrodesis subsequently becomes necessary. A popular modification of this procedure uses a split EHL transfer that leaves one-half of the EHL tendon intact to control the IP joint and thus eliminates the need for an IP joint arthrodesis.[30]

Another soft-tissue procedure to correct hallux varus uses the extensor hallucis brevis (EHB) tendon instead of the EHL. The distal insertion of the EHB is left intact, and the proximal portion of the tendon is transected. The proximal end of the tendon is passed deep to the transverse metatarsal ligament and secured under tension to the first metatarsal head to create a static tenodesis that corrects the varus deformity. A small incision technique for both EHL and EHB tendon transfers has been described.[31] Both tendon transfer techniques require an adequate release of the contracted medial structures including the capsule and the abductor hallucis tendon.

Bony correction is often required if the hallux varus deformity resulted from excessive correction during a first metatarsal osteotomy, resulting in a narrow or negative intermetatarsal angle. A proximal metatarsal osteotomy or first TMT arthrodesis to restore a normal intermetatarsal angle is a reliable option. A reverse distal chevron osteotomy has also been described as an alternative.[32] The bony procedure is combined with distal soft-tissue realignment.

Suture suspension has also been proposed for correcting hallux varus.[33] A suture suspensory device is passed first from medial to lateral through the hallux proximal phalanx and then from lateral to medial through the first metatarsal head to replicate the path of the EHB tendon transfer. As the suture is tensioned, it becomes a static tether that corrects the varus deformity.

HALLUX RIGIDUS

The term hallux rigidus is used to describe a painful degenerative condition of the hallux MTP joint. Hallux rigidus is characterized by progressive loss of joint motion, joint space narrowing, and osteophyte formation, which lead to pain and declining physical function. The condition was first reported in 1887 as a plantar-flexed hallux at the first MTP joint with degenerative arthritis.[34]

Etiology and Pathophysiology

Hallux rigidus is thought to be incited by a traumatic event to the hallux, as in an intra-articular fracture or a turf toe injury, or by repetitive, cumulative micro-injury.[35,36] Any loading injury to the hallux can cause compression or shear forces across the joint and, in association with hyperdorsiflexion or plantar flexion, can cause acute chondral or osteochondral injury. Not all patients recall such an injury, however. In other cases, an acute injury to the hallux may uncover long-standing but previously asymptomatic degenerative changes.

In addition to trauma, several factors are thought to be related to the etiology of hallux rigidus or a predisposition to the condition. These include female sex, family history, hallux valgus interphalangeus, metatarsus adductus, and metatarsal head morphology.[36] Hallux rigidus has long been associated with metatarsus primus elevatus, although this condition was found to be a compensatory deformity often corrected by surgical management of hallux rigidus. Another study found no relationship between the two conditions.[37] No association has been found between hallux rigidus and hindfoot contracture, abnormal foot posture, first ray hypermobility, metatarsal length, or the patient's occupation or shoe wear.[36,38]

The differential diagnosis includes crystalline disorders such as gout and pseudogout, rheumatoid arthritis, other types of inflammatory arthritis, and septic arthritis. Sesamoiditis, sesamoid fracture, turf toe injury, acute isolated osteochondral injury to the hallux MTP joint, hallux varus, and hallux valgus can cause pain around the joint but typically do not lead to joint space narrowing or other radiographic signs of arthritis of the hallux MTP joint.

Physical Examination

Patients will report pain and physical limitation, though patients with mild hallux rigidus will typically only have pain during activities requiring an increase in loading of the first MTP joint. As disease progresses and there is progressive loss of joint space and motion, activities of daily living become more difficult. With dorsal osteophyte formation, painful impingement causes increasing difficulty with shoe wear.

On physical examination, patients will have pain with palpation over the MTP joint. Mild erythema may be present, although typically not the cherry-red hyperemic inflammation characteristic of an acute gout flare-up. Range of motion (ROM) restriction depends on the stage of the disease: early stages will only have pain with terminal dorsiflexion and plantar flexion, whereas later in the disease process, pain will be throughout the ROM. Pain during midrange motion or gentle loading of the MTP joint (grind test) indicates a more profound joint cartilage loss.

Radiographic Examination and Classification

Plain radiographs (AP, lateral, and oblique views of the foot) reveal joint asymmetry, joint space narrowing, sclerosis, subchondral cyst formation, osteophyte formation, and toe deviation at the MTP joint (**Figure 7**). The oblique view may be helpful in assessing patients with primarily dorsal cartilage loss but retained plantar joint space. MRI or CT is rarely required for diagnosis but may be useful if the differential diagnosis is unclear. Similarly, laboratory studies or joint aspiration can be useful to rule out crystalline disorders but typically are not required unless the diagnosis of hallux rigidus is unclear.

The Coughlin grading system (**Table 3**) is commonly used to guide treatment in conjunction with clinical findings.[39] The grading system ranges from 0 to 4, with grade 4 indicating the most severe disease. The grading system includes both physical examination and radiographic findings and has historically been used to guide treatment of hallux rigidus.

Nonsurgical Treatment

The nonsurgical treatment of hallux rigidus is similar to that of other degenerative arthritides and consists of the use of NSAIDs, injections, immobilization, stiff carbon fiber inserts (Morton extension), shoewear modification, and activity modification. The decision to manage hallux rigidus nonsurgically depends mainly on the patient's symptoms, limitations, and activity level because radiographic grade has been shown to correlate poorly with symptoms.[40]

Nonsurgical treatment has been found to be effective. At a mean 14.4-year follow-up of nonsurgical treatment in 22 patients (24 feet), patients agreed with the earlier decision not to have surgery for 18 of the feet (75%), despite an overall lack of symptom improvement and worsening radiographic findings.[41]

Intra-articular cortisone can be used, but there are concerns of both safety and efficacy of the injection. Given the small space in the MTP joint, imaging should be used to guide the injection. Furthermore, cortisone may have adverse effects on the soft tissues (thinning and impaired wound healing), which should be considered if surgical intervention is being considered. In one series, intra-articular steroid injection into the MTP joint and gentle joint manipulation led to clinical improvement of 6 months' duration in patients with mild to moderate

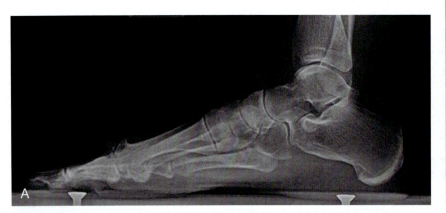
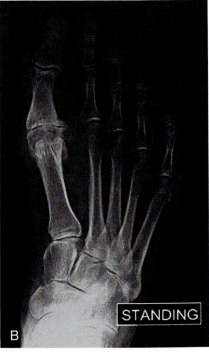

FIGURE 7 Weight-bearing lateral (**A**) and AP (**B**) foot radiographs showing grade 3 hallux rigidus.

Table 3

Coughlin Classification of Hallux Rigidus

Grade	Examination Findings	Radiographic Findings
0	Stiffness of the first MTP joint	Normal
1	Mild pain at the extremes of ROM Mild loss of ROM	Small dorsal osteophyte Normal to minimal joint space narrowing
2	Moderate pain with ROM Consistent pain	Moderate dorsal osteophyte <50% joint space narrowing
3	Significant stiffness Pain at extremes of ROM No pain with midrange motion	Severe dorsal osteophyte >50% joint space narrowing
4	Significant stiffness Pain at extremes of ROM Pain with midrange motion	Severe dorsal osteophyte >50% joint space narrowing

MTP = metatarsophalangeal, ROM = range of motion

hallux rigidus.[42] However, patients with severe hallux rigidus had little symptomatic relief and required surgical treatment.

Surgical Treatment

As with all arthritic conditions, the decision to undertake surgical treatment is based on the patient's symptoms, the effect of the disease on their quality of life, and their response to nonsurgical treatment. Few level I studies have compared the available surgical modalities, and a Cochrane review identified only one clinical study that met the inclusion criteria.[43] More robust randomized controlled studies are needed to determine the efficacy of interventions for the treatment of hallux rigidus. A review of evidence-based reports found that no definitive conclusions could be drawn from adequately powered studies using appropriately validated outcome measures.[44]

Available procedures are characterized as joint-modifying or joint ablation procedures.

Joint-Modifying Procedures

The joint-modifying procedures include cheilectomy, osteotomy, and MTP joint arthroscopy. Often these procedures are used in combination.

Cheilectomy

First described in 1930, cheilectomy is the most common joint-modifying procedure, which is excision of the dorsal osteophyte and the degenerative dorsal portion of the articular surface[45] (**Figure 8**). Typically, the dorsal 25% to 30% of the first metatarsal head is resected to facilitate clearance of the proximal phalanx during MTP dorsiflexion, with the goal of achieving approximately

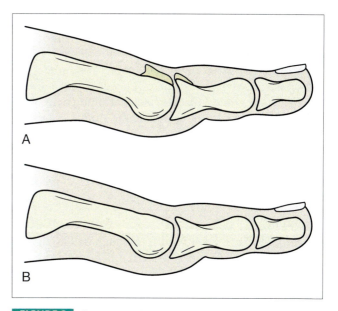

FIGURE 8 Illustration showing a cheilectomy. **A**, Dark gray areas demonstrate the planned bony areas to be resected by cheilectomy. **B**, The hallux metatarsophalangeal joint is shown after cheilectomy. (Reprinted from Seibert NR, Kadakia AR: Surgical management of hallux rigidus: Cheilectomy and osteotomy (phalanx and metatarsal). *Foot Ankle Clin* 2009;14[1]:9-22. Copyright 2009, with permission from Elsevier.)

90° of dorsiflexion intraoperatively. Cheilectomy is most effective for relieving symptoms directly over the dorsal spur and for limitations in motion from a bony block.

In general, cheilectomy has been found effective for patients with low-grade hallux rigidus. One study reported that, at a mean 56-month follow-up of 25 patients, none required additional surgical intervention after cheilectomy, and only 3 patients reported minimal discomfort.[45] In a study of 20 patients treated with isolated cheilectomy over a 6-year period, 18 (90%) reported near-complete pain relief; 16 (74%) had improvement in ROM, and 13 (68%) had more than 30° of dorsiflexion with minimal progression of the degenerative process.[46] In another clinical study, 42 patients treated with cheilectomy had subsequent improvement in ROM, return to previous level of activity, dissipation of pain (within 3 months), and a high level of satisfaction.[47]

Simple cheilectomy appears to be less effective in patients with advancing disease. A review of 58 cheilectomies in 53 patients found that 53% of patients had a satisfactory result, 19% had a satisfactory result with reservations, and 28% had an unsatisfactory result.[48] When clinical results were correlated with the radiographic grade of the joint, the researchers found an unsatisfactory result in 15% of patients with grade 1 disease, 31.8% of those with grade 2 disease, and 37.5% of those with grade 3 disease. A separate study of 52 patients who underwent a dorsal cheilectomy through a medial approach found a 90% satisfaction rate at a mean 63-month follow-up, improved patient-reported outcomes scores, and an increase in dorsiflexion ROM from 19° to 39°. None of the 82% of feet with grade 1 or 2 disease required a subsequent procedure, but most of the 18% with grade 3 disease had continuing pain, with 25% requiring arthrodesis during the study period.[49]

An isolated cheilectomy is an excellent treatment option that typically is reserved for low-grade hallux rigidus, although it appears to have some benefit in more advanced disease. Careful patient selection and preoperative counseling regarding expectations are important.

Osteotomy

Osteotomies have been used to manage hallux rigidus when joint preservation is preferred. These joint-modifying procedures include osteotomies of the proximal phalanx and distal first metatarsal. Proximal osteotomies of the first metatarsal have been described primarily for the management of metatarsus primus elevatus.

The Moberg osteotomy, a dorsiflexion osteotomy of the proximal phalanx, can be beneficial for patients with hallux rigidus (**Figure 9**). As hallux rigidus advances, dorsiflexion is limited to a greater extent than plantar flexion. The use of a dorsal closing wedge osteotomy of the proximal phalanx repositions the toe into an extended position, thus altering and improving the arc of motion. This procedure typically is performed in conjunction with cheilectomy and was first used in pediatric patients with painful hallux rigidus. The role of cheilectomy and proximal phalangeal extension osteotomy in treating advanced disease was examined in 81 patients. At a mean 4.3-year follow-up, the mean

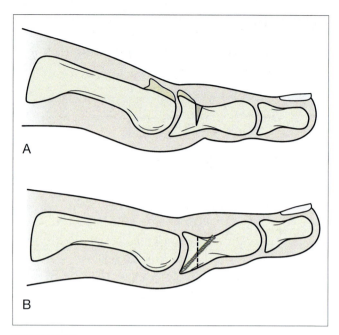

FIGURE 9 Illustration showing a Moberg osteotomy. **A**, Planned resection and osteotomies are shown. **B**, Postoperative appearance. (Reprinted from Seibert NR, Kadakia AR: Surgical management of hallux rigidus: Cheilectomy and osteotomy (phalanx and metatarsal). *Foot Ankle Clin* 2009;14[1]:9-22. Copyright 2009, with permission from Elsevier.)

dorsiflexion of the first MTP joint had improved 27°. The average American Orthopaedic Foot and Ankle Society (AOFAS) score had improved from 67.2 points to 88.7 points. Radiographs of the IP joint showed no evidence of IP joint arthritis. Sixty-nine patients (85%) were satisfied with the results of treatment; four patients (5%) subsequently underwent arthrodesis to treat persistent symptoms at the first MTP joint.[50]

The effectiveness of distal first metatarsal osteotomy has been examined for the treatment of hallux rigidus and associated conditions such as metatarsus primus elevatus.[51] These osteotomies are focused on reorientation of the proximal portion of the first MTP joint to improve the functional ROM and to treat dorsal articular wear. The goal of a dorsal closing wedge trapezoidal osteotomy of the distal metaphysis of the first metatarsal is to reorient intact articular cartilage on the plantar surface of the metatarsal head into a more functional position. A study of 42 toes with a mean 60-month follow-up demonstrated improvement in AOFAS scores from 56.4 preoperatively to 87.6 postoperatively after first metatarsal dorsiflexion osteotomy for hallux rigidus. Dorsiflexion increased from 14.8° before surgery to 35.5° after surgery. Four cases were converted to fusion.[51] Notably, it can be difficult to interpret published studies on the use of distal first metatarsal osteotomies to treat hallux rigidus for two primary reasons: the concomitant performance of cheilectomy in most patients and lack of clarity regarding whether patients' symptoms were caused by hallux rigidus, metatarsus primus elevatus, or a combination of the two conditions.

Arthroscopy

Arthroscopy for the treatment of hallux rigidus has been reported, but there are no comparative studies, and the therapeutic benefit is unclear. Arthroscopy has been used for the treatment of osteochondritis dissecans lesions of the first metatarsal head.[52] A study published in 2020 reported on the outcomes of minimally invasive cheilectomy and MTP arthroscopy in 20 patients with 16.5-month follow-up. The average visual analog scale (VAS) score improved from 7.05 preoperatively to 0.75 postoperatively, and average dorsiflexion improved from 32° to 48°. Only one patient required revision to fusion, 3 years after their index procedure.[53] The indications for arthroscopy and its effectiveness are unclear, and it is not commonly used for the management of hallux rigidus.

Joint Ablation Procedures

Joint ablation procedures include resection arthroplasty, interposition arthroplasty, allograft MTP resurfacing, hemiarthroplasty, total joint arthroplasty, and arthrodesis.

Resection and Interposition Arthroplasty

Resection arthroplasty was first reported in 1904, and it continues to be a treatment option for end-stage hallux rigidus in low-demand patients.[54] Although modifications have been made to the original procedure and interpositional techniques have been added, the basic procedure still entails resection of the base of the proximal phalanx with an associated cheilectomy and/or medial eminence resection to decompress the joint. Because of the functional sequelae and the difficulty of salvage surgery, Keller resection arthroplasty and interposition techniques are best reserved for older patients who have low physical demands.[55] Common sequelae of the Keller arthroplasty include flail hallux, cock-up or deviational deformities, hammer toes, transfer metatarsalgia, toe shortening, push-off weakness, and poor cosmesis.[56]

In a long-term study of 104 patients who underwent a Keller resection arthroplasty, 32 patients (42 feet) were available at a mean 7.6-year follow-up. Of the 32 patients, 76% were completely satisfied, 21.5% were satisfied with reservations, and 2.5% were dissatisfied. Ninety-five percent reported improvement in their symptoms, but 9.5% reported transfer metatarsalgia, and 19%, all of whom were female, were not happy with the cosmetic appearance of the foot.[57]

Modifications of the Keller procedure with interposition arthroplasty have improved the results. The modifications include oblique proximal phalangeal osteotomies to preserve the flexor hallucis brevis insertion and interposition of the EHB or another autograft or allograft material. In a series of young, active patients with end-stage hallux rigidus who underwent a Keller procedure with both cheilectomy and interposition arthroplasty, as well as a tenodesis of the EHB to the flexor hallucis brevis tendon, 94% had a good to excellent result.[58,59] At a mean 38-month follow-up after interposition arthroplasty in 18 patients, the hallux MTP joint ROM had increased a mean of 37°, most patients had substantial pain relief, and 17 patients stated they would choose to have the procedure again.[60] The researchers concluded that interposition arthroplasty was a reasonable treatment option for end-stage hallux rigidus and was associated with fewer complications than previously reported.

Bipolar Allograft MTP Resurfacing

Bipolar fresh osteochondral allograft resurfacing of the first MTP joint has been described as a means of retaining motion in cases of advanced hallux rigidus. Results are limited to small case series and no large or comparative studies have been performed to date. Allograft bipolar osteochondral MTP resurfacing was performed on six feet with a mean follow-up of 72 months. There were two failures because of infection. The remaining four feet demonstrated improvement in AOFAS scores from 27.8 preoperatively to 87.2 postoperatively; however, mild joint space narrowing between immediate postoperative and final postoperative radiographs was developed in all transplanted MTP joints.[61]

Hemiarthroplasty and Total Joint Arthroplasty

The potential benefits of prosthetic replacement include pain relief, restoration of joint motion, better function than with arthrodesis, and prevention of adjacent-joint degeneration or transfer loading. The design of prosthetic implants used to manage hallux rigidus, such as implants for total knee and hip arthroplasty, has undergone an evolution. Early implant failures and difficult salvage reconstruction after unsuccessful arthroplasty led to infrequent use of the procedure, but changes in implant design and the theoretical advantages of arthroplasty over arthrodesis have led to renewed enthusiasm. Few studies have compared the benefits of prosthetic replacement with those of arthrodesis, which has long been considered the benchmark.

The first widely used implant designs were intended to preserve length while allowing MTP joint motion through an articulation with a Silastic-based hemiarthroplasty. These designs were abandoned because of high rates of implant failure and osteolysis as well as difficulty in reconstruction. A 10% rate of implant failure was found in 66 patients and as many as one-third of patients had osteolytic changes.[62]

Subsequent implant designs used metal as a surface replacement bearing.[63] The early hemiarthroplasty designs used a cobalt-chromium alloy that allowed resurfacing of the proximal phalanx of the great toe. A study of 279 patients treated for hallux rigidus, rheumatoid arthritis, or unsuccessful bunion surgery found that 95% had a good or excellent clinical result at follow-up of as much as 33 years.[63] However, other studies had difficulty replicating these encouraging results. A comparison of the Townley hemiarthroplasty with arthrodesis concluded that arthrodesis more predictably alleviated symptoms and restored function.[64]

Resurfacing of the metatarsal rather than the proximal phalanx was introduced in 2005, using technology and an implant design similar to implants used in knee and shoulder arthritis. Early results have been promising. Thirty patients treated using the HemiCAP implant (Arthrosurface) had significant improvements in ROM, AOFAS scores, and Medical Outcomes Study 36-Item Short Form (SF-36) scores at a mean 27-month follow-up. All patients reported excellent satisfaction. Implant survivorship was 87% at 5-year follow-up.[65] In 2021, a study of the midterm results of 116 HemiCAP procedures found a survivorship of 87%, 83%, and 81% at 2, 4, and 6 years, respectively. The indication for all revisions was pain. However, patients with retained implants had less pain, increased ROM, and improved foot and ankle function compared with their preoperative scores.[66]

Polyvinyl alcohol hydrogel synthetic cartilage implants were developed for the management of osteochondral defects of the knee, talus, and first MTP joint. Proposed advantages of the implant (Cartiva) include good biocompatibility, water content, and tensile strength comparable with healthy human articular cartilage, and less wear debris than metal articulated prostheses.[67] A prospective randomized controlled trial of 205 patients randomized to either first MTP hemiarthroplasty with the Cartiva implant or first MTP arthrodesis demonstrated noninferiority of the implant at 2-year follow-up[68] (**Figure 10**). Significant improvements in VAS pain and Foot and Ankle Ability Measure scores were demonstrated for both the hemiarthroplasty and arthrodesis cohorts, with no significant difference between the two at final follow-up. Implant survivorship was 90.8% at 2 years. All failed implants were removed because of persistent pain and successfully converted to arthrodesis. There were no cases of implant wear, fragmentation, or osteolysis. The authors concluded that the Cartiva implant outcomes were equivalent to those of first MTP fusion. Five-year midterm outcomes were reported on a subset of patients from the original study and 95% survivorship in 26 patients was demonstrated. Patients demonstrated significant improvements in ROM, VAS pain, SF-36, and Foot and Ankle Ability Measure scores.[69] Potential adverse events related to Cartiva include malpositioning, loosening, implant wear or complete failure, erosion into the proximal phalanx, and continued pain and stiffness.

Modern total joint arthroplasty implant designs are typically a metal-on-polyethylene bearing and are either press fit or cemented. The available studies primarily

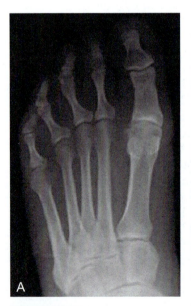
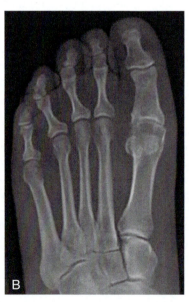
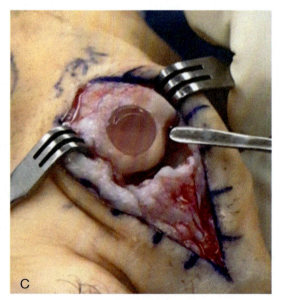

FIGURE 10 AP radiographs demonstrating an arthritic first metatarsophalangeal joint before (**A**) and after (**B**) placement of a polyvinyl alcohol hydrogel implant. **C**, Intraoperative photograph demonstrating correct positioning of the implant in the first metatarsal. (Panels B and C, Cartiva SCI, Stryker.)

focused on specific implant designs, and few comparative or prospective studies have been completed. Across most studies, long-term results continue to demonstrate superior pain and functional scores in patients who underwent arthrodesis versus arthroplasty.

Overall, published studies show that the use of prosthetic implants may be a viable option, but there are few comparative studies, and high complication rates were reported in multiple studies. As implant designs evolve and high-quality prospective randomized studies are performed, the use of prosthetic implants may appear more promising.

Arthrodesis

Arthrodesis of the first MTP joint is an effective treatment option for patients with high-grade hallux rigidus and is considered the gold standard of treatment. The primary indication for arthrodesis is end-stage arthritis in a patient in whom nonsurgical management has failed.

Although pain relief is the primary objective of arthrodesis, fusion of the first MTP joint has biomechanical and functional consequences. A gait study comparing pedobarographs before and after arthrodesis demonstrated restoration of weight bearing on the hallux and medial column; however, there were subtle changes in normal ankle kinematics (loss in the ankle plantar flexion moment and ankle power at toe-off) in compensation for the loss of first MTP motion.[70] Other studies found no observable change in the gait pattern of patients who underwent hallux MTP arthrodesis.

As with any arthrodesis procedure, patients are concerned about the effect on their ability to perform activities of daily living and participate in recreational activities after surgery. A 2019 study of return to activities after first MTP arthrodesis reported that 96% of patients were satisfied with their level of activity postoperatively, and no activities were discontinued after surgery.[71]

Typically, the hallux is fused in a functional position; the most recommended position approximates 20° of dorsiflexion in comparison with the long axis of the first metatarsal shaft and 5° to 15° of valgus positioning with neutral rotation.[72] Malpositioning of the hallux can lead to significant difficulties. Excessive dorsiflexion (**Figure 11**) can cause irritation of the tip of the hallux during shoe wear, compensatory loading of the IP joint, and transfer metatarsalgia. Excessive plantar flexion can lead to gait abnormalities because of a stiff toe-off, compensatory loading of the IP joint, and plantar distal overloading of the toe. Varus malpositioning can lead to impingement of the toe against the shoe toe box and can also accelerate IP joint arthritis. Excessive valgus position can lead to painful impingement against the second toe. Rotational

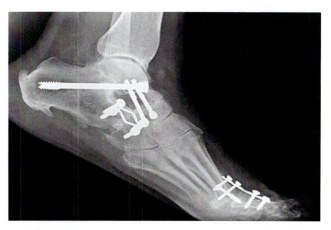

FIGURE 11 Lateral radiograph showing a malpositioned first metatarsophalangeal arthrodesis.

alignment is best evaluated by observing the position of the hallux nail bed relative to the lesser toes. A neutral alignment is preferred, although any iatrogenic rotational malpositioning in a well-positioned arthrodesis is more of a cosmetic than functional concern.

The reported means of fixation include Kirschner wires, crossed screws, staples, external fixation devices, locking and nonlocking plates, and screw constructs[73] (**Figure 12**). Evidence exists to support

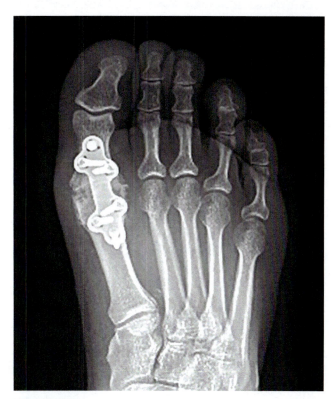

FIGURE 12 AP radiograph showing a first metatarsophalangeal arthrodesis using a locked plate-and-screw construct.

Section 4: The Forefoot

the effectiveness of each technique, and the choice often is based on surgeon preference. Regardless of fixation technique, proper positioning of the arthrodesis is paramount for restoring function and avoiding compensatory changes.

Rates of fusion after arthrodesis are reported to be 90% to 100%, with excellent overall functional outcomes. A 94% fusion rate and good or excellent results were found in all 34 patients with advanced hallux rigidus at a mean 6.7-year follow-up.[39] A 100% fusion rate was reported in 56 feet with a mean 40-month follow-up. The Foot and Ankle Outcome Survey results improved from 54.4 preoperatively to 82.6 postoperatively, and SF-36/12 scores increased from 65.7 to 81.3 after surgery. Satisfaction rate was 85%, and 81% of patients stated they would have the procedure performed again.[74]

A 2019 meta-analysis evaluating arthrodesis and implant arthroplasty found seven comparative studies that were eligible for inclusion. Overall, there was no difference between the groups regarding AOFAS–hallux MTP-IP score, patient satisfaction, revision surgery, or complication rate. However, the VAS score was lower in the arthrodesis group.[75]

SUMMARY

Hallux valgus is a common disorder that is a result of both intrinsic and extrinsic patient factors. If nonsurgical management is unsuccessful, choosing the correct surgical procedure requires a detailed physical examination and careful evaluation of the radiographs. Congruity of the first MTP joint, severity of the hallux valgus deformity, and the presence of arthritis or stiffness should be considered. Hallux varus most commonly occurs as a complication following hallux valgus surgery. If nonsurgical management is unsuccessful, it is important to understand the underlying etiology of the iatrogenic deformity when selecting a reconstruction procedure. The surgical options to realign the varus deformity include both soft-tissue and bony procedures. Hallux rigidus is a painful degenerative condition of the first MTP joint characterized by progressive loss of joint motion, joint space narrowing, and osteophyte formation. Nonsurgical modalities are tried before surgical treatment is considered. The choice of surgical option depends on the patient's symptoms, goals, and expectations. Long-term comparison studies are required to determine the optimal surgical treatment of end-stage hallux rigidus.

KEY STUDY POINTS

- Hallux valgus is caused by both intrinsic and extrinsic patient factors, and surgical decision making requires careful assessment of the deformity.
- Hallux varus is typically seen as a complication of hallux valgus surgery.
- Nonsurgical management of hallux rigidus includes activity and shoe wear modifications, carbon fiber inserts, NSAIDs, and steroid injections.
- Surgical options for hallux rigidus include cheilectomy, hemiarthroplasty, total joint arthroplasty, and arthrodesis.
- Arthrodesis remains the gold standard for end-stage disease, but midterm results of implant arthroplasty are promising.

ANNOTATED REFERENCES

1. Perera AM, Mason L, Stephens MM: The pathogenesis of hallux valgus. *J Bone Joint Surg Am* 2011;93(17): 1650-1661.

2. Nery C, Coughlin MJ, Baumfeld D, Ballerini FJ, Kobata S: Hallux valgus in males--part 1: Demographics, etiology, and comparative radiology. *Foot Ankle Int* 2013;34(5): 629-635.

3. Kim JS, Young KW: Sesamoid position in hallux valgus in relation to the coronal rotation of the first metatarsal. *Foot Ankle Clin* 2018;23(2):219-230.

4. Van Beek C, Greisberg J: Mobility of the first ray: Review article. *Foot Ankle Int* 2011;32(9):917-922.

5. Kim JY, Park JS, Hwang SK, Young KW, Sung IH: Mobility changes of the first ray after hallux valgus surgery: Clinical results after proximal metatarsal chevron osteotomy and distal soft tissue procedure. *Foot Ankle Int* 2008;29(5):468-472.

6. Dietze A, Bahlke U, Martin H, Mittlmeier T: First ray instability in hallux valgus deformity: A radiokinematic and pedobarographic analysis. *Foot Ankle Int* 2013;34(1):124-130.

7. Kimura T, Kubota M, Taguchi T, Suzuki N, Hattori A, Marumo K: Evaluation of first-ray mobility in patients with hallux valgus using weight-bearing CT and a 3-D analysis system: A comparison with normal feet. *J Bone Joint Surg Am* 2017;99(3):247-255.

8. Kimura T, Kubota M, Suzuki N, Hattori A, Marumo K: Comparison of intercuneiform 1-2 joint mobility between hallux valgus and normal feet using weightbearing computed tomography and 3-dimensional analysis. *Foot Ankle Int* 2018;39(3):355-360.

9. de Cesar Netto C, Richter M: Use of advanced weightbearing imaging in evaluation of hallux valgus. *Foot Ankle Clin* 2020;25(1):31-45.

© 2025 American Academy of Orthopaedic Surgeons

Orthopaedic Knowledge Update®: Foot and Ankle 7

This review study highlights the importance of the use of weight-bearing CT in the evaluation of patients with hallux valgus.

10. Steadman J, Barg A, Saltzman CL: First metatarsal rotation in hallux valgus deformity. *Foot Ankle Int* 2021;42(4):510-522.

    This systematic review of the literature on first metatarsal rotation in hallux valgus deformities summarizes history, current imaging methods, and surgical techniques. Level of evidence: III.

11. Hardy RH, Clapham JC: Observations on hallux valgus; based on a controlled series. *J Bone Joint Surg Br* 1951;33-B(3):376-391.

12. Okuda R, Kinoshita M, Yasuda T, Jotoku T, Kitano N, Shima H: Postoperative incomplete reduction of the sesamoids as a risk factor for recurrence of hallux valgus. *J Bone Joint Surg Am* 2009;91(7):1637-1645.

13. Park CH, Lee WC: Recurrence of hallux valgus can be predicted from immediate postoperative non-weight-bearing radiographs. *J Bone Joint Surg Am* 2017;99(14):1190-1197.

14. Park YB, Lee KB, Kim SK, Seon JK, Lee JY: Comparison of distal soft-tissue procedures combined with a distal chevron osteotomy for moderate to severe hallux valgus: First web-space versus transarticular approach. *J Bone Joint Surg Am* 2013;95(21):e158.

15. Holmes GB: Correction of hallux valgus deformity using the mini tightrope device. *Tech Foot Ankle Surg* 2008;7(1):9-16.

16. Holmes GB, Hsu AR: Correction of intermetatarsal angle in hallux valgus using small suture button device. *Foot Ankle Int* 2013;34(4):543-549.

17. Kemp TJ, Hirose CB, Coughlin MJ: Fracture of the second metatarsal following suture button fixation device in the correction of hallux valgus. *Foot Ankle Int* 2010;31(8):712-716.

18. Shurnas PS, Watson TS, Crislip TW: Proximal first metatarsal opening wedge osteotomy with a low profile plate. *Foot Ankle Int* 2009;30(9):865-872.

19. Singh D, Dudkiewicz I: Lengthening of the shortened first metatarsal after Wilson's osteotomy for hallux valgus. *J Bone Joint Surg Br* 2009;91(12):1583-1586.

20. Bock P, Kluger R, Kristen KH, Mittlböck M, Schuh R, Trnka HJ: The scarf osteotomy with minimally invasive lateral release for treatment of hallux valgus deformity: Intermediate and long-term results. *J Bone Joint Surg Am* 2015;97(15):1238-1245.

21. DeVries JG, Granata JD, Hyer CF: Fixation of first tarsometatarsal arthrodesis: A retrospective comparative cohort of two techniques. *Foot Ankle Int* 2011;32(2):158-162.

22. Hunt KJ, Barr CR, Lindsey DP, Chou LB: Locked versus nonlocked plate fixation for first metatarsophalangeal arthrodesis: A biomechanical investigation. *Foot Ankle Int* 2012;33(11):984-990.

23. Pydah SK, Toh EM, Sirikonda SP, Walker CR: Intermetatarsal angular change following fusion of the first metatarsophalangeal joint. *Foot Ankle Int* 2009;30(5):415-418.

24. McKean RM, Bergin PF, Watson G, Mehta SK, Tarquinio TA: Radiographic evaluation of intermetatarsal angle correction following first MTP joint arthrodesis for severe hallux valgus. *Foot Ankle Int* 2016;37(11):1183-1186.

25. Chen L, Lyman S, Do H, et al: Validation of foot and ankle outcome score for hallux valgus. *Foot Ankle Int* 2012;33(12):1145-1155.

26. Chen JY, Ang BF, Jiang L, Yeo NE, Koo K, Singh Rikhraj I: Pain resolution after hallux valgus surgery. *Foot Ankle Int* 2016;37(10):1071-1075.

27. Devos Bevernage B, Leemrijse T: Hallux varus: Classification and treatment. *Foot Ankle Clin* 2009;14(1):51-65.

28. Geaney LE, Myerson MS: Radiographic results after hallux metatarsophalangeal joint arthrodesis for hallux varus. *Foot Ankle Int* 2015;36(4):391-394.

29. Johnson KA, Spiegl PV: Extensor hallucis longus transfer for hallux varus deformity. *J Bone Joint Surg Am* 1984;66(5):681-686.

30. Lau JT, Myerson MS: Modified split extensor hallucis longus tendon transfer for correction of hallux varus. *Foot Ankle Int* 2002;23(12):1138-1140.

31. Lui TH: Technique tip: Minimally invasive approach of tendon transfer for correction of hallux varus. *Foot Ankle Int* 2009;30(10):1018-1021.

32. Lee KT, Park YU, Young KW, Kim JS, Kim KC, Kim JB: Reverse distal chevron osteotomy to treat iatrogenic hallux varus after overcorrection of the intermetatarsal 1-2 angle: Technique tip. *Foot Ankle Int* 2011;32(1):89-91.

33. Pappas AJ, Anderson RB: Management of acquired hallux varus with an endobutton. *Tech Foot Ankle Surg* 2008;7(2):134-138.

34. Colley ND: Contraction of the metatarsophalangeal joint of the great toe. *Br Med J* 1887;1:728.

35. Coughlin M: Conditions of the forefoot, in DeLee J, Drez D, eds: *Orthopaedic Sports Medicine: Principles and Practice.* WB Saunders, 1994, pp 221-224.

36. Coughlin MJ, Shurnas PS: Hallux rigidus: Demographics, etiology, and radiographic assessment. *Foot Ankle Int* 2003;24(10):731-743.

37. Horton GA, Park YW, Myerson MS: Role of metatarsus primus elevatus in the pathogenesis of hallux rigidus. *Foot Ankle Int* 1999;20(12):777-780.

38. Coughlin MJ, Shurnas PJ: Soft-tissue arthroplasty for hallux rigidus. *Foot Ankle Int* 2003;24(9):661-672.

39. Coughlin MJ, Shurnas PS: Hallux rigidus. Grading and long-term results of operative treatment. *J Bone Joint Surg Am* 2003;85(11):2072-2088.

40. Nixon DC, Lorbeer KF, McCormick JJ, Klein SE, Johnson JE: Hallux rigidus grade does not correlate with foot and ankle ability measure score. *J Am Acad Orthop Surg* 2017;25(9):648-653.

41. Smith RW, Katchis SD, Ayson LC: Outcomes in hallux rigidus patients treated nonoperatively: A long-term follow-up study. *Foot Ankle Int* 2000;21(11):906-913.

42. Solan MC, Calder JD, Bendall SP: Manipulation and injection for hallux rigidus. *J Bone Joint Surg Br* 2001;83(5):706-708.

43. Zammit GV, Menz HB, Munteanu SE, Landorf KB, Gilheany MF: Interventions for treating osteoarthritis of the big toe joint. *Cochrane Database Syst Rev* 2010;9:CD007809.

44. McNeil DS, Baumhauer JF, Glazebrook MA: Evidence-based analysis of the efficacy for operative treatment of hallux rigidus. *Foot Ankle Int* 2013;34(1):15-32.

45. Mann RA, Clanton TO: Hallux rigidus: Treatment by cheilectomy. *J Bone Joint Surg Am* 1988;70(3):400-406.

46. Mann RA, Coughlin MJ, DuVries HL: Hallux rigidus: A review of the literature and a method of treatment. *Clin Orthop Relat Res* 1979;142:57-63.

47. Gould N: Hallux rigidus: Cheilotomy or implant? *Foot Ankle* 1981;1(6):315-320.

48. Hattrup SJ, Johnson KA: Subjective results of hallux rigidus following treatment with cheilectomy. *Clin Orthop Relat Res* 1988;226:182-191.

49. Easley ME, Davis WH, Anderson RB: Intermediate to long-term follow-up of medial-approach dorsal cheilectomy for hallux rigidus. *Foot Ankle Int* 1999;20(3):147-152.

50. O'Malley MJ, Basran HS, Gu Y, Sayres S, Deland JT: Treatment of advanced stages of hallux rigidus with cheilectomy and phalangeal osteotomy. *J Bone Joint Surg Am* 2013;95(7):606-610.

51. Cho BK, Park KJ, Park JK, SooHoo NF: Outcomes of the distal metatarsal dorsiflexion osteotomy for advanced hallux rigidus. *Foot Ankle Int* 2017;38(5):541-550.

52. Bartlett DH: Arthroscopic management of osteochondritis dissecans of the first metatarsal head. *Arthroscopy* 1988;4(1):51-54.

53. Glenn RL, Gonzalez TA, Peterson AB, Kaplan J: Minimally invasive dorsal cheilectomy and hallux metatarsal phalangeal joint arthroscopy for the treatment of hallux rigidus. *Foot Ankle Orthop* 2021;6(1):2473011421993103.

    This is a retrospective review of 20 patients who underwent a minimally invasive cheilectomy with MTP arthroscopy between November 2017 and July 2020. Average follow-up was 16.5 months. The average VAS score improved from 7.05 preoperatively to 0.75 postoperatively (*P* < 0.05). Average ROM in dorsiflexion increased from 32° to 48° (*P* < 0.05) and plantar flexion increased from 15° to 19° (*P* < 0.05). Only one patient underwent revision fusion 3 years after their index procedure. Level of evidence: IV.

54. Keller W: The surgical treatment of bunions and hallux valgus. *NY Med J* 1904;80:741-742.

55. Schenk S, Meizer R, Kramer R, Aigner N, Landsiedl F, Steinboeck G: Resection arthroplasty with and without capsular interposition for treatment of severe hallux rigidus. *Int Orthop* 2009;33(1):145-150.

56. Fuhrmann R, Anders J: The long-term results of resection arthroplasties of the first metatarsophalangeal joint in rheumatoid arthritis. *Int Orthop* 2001;25(5):312-316.

57. Coutts A, Kilmartin TE, Ellis MJ: The long-term patient focused outcomes of the Keller's arthroplasty for the treatment of hallux rigidus. *Foot (Edinb)* 2012;22(3):167-171.

58. Hamilton WG, O'Malley MJ, Thompson FM, Kovatis PE: Roger Mann Award 1995. Capsular interposition arthroplasty for severe hallux rigidus. *Foot Ankle Int* 1997;18(2):68-70.

59. Hamilton WG, Hubbard CE: Hallux rigidus. Excisional arthroplasty. *Foot Ankle Clin* 2000;5(3):663-671.

60. Kennedy JG, Chow FY, Dines J, Gardner M, Bohne WH: Outcomes after interposition arthroplasty for treatment of hallux rigidus. *Clin Orthop Relat Res* 2006;445:210-215.

61. Giannini S, Buda R, Ruffilli A, Pagliazzi G, Vannini F: Bipolar fresh osteochondral allograft for the treatment of hallux rigidus. *Foot Ankle Int* 2013;34(6):908-911.

62. Cracchiolo A, Weltmer JB, Lian G, Dalseth T, Dorey F: Arthroplasty of the first metatarsophalangeal joint with a double-stem silicone implant. Results in patients who have degenerative joint disease failure of previous operations, or rheumatoid arthritis. *J Bone Joint Surg Am* 1992;74(4):552-563.

63. Townley CO, Taranow WS: A metallic hemiarthroplasty resurfacing prosthesis for the hallux metatarsophalangeal joint. *Foot Ankle Int* 1994;15(11):575-580.

64. Raikin SM, Ahmad J, Pour AE, Abidi N: Comparison of arthrodesis and metallic hemiarthroplasty of the hallux metatarsophalangeal joint. *J Bone Joint Surg Am* 2007;89(9):1979-1985.

65. Kline AJ, Hasselman CT: Metatarsal head resurfacing for advanced hallux rigidus. *Foot Ankle Int* 2013;34(5):716-725.

66. Jørsboe PH, Pedersen MS, Benyahia M, Kallemose T, Penny JØ: Mid-term functionality and survival of 116 HemiCAP® implants for hallux rigidus. *J Foot Ankle Surg* 2021;60(2):322-327.

    In this retrospective review of patients who underwent a HemiCAP procedure between 2006 and 2014, 105 patients with 116 HemiCAP procedures were identified. Implant survivorship was 87%, 83%, and 81% at 2, 4, and 6 years, respectively. All revisions were performed secondary to pain. At a mean 5-year follow-up, average ROM was 45°, AOFAS score was 87.2, and VAS score was 2. Level of evidence: III.

67. Baker MI, Walsh SP, Schwartz Z, Boyan BD: A review of polyvinyl alcohol and its uses in cartilage and orthopedic applications. *J Biomed Mater Res B Appl Biomater* 2012;100(5):1451-1457.

68. Baumhauer JF, Singh D, Glazebrook M, et al: Prospective, randomized, multi-centered clinical trial assessing safety and efficacy of a synthetic cartilage implant versus first metatarsophalangeal arthrodesis in advanced hallux rigidus. *Foot Ankle Int* 2016;37(5):457-469.

69. Daniels TR, Younger AS, Penner MJ, et al: Midterm outcomes of polyvinyl alcohol hydrogel hemiarthroplasty of the first metatarsophalangeal joint in advanced hallux rigidus. *Foot Ankle Int* 2017;38(3):243-247.

70. DeFrino PF, Brodsky JW, Pollo FE, Crenshaw SJ, Beischer AD: First metatarsophalangeal arthrodesis: A clinical, pedobarographic and gait analysis study. *Foot Ankle Int* 2002;23(6):496-502.

71. Da Cunha RJ, MacMahon A, Jones MT, et al: Return to sports and physical activities after first metatarsophalangeal joint arthrodesis in young patients. *Foot Ankle Int* 2019;40(7):745-752.

    This retrospective case series focused on the return to sports and physical activity in young patients after first MTP arthrodesis. Seventy-three eligible patients between the ages of 18 and 55 years were identified and surveys were obtained from 50 patients (68%). They reported 22 different sports/activities that patients participated in. In 6 months, 44.6% of patients had returned to preoperative activities, with maximum participation of 88.6%. Ninety-six percent of patients were satisfied with their level of activity. Level of evidence: IV.

72. Harper MC: Positioning of the hallux for first metatarsophalangeal joint arthrodesis. *Foot Ankle Int* 1997;18(12):827.

73. Kelikian AS: Technical considerations in hallux metatarsalphalangeal arthrodesis. *Foot Ankle Clin* 2005;10(1):167-190.

74. DeSandis B, Pino A, Levine DS, et al: Functional outcomes following first metatarsophalangeal arthrodesis. *Foot Ankle Int* 2016;37(7):715-721.

75. Park YH, Jung JH, Kang SH, Choi GW, Kim HJ: Implant arthroplasty versus arthrodesis for the treatment of advanced hallux rigidus: A meta-analysis of comparative studies. *J Foot Ankle Surg* 2019;58(1):137-143.

    A meta-analysis of comparative studies looking at implant arthroplasty or arthrodesis for hallux rigidus identified seven eligible studies. Overall, the AOFAS–MTP-IP score, patient satisfaction rate, reoperation rate, and complication rate were similar between the groups. The VAS score for pain was significantly lower in the arthrodesis group. Level of evidence: III.

CHAPTER 13

Lesser Toe Deformities and Metatarsalgia

LAUREN E. GEANEY, MD, FAAOS

ABSTRACT

Lesser toe deformities and metatarsalgia can cause patients significant pain, difficulty with shoe wear, and functional limitations. Correctly identifying the location of the deformity or deformities and the cause of the pain, and understanding the pathophysiology are keys to guiding treatment. Treatment spans from nonsurgical modalities and shoe wear modifications to surgical options. Successful results are common in the treatment of lesser toe deformities when the correct pathology is identified. It is important to provide an in-depth review of hammer toes and the most common etiologies that can result in metatarsalgia including Freiberg disease, intractable plantar keratosis, lesser metatarsophalangeal synovitis, stress fracture, Morton (interdigital) neuroma, sesamoid pathology, transfer metatarsalgia (insufficient loading through the first ray), and equinus contracture.

Keywords: Freiberg infraction; hammer toe; metatarsalgia; Morton neuroma; sesamoiditis

Dr. Geaney or an immediate family member has received royalties from Paragon 28; serves as a paid consultant to or is an employee of Novastep, Paragon 28, Smith & Nephew, and Vilex LLC; has received research or institutional support from Arthrex, Inc.; and serves as a board member, owner, officer, or committee member of American Orthopaedic Foot and Ankle Society and Connecticut Orthopaedic Society.

INTRODUCTION

Forefoot pain related to hammer toes and metatarsalgia can have a substantial effect on a patient's daily life by causing pain with ambulation. Lesser toe deformities and metatarsalgia can be caused by trauma, intrinsic muscle imbalance, neurologic disorders, inflammatory disorders, ill-fitting shoe wear, diabetes, or deformity. Although the term metatarsalgia generally is used to describe pain in the forefoot, it is better suited to describe the location of pain rather than a specific diagnosis. There are numerous nonsurgical treatment modalities for lesser toe deformities. However, nonsurgical management will fail in some patients. There are multiple surgical options that can lead to successful restoration of toe alignment and decrease in forefoot pain. The physician must carefully consider the entire foot and ankle to appropriately diagnose and treat the patient's disease process.

MALLET TOE, HAMMER TOE, AND CLAW TOE

Pathoanatomy and Etiology

An understanding of the anatomy of the lesser toes is important to appreciate the pathologic changes that occur with deformity. The lesser toes serve to distribute pressure and balance the foot. Deformities can lead to pain, callus formation, transfer lesions, and compensatory gait changes. The deformity initially is flexible, but it may become more rigid as it progresses. The terms that are used to describe deformities of the lesser toes are often used incorrectly. This can lead to misunderstandings about the exact pathophysiology and treatment.

A mallet toe is defined as an isolated flexion deformity of the distal interphalangeal (DIP) joint. A hammer toe

This chapter is adapted from Jackson JB III, Bemenderfer TB, Ellington JK: Lesser toe deformities and Patel MS, Kadakia AR: Metatarsalgia, in Chou LB, ed: Orthopaedic Knowledge Update®: Foot and Ankle 6. American Academy of Orthopaedic Surgeons, 2020, pp 205-227.

© 2025 American Academy of Orthopaedic Surgeons

is a flexion deformity of the proximal interphalangeal (PIP) joint, with or without DIP joint involvement. A claw toe deformity is an extension of the metatarsophalangeal (MTP) joint with flexion of the PIP and DIP joints. Claw toes often are frequently associated with neuromuscular conditions and typically involve multiple lesser toes and both feet. A hammer toe, however, can occur in isolation; the second toe is most commonly affected.[1]

The static stabilizers of the lesser toes include the plantar plate, joint capsule, plantar aponeurosis, and the proper and accessory collateral ligaments. The dynamic stabilizers include the extrinsic muscles (extensor digitorum longus and flexor digitorum longus [FDL]) and the intrinsic muscles (extensor digitorum brevis and flexor digitorum brevis, lumbricals, and interossei). The FDL tendon inserts on the distal phalanx and flexes the DIP joint. The flexor digitorum brevis tendon inserts on the middle phalanx and flexes the PIP joint. Because there is no direct flexor insertion on the proximal phalanx, the MTP joint in the extended position lacks antagonists, resulting in flexion in the PIP and DIP joints. The extensor digitorum longus tendon divides into three slips over the proximal phalanx (**Figure 1**); the middle slip inserts onto the base of the middle phalanx, and the medial and lateral slips pass laterally and converge to form the terminal tendon that inserts on the base of the distal phalanx. The transverse metatarsal ligament divides the intrinsic musculature, with the interossei dorsal and the lumbricals plantar to the ligament. Both muscles are plantar to the MTP joint axis and provide flexion of the MTP joint. The intrinsic muscles pass dorsal to the PIP and DIP joint axes to extend these joints.[2] Hammer toe and claw toe deformities occur as a result of muscle imbalance, with extrinsic musculature overpowering the weaker intrinsic musculature. The simultaneous contracture of the long flexors and extensors of the toe results in the deformity seen at the PIP and DIP joints.[3]

The MTP joint often is involved in these deformities. It is stabilized by collateral ligaments and the plantar plate. The metatarsal fat pad is attached to the base of the proximal phalanx. As the deformity progresses, attenuation of the plantar plate leads to subluxation of the proximal phalanx dorsally onto the metatarsal head. When the MTP joint is dorsiflexed, the metatarsal fat pad is pulled distally, and the metatarsal head is depressed plantarly, often leading to metatarsalgia. These are often associated with chronic attenuation of the plantar plate but may also be caused by acute injuries to the plantar plate.

Clinical Evaluation

Patients commonly report pain as well as callus formation. Calluses may occur over the PIP joint at the tip of the toe or under the metatarsal head. In some cases, pain is exacerbated by shoe wear, as is common for dorsal PIP irritation. Alternatively plantar pain is often relieved by shoe wear and more pronounced while walking barefoot. In addition, the patient may have pain and callosity under the MTP joint. A standing and seated foot examination is imperative. Many deformities cannot be truly appreciated during the seated examination alone. The position of the hallux should be evaluated as a possible contributor to lesser toe deformity. A careful examination of the patient's neurovascular status is important because a neurologic condition may be the underlying etiology. If surgery is being considered, it is necessary to ensure that tissue perfusion is adequate for successful healing.

Standing Examination
- Hindfoot, midfoot alignment
- Areas of callus or ulcer
- Alignment of the hallux
- Alignment of the lesser toes and specific joint(s) that have deformity
- Ability to perform a double and single limb heel rise

Seated Examination
- Ability to passively correct deformity or deformities of the lesser toes (flexible versus rigid)
- Areas of tenderness to palpation
- Neurologic and vascular examination
- Notation of any prior surgical incisions
- Vertical drawer (Lachman) examination of the lesser toes
- Web space ulcers, lesions, or infection

The seated examination determines whether the deformity is flexible or rigid. A flexible toe deformity will be corrected when the ankle is passively placed into plantar flexion, but a rigid deformity will not be corrected. It is critical that the flexibility is assessed with the ankle in a dorsiflexed position. In this position, the FDL and flexor digitorum brevis are taut and best simulate a weight-bearing situation. The stability of the MTP joint should be tested using the vertical drawer test or Lachman test and should be compared with the opposite extremity. Pain with this examination can indicate a partial plantar plate tear, where significant subluxation or dislocation of the MTP joint can indicate a complete tear of the plantar plate. Standard weight-bearing radiographs of the foot are required to evaluate overall forefoot alignment and identify hallux valgus, metatarsus adductus, and the relative lengths of the lesser metatarsals. Severe flexion deformities of the lesser toes are readily observed on radiographs, often as a so-called gun barrel sign on the AP radiograph.

Chapter 13: Lesser Toe Deformities and Metatarsalgia

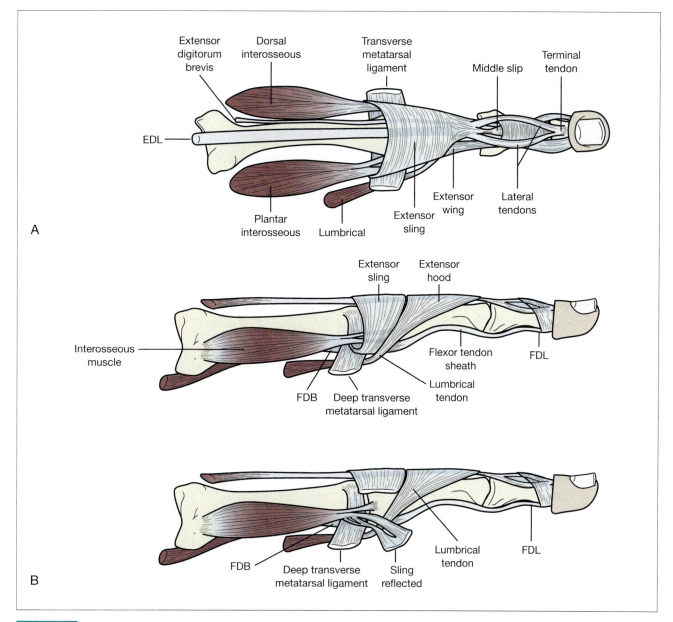

FIGURE 1 Schematics showing the anatomy of a lesser toe. **A**, The dorsal extrinsic and intrinsic musculature. The extensor digitorum longus (EDL) tendon traverses the metatarsophalangeal (MTP) joint dorsally and splits into three parts. The middle slip extends the proximal interphalangeal joint. The lateral and medial slips form the terminal tendon and extend the distal interphalangeal joint (DIP). The tendon extends the MTP joint through the extensor sling, which is composed of medial and lateral fibroaponeurotic bands that originate on each side of the EDL tendon. **B**, The lateral extrinsic (top) and intrinsic (bottom) musculature. The flexor digitorum longus (FDL) tendon inserts onto the plantar base of the distal phalanx and flexes the DIP joint. The flexor digitorum brevis (FDB) tendon is split by the central FDL tendon into medial and lateral slips that insert onto the plantar base of the middle phalanx; this tendon is responsible for proximal interphalangeal joint flexion.

Nonsurgical Treatment

In most patients, the initial treatment is nonsurgical. The patient is encouraged to wear shoes with a wide and deep toe box to accommodate the deformity and alleviate impingement of the digits. Metatarsal pads placed proximal to the metatarsal heads may be used to alleviate plantar forefoot pain. High-heeled shoes can exacerbate symptoms of metatarsalgia, and patients can be counseled on this. Periodic trimming or shaving of painful calluses may be helpful. If the affected toes are flexible, taping or strapping or use of a Budin splint may improve their alignment. However, these techniques do

Section 4: The Forefoot

not provide a permanent solution. Padding painful calluses with felt or silicone gel pads, such as a toe sleeve, can relieve impingement over bony prominences, but often the padding is too cumbersome for routine use.

Surgical Treatment

Several surgical options are available to correct lesser toe deformity, including soft-tissue releases, bony procedures, and a combination of these two options. The decision to undertake surgical intervention is based on a discussion with the patient regarding pain and disability related to their deformity as well as a clear understanding of goals and expectations afterward. A thorough preoperative discussion with the patient is necessary to explain that a normally functioning toe is usually not achievable. Some stiffness and shorting of the toe or toes are expected after surgery, and the patient should be counseled about this preoperatively. A floating toe is another common complication after lesser toe deformity correction that may warrant specific preoperative discussion with the patient. Recurrent deformity, incomplete correction, or vascular injury requiring amputation can occur.[4]

Mallet Toe

A mallet toe deformity is uncommon but often causes pain and a callus at the tip of the affected toe. If the toe is flexible, the condition is easily correctable with a percutaneous flexor tenotomy at the DIP joint with or without pinning for 4 to 6 weeks afterward. If not using a pin, this procedure can be done in the office setting using a digital block. A rigid deformity requires correction of the DIP joint with a DIP arthrodesis or arthroplasty. A dorsal central longitudinal incision or a horizontal elliptical incision can be used. The elliptical incision offers the advantage of removing redundant, often callused skin. The extensor tendon, joint capsule, and collateral ligaments are released. The FDL is released through the incision. The cartilage from both sides of the joint is removed and the subchondral bone is prepared for fusion either by resection of part of the phalanx or by perforating the bone. The options for fixation range from a simple Kirschner wire (K-wire) (which may require crossing the PIP joint to obtain proximal purchase and removed 4 to 6 weeks after surgery) to an intramedullary implant or screw.[5,6]

Hammer Toe

Characterization of a hammer toe deformity as flexible or rigid is important in the surgical decision-making process. A flexible deformity is present during the standing examination but is corrected during passive manipulation of the PIP joint or with ankle plantar flexion. Conversely, a fixed deformity is not able to be passively corrected.

A flexible deformity can be surgically corrected with an FDL tendon transfer into the extensors, but a fixed deformity requires PIP arthroplasty or arthrodesis.

Many procedures have been described for correcting the PIP joint, including soft-tissue capsulotomy, tendon release or transfer, proximal phalangeal condylectomy, PIP arthroplasty, PIP arthrodesis, diaphysectomy, silicone implant, amputation, and partial proximal phalangectomy. In addition, numerous fixation techniques are available, using pins, wires, screws, bone dowels, bioabsorbable pins, digital implants, or intramedullary implants.[7-12]

For flexible deformities, a split FDL tendon transfer to the extensor hood at the proximal phalanx, also known as the Girdlestone-Taylor procedure, allows realignment with limited retention of motion.[13] This technique sometimes can be used in combination with a PIP arthroplasty or arthrodesis. The tendon transfer is used to prevent further and/or progressive dorsiflexion of the toe, which is common with hammer toe correction. The surgical technique includes exposing the FDL tendon at the plantar base of the toe. The FDL tendon is percutaneously released from the distal phalanx and delivered in the plantar proximal wound. The tendon is split longitudinally, and its lateral and medial slips are passed dorsally around the base of the proximal phalanx. Care must be taken to ensure that the transfer is deep to the neurovascular bundle but superficial to the extensor hood. A dorsal incision is made, and the limbs of the FDL are sutured to the extensor hood and each other, with the toe in slight plantar flexion to obtain the correct tension.

Fixed deformities require bone removal to obtain correction. A PIP arthroplasty or arthrodesis can be performed with a dorsal longitudinal incision or a horizontal (elliptical) incision centered over the PIP joint. In resection arthroplasty, half of the joint is removed to allow postoperative motion; in arthrodesis, both ends of the joint are removed to achieve fusion[5-9,11,12] (**Figure 2**). The extensor hood is split longitudinally and then removed. Next, the distal condyle of the proximal phalanx is resected at the proximal margin of the articular cartilage with a microsagittal saw or bone cutter perpendicular to the shaft and parallel to the joint. Finally, if the toe is being fused, the base of the middle phalanx is denuded of articular cartilage with a rongeur or a microsagittal saw cut perpendicular to the shaft and parallel to the joint at the margin of the articular cartilage and the bone.

After joint preparation, the PIP joint is stabilized. Most commonly, a K-wire is driven anterograde out through the tip of the toe, then retrograde across the PIP joint (**Figure 3**). The use of a K-wire has the potential risk of breakage, migration, accidental removal, or infection associated with the exposed wire.[14,15] Studies

206 © 2025 American Academy of Orthopaedic Surgeons

Orthopaedic Knowledge Update®: Foot and Ankle 7

Chapter 13: Lesser Toe Deformities and Metatarsalgia

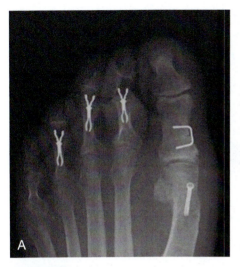 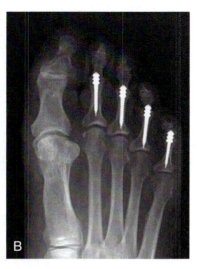 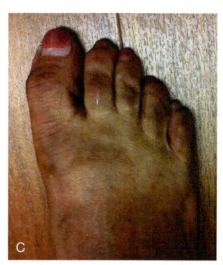

FIGURE 2 Images showing hammer toe fixation with an intramedullary proximal interphalangeal implant. **A**, AP radiograph showing the HAMMERLOCK device (DePuy Synthes, Inc. HAMMERLOCK is a trademark of DePuy Synthes, Inc.). **B**, AP radiograph showing the PRO-TOE device (Stryker). **C**, Postoperative clinical photograph of the foot shown in **B**.

show relatively good outcomes using K-wires with improvement in visual analog scale (VAS) and Short Form 36 scores between baseline and both 6 and 12 months postoperatively. Complications occurred in 10% to 13% of patients, including valgus malalignment, deep vein thrombosis, pain, and recurrence.[16] Several alternatives have been developed. These techniques use pins, wires, screws, bone dowels, bioabsorbable pins, straight or angled intramedullary devices, or digital implants.[7-12] Risks of these implants include breakage, bone destruction, incorrect placement, and increased cost. A 2020 study showed that patients with more comorbidities had a higher rate of postoperative complications.[17] A 2020 systematic review showed that although there may be a higher rate of union with intramedullary devices, there was no specific benefit to intramedullary devices over K-wires when evaluating clinical parameters.[18] Based on a 2020 study, risk factors for failure after hammer toe surgery include increased preoperative deformity, surgery on the second toe, use of a phalangeal osteotomy to correct the deformity, and use of less common surgical techniques to reduce the PIP joint. Performing surgical treatment on the first ray was protective against recurrence.[19]

Claw Toe

By definition, claw toes have pathology at the MTP joint. Correction of the PIP and/or DIP joint is done as previously described for mallet toes and hammer toes. To fully correct a claw toe, however, the MTP joint also must be corrected. A stepwise approach allows for correction of each of the pathologic structures. A longitudinal incision is made over the MTP joint. During the dissection the extensor tendons are protected. However, if there is a contracture, which is common, the tendons are either released or Z-lengthened. Next, an intraoperative examination of the MTP dorsal capsule, collateral ligaments, and/or plantar plate will determine which structures need to be released or reconstructed. A plantar plate repair has

FIGURE 3 AP radiograph showing a hammer toe fixed with a Kirschner wire.

become increasingly used with or without a metatarsal osteotomy to add static plantar stabilization.[20,21] For a crossover deformity, the extensor digitorum brevis can be cut proximally, rerouted deep to the transverse intermetatarsal ligament, and transferred as an additional static stabilizer onto the side with laxity.

Residual deformity at the MTP joint, which is not corrected by a soft-tissue release alone, may be addressed with a horizontal oblique metatarsal osteotomy (**Figure 4**). Regardless of attention to detail, the lesser toes will frequently drift upward at the MTP joint over the next several months and the resultant floating toe can be a source of cosmetic displeasure or a source of persistent pain and functional loss. Floating toes develop as a result of translating the center of rotation of the MTP plantarly as the metatarsal is shortened. As a result, the pull of the interosseous tendons translate from being plantar to the center of rotation to dorsal, causing a dorsiflexion force of the MTP joint. To help to prevent this occurrence, the MTP joint can be pinned in slight plantar flexion, or a splint/taping can be used after surgical treatment.

Plantar plate instability recently has received increased attention and is important to consider in diagnosing and treating claw toe deformity. Novel techniques and devices have been developed for use in direct anatomic repair of the plantar plate in which the plantar plate is grasped and secured to the base of the proximal phalanx through drill holes (**Figure 5**).

BUNIONETTE

A bunionette, also known as a tailor's bunion, historically is related to the lateral pressure placed on a tailor's foot while sitting and working.

Pathoanatomy and Etiology

Physiologically a bunionette is related to a prominence over the fifth metatarsal head. As the deformity progresses, the lateral structures are stretched. In severe and/or long-standing deformities, a dorsal contracture of the MTP joint and distal translation of the plantar fat pad develops, leading to pain under the fifth metatarsal head.

A bunionette is classified as type I, enlargement of the metatarsal head; type II, lateral bowing of the fifth metatarsal; type III, widening of the fourth-fifth intermetatarsal angle; or type IV, a combination of types I, II, and III.

Clinical Evaluation

When bunionettes become painful, patients present with pain and irritation of the lateral fifth metatarsal head. This is often aggravated by shoe wear and relieved when removing shoes. On physical examination, patients have

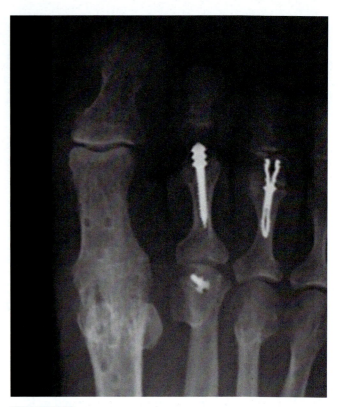

FIGURE 4 AP radiograph showing a Weil osteotomy.

pain and erythema over the lateral fifth metatarsal head. Calluses may develop either plantarly or laterally over the prominence.

Standard weight-bearing radiographs are required to evaluate a bunionette deformity. The fourth-fifth intermetatarsal angle and fifth MTP joint angle are used to measure the deformity (**Figure 6**). The average normal fourth-fifth intermetatarsal angle is 9.1°, but is 10.7° in

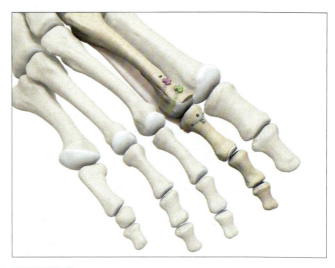

FIGURE 5 Three-dimensional drawing showing a repair of the plantar plate.

Chapter 13: Lesser Toe Deformities and Metatarsalgia

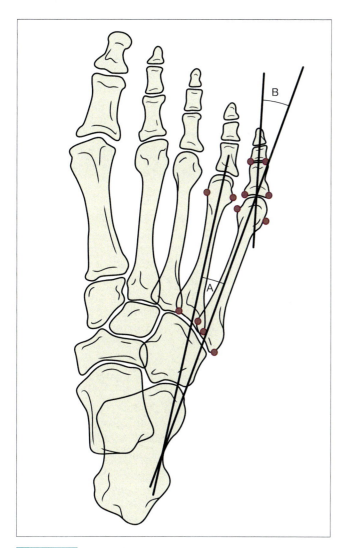

FIGURE 6 Schematic showing the use of the fourth-fifth intermetatarsal angle (**A**) and the fifth metatarsophalangeal joint angle (**B**) to measure bunionette deformity.

patients with a bunionette.[22] The average normal fifth MTP joint angle is 10.2°, but it is 16.6° in patients with a bunionette.

Nonsurgical Treatment
The nonsurgical treatment of a bunionette deformity is directed toward pain relief and includes shoe wear modification, silicone toe sleeves, and/or pads over the painful areas. Topical anti-inflammatory creams may also be applied to address the pain and bursitis.

Surgical Treatment
Surgical treatment of bunionette deformities is related to the type of deformity. In type I bunionette with an enlarged metatarsal head, a simple resection of the lateral eminence may be performed. Aggressive resection of the fifth metatarsal head can destabilize the fifth MTP joint.

Fifth metatarsal osteotomy is the preferred technique for correcting a type II or type III bunionette deformity. Many procedures have been described. A distal chevron or Weil osteotomy is commonly used for a mild to moderate deformity (**Figure 7**) and deformities related to a widened fourth-fifth intermetatarsal angle. More proximal osteotomies should be considered for patients with a type II deformity with a large 4,5 IMA. Fixation is completed with a small screw or K-wire. Fifth metatarsal osteotomy can reduce the fourth-fifth intermetatarsal angle by 2.6°, the MTP angle by 7.9°, and forefoot width by 3 mm.[23] A diaphyseal or proximal osteotomy can be used for a large deformity or after an unsuccessful distal osteotomy. However, these osteotomies are technically demanding and nonunions have been reported.[24] Resection of the fifth metatarsal head is not recommended; at long-term follow-up, recurrence, pain, fourth transfer metatarsalgia, cock-up deformity, and substantial shortening were noted.[25] More recently, percutaneous bunionette correction with or without hardware has been described with improvement in patient-reported outcomes and radiographic outcomes with minimal complications.[26,27]

METATARSALGIA

Pathoanatomy and Etiology
Freiberg Infraction
Freiberg infraction is an osteochondrosis of a lesser metatarsal head. The second metatarsal is affected in 68% of

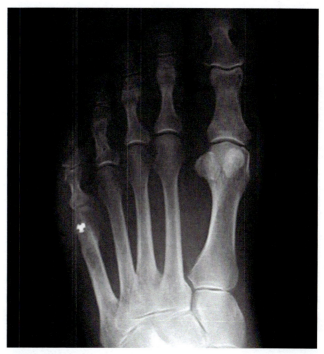

FIGURE 7 AP radiograph showing correction of a bunionette deformity using a snap-off screw osteotomy.

Section 4: The Forefoot

patients, and the third metatarsal is affected in 27%.[28] The disease most commonly affects females and is most prevalent during adolescence. Repetitive minor trauma is commonly but not universally associated with the condition. Recurrent microtrauma or overloading of the metatarsal can lead to interruption of the blood supply to the metatarsal head, with resulting ischemia, bone resorption, and collapse. The entire foot must be examined to determine the factors contributing to lesser metatarsal overload in a patient with Freiberg disease. These factors can include a gastrocnemius contracture, an unstable first ray, and relatively long lesser metatarsals.

Intractable Plantar Keratosis

An intractable plantar keratosis (IPK) is a painful callus on the plantar aspect of the foot secondary to excess pressure from the metatarsal head or sesamoid (**Figure 8**). There are two forms, which are treated differently. The discrete form of IPK affects a single metatarsal and has a keratotic core. The diffuse form of IPK appears as a thickening of the skin under an entire metatarsal head or multiple metatarsal heads, and it does not have a discrete keratotic core. In IPK primarily involving the second metatarsal, the overloading is caused by an incompetent first metatarsal and may involve first tarsometatarsal instability, hallux valgus, or an iatrogenically short first metatarsal.[29] An equinus contracture may be the sole underlying etiology if the callus is present over multiple metatarsals including the first ray. An equinus contracture can occur with both the discrete and diffuse forms and must be assessed in every patient. Alternate diagnoses include plantar warts, a foreign body reaction, and epidermal inclusion cysts.

Morton Neuroma

A Morton (interdigital) neuroma is thought to develop as an entrapment neuropathy of the digital nerve. Chronic pressure on the digital nerve as it courses beneath the transverse intermetatarsal ligament leads to perineural and endoneural fibrosis. Degeneration of the myelinated fibers is common and must be histologically verified. The anatomy of the digital nerves formerly was thought to create a predisposition to a Morton neuroma in the third web space. Branches from the lateral and medial plantar nerves enter the web spaces as common digital nerves; it was thought that both the lateral and medial plantar nerves have branches extending to the third web space, thus creating a relatively thick nerve predisposed to microtrauma. The medial communicating branch to the third web space is present in only 27% of the population, however, and if present, the common interdigital nerve is no thicker than other interdigital nerves.[30]

Wearing narrow-toed shoes or high heels may contribute to neuroma formation. Dorsiflexion of the MTP joints causes plantar flexion of the metatarsal heads, making the nerve subject to repetitive trauma through increased compression of the metatarsal heads and stretching under the intermetatarsal ligament. Extrinsic factors also can influence neuroma formation. Ganglions or synovial cysts arising from the MTP joint may cause direct pressure on the digital nerve. Degeneration of the MTP joint capsule in a patient with an inflammatory condition such as rheumatoid arthritis often causes subluxation of the joint and stretches the nerve. Similarly, hammer toes with dorsiflexion at the MTP joint can cause secondary neuritis from traction on the digital nerves. Distortion of the MTP joint also can compress the bursae surrounding the ligament, increasing pressure on the surrounding tissues.

Sesamoiditis

The sesamoids are primary load-bearing structures of the forefoot, in addition to their function in decreasing friction and increasing the mechanical advantage of the flexor hallucis brevis. The importance of these structures is underscored by their absorption of as much as 32% of the energy generated during the stance phase of sprinting.

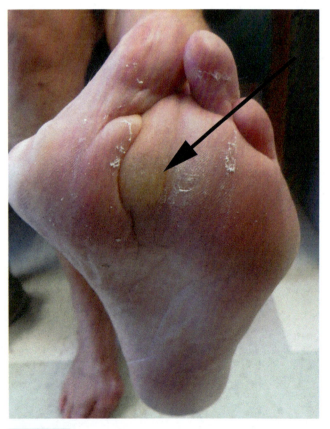

FIGURE 8 Photograph showing a discrete intractable plantar keratosis (arrow) in a patient with concomitant severe hallux valgus.

Sesamoiditis is inflammation and pain affecting the sesamoids resulting from arthrosis, osteonecrosis, acute fracture, stress fracture, or mechanical overloading. The medial (tibial) sesamoid is most commonly involved because of the increased load on the medial aspect of the foot during gait. Bipartite sesamoids occur in 10% to 30% of the population and should not be confused with acute fracture. Eighty-five percent of these individuals have bipartite sesamoids in both feet; therefore, a normal contralateral radiograph is not sufficient to determine the presence of an acute fracture. These injuries commonly occur in athletes and must be aggressively treated to prevent long-term disability. Unlike lesser metatarsal pain, which can be secondary to an unstable first ray, sesamoid pain may be associated with a plantarflexed rigid first ray (as in a cavus foot).

Transfer Metatarsalgia

Incompetence of the medial column during the load-bearing phases of gait increases stress on the lesser metatarsals.[31] This phenomenon may be a factor in Freiberg disease, IPK, and Morton neuroma as well as stress fracture, synovitis, and joint subluxation, and it must be considered in all patients with lesser metatarsalgia. Hallux valgus with associated first tarsometatarsal instability is a common cause of stress transfer. Iatrogenic shortening or elevation of the first ray also must be considered. The weight-bearing function of the medial column must be restored during an isolated lesser metatarsal correction to avoid increasing the risk of recurrent pain and deformity.

CLINICAL AND RADIOGRAPHIC EVALUATION

Clinical Evaluation

The inciting factors and the location of a patient's forefoot pain are critical for determining the underlying cause.

Weight-bearing activities, in particular those associated with running, are a common inciting factor in all forefoot pathologies. Taking a careful history of a patient's symptoms with different types of shoes can aid in diagnosing metatarsalgia. Symptoms that worsen with constrictive shoe wear are associated with Freiberg disease or a Morton neuroma. Wearing shoes with very high heels (4 inches or higher) universally exacerbates forefoot pain; patients having an underlying gastrocnemius contracture will have relief from pain in shoes with a 1- to 2-inch heel. Ambulation without shoes typically reduces pain in patients with neuroma but worsens the discomfort in patients with another etiology. The use of a cushioned insole is common but offers little relief to patients with Freiberg disease or a Morton neuroma.

The location of a patient's symptoms is the most helpful component of the history in diagnosing metatarsalgia. In Freiberg disease, the pain is limited to one lesser MTP joint but never is associated with the first or fifth metatarsal. The primary location is the dorsal aspect of the affected joint. Plantar pain directly over a callus is associated with an IPK. A callus over both the first and fifth metatarsal heads suggests a cavus foot deformity. Pain in multiple lesser metatarsals may be secondary to a Morton neuroma, transfer metatarsalgia, or gastrocnemius contracture. A history of a burning sensation, tingling, or numbness ideally should be elicited before a Morton neuroma is diagnosed. Isolated pain over the plantar aspect of the first metatarsal without an associated callus probably is secondary to sesamoid pathology. Lesser metatarsal symptoms that arise after hallux valgus correction suggest transfer metatarsalgia rather than an isolated lesser metatarsal condition.

The physical examination should begin with a standing examination of the alignment of the foot, with a focus on the medial column. A forefoot-driven cavovarus deformity (a plantarflexed first ray) will contribute to sesamoid pain and possibly to isolated discrete IPK, whereas a midfoot cavus deformity leads to a diffuse IPK. Medial column instability, as may occur in hallux valgus deformity, contributes to lesser metatarsal symptoms. Iatrogenic dorsal elevation of the medial column may be noted clinically if the condition is severe but is more easily identified radiographically. Compression during shoe wear can exacerbate neuroma symptoms in a splay foot with hallux valgus or a bunionette deformity. These associated deformities must be treated if nonsurgical or surgical treatment is to be successful.

Inspection of the soft tissues will reveal gastrocnemius contracture, transfer metatarsalgia, calluses in IPK, or swelling in Freiberg disease. The Silfverskiöld test should be used to assess for isolated contracture of the gastrocnemius in all patients. In this test, ankle dorsiflexion is assessed with the knee in full extension and in 90° of flexion (**Figure 9**). The foot must be locked in subtalar neutral position. Lack of dorsiflexion past neutral is consistent with an equinus contracture. An increase in dorsiflexion with the knee in flexion is indicative of an isolated gastrocnemius contracture.

Palpation for tenderness is useful for determining the source of the pain and narrowing the differential diagnosis. Localizing pain to the plantar metatarsal head or MTP joint versus the interspace can help differentiate pain from the MTP joint (synovitis, stress fracture, plantar plate injury) from pain from a Morton neuroma. In Freiberg disease, there is tenderness to palpation at the affected joint when a plantar-directed force is applied from the dorsal surface. Isolated dorsal-directed pressure from the plantar surface typically is painless unless the

Section 4: The Forefoot

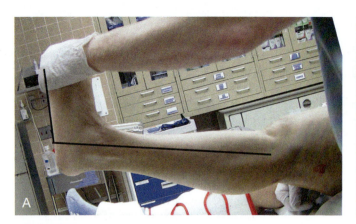 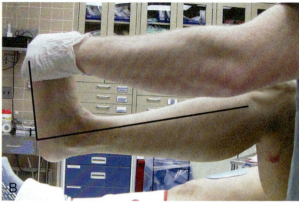

FIGURE 9 Photographs showing the Silfverskiöld test. **A**, An equinus contracture with the knee in extension denoted by the angle formed by the tibia and the plantar aspect of the foot (black lines). **B**, Dorsiflexion past neutral with 90° flexion of the knee, denoting an isolated gastrocnemius contracture.

patient has an IPK. Compression of the joint elicits pain in patients with MTP synovitis or Freiberg disease. To mitigate confounding pain from an IPK, care must be taken to avoid placing pressure on any callus during this test while compressing the joint. The presence of a palpable dorsal osteophyte allows Freiberg disease to be easily differentiated from MTP synovitis. Provocative testing for a neuroma is done by compressing the forefoot while alternating plantar and dorsal pressure at the affected web space. This test may elicit a palpable click (the Mulder click) when the nerve and bursal tissue snap between the metatarsal heads. The Mulder click without pain also may be present in patients without foot pathology, however. A positive Mulder sign requires the click to be accompanied by pain radiating into the affected toes, and it is diagnostic for interdigital neuritis. The compression should be applied proximal to the metatarsal head to avoid irritating the joint, possibly leading to a false-positive test in the setting of MTP synovitis or Freiberg infraction. The range of motion of the toe typically is normal unless the patient has Freiberg infraction, in which the range of motion gradually becomes limited, with progressive articular collapse and osteophyte formation. Absolute dorsiflexion varies, and a comparison with the contralateral foot or the unaffected lesser toes provides a reliable reference. Deformity of the phalanx, as seen with hammer toes, claw toes, or a crossover toe, requires a different treatment algorithm. The vertical drawer test is 99.8% specific and should be performed to rule out the presence of a plantar plate injury.[32] Dorsally directed pressure placed directly along the sesamoids will reproduce pain in patients with sesamoid pathology. Identification of the affected sesamoid is critical because resection of only a single sesamoid can be done without creating a cock-up toe deformity. Metatarsosesamoid pain may be relieved with plantar flexion of the first MTP joint but is exacerbated with dorsiflexion of the joint, which engages the sesamoids onto the plantar aspect of the metatarsal head.

Radiologic Evaluation

Three weight-bearing radiographic views of the foot are necessary to identify a pathologic process of the MTP joint, depression or elevation of the first metatarsal, or an abnormal relative length of the lesser metatarsals.

Common radiographic findings in Freiberg disease include resorption of the central metatarsal bone adjacent to the articular surface, flattening of the metatarsal head, and osteochondral loose bodies (**Figure 10**). In late-stage disease, joint space narrowing with osteophyte formation

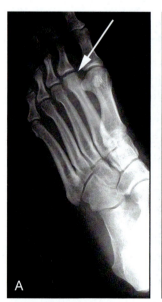 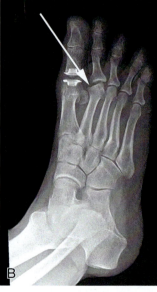

FIGURE 10 Oblique radiographs of the foot showing resorption of the central metatarsal head with resultant flattening of the articular surface (arrows). The condition is worse in **A** than in **B**. These findings are consistent with Freiberg disease.

and collapse of the articular surface can be seen (**Figure 11**). An axial view of the forefoot with dorsiflexion of the MTP joints may reveal relative prominence of the fibular condyle in patients with a discrete IPK. A non–weight-bearing medial oblique view and an axial sesamoid view are recommended for patients with suspected sesamoid pathology (**Figure 12**). Radiographs typically show no abnormality in patients with Morton neuroma, but a malunited metatarsal fracture with narrowing of the intermetatarsal space is seen in rare instances. The possibility of a shortened or elevated first metatarsal should be evaluated in all patients and specifically in patients who have had surgery. This deformity may result in transfer metatarsalgia or may be associated with Freiberg disease, and it may require correction in addition to treatment of osteonecrosis of the lesser metatarsal.

Additional imaging is not routinely required for the diagnosis of metatarsalgia. In a patient with Freiberg disease, T1-weighted MRI will show low fat saturation in the subchondral bone of the metatarsal head and T2-weighted MRI will show variable fat saturation, and flattening of the metatarsal head is seen. With eventual fragmentation of the bone, intra-articular loose bodies

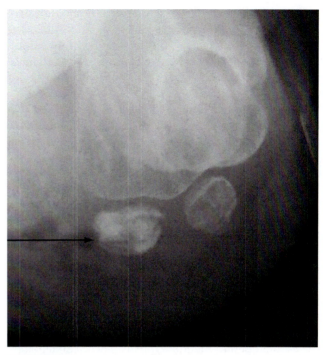

FIGURE 12 Sesamoid radiograph showing the metatarsosesamoid articulation. Sclerosis (arrow), flattening, arthritis, and fracture can be seen.

are formed. Arthritis in late-stage disease is indicated by subchondral bone marrow edema involving both the metatarsal and the phalanx (seen as high signal on T2-weighted MRI). The use of MRI in the diagnosis of Morton neuroma is controversial. Before the development of high-resolution scanners, the predictive value of MRI was low. Currently, MRI can detect aberrant pathology such as a cyst or ganglion, but its usefulness for detecting and diagnosing an interdigital neuroma remains open to debate.

Ultrasonography has high sensitivity and variable specificity in the diagnosis of a neuroma. One study found that ultrasonography accurately predicted the size and location of the neuroma in 98% of 55 neuromas, with no false-positive readings, but other studies found 95% sensitivity and only 65% specificity.[33] Routine use of ultrasonography is not required because neuroma is a clinical diagnosis.

NONSURGICAL TREATMENT

The term metatarsalgia is relevant when considering treatment to relieve a patient's pain, despite the many underlying pathologies, because several of these diagnoses can be treated similarly. The patient is instructed to cease any activities that increase the load on the forefoot, such as running, jumping, ballroom dancing, or impact sports. Nonimpact activities such as biking, elliptical

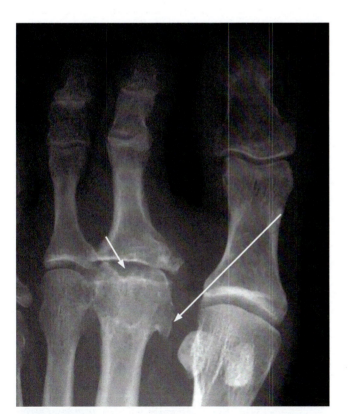

FIGURE 11 Coned-down AP radiograph of the forefoot showing the natural history and long-term sequelae of untreated Freiberg disease. The significant subchondral cysts (short arrow) and osteophyte formation (long arrow) indicate osteoarthritis.

equipment exercise, and swimming are encouraged. NSAIDs are useful for minimizing pain and inflammation but require consideration of the gastrointestinal, renal, and hepatic system complications related to long-term use. The use of narcotic pain medication is not encouraged.

Shoe wear modification and the use of orthotic devices are the mainstay treatments of the underlying conditions and the primary means of achieving long-term pain relief without medication. A stiff-soled shoe, such as a walking shoe, minimizes the force placed on the forefoot and prevents the MTP dorsiflexion that increases the stress and pain within the forefoot. For patients with lesser metatarsalgia, the use of a rigid insert that extends beneath the hallux, known as a Morton extension, can provide relief by effectively creating a stiff-soled shoe without placing extra pressure on the metatarsal heads. A Morton extension is a good alternative if the patient wants to avoid modifying shoe wear. Wearing shoes with a wide toe box is especially helpful in patients with a neuroma to minimize compressive force on the nerve in the coronal plane. Metatarsal pads placed immediately proximal to the metatarsal heads elevate the metatarsal head and thereby stabilize and offload the MTP joint. Silicone pads placed directly beneath a painful callus may decrease pain in patients with IPK. In patients with sesamoid pain, a so-called dancer's pad is an effective orthotic device. This C-shaped pad has a recess for the sesamoid that is effective at reducing the pressure and pain of sesamoid pathology. Patients with an equinus contracture may achieve pain relief by using a half-inch heel lift or shoes with a 1- to 2-inch heel. This heel height is contrary to conventional beliefs on forefoot pain but is appropriate for treating an equinus contracture. This mild heel elevation positions the ankle to allow a more functional range of motion and to minimize the effects of the equinus contracture on forefoot pressure during the stance phase of gait. Custom orthotic devices are most appropriate for patients who have had relief while using a simple over-the-counter device and want to achieve long-term nonsurgical relief. Given the cost of a custom orthotic device, it is important to determine that the patient has a reasonable chance of achieving pain relief from a mechanical alteration in foot pressure. A full-length orthotic device with recesses for the affected metatarsal heads is effective. The addition of a metatarsal bar just proximal to the lesser metatarsal heads can also effectively relieve pressure. Pain relief can also be aided by the use of a removable carbon fiber plate with the orthotic device. Although this combination is bulky, it can provide significant relief if the patient is willing to wear athletic or walking shoes. For patients with sesamoid pain, a full-length orthotic device with a built-in dancer's pad and a reverse Morton extension is effective.

Intra-articular injections can be effective but should be used with caution because they can cause further articular damage in Freiberg disease, weaken the surrounding capsular restraints, and lead to an iatrogenic crossover toe. A cortisone injection can be used as both a diagnostic and a therapeutic tool for Morton neuroma. The reported success rates of cortisone injection vary. Medium-term follow-up of a randomized controlled trial showed that at an average of 4.8 years after an injection, the original cortisone injection remained effective in 26% of patients. Eleven patients underwent a second injection and all of those patients were asymptomatic in the medium term. Overall 44% of patients ultimately underwent surgical excision.[34] A single cortisone injection is appropriate during the diagnostic workup and management of a neuroma, and it has the potential to provide long-term pain relief with a low risk of complications. However, multiple injections can lead to fat pad atrophy and soft-tissue disruption, and they should be used with caution.

Multiple ethanol injections also have been used as a surgical alternative. The basis for intralesional alcohol injection is the ability of 20% dehydrated alcohol to inhibit neuron cell function in vitro. Mechanism of action and efficacy of this agent is somewhat controversial. Given the variability in reported relief and the discomfort associated with multiple ethanol injections, these injections cannot be recommended. Other options such as radiofrequency ablation, cryoablation, and shockwave therapy have been described but a 2020 systematic review did not find enough evidence to currently support these therapies.[35]

Recently, hyaluronic acid injections have shown promising short-term results. A retrospective case study with 83 patients who received a series of three weekly ultrasound-guided injections of hyaluronic acid around the neuroma achieved significant improvement in VAS and American Orthopaedic Foot and Ankle Society (AOFAS) scores at 2 months and its effects continued until 12 months. No complications were reported.[36]

SURGICAL TREATMENT

Freiberg Infraction

Joint débridement, in which all synovitis, osteophytes, and loose bodies are débrided through a dorsal incision, should be considered for patients with early-stage Freiberg infraction after unsuccessful nonsurgical management. Candidates for simple débridement should have relatively good articular surface congruity and minimal metatarsal deformity. Many studies have reported good results after a dorsal closing-wedge metaphyseal osteotomy of the affected metatarsal in conjunction with a thorough débridement of synovitis, abnormal cartilage, osteophytes, and necrotic bone (**Figure 13**). The osteotomy serves to rotate the plantar aspect of the articular surface, which typically is well preserved, to a more superior position where it articulates with the phalanx. The metatarsal is shortened by several millimeters to help offloading. Dorsal closing-wedge metatarsal osteotomy has demonstrated improved outcome in 20 patients with a mean follow-up of 23.4 years. AOFAS score of 96.8 at final follow-up provides evidence that results can be sustained long term.[37] A 2021 systematic review of surgical interventions of Freiberg disease notes overall poor evidence in support of any one surgical intervention over another and encourages future studies.[38]

The use of an extra-articular osteotomy has been described, with recent results showing a mean improvement from 7.5 to 1 on the VAS and a 6.2° improvement in motion in 12 patients.[39] The benefit of the osteotomy was thought to derive from simple fixation with crossed K-wires that were removed 4 to 8 weeks after surgery. A concomitant débridement was performed without excision of the lesion itself. The amount of the excision was calculated before surgery based on MRI findings. The plantar cartilage was successfully rotated to the center of the joint.

Excisional arthroplasty of the metatarsal head has been used, but the results have been poorer than those of osteotomy. The results were better after interpositional arthroplasty using the extensor digitorum brevis tendon.[40] Another potential option for surgical management is osteochondral autologous transplantation. In this technique, a plug of healthy cartilage is harvested from the lateral edge of the lateral trochlea of the ipsilateral knee and transplanted into the same sized defect in the metatarsal head. A 2019 randomized controlled trial that compared this technique with a distal dorsal closing-wedge osteotomy concluded that the osteochondral autologous transplantation procedure was equivalent to the dorsal closing-wedge osteotomy.[41] Similarly, another group demonstrated the effectiveness of osteochondral autograft transplantation in 13 patients with more than 5-year follow-up. All 13 patients experienced improvement in symptoms and function. The mean AOFAS score improved from 66.9 to 93 and VAS score improved from 72.7 to 10.3. Mean dorsiflexion increased from 27.3° to 50.4°. MRI at 5-year follow-up in six patients demonstrated consolidation of the graft with smooth configuration and preservation of the transplanted cartilage.[42] Replacement arthroplasty with a silicone prosthesis should be avoided because of the risk of complications. The use of metallic and ceramic implants is being investigated, but adequate evidence is not yet available to recommend their use. Currently, the best evidence is for the use of débridement and dorsal closing-wedge osteotomy.

Intractable Plantar Keratosis

Discrete IPK resulting from a prominent metatarsal head fibular condyle is managed with a plantar condylectomy in which 20% to 30% of the plantar metatarsal head is removed (**Figure 14**). Care must be taken to avoid notching the plantar cortex by making the cut parallel to the metatarsal shaft.[43] For a discrete IPK inferior to a sesamoid, excision of the plantar 50% of the sesamoid leaving the articular surface intact can be performed to decrease the focal pressure (**Figure 15**).

The focus of treatment of diffuse IPKs should be on the overall deformity rather than narrowly on the metatarsal head. If the IPK is secondary to a relatively long metatarsal, a metatarsal shortening osteotomy can be considered. A gastrocnemius contracture may be managed with a gastrocnemius recession and can be particularly helpful in patients with more diffuse IPK. A gastrocnemius recession is a less invasive treatment than multiple metatarsal osteotomies. Any associated deformities, such as a midfoot cavus or an unstable or elevated first ray, should be managed concomitantly. A retrospective study of patients with foot pain found that the use of a gastrocnemius recession to treat isolated metatarsalgia with no other underlying deformity was successful.[44] Six of the 34 feet in this study underwent treatment for metatarsalgia; the patients had improvement on the VAS score from 7.5 to 2.2 at a mean 28-week follow-up. This improvement is encouraging but should be interpreted in the setting of the small number of patients, short follow-up time, and lack of a control group.

Morton Neuroma

Surgical excision of a Morton neuroma should be considered if nonsurgical treatment is unsuccessful (**Figure 16**). Long-term follow-up of surgical excision at 15.3 years demonstrates good to excellent results in 76.5%.[45]

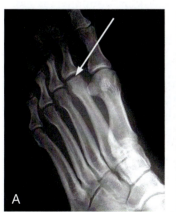
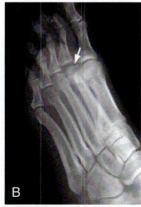

FIGURE 13 Oblique radiographs showing the characteristic flattening of the metatarsal head (long arrow) in Freiberg disease before (**A**) and after (**B**) treatment with a dorsal closing-wedge osteotomy. The contour of the metatarsal head has been re-created (short arrow).

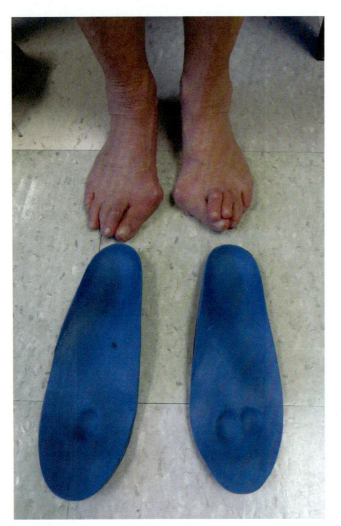

FIGURE 14 Photograph showing multiple foot deformities including hallux valgus and claw toes. Intractable plantar keratoses were diagnosed bilaterally under the second metatarsal head and on the left foot under the third metatarsal. The patient had unrelieved pain for 5 years before evaluation. The use of orthotic devices with metatarsal pads and recesses for the affected metatarsals provided significant relief and mitigated the need for surgical intervention.

Isolated release of the intermetatarsal ligament alone without nerve resection should not be done secondary to the histopathologic changes known to occur with a Morton neuroma. Release of the ligament does not correct the underlying pathologic process and therefore may not lead to pain relief. Metatarsal shortening osteotomy with release of the intermetatarsal ligament may be considered as an alternative to resection, however. In patients with two adjacent neuromas, excision of one neuroma and transection of the intermetatarsal ligament in the neighboring web space with a macroscopically normal-appearing nerve can prevent anesthesia of the middle digit. If both nerves appear thickened and abnormal, resection should be performed.

Both the dorsal and plantar approaches to resect Morton neuroma have been successful. A prospective, randomized study demonstrated 87% and 83% clinically good results using a plantar or dorsal approach, respectively, with no significant difference in regard to pain, restrictions in daily activities, and scar tenderness at 34-month follow-up.[46] Results in 125 patients were retrospectively reviewed 2 years after neuroma resection using a dorsal or plantar approach.[47] The intermetatarsal ligament was transected when the dorsal approach was used and was left intact with the plantar approach. Neuroma resection was histologically confirmed in all patients. No significant between-group difference in overall satisfaction was identified, but the patients who underwent surgery with a plantar approach had a substantially lower complication rate, less sensory loss, and a shorter recovery time. There was a 5% rate of missed neuromas with a dorsal approach and a 5% rate of hypertrophic painful scar formation with a plantar approach. Given the similar rates of patient satisfaction, the choice of a dorsal or plantar approach to treating a primary neuroma should be based on the surgeon's comfort level.

A plantar approach is preferable for revision surgery because it allows superior visualization and a more proximal resection. If a plantar approach is used, the incision should be placed off the weight-bearing bone to minimize risk for a painful plantar scar. Advanced imaging studies can be obtained before surgical intervention if the patient has undergone unsuccessful nonsurgical management or has an atypical Morton neuroma.

A 2021 prospective observational study of 44 patients treated nonsurgically and 94 patients treated surgically evaluated the patient related outcome measures after 12 months. A statistically significant improvement in the Manchester-Oxford Foot Questionnaire for pain, EuroQoL time trade-off, and EuroQol VAS was found in both groups.[48]

Sesamoiditis

A patient with sesamoiditis who has undergone unsuccessful nonsurgical management, generally for at least 6 months, may be a candidate for surgical treatment. The surgical options include tibial or fibular sesamoidectomy as well as sesamoid shaving. Removal of both tibial and fibular sesamoids is rarely indicated because it predictably leads to development of a cock-up and intrinsic-minus deformity of the hallux. After 26 tibial or fibular sesamoidectomies, all 20 patients returned to sporting activity at a mean of 12 weeks, as reported at a mean 86-month follow-up.[49] The complication rate was 19%, however, with two cases of iatrogenic hallux

Chapter 13: Lesser Toe Deformities and Metatarsalgia

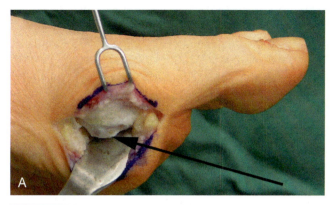
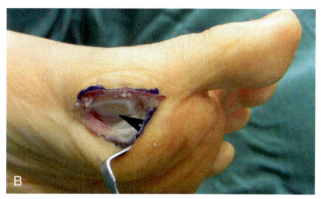

FIGURE 15 Intraoperative photographs showing a prominent tibial sesamoid (arrow) that caused a discrete intractable plantar keratosis before (**A**) and after (**B**) excision of its plantar 50%. The resultant smooth plantar surface (arrowhead) decreased plantar pressure and maintained the integrity of the flexor hallucis brevis.

valgus, one of hallux varus, and two with postoperative scarring and neuroma-type symptoms. After isolated tibial sesamoidectomy for recalcitrant sesamoid pain, 29 of the 32 patients (90%) were able to return to preoperative levels of activity and said they would choose to have the same surgery again.[50] Ten patients (30%) had extreme difficulty standing on their toes, and seven patients (21%) had transfer metatarsalgia or plantar cutaneous neuritis. It is important to be careful during the exposure to avoid damage to the plantar digital nerve and to ensure repair of the flexor hallucis brevis so as to decrease the risk of hallux varus or hallux valgus after resection of the fibular or tibial sesamoid, respectively.

Transfer Metatarsalgia

Correction of the deformity of the first metatarsal is the focus of treatment for patients with transfer metatarsalgia because first metatarsal deformity is primarily responsible for the transfer metatarsalgia. Elevation of the first metatarsal should be treated with a plantar flexion osteotomy to restore the normal weight-bearing forces. Hallux valgus and associated first ray instability are associated with weight transfer to the central metatarsals. Correction of the hallux valgus deformity alone with a first metatarsal proximal osteotomy led to resolution of lesser metatarsal plantar pain and callosity in 32 of 40 patients (80%), with no secondary surgery.[51] A Lapidus procedure with plantar flexion of the first metatarsal also is effective if the patient is known to have first tarsometatarsal instability and lesser metatarsalgia. However, the surgery will produce shortening of the medial column that may exacerbate the metatarsalgia.

Treating the excessive relative length of the lesser metatarsals using lesser metatarsal osteotomies has been found to relieve metatarsalgia, but this is commonly combined with first ray procedures when transfer metatarsalgia is suspected. In a retrospective review of propulsive metatarsalgia treated with lesser metatarsal osteotomies, 71 of the 82 patients (86%) were found to require additional surgery.[52] Most of the additional procedures were scarf osteotomies for correction of hallux valgus, and therefore it was difficult to isolate

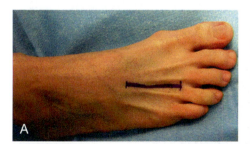
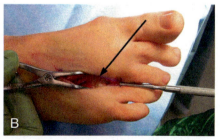
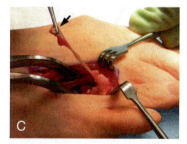

FIGURE 16 Photographs showing resection of an interdigital neuroma. **A**, The marking for a dorsal approach, showing the proximal extent of the incision required to obtain adequate exposure. **B**, Exposure of the intermetatarsal ligament (arrow) is facilitated by placing a lamina spreader between the metatarsals. **C**, The neuroma is excised from proximal (arrowhead) to distal to ensure that both branches of the nerve are excised distally.

© 2025 American Academy of Orthopaedic Surgeons · Orthopaedic Knowledge Update®: Foot and Ankle 7 · 217 the effect of the lesser metatarsal osteotomy. The patient satisfaction rate was 80% in patients treated with the Weil or triple Weil osteotomy technique, but the complication rate was relatively high. Recurrence occurred in 4.3% of patients, stiffness in 60.2%, floating toes in 4.3%, and delayed union in 7.5%. The use of a metatarsal shaft osteotomy may mitigate the complications associated with intra-articular osteotomy but requires significant soft-tissue dissection and, because of the diaphyseal nature of the osteotomy, is associated with a higher nonunion rate than distal metatarsal osteotomy. A study comparing a double and triple osteotomy recommended performing a triple osteotomy if the patient required more than or equal to 3 mm of shortening to avoid a floating toe.[53]

In patients with mechanical metatarsalgia, where bony pathology is not apparent, gastrocnemius release is an option to alleviate pain. Proximal gastrocnemius release has shown to improve VAS score from 7.4 to 3.5 and AOFAS score from 46.8 to 83.6 at 6 months. The most common complication was bruising and skin discoloration distal to the surgical site in 21 of 78 patients, which resolved spontaneously without complication.[54]

As technology advances, patients expect to be treated with newer techniques and technology with faster recovery. Minimally invasive distal metatarsal metaphyseal osteotomy for mechanical metatarsalgia is becoming more popular, but it has a steep learning curve and is associated with complications such as nonunion, malunion, transfer metatarsalgia, and soft-tissue ossification.

To correct a rarely occurring severe iatrogenic shortening of the first metatarsal, lengthening can be done with a one-stage bone block or gradually with a mini-external fixator. Long-term longitudinal studies are lacking to determine the efficacy of lengthening, but it can be considered if significant shortening of multiple lesser metatarsals would otherwise be necessary to re-create a neutral arc of the forefoot.

SUMMARY

Understanding the pathophysiology of a lesser toe deformity and metatarsalgia is important to the success of nonsurgical or surgical treatment. The patient must be thoroughly evaluated, and treatment should be tailored to the patient's deformity, comorbidities, and expectations as well as the surgeon's experience. The goals of treatment are to decrease pain, improve toe alignment and function, and increase the patient's shoe wear options. No single surgical procedure can treat all deformity and metatarsalgia, and often multiple different procedures are required.

KEY STUDY POINTS

- Nonsurgical management of hammer toes is limited to shoe wear modifications with extra-depth shoes, taping the toes, using Budin splints, or using toe sleeves or cushioning.
- Hammer toes can be successfully managed surgically with PIP arthroplasty or arthrodesis with intramedullary or K-wire fixation.
- Metatarsalgia is a general term for pain in forefoot that can be caused by direct or indirect pathology. Appropriate workup is warranted to narrow down to the correct etiology.
- The differential diagnosis of plantar forefoot pain include Freiberg infraction, Morton neuroma, intractable plantar keratosis, sesamoiditis, stress fractures, plantar plate injuries, or hammer toes.
- Current nonsurgical management of metatarsalgia is dependent on shoe wear modification, shoe orthoses/inserts, activity modification, and selective injections.

ANNOTATED REFERENCES

1. Coughlin MJ, Dorris J, Polk E: Operative repair of the fixed hammertoe deformity. *Foot Ankle Int* 2000;21(2):94-104.

2. Ellington JK: Hammertoes and clawtoes: Proximal interphalangeal joint correction. *Foot Ankle Clin* 2011;16(4):547-558.

3. Sarrafian SK, Topouzian LK: Anatomy and physiology of the extensor apparatus of the toes. *J Bone Joint Surg Am* 1969;51(4):669-679.

4. Femino JE, Mueller K: Complications of lesser toe surgery. *Clin Orthop Relat Res* 2001;391:72-88.

5. Caterini R, Farsetti P, Tarantino U, Potenza V, Ippolito E: Arthrodesis of the toe joints with an intramedullary cannulated screw for correction of hammertoe deformity. *Foot Ankle Int* 2004;25(4):256-261.

6. Coughlin MJ: Lesser toe deformities. *Orthopedics* 1987;10(1):63-75.

7. Ellington JK, Anderson RB, Davis WH, Cohen BE, Jones CP: Radiographic analysis of proximal interphalangeal joint arthrodesis with an intramedullary fusion device for lesser toe deformities. *Foot Ankle Int* 2010;31(5):372-376.

8. Chadwick C, Saxby TS: Hammertoes/clawtoes: Metatarsophalangeal joint correction. *Foot Ankle Clin* 2011;16(4):559-571.

9. Fernández CS, Wagner E, Ortiz C: Lesser toes proximal interphalangeal joint fusion in rigid claw toes. *Foot Ankle Clin* 2012;17(3):473-480.

10. Atinga M, Dodd L, Foote J, Palmer S: Prospective review of medium term outcomes following interpositional arthroplasty for hammer toe deformity correction. *Foot Ankle Surg* 2011;17(4):256-258.

11. Edwards WH, Beischer AD: Interphalangeal joint arthrodesis of the lesser toes. *Foot Ankle Clin* 2002;7(1): 43-48.

12. Schrier JC, Keijsers NL, Matricali GA, Louwerens JW, Verheyen CC: Lesser toe PIP joint resection versus PIP joint fusion: A randomized clinical trial. *Foot Ankle Int* 2016;37(6):569-575.

13. Taylor RG: The treatment of claw toes by multiple transfers of flexor into extensor tendons. *J Bone Joint Surg Br* 1951;33-B(4):539-542.

14. Kramer WC, Parman M, Marks RM: Hammertoe correction with K-wire fixation. *Foot Ankle Int* 2015;36(5):494-502.

15. Richman SH, Siqueira MB, McCullough KA, Berkowitz MJ: Correction of hammertoe deformity with novel intramedullary PIP fusion device versus K-wire fixation. *Foot Ankle Int* 2017;38(2):174-180.

16. Obrador C, Losa-Iglesias M, Becerro-de-Bengoa-Vallejo R, Kabbash CA: Comparative study of intramedullary hammertoe fixation. *Foot Ankle Int* 2018;39(4):415-425.

17. Maidman SD, Nash AE, Manz WJ, et al: Comorbidities associated with poor outcomes following operative hammertoe correction in a geriatric population. *Foot Ankle Orthop* 2020;5(4):1-6.

    This was a prospective study of 78 patients older than 60 years who underwent correction of hammer toe deformities. The authors found that patients with two or more comorbidities had an adjusted odds ratio for superficial wound infection of 4.18 and for deformity recurrence requiring surgery of 12.15. Level of evidence: III.

18. Wei RXZ, Ling SKK, Lui TH, Yung PSH: Ideal implant choice for proximal interphalangeal joint arthrodesis in hammer toe/claw toe deformity correction: A systematic review. *J Orthop Surg* 2020;28(1):1-9.

    This systematic review was designed to compare the clinical outcomes of intramedullary devices with those of K-wire devices. The authors included five level I, II, and III studies and determined that the union rate may be higher using intramedullary devices, but there was no difference in pain scores, patient satisfaction, foot-related function, or surgical complication rates. Level of evidence: II.

19. Albright RH, Hassan M, Randich J, et al: Risk factors for failure in hammertoe surgery. *Foot Ankle Int* 2020;41(5):562-571.

    This was a prospective study of 152 consecutive patients (311 toes) who underwent hammer toe correction with 6 months of follow-up. Treatment failed in 68 toes at an average of 16 months after surgery. A greater transverse plane deformity, operating on the second toe, use of a phalangeal osteotomy, and using less common surgical techniques to reduce the PIP joint were associated with a higher rate of failure. Concomitant surgery on the first ray was protective by 50%. Level of evidence: III.

20. Flint WW, Macias DM, Jastifer JR, Doty JF, Hirose CB, Coughlin MJ: Plantar plate repair for lesser metatarsophalangeal joint instability. *Foot Ankle Int* 2017;38(3):234-242.

21. Watson TS, Reid DY, Frerichs TL: Dorsal approach for plantar plate repair with Weil osteotomy: Operative technique. *Foot Ankle Int* 2014;35(7):730-739.

22. Nestor BJ, Kitaoka HB, Ilstrup DM, Berquist TH, Bergmann AD: Radiologic anatomy of the painful bunionette. *Foot Ankle* 1990;11(1):6-11.

23. Moran MM, Claridge RJ: Chevron osteotomy for bunionette. *Foot Ankle Int* 1994;15(12):684-688.

24. Lee D, Netto C, Staggers J, et al: Clinical and radiographic outcomes of the Kramer osteotomy in the treatment of bunionette deformity. *Foot Ankle Surg* 2018;24(6):530-534.

25. Kitaoka HB, Holiday AD: Metatarsal head resection for bunionette: Long-term follow-up. *Foot Ankle* 1991;11(6):345-349.

26. Nunes G, Baumfeld T, Nery C, Baumfeld D, Carvalho P, Cordier G: Percutaneous bunionette correction: Retrospective case series. *Foot Ankle Spec* 2022;15(1):36-42.

    A retrospective case series of 18 patients with 25 bunionettes treated with a percutaneous, minimally invasive technique was recently published. At an average follow-up of 15.9 months, the AOFAS score increased from 49.6 to 92.4, and the VAS decreased from 7.7 to 1.2. The fourth-fifth intermetatarsal angle decreased from 9.1° to 3.3° and the average fifth toe metatarsophalangeal angle decreased from 15° to 2.7°, which was all statistically significant. Level of evidence: III.

27. Ferreira GF, Ferreira dos Santos T, Oksman D, Filho MVP: Percutaneous oblique distal osteotomy of the fifth metatarsal for bunionette correction. *Foot Ankle Int* 2020;41(7):811-817.

    This was a prospective evaluation of 31 consecutive patients with 42 feet with bunionette deformity and underwent percutaneous distal osteotomy for correction. After an average follow-up of 13.1 months, there was a decrease in VAS score of 6.6 points and an increase in the AOFAS score of 34.9 points. The fourth-fifth intermetatarsal angle improved from 11.4° to 3.7° and the metatarsophalangeal angle increased from 16.5° to 4.8°. There were three complications including one superficial infection and two asymptomatic nonunions. Level of evidence: II.

28. Carmont MR, Rees RJ, Blundell CM: Current concepts review: Freiberg's disease. *Foot Ankle Int* 2009;30(2):167-176.

29. Lee KB, Park JK, Park YH, Seo HY, Kim MS: Prognosis of painful plantar callosity after hallux valgus correction without lesser metatarsal osteotomy. *Foot Ankle Int* 2009;30(11):1048-1052.

30. Levitsky KA, Alman BA, Jevsevar DS, Morehead J: Digital nerves of the foot: Anatomic variations and implications regarding the pathogenesis of interdigital neuroma. *Foot Ankle* 1993;14(4):208-214.

31. Dietze A, Bahlke U, Martin H, Mittlmeier T: First ray instability in hallux valgus deformity: A radiokinematic and pedobarographic analysis. *Foot Ankle Int* 2013;34(1):124-130.

32. Klein EE, Weil L Jr, Weil LS Sr, Coughlin MJ, Knight J: Clinical examination of plantar plate abnormality: A diagnostic perspective. *Foot Ankle Int* 2013;34(6):800-804.

33. Read JW, Noakes JB, Kerr D, Crichton KJ, Slater HK, Bonar F: Morton's metatarsalgia: Sonographic findings and correlated histopathology. *Foot Ankle Int* 1999;20(3):153-161.

34. Hau MYT, Thomson L, Aujla R, Madhadevan D, Bhatia M: Medium-term results of corticosteroid injections for Morton's neuroma. *Foot Ankle Int* 2021;42(4):464-468.

This was a prospective follow-up of a previous randomized controlled trial following patients an average of 4.8 years from their original corticosteroid injections. The original injection was still effective in 46% of patients. Eleven patients were reinjected and remained asymptomatic at follow-up. Forty-four percent of patients underwent surgical intervention. Level of evidence: II.

35. Thomson L, Aujla RS, Divall P, Bhatia M: Non-surgical treatments for Morton's neuroma: A systematic review. *Foot Ankle Surg* 2020;26:736-743.

This was a systematic review of nonsurgical treatment for Morton neuromas. The authors determined that corticosteroid remains the mainstay of treatment with excellent or good satisfaction overall and can be successfully performed without ultrasound guidance. They noted the potential for post-injection pain and subsequent surgical excision in patients treated with alcohol injection. Level of evidence: III.

36. Lee K, Hwang IY, Ryu CH, Lee JW, Kang SW: Ultrasound-guided hyaluronic acid injection for the management of Morton's neuroma. *Foot Ankle Int* 2018;39(2):201-204.

37. Pereira BS, Frada T, Freitas D, et al: Long-term follow-up of dorsal wedge osteotomy for pediatric Freiberg disease. *Foot Ankle Int* 2016;37(1):90-95.

38. Alhadhoud MA, Alsiri NF, Daniels TR, Glazebrook MA: Surgical interventions of Freiberg's disease: A systematic review. *Foot Ankle Surg* 2021;27:606-614.

This was a systematic review of the literature on Freiberg disease. The authors reviewed 50 articles, including two level III papers and the rest level IV to V studies and found poor evidence to support surgical intervention. They concluded that more studies of higher level of evidence should be conducted. Level of evidence: III.

39. Lee HJ, Kim JW, Min WK: Operative treatment of Freiberg disease using extra-articular dorsal closing-wedge osteotomy: Technical tip and clinical outcomes in 13 patients. *Foot Ankle Int* 2013;34(1):111-116.

40. Özkan Y, Ozturk A, Ozdemir R, Aykut S, Yalçin N: Interpositional arthroplasty with extensor digitorum brevis tendon in Freiberg's disease: A new surgical technique. *Foot Ankle Int* 2008;29(5):488-492.

41. Georgiannos D, Tsikopoulos K, Kitridis D, Givisis P, Bisbinas I: Osteotochondral autologous transplantation versus dorsal closing wedge osteotomy for the treatment of Freiberg infraction in athletes: A randomized controlled study with 3-year follow up. *Am J Sports Med* 2019;47(10):2367-2373.

In this study, 27 consecutive athletes with Freiberg infraction were randomized into a dorsal closing-wedge osteotomy or a osteochondral autologous transplantation procedure with harvest from the ipsilateral knee. At a mean follow-up of 46 months, the mean AOFAS–lesser metatarsophalangeal-interphalangeal score increased in both groups. The differences in the AOFAS–lesser metatarsophalangeal-interphalangeal scores favoring the osteochondral autologous transplantation group at 1 and 3 years reached statistical but not clinical significance. The mean VAS score improved significantly in both groups as well. Patients were able to return to full sport at 10 weeks in the osteochondral autologous transplantation group and 13 weeks in the osteotomy group. Level of evidence: II.

42. Miyamoto W, Takao M, Miki S, Kawano H: Midterm clinical results of osteochondral autograft transplantation for advanced stage Freiberg disease. *Int Orthop* 2016;40(5):959-964.

43. Mann RA, Mann JA: Keratotic disorders of the plantar skin, in Coughlin MJ, Mann RA, Saltzman CL, eds: *Surgery of the Foot and Ankle*, ed 8. Mosby Elsevier, 2007, pp 465-490.

44. Maskill JD, Bohay DR, Anderson JG: Gastrocnemius recession to treat isolated foot pain. *Foot Ankle Int* 2010;31(1):19-23.

45. Kasparek M, Schneider W: Surgical treatment of Morton's neuroma: Clinical results after open excision. *Int Orthop* 2013;37(9):1857-1861.

46. Akermark C, Crone H, Skoog A, Weidenhielm L: A prospective randomized controlled trial of plantar versus dorsal incisions for operative treatment of primary Morton's neuroma. *Foot Ankle Int* 2013;34(9):1198-1204.

47. Åkermark C, Crone H, Saartok T, Zuber Z: Plantar versus dorsal incision in the treatment of primary intermetatarsal Morton's neuroma. *Foot Ankle Int* 2008;29(2):136-141.

48. Faulkner A, Mayne A, Davies P, Ridley D, Harrold F: Patient-related outcome measures (PROMs) with nonoperative and operative management of Morton's neuroma. *Foot Ankle Int* 2021;42(2):151-156.

Patients with a new diagnosis of Morton neuroma were prospectively observed in this study. This study evaluated 44 patients treated nonsurgically and 94 patients treated surgically for the patient-related outcome measures after 12 months. The authors found a statistically significant improvement in the Manchester-Oxford Foot Questionnaire for pain, EuroQoL time trade-off, and EuroQol VAS in both groups. Level of evidence: III.

49. Saxena A, Krisdakumtorn T: Return to activity after sesamoidectomy in athletically active individuals. *Foot Ankle Int* 2003;24(5):415-419.

50. Lee S, James WC, Cohen BE, Davis WH, Anderson RB: Evaluation of hallux alignment and functional outcome after isolated tibial sesamoidectomy. *Foot Ankle Int* 2005;26(10):803-809.

51. Greisberg J, Prince D, Sperber L: First ray mobility increase in patients with metatarsalgia. *Foot Ankle Int* 2010;31(11):954-958.

52. Pérez-Muñoz I, Escobar-Antón D, Sanz-Gómez TA: The role of Weil and triple Weil osteotomies in the treatment of propulsive metatarsalgia. *Foot Ankle Int* 2012;33(6):501-506.

53. Bougiouklis D, Tyllianakis M, Deligianni D, Panagiotopoulos E: Comparison of the Weil and triple Weil osteotomies: A clinical retrospective study. *Cureus* 2022;14(2):1-15.

Seventy-one patients were retrospectively reviewed in this study. Patients who required more than 3 mm of shortening based on their parabolic curves were indicated for a triple Weil osteotomy and those with less shortening underwent a traditional Weil osteotomy. AOFAS scores and VAS scores improved in both groups. Floating toe occurred in 28.3% of patients treated with a traditional Weil osteotomy versus 6.8% in those with the triple Weil osteotomy. Level of evidence: III.

54. Morales-Muñoz P, De Los Santos Real R, Barrio Sanz P, Pérez JL, Varas Navas J, Escalera Alonso J: Proximal gastrocnemius release in the treatment of mechanical metatarsalgia. *Foot Ankle Int* 2016;37(7):782-789.

SECTION 5

Special Problems of the Foot and Ankle

Section Editor:
Sheldon S. Lin, MD, FAAOS

CHAPTER 14

Nondiabetic Foot Infections

MEGHAN KELLY, MD, PhD • A. SAMUEL FLEMISTER Jr, MD, FAAOS

ABSTRACT

Foot and ankle infections in patients who do not have diabetes are relatively uncommon. However, it is important to recognize these infections using a thorough history and physical examination, and appropriate laboratory and imaging studies, along with a high index of suspicion. In the setting of many deep infections, prompt administration of antibiotics and surgical débridement to remove infected tissue are essential. In addition, the biomechanics and weight-bearing characteristics of the foot and ankle should be considered during surgical débridement. Finally, the role of utilization of perioperative antibiotics has recently been challenged and may not be required in patients without significant risk factors.

Keywords: neuropathy; nondiabetic; osteomyelitis; surgical site infection

INTRODUCTION

Although most foot and ankle infections occur in patients with diabetic neuropathy, infections can develop in patients who do not have diabetes and often occurs in the setting of penetrating trauma, repetitive microtrauma, compromised postoperative wound, or

---

Dr. Kelly or an immediate family member serves as a board member, owner, officer, or committee member of American Academy of Orthopaedic Surgeons and American Orthopaedic Foot and Ankle Society. Dr. Flemister or an immediate family member serves as a board member, owner, officer, or committee member of American Orthopaedic Foot and Ankle Society and New York State Society of Orthopaedic Surgeons.

hematogenous spread. The results of a foot or ankle infection can be devastating, potentially resulting in limb loss or permanent dysfunction regardless of whether the patient has diabetes. Prompt diagnosis and treatment are essential to prevent significant morbidity and prolonged disability.

HISTORY AND PHYSICAL EXAMINATION

Patients with a foot or ankle infection have some combination of pain, swelling, and erythema, with or without an obvious wound. It is important to determine the duration of symptoms, the severity of pain, and the presence of constitutional symptoms such as fevers, chills, and malaise. In addition to immunodeficiency disorders, such as HIV, diseases such as chronic renal insufficiency, diabetes mellitus, inflammatory arthropathy or a history of organ transplantation can all result in a compromised immune system inhibiting the ability to fight an infection and may have atypical presentations of infection. Current tobacco use and peripheral vascular disease can negatively affect soft-tissue healing because of compromised blood flow.[1-3] Finally, it is important to determine whether the patient has a history of gout or pseudogout, as the symptoms of these conditions can mimic infection.

The physical examination begins with the patient's vital signs, including temperature, heart rate, and blood pressure. The patient's overall mental status must be assessed. Tachycardia, hypotension, fever, and altered mental status should alert the clinician to the possibility of early sepsis. The affected limb should be inspected for overall alignment, deformity, swelling, and erythema and compared with the contralateral limb.

If the limb is erythematous, it should first be elevated for 15 to 20 minutes; if the erythema persists, there is the suggestion of an infection, such as cellulitis.[4] The skin and interdigital areas of the foot must

---

© 2025 American Academy of Orthopaedic Surgeons

Orthopaedic Knowledge Update®: Foot and Ankle 7

225

be closely inspected for calluses, blisters, fissures, and open wounds. The size and depth of a wound should be assessed as well as the presence, amount, and consistency of drainage. If the wound can be probed to bone, there is a significant risk in developing osteomyelitis.[5] Exposed tendons, ligaments, and other structures should be identified. Fluctuant areas should be identified by palpation, with specific attention to gaslike crepitus, regardless of the presence of a wound. Careful inspection and palpation of the surrounding joints are essential to assessing joint range of motion and stability. Diminished range of motion or instability that compromises normal foot mechanics can lead to overloading of other areas of the foot resulting in repetitive microtrauma increasing the risk of skin breakdown. Swollen and painful joints with suspected effusion suggest septic arthritis and may require aspiration.

A thorough neurovascular examination is essential. Although diabetes mellitus is the common known cause of peripheral neuropathy in the United States, neuropathy can develop in patients without diabetes as a result of idiopathic factors or other known causes, such as alcohol abuse, chemotherapy, genetic disorders such as Charcot-Marie-Tooth, a viral infection, or a vitamin deficiency. It is essential to determine the patient's gross sensation to light touch and the ability to feel a Semmes-Weinstein 5.07 monofilament.[6] Motor function should be carefully evaluated. If pulses are not palpable, the ankle-brachial index and toe pressure should be measured. An ankle-brachial index of less than 0.45 and an absolute toe pressure of 40 mm Hg or less suggest that the patient is at risk for poor wound healing and should obtain a more extensive vascular workup.[7]

IMAGING STUDIES

Plain radiography of the foot and ankle is the primary screening tool for infection. If possible, weight-bearing studies should be obtained to best evaluate bone and joint alignment. Radiographs may show soft-tissue gas or densities representing localized edema, gas gangrene, or abscess. Furthermore, weight-bearing views can indicate altered bony alignment resulting in pressure overload on the plantar aspect of the foot that may result in wound development. Bone changes such as erosion, periosteal reaction, and frank destruction are late changes and can indicate osteomyelitis, especially with heightened clinical suspicion. However, bone erosions can also be seen in chronic rheumatologic conditions such as gout or pseudogout, highlighting the necessity of a thorough medical history and comparison radiographs, if available. In addition, it is important to note that negative plain

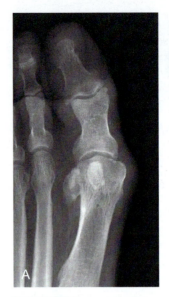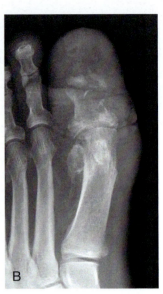

FIGURE 1 AP radiographs of the great toe showing a dorsal proximal interphalangeal ulcer in a 60-year-old patient (**A**) and destructive osteomyelitis 3 weeks later (**B**).

radiographs do not eliminate the possibility of osteomyelitis.[5] Bony change may not appear radiographically during the first 2 to 4 weeks of the acute stage of osteomyelitis (**Figure 1**).

CT is more sensitive than plain radiography for detecting early-stage bony erosion or destruction. In addition, CT can also show the presence of air in the soft tissues and the presence of an abscess and is commonly used if MRI is contraindicated. If there is a high suspicion for gout or pseudogout, a dual-energy CT can evaluate for the presence of monosodium urate and calcium phosphate crystals with high sensitivity and specificity.[8] Ultrasonography can also be useful for detecting soft-tissue abscesses and can be used for image-guided aspiration. Finally, MRI is an effective imaging study for evaluation of soft tissues, and it is the study of choice for detection of a fluid pocket such as an abscess. In addition, MRI also readily detects bone edema as evidenced by increased signal with T2 weighting and decreased signal with T1 weighting. However, it should be noted that bone marrow edema is a nonspecific finding that also is seen in fracture, tumor, Charcot arthropathy, or bony overload related to poor mechanics. The sensitivity and specificity of MRI for detecting osteomyelitis varies among studies.[5,9-12]

Nuclear imaging can provide valuable information about the presence or absence of osteomyelitis.[9,11,13] Triple-phase technetium Tc-99m bone scanning detects even subtle bony destruction, but is also positive in the setting of fracture, Charcot arthropathy, or stress reactions. The addition of an indium-111-labeled white blood cell (WBC) scan can increase the specificity and sensitivity of this testing for chronic osteomyelitis.[13]

LABORATORY STUDIES

Laboratory studies are an important adjuvant in the diagnosis and treatment of infection. A complete WBC count with differential, erythrocyte sedimentation rate (ESR), and C-reactive protein (CRP) level should be obtained.[14] In an acute infection, the WBC count is elevated accompanied by an increase in neutrophils with left shift; however, this may not be seen in patients older than 65 years or those who are immunocompromised. An elevated ESR and CRP level is often seen in the setting of an infection; however, it should be noted that they are general markers and be elevated in the setting of any inflammatory process such as rheumatologic conditions and are often elevated after surgery. An elevated ESR can persist for several weeks after surgery, whereas an elevated CRP often declines to normal levels within days. However, these markers are also useful for monitoring the patient's response to treatment because typically they return to normal with effective treatment of the infection.[14] The CRP level declines rapidly, but the ESR tends to remain somewhat elevated for several weeks, even with effective treatment.[14] Finally, the patient's nutritional status can have a substantial effect on the response to treatment. Albumin, prealbumin, and transferrin levels all are measures of the patient's nutritional status and should be obtained as part of the infection workup. A total lymphocyte count higher than 1,500 mm^3 is a useful indicator of general health. A patient found to be nutritionally depleted should take nutritional supplements.[15]

The preferred tissue for culturing contains débrided soft tissue or fluid rather than tissue from a simple wound swab because a single swab will often give confounding results because of the presence of skin flora.[16] If there is concern for a joint infection, the joint should be aspirated and the fluid sent for Gram staining and cultured for aerobic and anaerobic bacteria as well as fungi and acid-fast bacilli. In addition, it should be sent for WBC count and the presence of crystals.[3,17] A WBC count higher than 50,000 mL generally indicates an infection but may have to be repeated if this is early in onset of septic joint. An elevated WBC count can be seen in the setting of gout or pseudogout; however, Gram stain and cultures should still be evaluated as there is the possibility for a concurrent septic joint in the setting of gout. Finally, according to a 2019 study, if the patient has a total ankle arthroplasty, testing synovial fluid for alpha defensin has a high sensitivity and specificity (100%, 93.5%, respectively) for the presence of a late prosthetic joint infection.[18]

NAIL DISORDERS

Infection surrounding the toenail bed is classified as an infected ingrown nail (paronychia), felon, or onychomycosis. An ingrown toenail is caused by a deformity of the nail bed or improper trimming. The irritated surrounding soft tissues become colonized with bacteria. Numerous bacteria have been implicated in such infections, including *Staphylococcus aureus, Streptococcus,* and *Pseudomonas.*[19] Patients have a red, swollen, and draining area adjacent to the medial or lateral nail fold. Initial radiographs are taken to evaluate for osteomyelitis. In most patients, an early infection responds to local nail débridement. The use of oral antibiotics is not helpful. A resistant or recurrent infection may require partial or complete nail removal for permanent ablation.[19,20]

Felon is a deeper infection occurring in the tissue septi of the distal pulp of the toe, with *S aureus* being the most common organism. Patients have a red, swollen, fluctuant area at the distal aspect of the toe. Surgical drainage is essential, followed by culture-specific antibiotic therapy. The wound should be left open and packed as needed, depending on its size. Commonly, these infections respond to an antibiotic that covers gram-positive organisms.

Onychomycosis is one of the most common diseases of the nails. The nails become thickened, discolored, and often brittle. The pathogens most often responsible for onychomycosis are dermatophytes, including *Trichophyton rubrum* and *Trichophyton mentagrophytes.*[21] *Candida* and molds are less common causal agents. Onychomycosis can be difficult to treat and often several months of treatment are required. The systemic antifungal agents carry a risk of liver toxicity, but the use of topical medications may lead to a recurrence after discontinuance. In a healthy patient, onychomycosis rarely is more than a cosmetic concern.[21] The thickened nails may catch on clothing and occasionally cause an ingrown toenail, but frequent débridement usually is sufficient for controlling such issues.

SOFT-TISSUE INFECTIONS

Cellulitis is an infection of skin and subcutaneous tissues. One common cause is contamination of an obviously open wound or small nondetectable wounds secondary to microtrauma. The incidence of cellulitis increases with patient age, and commonly seen in patients with compromised skin from lymphedema, chronic venous stasis, chronic steroid use, or chronic edema.[22] The foot and ankle are inherently predisposed to cellulitis because of their weight-bearing position, multiple bony prominences, and shoe wear requirements, all of which increase the risk of microtrauma to the surrounding soft tissues. Cellulitis appears as erythema, swelling, increasing pain, and induration. Patients may have fever or other constitutional symptoms. Lymphadenopathy may occur proximally at the knee or groin. Initial outlining of the involved area can be helpful in guiding the treatment response. If there is a low index of suspicion for an abscess, advanced imaging, such as MRI, may not be necessary as the rate of osteomyelitis in the setting of uncomplicated cellulitis is low.[12]

Methicillin-susceptible *S aureus* and streptococci are the most common organisms responsible for cellulitis. These organisms often reside in the interdigital toe spaces.[23] Usually cellulitis will respond to oral or intravenous antibiotic therapy within the first 1 to 2 days, depending on the severity of the condition, with antibiotics effective against methicillin-susceptible *S aureus* and streptococci. The patient should be closely followed as the symptoms resolve because fluctuant areas or painful joints may become evident, indicating the concomitant presence of an abscess or septic arthritis.[24]

Necrotizing fasciitis is an aggressive, rapidly spreading soft-tissue infection that travels along fascial planes. Necrotizing fasciitis is most common in the lower extremities and often starts with a traumatic wound. The foot is particularly at risk for this type of infection. The infection often is polymicrobial, involving both gram-negative and gram-positive species as well as aerobic and anaerobic organisms.[25,26] The commonly found organisms include group A and alpha-hemolytic streptococci, *S aureus*, *Escherichia coli*, and *Pseudomonas*. Many of these organisms secrete toxins, causing septic shock followed by multiple organ failure.[25-27] Patients who are immunocompromised, such as those with diabetes mellitus, are particularly at risk.

In the early stages of necrotizing fasciitis, the patient has vague muscle joint aches and pains. The symptoms can rapidly deteriorate, however, and the patient may have signs of systemic toxicity such as hypotension.[25] The affected limb rapidly becomes swollen and erythematous. Fluid-filled bullae may be present, signs of necrosis may ensue, and sepsis may progress rapidly.[25,26] A delayed diagnosis resulting from the insidious onset of symptoms can further compromise the outcome.

Emergency surgical débridement of all necrotic tissue including subcutaneous tissues, fascia, and skin is essential to eradicate the infection.[25-27] Multiple repeat débridement is required in a temporally staged manner and ultimate amputation may be required to avoid mortality. Often, large soft-tissue defects remain that ultimately require coverage using techniques such as negative pressure wound therapy, split-thickness skin grafting, or free flap coverage after the infection has been eradicated.[25,26] Recently the use of a regenerative dermal matrix has been described to assist with soft-tissue coverage; however, additional studies are required to evaluate the long-term outcomes of this treatment.[28]

DEEP INFECTIONS

The weight-bearing nature predisposes the foot to multiple forms of trauma, such as penetrating trauma and repetitive microtrauma. A deep infection of the foot may be manifested as a plantar space abscess, osteomyelitis, or septic arthritis. Penetrating trauma is commonly caused by a puncture injury, with *S aureus*, group A streptococci, and *Pseudomonas aeruginosa* as organisms most commonly identified after such a direct inoculation.[29,30] Most wounds initially can be managed with local irrigation and débridement as well as an oral antibiotic (usually a cephalosporin). A deeper infection may appear days or weeks after the initial injury and will require a thorough surgical débridement. Care should be taken to identify and remove all foreign material.[31]

Patients with peripheral neuropathy are especially prone to wounds secondary to repetitive microtrauma. Superficial ulceration is treated with local débridement and total-contact casting, as for a patient with diabetes. A deeper ulcer with exposed tendon, bone, or joint tissue requires more extensive débridement, followed by the total-contact cast protocol.

A plantar space abscess appears as a red, warm, and swollen foot with tenderness along the plantar surface. An obvious wound or fluctuant area may not be present. In the absence of an obvious abscess location, MRI is helpful for locating the infection and outlining the extent of the process. Surgical drainage, débridement of devitalized tissue, and culture-specific antibiotic therapy are required to eradicate the infection.

Osteomyelitis can result from direct inoculation of tissues in a traumatic or surgical wound or as a result of hematogenous spread. Hematogenous osteomyelitis is common in children and adults who are immunocompromised.[32] The patient has acute pain, redness, warmth, and tenderness over the affected area. In children, metaphyseal bone is particularly prone to hematogenous spread of infection because of its highly vascularized nature.[32] MRI is helpful in determining the extent of the disease and the presence of an intramedullary abscess. The presence of a concurrent ulcer increases the likelihood of osteomyelitis in the setting of cellulitis.[12] Deep infections in children can be adequately treated with intravenous antibiotics. A bone abscess must be drained, however, and an infection that does not respond to intravenous antibiotic therapy in a timely fashion requires surgical débridement.

Osteomyelitis that appears within the first few weeks of the surgical procedure or trauma is classified as acute. Acute osteomyelitis has the classic signs of infection:

erythema, warmth, tenderness, and usually systemic signs such as fevers, chills, and malaise. In contrast, chronic osteomyelitis commonly has an indolent course characterized by persistent or intermittent drainage from a wound or sinus tract. The consistency of the drainage can be serous, serosanguineous, cloudy, or purulent, depending on the extent of the infection. To eradicate chronic osteomyelitis, removal of infected and necrotic bone is required, followed by culture-specific antibiotic therapy.[33,34] If a sinus tract is present, this should also be excised and evaluated by pathology for the presence of a Marjolin ulcer, a rare squamous cell carcinoma that can arise in the setting of an unhealed wound. As described in a 2020 study, and acute malignant transformation can occur within 12 months of trauma; however, most occur 20 to 35 years after the initial injury.[35]

Once identified, acute osteomyelitis can be treated with culture-specific intravenous antibiotics based on an accurate culture from a bone biopsy.[33] Biopsy of the bone through an open wound can lead to contamination of the specimen, and therefore it is preferable to make an incision outside the wound to perform the biopsy; this can be performed in certain settings using CT guidance.[36] Multiple small bones of the foot often are involved, and obtaining an accurate biopsy specimen can be difficult. The optimal biopsy specimens are likely to be obtained during débridement to remove necrotic bone and compromised soft tissue. As discussed in a 2020 study, it is important to discern the presence of osteomyelitis versus a soft-tissue infection as those with osteomyelitis often require additional procedures and have a higher risk of amputation.[37] Biopsy samples should be sent for both cultures and histopathology to ensure an accurate diagnosis.

Septic arthritis appears as an acute onset of pain, swelling, warmth, and erythema as well as a diminished range of motion in the affected joint. Hematogenous spread is likely to occur in children and adults who are immunocompromised. If hematogenous spread is suspected, care should be taken to closely examine the patient to identify any other source of infection or area of spread. Septic arthritis from direct inoculation of the joint most commonly occurs with a puncture wound or foot ulcer around the metatarsophalangeal joints. The signs and symptoms of septic arthritis are similar to those of a crystalline arthropathy, such as gout, or another inflammatory arthropathy. Joint aspiration is essential for an accurate diagnosis.[17] The analysis of aspirates should include WBC count, Gram staining, culturing, and the presence of crystals. A WBC count of more than 50,000/mL is suspicious but not diagnostic for infection.[3,17] If the cell count is less than 50,000/mL, the results of the Gram stain should be used to determine whether there is an early infection.[3] When a diagnosis of septic arthritis is confirmed, surgical drainage should be

done on an urgent basis. A delay in treating septic arthritis can lead to early proteoglycan loss, cartilage damage, and severe joint destruction with spread of osteomyelitis to adjacent bones.[38] Open débridement, including an aggressive synovectomy, is required for most joints of the foot. A larger joint, such as the ankle or subtalar joint, can be treated with arthroscopic débridement, depending on the surgeon's level of comfort and possibly on the extent of the infection.

SURGICAL DÉBRIDEMENT OF THE FOOT AND ANKLE

The biomechanics and weight-bearing characteristics of the foot and ankle should be considered during surgical débridement. Because the plantar surface of the foot is designed for durability, plantar incisions that compromise the plantar skin and fat should be avoided, if possible. Fortunately, most anatomic structures of the foot can be exposed through a medial, lateral, dorsal, or combined incision.

OSTEOMYELITIS OF THE HALLUX AND LESSER TOES

Osteomyelitis of the great and lesser toes is best treated with removal of all involved bone, which may involve toe amputation. The optimal débridement of a lesser toe removes all infected bone and soft tissue and leaves a stable remnant. Leaving a stable residual portion of a lesser toe after débridement or amputation may prevent migration of the adjacent toes. However, leaving a floppy residual toe after metatarsal resection can lead to the formation of new wounds and can result in difficulty with shoe wear.

In the great toe, maintaining as much length as possible allows better function than amputation through the metatarsophalangeal joint. The balance of the sesamoid mechanism and relatively normal weight bearing are best preserved when at least 1 cm of the base of the proximal phalanx is maintained.[39] If an amputation through the metatarsophalangeal joint is necessary, the remaining sesamoid bones can be resected; these bones, will have no significant function and can be a source of recurrent ulceration or discomfort.

Ray resection (amputation of the toe with all or part of the metatarsal) is required if an infection involves both the metatarsal and phalanx of the toe. Ray resection is preferred even in the absence of infection in the toe itself, if it is necessary to avoid an excessively floppy residual toe. The foot remains functional and weight bearing even after resection of the lateral two rays. However, resection of the first ray is more likely to lead to ineffective weight transfer and a less-than-functional foot. The

Section 5: Special Problems of the Foot and Ankle

loss of weight-bearing function can be overcome with offloading and an appropriately molded insole, which are preferable to transmetatarsal amputation. However, resection of three or more central rays or the first and second medial rays invariably creates an unstable, poorly functioning foot, and transmetatarsal amputation may be the preferable treatment.[39]

INFECTION OF THE MIDFOOT, HINDFOOT, OR ANKLE

Infection about the midfoot, hindfoot, or ankle often involves multiple bones and joints. Multiple aggressive débridement usually is required to eradicate such an infection. Cavitary defects typically remain, which can be temporarily filled with antibiotic-impregnated cement beads, antibiotic biodegradable carrier, or spacers.[40,41] It is critical to determine the extent of bone loss and the relative stability of the bone. External fixation often is used when eradication of the infection leads to bony instability. The use of thin wires with a circular or semicircular frame has the advantage of minimizing soft-tissue trauma. A thin-wire external fixator maintains multiplanar stability and allows earlier weight bearing than a traditional large-pin external fixator.[42-44]

After the eradication of infection, the patient may require additional procedures to treat the bone loss. As such, careful preoperative evaluation before internal fixation is done to ensure the infection is eradicated. Autogenous bone graft is used in preference to allograft.[45] The soft-tissue envelope is relatively sparse around the foot and ankle, and surgical débridement often leaves soft-tissue defects that require a local flap or soft-tissue transfer for coverage.[45] Early consultation with a plastic surgeon is recommended.

Calcaneal osteomyelitis occurs as a consequence of a posttraumatic wound, heel pressure ulcer, or postsurgical infection.[46-48] Many calcaneal infections occur with delayed wound healing. Most postoperative infections follow open reduction and internal fixation of an intraarticular calcaneal fracture.[46] Irrigation and débridement with an attempt at retaining the hardware is initially indicated. If the infection cannot be controlled or an osteomyelitis has been detected, thorough débridement of bone and removal of all infected hardware is indicated. Cavitary defects typically remain and can be filled with antibiotic-impregnated cement. Débridement often creates soft-tissue defects that require flap coverage. The use of a vacuum-assisted device can be helpful for minimizing soft-tissue defects, but early consultation with a plastic surgeon again is recommended.[49] In patients whose calcaneal infection originated in a heel pressure ulcer, the osteomyelitis initially is restricted to the tuberosity. The use of partial or total calcanectomy as a limb-salvage procedure has not been well studied in patients who do not have diabetes, but early results in patients with diabetes were promising. Some studies found poor functional results and a high reamputation rate after calcanectomy in patients with diabetes.[50-52]

Infection about the ankle most commonly occurs as a complication after treatment of a severe talus or pilon fracture with soft-tissue compromise.[44,45] Total ankle arthroplasty has been done with increasing frequency in recent years, but the incidence of infection after unsuccessful procedures also has increased.[53] A 2020 review noted that the presence of inflammatory arthritis, prior ankle surgical treatment, age younger than 65 years, hypothyroidism, body mass index less than 19 kg/m^2, peripheral vascular disease, and chronic lung disease may all predispose a patient to a periprosthetic joint infection following total ankle arthroplasty.[54] Hematogenous spread of infection can occur, leading to septic ankle arthritis and subsequent osteomyelitis, especially in patients who are immunocompromised. Initial management of infection about the ankle involves multiple débridement until all compromised bone and soft tissue have been removed. If the infection occurs during the first weeks after fracture surgical treatment, attempts can be made to retain the hardware. However, infected bone should not be left in place in an effort to retain hardware. Cavitary defects can be filled with antibiotic cement or biodegradable carrier placed as a spacer to maintain height.[40,41] External fixation usually is also required to maintain stability. After the infection has been controlled, arthrodesis is indicated to treat postseptic arthrosis or bone loss. The method of fusion varies with the amount of bone loss, the bone involved, and the surgeon's preference.

For osteomyelitis after pilon fracture, a portion of the distal tibia along the joint line usually is left intact to maintain bone length. The defects resulting from tibial bone loss most often are filled with autogenous bone graft.[45] In the setting of large segmental defects in the tibia, bone transport with the use of a thin-wire external fixator can be used with or without internal fixation once the infection is eradicated, as discussed in a 2021 study.[55]

In the presence of an infected talar fracture, resection of the entire talar body may be required, leading to substantial shortening. The surgeon may decide to perform a tibiocalcaneal arthrodesis, using either internal or external fixation; however, this procedure has variable results and often results in functional deficits and gait abnormality.[44,56] In a 2020 study, the use of either a bulk femoral head allograft or a three-dimensional printed trabecular metal graft has been suggested to maintain height[57] (**Figure 2**).

Osteomyelitis of the fibula most commonly occurs in patients with a deformity of the foot, many of whom

Chapter 14: Nondiabetic Foot Infections

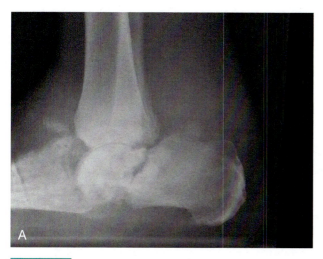
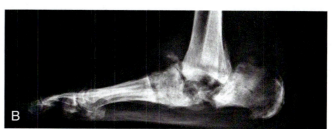

FIGURE 2 Lateral radiographs of the ankle showing osteomyelitis of the talus in a patient who had neuropathy but did not have diabetes, before (**A**) and 5 months after talectomy and arthrodesis with a circular external fixator (**B**). The patient had a stable plantigrade foot.

have neuropathy. Abnormal weight bearing on the fibula causes wound breakdown with subsequent infection. Excision of the infected fibula is required. If resection leads to tibiotalar instability, ankle arthrodesis can be done. Because resection of the involved fibula usually completely eradicates the osteomyelitis, a variety of internal or external fixation techniques can be used for arthrodesis (**Figure 3**).

SURGICAL SITE INFECTIONS

Surgical site wound complications are a common cause of nondiabetic foot and ankle infections. Risk factors for a surgical site infection include neuropathy with or without diabetes mellitus, advanced age, tobacco use, peripheral vascular disease, and prolonged tourniquet times.[58-60] Patients with neuropathy and without diabetes

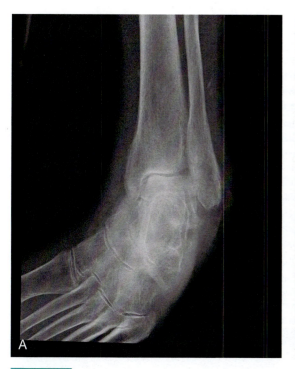
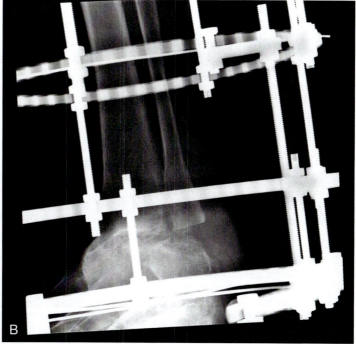

FIGURE 3 AP radiographs showing a fixed varus deformity in a 75-year-old patient with Charcot-Marie-Tooth disease, osteomyelitis of the fibula, and a 10-cm lateral ulcer before (**A**) and after resection of the involved fibula, partial talus resection, and arthrodesis (**B**). The patient's foot was placed in a static frame circular external fixator.

have a 4.72-fold increased risk of surgical site infection compared with patients without neuropathy and without diabetes.[58]

The use of postoperative antibiotics is controversial. However, postoperative antibiotics have been used by up to 75% of surgeons following elective foot and ankle surgical treatment.[61] Indications include previous infection, medical comorbidities, and previous wound healing difficulties. However, there is increasing evidence that postoperative antibiotics may not be necessary in patients without medical comorbidities, especially those isolated to the forefoot.[62-64]

Preoperative antibiotics are commonly used and should be administered any time within 60 minutes before a surgical procedure.[62] Recently, the need for preoperative antibiotics for some foot and ankle procedures has been questioned. A study looking at post-fracture hardware removal from the lower extremity showed no difference in surgical site infections whether preoperative antibiotics or placebo were administered before surgical treatment.[65] Other studies, however, have shown that bacterial growth following various standard preoperative skin preparations was found in 10.9% to 19% of specimens.[66] Wound-healing adjuncts such as the use of platelet-rich plasma or platelet-poor plasma have not been shown to decrease the rate of surgical site infection.[67]

MULTIDISCIPLINARY MANAGEMENT

The management of foot infection in patients who do not have diabetes can be complex. Often the infection involves significant trauma or severe postoperative infection. Many patients have multiple medical comorbidities or are immunocompromised. The foot or ankle infection is likely to involve soft-tissue compromise and to be polymicrobial. A team approach may be required, involving medical specialists, infectious disease specialists, plastic surgeons, and vascular surgeons.[33,68] The orthopaedic surgeon should not hesitate to involve the necessary subspecialists.

SUMMARY

The goal of managing a nondiabetic foot or ankle infection is to achieve a stable, plantigrade limb devoid of infection. Prompt diagnosis and treatment are required for a successful outcome. Although many superficial infections can be treated nonsurgically, a deep or complicated infection requires repeated aggressive surgical débridement, stabilization, and ultimately reconstruction.

KEY STUDY POINTS

- Although less common than diabetic infections, nondiabetic foot infections can lead to significant dysfunction and even limb loss.
- The biomechanics and weight-bearing characteristics of the foot and ankle should be considered during surgical débridement.
- Onychomycosis is a fungal infection that is one of the common diseases of the nails. The pathogens often responsible for onychomycosis are dermatophytes, including *T rubrum* and *T mentagrophytes*.
- Peripheral neuropathy is a significant risk factor for nondiabetic foot infections.
- Risk factors for surgical site infections in the nondiabetic patient include neuropathy, older age, peripheral vascular disease, host factors including nutrition, and tobacco use.

ANNOTATED REFERENCES

1. Wukich DK, McMillen RL, Lowery NJ, Frykberg RG: Surgical site infections after foot and ankle surgery: A comparison of patients with and without diabetes. *Diabetes Care* 2011;34(10):2211-2213.

2. Wukich DK, Lowery NJ, McMillen RL, Frykberg RG: Postoperative infection rates in foot and ankle surgery: A comparison of patients with and without diabetes mellitus. *J Bone Joint Surg Am* 2010;92(2):287-295.

3. Lee JJ, Patel R, Biermann JS, Dougherty PJ: The musculoskeletal effects of cigarette smoking. *J Bone Joint Surg Am* 2013;95(9):850-859.

4. Heidari N, Oh I, Li Y, et al: What is the best method to differentiate acute Charcot foot from acute infection? *Foot Ankle Int* 2019;40(1 suppl):39S-42S.

   Findings from Foot and Ankle Work Group of the 2018 International Consensus Meeting on Musculoskeletal Infection demonstrating moderate evidence and a strong consensus for the use of multiple diagnostic criteria for infection versus Charcot arthropathy including neuropathy, history, and physical and evidence of skin wounds. If unclear, use of laboratory studies and imaging may be beneficial. Level of evidence: V.

5. Butalia S, Palda VA, Sargeant RJ, Detsky AS, Mourad O: Does this patient with diabetes have osteomyelitis of the lower extremity? *J Am Med Assoc* 2008;299(7):806-813.

6. Kanji JN, Anglin RES, Hunt DL, Panju A: Does this patient with diabetes have large-fiber peripheral neuropathy? *J Am Med Assoc* 2010;303(15):1526-1532.

7. Apelqvist J, Castenfors J, Larsson J, Stenström A, Agardh CD: Prognostic value of systolic ankle and toe blood pressure levels in outcome of diabetic foot ulcer. *Diabetes Care* 1989;12(6):373-378.

8. Yu Z, Mao T, Xu Y, et al: Diagnostic accuracy of dual-energy CT in gout: A systematic review and meta-analysis. *Skeletal Radiol* 2018;47(12):1587-1593.

9. Dinh MT, Abad CL, Safdar N: Diagnostic accuracy of the physical examination and imaging tests for osteomyelitis underlying diabetic foot ulcers: Meta-analysis. *Clin Infect Dis* 2008;47(4):519-527.

10. Kapoor A, Page S, Lavalley M, Gale DR, Felson DT: Magnetic resonance imaging for diagnosing foot osteomyelitis: A meta-analysis. *Arch Intern Med* 2007;167(2):125-132.

11. Termaat MF, Raijmakers PG, Scholten HJ, Bakker FC, Patka P, Haarman HJ: The accuracy of diagnostic imaging for the assessment of chronic osteomyelitis: A systematic review and meta-analysis. *J Bone Joint Surg Am* 2005;87(11):2464-2471.

12. Klein DA, Lee BH, Bezhani H, Droukas DD, Stoffels G: The clinical utility of MRI in evaluating for osteomyelitis in patients presenting with uncomplicated cellulitis. *J Foot Ankle Surg* 2020;59(2):323-329.

    This is a retrospective analysis of 441 patients with MRI concerning for soft-tissue infection versus osteomyelitis. Presence of uncomplicated cellulitis (negative for abscesses, ulcers without medical comorbidities such as diabetes, hyperlipidemia, and peripheral vascular disease) was positive for osteomyelitis in only 11.8% of patients (versus 43.9%). Presence of an ulcer in the forefoot had a 5.6-fold increased risk for osteomyelitis. Level of evidence: III.

13. Johnson JE, Kennedy EJ, Shereff MJ, Patel NC, Collier BD: Prospective study of bone, indium-111-labeled white blood cell, and gallium-67 scanning for the evaluation of osteomyelitis in the diabetic foot. *Foot Ankle Int* 1996;17(1):10-16.

14. Michail M, Jude E, Liaskos C, et al: The performance of serum inflammatory markers for the diagnosis and follow-up of patients with osteomyelitis. *Int J Low Extrem Wounds* 2013;12(2):94-99.

15. Kavalukas SL, Barbul A: Nutrition and wound healing: An update. *Plast Reconstr Surg* 2011;127(suppl 1):38S-43S.

16. Aggarwal VK, Higuera C, Deirmengian G, Parvizi J, Austin MS: Swab cultures are not as effective as tissue cultures for diagnosis of periprosthetic joint infection. *Clin Orthop Relat Res* 2013;471(10):3196-3203.

17. Mathews CJ, Kingsley G, Field M, et al: Management of septic arthritis: A systematic review. *Ann Rheum Dis* 2007;66(4):440-445.

18. Thiesen DM, Koniker A, Gehrke T, et al: The impact of α-defensin test in diagnosing periprosthetic infection after total ankle arthroplasty. *J Foot Ankle Surg* 2019;58(6):1125-1128.

    This is a retrospective study of 33 patients who underwent aspiration because of pain or suspected loosening of total ankle arthroplasty. Testing for alpha defensin had 100% sensitivity, 93.5% specificity, 50% positive predictive value, and 100% negative predictive value. Level of evidence: IV.

19. Heidelbaugh JJ, Lee H: Management of the ingrown toenail. *Am Fam Physician* 2009;79(4):303-308.

20. Eekhof JA, Van Wijk B, Knuistingh Neven A, van der Wouden JC: Interventions for ingrowing toenails. *Cochrane Database Syst Rev* 2012;4:CD001541.

21. de Berker D: Clinical practice. Fungal nail disease. *N Engl J Med* 2009;360(20):2108-2116.

22. McNamara DR, Tleyjeh IM, Berbari EF, et al: Incidence of lower-extremity cellulitis: A population-based study in Olmsted county, Minnesota. *Mayo Clin Proc* 2007;82(7):817-821.

23. Hirschmann JV, Raugi GJ: Lower limb cellulitis and its mimics: Part I. Lower limb cellulitis. *J Am Acad Dermatol* 2012;67(2):163.

24. Picard D, Klein A, Grigioni S, Joly P: Risk factors for abscess formation in patients with superficial cellulitis (erysipelas) of the leg. *Br J Dermatol* 2013;168(4):859-863.

25. Endorf FW, Cancio LC, Klein MB: Necrotizing soft-tissue infections: Clinical guidelines. *J Burn Care Res* 2009;30(5):769-775.

26. Wong CH, Chang HC, Pasupathy S, Khin LW, Tan JL, Low CO: Necrotizing fasciitis: Clinical presentation, microbiology, and determinants of mortality. *J Bone Joint Surg Am* 2003;85(8):1454-1460.

27. Tsai YH, Hsu RW, Huang KC, Huang TJ: Laboratory indicators for early detection and surgical treatment of Vibrio necrotizing fasciitis. *Clin Orthop Relat Res* 2010;468(8):2230-2237.

28. Narayanan AS, Walley KC, Borenstein T, Luther GA, Jackson JB, Gonzalez TA: Surgical strategies: Necrotizing fasciitis of the foot and ankle treated with dermal regeneration matrix for limb salvage. *Foot Ankle Int* 2021;42(1):107-114.

    This study provides a technique tip regarding the treatment of large soft-tissue defects from necrotizing fasciitis with the use of a dermal matrix. Level of evidence: V.

29. Eidelman M, Bialik V, Miller Y, Kassis I: Plantar puncture wounds in children: Analysis of 80 hospitalized patients and late sequelae. *Isr Med Assoc J* 2003;5(4):268-271.

30. Gale DW, Scott R: Puncture wound of the foot? Persistent pain? Think of *Pseudomonas aeroginosa* osteomyelitis. *Injury* 1991;22(5):427-428.

31. Chang HC, Verhoeven W, Chay WM: Rubber foreign bodies in puncture wounds of the foot in patients wearing rubber-soled shoes. *Foot Ankle Int* 2001;22(5):409-414.

32. Bouchoucha S, Gafsi K, Trifa M, et al: Intravenous antibiotic therapy for acute hematogenous osteomyelitis in children: Short versus long course. *Arch Pediatr* 2013;20(5):464-469.

33. Rao N, Ziran BH, Lipsky BA: Treating osteomyelitis: Antibiotics and surgery. *Plast Reconstr Surg* 2011;127(suppl 1):177S-187S.

34. Conterno LO, Turchi MD: Antibiotics for treating chronic osteomyelitis in adults. *Cochrane Database Syst Rev* 2013;9:CD004439.

35. Khan K, Schafer C, Wood J: Marjolin ulcer: A comprehensive review. *Adv Skin Wound Care* 2020;33(12):629-634.

This review article discusses the epidemiology, etiology, pathogenesis, diagnosis, and treatment of Marjolin ulcers. Level of evidence: V.

36. Malone M, Bowling FL, Gannass A, Jude EB, Boulton AJ: Deep wound cultures correlate well with bone biopsy culture in diabetic foot osteomyelitis. *Diabetes Metab Res Rev* 2013;29(7):546-550.

37. Ryan EC, Crisologo PA, La Fontaine J, et al: Clinical outcomes of foot infections in patients without diabetes. *J Foot Ankle Surg* 2020;59(4):722-725.

    This is a retrospective study of 88 patients without diabetes and with either soft-tissue infection or osteomyelitis of the foot. Those with osteomyelitis had a higher number of procedures and higher rate of amputation without differences in reinfection, readmission, or duration of antibiotics after 1 year. Level of evidence: III.

38. Montgomery CO, Siegel E, Blasier RD, Suva LJ: Concurrent septic arthritis and osteomyelitis in children. *J Pediatr Orthop* 2013;33(4):464-467.

39. Ng VY, Berlet GC: Evolving techniques in foot and ankle amputation. *J Am Acad Orthop Surg* 2010;18(4):223-235.

40. Melamed EA, Peled E: Antibiotic impregnated cement spacer for salvage of diabetic osteomyelitis. *Foot Ankle Int* 2012;33(3):213-219.

41. Ferrao P, Myerson MS, Schuberth JM, McCourt MJ: Cement spacer as definitive management for postoperative ankle infection. *Foot Ankle Int* 2012;33(3):173-178.

42. Kugan R, Aslam N, Bose D, McNally MA: Outcome of arthrodesis of the hindfoot as a salvage procedure for complex ankle pathology using the Ilizarov technique. *Bone Joint J* 2013;95-B(3):371-377.

43. Pinzur MS, Gil J, Belmares J: Treatment of osteomyelitis in Charcot foot with single-stage resection of infection, correction of deformity, and maintenance with ring fixation. *Foot Ankle Int* 2012;33(12):1069-1074.

44. Rochman R, Jackson Hutson J, Alade O: Tibiocalcaneal arthrodesis using the Ilizarov technique in the presence of bone loss and infection of the talus. *Foot Ankle Int* 2008;29(10):1001-1008.

45. Zalavras CG, Patzakis MJ, Thordarson DB, Shah S, Sherman R, Holtom P: Infected fractures of the distal tibial metaphysis and plafond: Achievement of limb salvage with free muscle flaps, bone grafting, and ankle fusion. *Clin Orthop Relat Res* 2004;427:57-62.

46. Kline AJ, Anderson RB, Davis WH, Jones CP, Cohen BE: Minimally invasive technique versus an extensile lateral approach for intra-articular calcaneal fractures. *Foot Ankle Int* 2013;34(6):773-780.

47. Dickens JF, Kilcoyne KG, Kluk MW, Gordon WT, Shawen SB, Potter BK: Risk factors for infection and amputation following open, combat-related calcaneal fractures. *J Bone Joint Surg Am* 2013;95(5):e24.

48. Wiersema B, Brokaw D, Weber T, et al: Complications associated with open calcaneus fractures. *Foot Ankle Int* 2011;32(11):1052-1057.

49. Mendonca DA, Cosker T, Makwana NK: Vacuum-assisted closure to aid wound healing in foot and ankle surgery. *Foot Ankle Int* 2005;26(9):761-766.

50. Faglia E, Clerici G, Caminiti M, Curci V, Somalvico F: Influence of osteomyelitis location in the foot of diabetic patients with transtibial amputation. *Foot Ankle Int* 2013;34(2):222-227.

51. Brown ML, Tang W, Patel A, Baumhauer JF: Partial foot amputation in patients with diabetic foot ulcers. *Foot Ankle Int* 2012;33(9):707-716.

52. Bollinger M, Thordarson DB: Partial calcanectomy: An alternative to below knee amputation. *Foot Ankle Int* 2002;23(10):927-932.

53. Jeng CL, Campbell JT, Tang EY, Cerrato RA, Myerson MS: Tibiotalocalcaneal arthrodesis with bulk femoral head allograft for salvage of large defects in the ankle. *Foot Ankle Int* 2013;34(9):1256-1266.

54. Smyth NA, Kennedy JG, Parvizi J, Schon LC, Aiyer AA: Risk factors for periprosthetic joint infection following total ankle replacement. *Foot Ankle Surg* 2020;26(5):591-595.

    This is a systemic review of eight observational studies examining risk factors for periprosthetic joint infection in total ankle arthroplasty. Limited recommendation that presence of inflammatory arthritis, prior ankle surgery, age younger than 65 years, body mass index less than 19, peripheral vascular disease, chronic lung disease, hypothyroidism, and low preoperative American Orthopaedic Foot and Ankle Society hindfoot scores correlates with increased risk of periprosthetic joint infection. Level of evidence: II.

55. Rosteius T, Pätzholz S, Rausch V, et al: Ilizarov bone transport using an intramedullary cable transportation system in the treatment of tibial bone defects. *Injury* 2021;52(6):1606-1613.

    This is a retrospective study of 42 patients with large segmental tibial defects (mean 7.7 + 3.4 cm) treated with Ilizarov bone transport with cable transportation system. This was successful in 76% of patients, with 84% of them having excellent or good functional scores. Level of evidence: IV.

56. DeVries JG, Berlet GC, Hyer CF: Predictive risk assessment for major amputation after tibiotalocalcaneal arthrodesis. *Foot Ankle Int* 2013;34(6):846-850.

57. Steele JR, Kadakia RJ, Cunningham DJ, Dekker TJ, Kildow BJ, Adams SB: Comparison of 3D printed spherical implants versus femoral head allografts for tibiotalocalcaneal arthrodesis. *J Foot Ankle Surg* 2020;59(6):1167-1170.

    This is a retrospective study of 15 patients who underwent either three-dimensional spherical implant or femoral head allograft with a tibiotalocalcaneal arthrodesis. The three-dimensional sphere group had a higher rate of total fused articulations (92% versus 62%) and a lower rate of graft resorption (zero versus 57%). Level of evidence: III.

58. Wukich DK, Crim BE, Frykberg RG, Rosario BL: Neuropathy and poorly controlled diabetes increase the rate of surgical site infection after foot and ankle surgery. *J Bone Joint Surg Am* 2014;96(10):832-839.

59. Wiewiorski M, Barg A, Hoerterer H, Voellmy T, Henninger HB, Valderrabano V: Risk factors for wound complications in patients after elective orthopedic foot and ankle surgery. *Foot Ankle Int* 2015;36(5):479-487.

60. Conti MS, Savenkov O, Ellis SJ: Association of peripheral vascular disease with complications after total ankle arthroplasty. *Foot Ankle Orthop* 2019;4(2):2473011419843379.

    This is a retrospective study of 334 patients in whom a postoperative infection developed within 90 days of a total ankle arthroplasty. Patients with peripheral vascular disease had an increased risk of developing a postoperative infection (OR, 2.85), requiring an incision and drainage (OR, 4.87), or total ankle arthroplasty failure at any time (OR, 2.51). Level of evidence: III.

61. Ruta DJ, Kadakia AR, Irwin TA: What are the patterns of prophylactic postoperative oral antibiotic use after foot and ankle surgery? *Clin Orthop Relat Res* 2014;472(10):3204-3213.

62. Tantigate D, Jang E, Seetharaman M, et al: Timing of antibiotic prophylaxis for preventing surgical site infections in foot and ankle surgery. *Foot Ankle Int* 2017;38(3):283-288.

63. Oh I, Englund K: Are prophylactic perioperative antibiotics required for isolated forefoot procedures, such as hammertoes? *Foot Ankle Int* 2019;40(1 suppl):17S-18S.

    Findings from Foot and Ankle Work Group of the 2018 International Consensus Meeting on Musculoskeletal Infection demonstrated moderate evidence and a weak consensus for the use of administration of perioperative antibiotics for isolated forefoot procedures in the absence of risk factors. Level of evidence: V.

64. Carl J, Shelton TJ, Nguyen K, et al: Effect of postoperative oral antibiotics on infections and wound healing following foot and ankle surgery. *Foot Ankle Int* 2020;41(12):1466-1473.

    This is a retrospective study of 631 patients who underwent elective foot and ankle surgery who either did or did not receive postoperative antibiotics. There was no significant difference in the rate of wound infections, wound healing, or superficial infections. Risk factors for infections include increased age, hypertension, neoplastic history, or higher aspirin (ASA) class. Level of evidence: III.

65. Backes M, Dingemans SA, Dijkgraaf MGW, et al: Effect of antibiotic prophylaxis on surgical site infections following removal of orthopedic implants used for treatment of foot, ankle, and lower leg fractures: A randomized clinical trial. *J Am Med Assoc* 2017;318(24):2438-2445.

66. Hunter JG, Dawson LK, Soin SP, Baumhauer JF: Randomized, prospective study of the order of preoperative preparation solutions for patients undergoing foot and ankle orthopedic surgery. *Foot Ankle Int* 2016;37(5):478-482.

67. SanGiovanni TP, Kiebzak GM: Prospective randomized evaluation of intraoperative application of autologous platelet-rich plasma on surgical site infection or delayed wound healing. *Foot Ankle Int* 2016;37(5):470-477.

68. Copley LA, Kinsler MA, Gheen T, Shar A, Sun D, Browne R: The impact of evidence-based clinical practice guidelines applied by a multidisciplinary team for the care of children with osteomyelitis. *J Bone Joint Surg Am* 2013;95(8):686-693.

CHAPTER 15

Plantar Heel Pain

DAVID J. CIUFO, MD • BENEDICT F. DIGIOVANNI, MD, FAAOS, FAOA

ABSTRACT

Plantar heel pain affects a vast number of individuals in the general population and can be quite debilitating to everyday functioning. Although plantar fasciitis is the one common etiologic agent of plantar heel pain, other common causes can include plantar fascia rupture, plantar fasciitis with nerve entrapment (distal tarsal tunnel syndrome), and calcaneal stress fractures. For a typical patient with isolated plantar fasciitis, tissue conditioning and stretching are the preferred first-line treatment, with evidence supporting plantar fascia–specific stretching and Achilles tendon/gastrocnemius stretching. Other nonsurgical treatments include the more traditional corticosteroid injection and the more contemporary biologic treatments such as platelet-rich plasma injections. These options have the drawbacks of putting patients at a higher risk for future plantar fascia rupture and being quite expensive, respectively. For chronic persistent symptoms, a number of surgical options exist. Plantar fascia release, typically with nerve entrapment release, is a preferred treatment approach. Successful evaluation and management of plantar heel pain depends on a thorough history and physical examination, an accurate diagnosis, and an evidence-based treatment approach.

Keywords: calcaneal stress fracture; heel pain; plantar fascia–specific stretching; plantar fasciitis; tarsal tunnel syndrome

INTRODUCTION

Pain on the plantar aspect of the heel is common and has multiple etiologies. Plantar heel pain is distinguished from pain in the posterior heel, as occurs at the Achilles tendon insertion or in the retrocalcaneal space. Plantar fasciitis is the commonly diagnosed condition, but a host of other disorders also can be responsible for a patient's symptoms. A careful history and physical examination are essential to accurate diagnosis and treatment.

THE DIAGNOSIS

It is important to determine the history and circumstances of the onset of symptoms as well as the details of current symptoms. The physical examination requires precise knowledge of the surface anatomy of the foot. Ancillary testing is helpful for documentation and elimination of some of the possible diagnoses but can be misleading in the absence of a careful history and examination.[1]

The history is useful for determining whether the etiology is mechanical, neurogenic, oncologic, infection

---

Dr. DiGiovanni or an immediate family member serves as a board member, owner, officer, or committee member of American Board of Orthopaedic Surgery, Inc. and American Orthopaedic Foot and Ankle Society. Neither Dr. Ciufo nor any immediate family member has received anything of value from or has stock or stock options held in a commercial company or institution related directly or indirectly to the subject of this chapter.

This chapter is adapted from Prong ML, Gould JS: Plantar heel pain, in Chou LB, ed: *Orthopaedic Knowledge Update®: Foot and Ankle 6*. American Academy of Orthopaedic Surgeons, 2020, pp 241-252.

Section 5: Special Problems of the Foot and Ankle

Section 5: Special Problems of the Foot and Ankle

Table 1

Etiologies of Plantar Heel Pain

Nerve syndromes (entrapments and neuromas)

Tarsal tunnel syndrome

Tarsal tunnel syndrome with chronic plantar fasciitis

Lateral plantar nerve entrapment

First branch of the lateral plantar nerve involvement (central heel pad syndrome)

Medial plantar nerve entrapment

Calcaneal nerve lesion

Sural nerve lesion

Osteomyelitis of the calcaneus

Plantar fasciitis

Ruptured plantar fascia

Skin lesion or foreign body of the heel pad

Stress fracture of the calcaneus

Tumor of the heel

based, or traumatic. The possible etiologies are listed in **Table 1**. The patient may report a remote or recent acute traumatic event. An injury can affect the skin, fat pad, fascia, nerve, vascular system, or bone, or it can introduce a foreign body that causes an infection. The traumatic event is not always related to the disorder, however. Often, an increasingly intense program of walking, running, or weight-bearing activity can strain the plantar tissues, cause repetitive microtrauma, and compress neurologic structures, leading to the spontaneous development of pain.[2]

The nature of the patient's current symptoms is useful for determining the responsible anatomic system. The patient should be asked whether the pain begins with the first step in the morning, disappears with further walking, and reappears when arising after sitting; or is the pain made worse by standing or walking? Does the pain occur at night and wake the patient from sleep? It is also helpful to ask the patient to describe the exact location of the pain: Is it in the medial, central, or lateral heel? Does the pain radiate, and, if so, where? Is the pain based on foot position or footwear? Such information should allow the physician to determine the anatomic system or systems involved in the patient's pain.

During the physical examination, the physician locates the precise area of tenderness and often can determine the site of the pathology. The pain may be over the central heel pad, at the medial soft spot where the neurovascular bundle enters the foot, or over the medial tubercle of the calcaneus at the origin of the plantar fascia. Palpation

may reveal a subcutaneous foreign body or a lack of prominence of the medial border of the plantar fascia. Dorsiflexion of the ankle and the great toe (the provocative test for a competent plantar fascia) may reveal a structural defect.

The history and physical examination should provide the physician with the information necessary to determine the type of pain, the anatomy involved, and the ideal means of proceeding to a final diagnosis.[3] The basic ancillary test is the plain radiograph. Any additional imaging is based on the history and physical examination findings. MRI is widely used and quite sensitive, but it is expensive and not particularly specific. Soft-tissue lesions of the heel, such as tumors, foreign bodies, and plantar fascia defects, can be seen with the use of less expensive ultrasonography as well as with MRI. However, the area that can be examined with ultrasonography is more limited, and interpretation of the test results is more difficult than with MRI.

On MRI, a change in signal in the calcaneus is nonspecific and can indicate a stress reaction, stress fracture, osteomyelitis, a bone bruise, or simply plantar fasciitis at the bony origin. If the history suggests infection, blood tests for infection markers should be considered; these should include white blood cell count and differential, erythrocyte sedimentation rate, C-reactive protein level, and labeled white blood cell scan. If a stress fracture is suspected, a healing response with a radiodense area may be noted on lateral radiographs.

PLANTAR HEEL DISORDERS AND THEIR TREATMENT

Plantar Fasciitis

Acute proximal plantar fasciitis is a specific entity that involves the origin of the plantar fascia on the medial tubercle of the calcaneus and for convenience is typically referred to as plantar fasciitis. Mid arch pain along the plantar fascia is a distinct and separate disorder and represents strain and inflammation of the mid plantar fascia. Classic plantar fasciitis is an enthesopathy caused by repeated minor trauma to the fascial origin, which lies plantar (superficial) to the origin of the flexor digitorum brevis. A broad ledge of bone may extend into this muscle origin, but the bone itself does not cause heel pain, despite the reputation, and patient focus, of the so-called heel spur.

Plantar fasciitis typically develops with an increase in activity related to weight bearing or a change in footwear. Sometimes the symptoms arise spontaneously, however.[4] The classic symptoms are pain in the heel during the first step in the morning that disappears after a few steps but may reoccur with standing or walking after sitting.

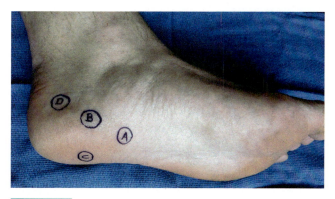

FIGURE 1 Labeled clinical photograph of medial foot demonstrating the most common tender areas in heel pain. **A,** Medial tubercle of calcaneus in plantar fasciitis. **B,** Soft spot where tibial nerve passes into foot, plantar nerve entrapment. **C,** Central fat pad/heel pain. **D,** Calcaneal body, region of positive squeeze test in stress fracture.

The pain does not occur at night or before arising in the morning. It does not become worse with activity. A variation on this history of the symptoms suggests a different diagnosis, which may involve a progression of plantar fasciitis into another entity.

The physical examination reveals specific tenderness limited to the origin of the plantar fascia, and provocative testing determines that the plantar fascia is intact (**Figure 1**). The plain radiograph is normal, although the so-called spur may be present on lateral views. Although MRI is not typically indicated, the MRI of the ankle shows reaction in the plantar fascial origin and often in the adjacent bone.

Myriad treatments have been suggested. Some are used indiscriminately for both the acute condition and recalcitrant symptoms that are presumed to represent persistent plantar fasciitis.[5] Many such treatments appear to be successful because of spontaneous remission, which is common in plantar fasciitis, or because the treatment was administered in combination with tissue-specific plantar fascial stretching, which is the fundamental effective treatment.[6] It has been hypothesized that because the Achilles tendon and the plantar fascia are anatomically connected, stretching the Achilles tendon and gastrocnemius will help with symptoms of plantar fasciitis. Indeed, very strong association exists between patients with plantar fasciitis and those with isolated gastrocnemius tightness, suggesting that managing gastrocnemius tightness may be effective at alleviating symptoms of plantar fasciitis.[7] A 2020 study demonstrated significant improvements in plantar heel pain as ankle dorsiflexion improves with a stretching program.[8] Although Achilles tendon stretching programs alone may provide some symptom relief, tissue-specific plantar fascia stretching programs in combination with Achilles tendon stretching programs are markedly more effective at improving plantar fasciitis symptoms.[9,10] Furthermore, a tissue-specific plantar fascial stretching program, on its own, has been demonstrated to be more effective in relieving pain symptoms and improving function than an Achilles tendon stretching program alone among patients with chronic plantar fasciitis.[6,11] Custom orthoses are not required for most patients, and the use of a soft, accommodative over-the-counter orthotic device can provide symptomatic relief by splinting the plantar fascia and gathering the heel pad fat, thereby decreasing the contact of the irritated plantar fascia with the weight-bearing surface.[12] Oral NSAIDs also are helpful for symptom relief.

Various injections have been explored as potential treatments for the symptoms of plantar fasciitis. Corticosteroid injections have been perhaps the historically widespread of these approaches, contributing to significant improvements in pain symptoms in many studies, with some studies comparing efficacy of corticosteroids versus platelet-rich plasma (PRP).[13-15] However, corticosteroid injections are associated with a markedly increased risk of subsequent plantar fascia rupture and should, therefore, be administered with caution.[16] Corticosteroid injections are also associated with fat pad atrophy and relatively short-term symptom relief. Some studies have reported that patients' pain often returns within 3 to 6 months and progresses to their baseline level within 1 year, in comparison with joint mobilization and stretching exercises, which can result in a more permanent resolution of symptoms and improved outcomes at 12 weeks to 1 year and beyond.[14,17]

In recent years, PRP injections and other biologics have been optimistically investigated as alternatives to corticosteroid injections. Several studies provide grounds for continued optimism, demonstrating PRP as equally or more effective than corticosteroids at managing symptoms of chronic plantar fasciitis.[18-20] In contrast, however, several studies also demonstrate no improvement with PRP when compared with corticosteroids or saline placebo. Similar results have been seen with amniotic membrane and other allogeneic growth factor injections.[21,22] Botulinum toxin injections have shown some benefit, with injection into either the heel itself or into the gastrocnemius muscle, but these studies often lack comparison groups or long-term follow-up.[23,24] Other recent studies have failed to corroborate these findings and show no notable differences in outcome.[25]

Nonsurgical treatments for plantar fasciitis have been the mainstay of treating the acute condition, with high-level evidence-based studies available to guide appropriate treatment for acute plantar fasciitis.[9] When these treatments are not sufficient to alleviate symptoms and restore function, surgical approaches may be considered. Yet high-level evidence-based studies for surgical treatment outcomes are limited.[9] Historically, open surgical release of the plantar fascia has been used to treat persistent symptoms, with or without removal of the so-called heel spur. Heel spur removal is no longer recommended. More contemporary studies including some from the past several years have revealed variable postsurgical outcomes, ranging from symptom relief in nearly three-fourths of patients receiving open or endoscopic plantar fasciotomies on the one hand to persistent pain and further complications on the other.[2] Treatment of gastrocnemius contracture with open gastrocnemius recession has shown some benefit as part of the surgical plan, as discussed in a 2021 study.[26] Postoperatively, patients who undergo a gastrocnemius recession do not experience significant loss of strength, and in some cases are stronger than preoperative testing by 6 months.[27,28] Further studies have reported suboptimal outcomes following isolated surgical plantar fascia release including persistent and worsening pain, pain on the lateral border and dorsum of the foot, inability to return to desired activity levels, and classic neurogenic symptoms.[9,29,30] In addition, preoperative steroid injections may be associated with patients reporting worse long-term outcomes following an open plantar fascia release.[29] The variable postsurgical outcomes combined with the potential for worse outcomes following some standard nonsurgical treatment suggest that the clinical value of treating plantar fasciitis through an isolated open partial or complete release is uncertain.[29] Denervation of the heel, including division of the calcaneal nerves, also has been attempted. Division of only the medial plantar fascia has had variable outcomes. With the advent of endoscopy, partial release of the plantar fascia has been recommended but can lead to complications including laceration of the tibial nerve or vascular structures.[31]

Other innovative treatment approaches have been investigated more recently and may be of benefit. The addition of acupuncture was found to add some benefit to a standard protocol using ice, NSAIDs, and stretching.[32] An isolated gastrocnemius contracture has been associated with acute and chronic plantar fasciitis. A 57% incidence of isolated gastrocnemius contracture was found in patients with plantar fasciitis.[33] Patients with chronic foot pain, including pain from plantar fasciitis, had a 93% success rate after gastrocnemius recession for an isolated contracture.[34] Proximal medial gastrocnemius release for patients with recalcitrant plantar fasciitis and a gastrocnemius contracture led to pain relief in 81% of patients.[35] The use of a full-length silicone insole was compared with an ultrasound-guided steroid injection to the origin of the plantar fascia in 42 randomly chosen patients.[36] One month after the procedure, the results were equivalent with respect to heel tenderness and pain relief. Patients who received an injection had less thickness of the fascia. The researchers recommended the use of insoles as primary management. Extracorporeal shock wave therapy is effective at treating recalcitrant plantar fasciitis, with one multicenter randomized clinical trial noting the success rate of heel pain reduction was between 50% and 65%.[37] In another randomized controlled study of radial extracorporeal shock wave therapy in 245 patients with chronic plantar fasciitis, the success rate was 61%, compared with 42% in those treated with a placebo.[38]

A nonsurgical protocol is recommended for management of acute plantar fasciitis, less than 9 months symptom duration.[6] Most patients with acute plantar fasciitis will have resolution of symptoms in 3 to 6 months. The authors use a treatment protocol using plantar fascia–specific stretching, Achilles tendon/gastrocnemius stretching, ice, NSAIDs, and an over-the-counter full-length soft orthotic device. Corticosteroid injections or physical therapy is reserved for recalcitrant cases, and oral steroids are not typically used.

Ruptured Plantar Fascia

Sudden tearing of the plantar fascia during an acute dorsiflexion stretch can occur regardless of whether the patient has a history of plantar fasciitis. Often the tear is associated with a history of steroid injections.[16] The patient reports acute pain in the heel and arch, aching on the lateral border of the foot and in the dorsal arch, and sometimes neurogenic symptoms in the tibial nerve distribution. A sensation of popping or suddenly giving way is classic. The physical findings are acute tenderness in the proximal fascia, midfoot ecchymosis, and a fascial defect. A subtle tear can be confirmed using ultrasonography or MRI, but advanced imaging is not typically needed.

The usual treatment is immobilization with partial weight bearing in a cast or walking boot with a soft orthotic for 2 to 3 weeks as well as ice and NSAIDs. A custom-molded orthotic device with posting of the longitudinal arch can be used for an extended period of time. Hypertrophic scarring of the plantar fascia may be palpable at the site of the rupture. Many patients continue to be symptomatic indefinitely after the rupture.[39] Typically, the medial border of the plantar fascia is ruptured, but the central and lateral portions may be left intact. Complete release of the remaining fascia can relieve the mechanical symptoms. If neurogenic symptoms ensue, the recommended treatment is a complete release of the remaining plantar fascia and tarsal tunnel.

Nerve Syndromes

Tarsal Tunnel Syndrome

Tarsal tunnel syndrome can be divided into proximal tarsal tunnel syndrome and distal tarsal tunnel syndrome. Proximal tarsal tunnel syndrome can occur in isolation, whereas distal tarsal syndrome most commonly occurs in association with chronic plantar fasciitis. The classic or proximal tarsal tunnel syndrome is described as compression of the tibial nerve under the flexor retinaculum (laciniate ligament).[40,41] The compression has variously been attributed to a ganglion, a lipoma, a neurilemoma, a fibroma, a varicose vein, an accessory muscle belly, or a displaced bone after fracture. The results of simple decompression of the flexor retinaculum are quite variable.

The patient has a subtle, spontaneous onset of pain in the heel and medial border of the ankle, and occasionally radiating along the medial and plantar foot. The symptoms typically are made worse with activity and slowly relieved by rest, but they may occur at night or at rest. The pain often is described as a burning or aching sensation. Tenderness exists over the medial retinaculum of the ankle and/or over the abductor hallucis, and Tinel sign can be positive. Nerve conduction velocity studies only occasionally are positive. The inciting lesion may be seen on MRI or ultrasonography.[42]

If there is a discrete lesion, excision with release of the retinaculum is often successful at decreasing foot pain (**Figure 2**). The outcome is less predictable if an accessory muscle or varicose vein is the source of compression.[43]

Distal tarsal tunnel syndrome is now recognized as a traction neuropathy of the tibial nerve and its branches[44,45] (**Figure 3**). This condition may be associated

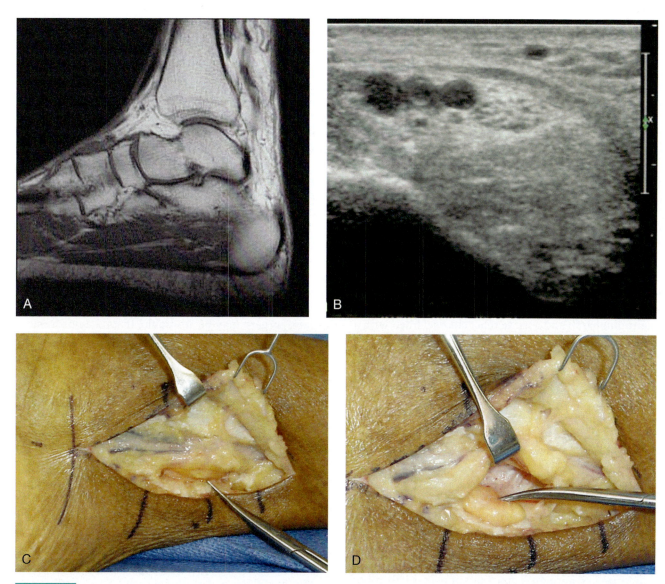

FIGURE 2 Lipoma in the tarsal tunnel. **A**, Magnetic resonance image showing a lipoma lying under the tibial nerve in the tarsal tunnel. **B**, Ultrasonogram showing a lipoma under the nerve. **C** and **D**, Intraoperative photographs in which the lipoma can be seen at the scissors tip. **C**, The flexor retinaculum has been released and the lipoma is dissected from under the nerve. **D**, The lipoma is dissected free from the nerve. (Panels **B**, **C**, and **D** reprinted from Gould JS: Tarsal tunnel syndrome. *Foot Ankle Clin* 2011;16[2]:275-286. Copyright 2011, with permission from Elsevier.)

Section 5: Special Problems of the Foot and Ankle

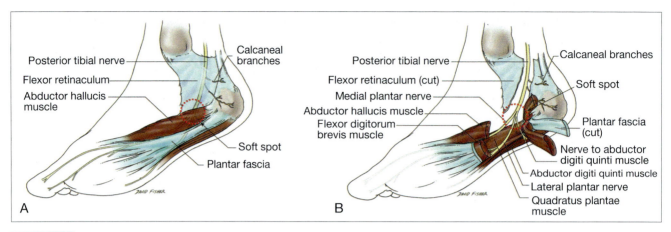

FIGURE 3 Schematics showing the anatomy of the tibial nerve in the tarsal tunnel before (**A**) and after (**B**) release of the flexor retinaculum (the laciniate ligament), plantar fascia, abductor hallucis, and flexor digitorum brevis. (Reprinted from Gould JS: Tarsal tunnel syndrome. *Foot Ankle Clin* 2011;16[2]:275-286. Copyright 2011, with permission from Elsevier.)

with chronic plantar fasciitis, attenuation of the plantar fascia, or unilateral flatfoot secondary to collapse of the medial structures and attenuation of the posterior tibial tendon.[46,47] The patient has a history of heel and medial ankle neurogenic pain made worse with activity and slowly relieved by rest. The pain may occur at rest and at night, however. The onset is gradual and often progressive. Tenderness occurs over the distal edge of the abductor hallucis at the soft spot where the neurovascular bundle enters the foot. Objective testing may not be helpful. Typical electromyographic testing does not show a conduction delay, but there may be signal abnormalities in the abductor hallucis and the abductor digiti quinti.[48] There may be associated weakness in abduction of the fifth toe. The condition is treated using a specially constructed total-contact orthotic shoe insert with a posted longitudinal arch and a nerve relief channel filled with a viscoelastic polymer that follows the posteromedial and plantar course of the tibial and lateral plantar nerves[43,49] (**Figure 4**). After treatment, the neurogenic symptoms often are relieved without the need for a nerve release.

Tarsal Tunnel Syndrome With Chronic Plantar Fasciitis

Plantar fasciitis usually is resolved in 3 to 6 months and often more rapidly with appropriate nonsurgical treatment. In some patients, the condition persists, however, and the symptoms change. The pain begins to resolve less quickly after taking the first step in the morning or arising during the day. Symptoms may include more prolonged after-burn sensation and pain characterized as sharp, aching, burning, or intensely itching develops after prolonged standing or walking. Pain may occur while sitting or at night. Some but not necessarily all of the elements of neurogenic pain may be present, such as the prolonged after-burn and first-step pain characteristic of plantar fasciitis. Tenderness occurs over the nerve at

the plantar edge of the abductor hallucis and the medial edge of the plantar fascia (the so-called soft spot), perhaps along the course of the nerve, and at the origin of the plantar fascia on the medial tubercle. During the ankle and great toe provocative dorsiflexion test, loss of definition of the medial border of the plantar fascia is common, indicating attenuation or rupture of the structure.[43] Electromyographic changes in the intrinsic musculature are more likely than with normally resolving plantar fasciitis.[48]

The nonsurgical treatment includes plantar fascia–specific stretching exercises, Achilles tendon/gastrocnemius stretching exercises, ice/NSAIDs, and use of a custom orthotic device with a soft posteromedial nerve channel. If there is no improvement after 6 months for patients with plantar fasciitis and tarsal tunnel syndrome, surgery may be advisable. If some improvement occurs, the orthotic device should be used until the patient reaches a satisfactory resolution of symptoms,

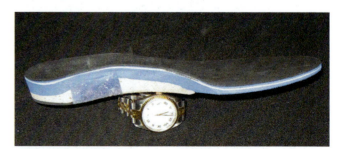

FIGURE 4 Photograph showing the total-contact orthotic shoe insert (medial view), with a posteromedial and plantar nerve relief channel. (The wristwatch is used to prop up the medial side of the insert to show the nerve relief channel filled with the viscoelastic polymer.) (Reprinted from Gould JS: Recurrent tarsal tunnel syndrome. *Foot Ankle Clin* 2014;19[3]:451-467. Copyright 2014, with permission from Elsevier.)

completely recovers, or decides to undergo surgical intervention after inadequate improvement.

The preferred surgical procedure is a partial or complete release of the plantar fascia with decompression of the entire tarsal tunnel (**Figure 5**). This may be combined with a gastrocnemius recession based on the results of Silfverskiöld testing. A posteromedial incision is begun midway between the posterior edge of the medial malleolus and the medial edge of the Achilles tendon. The incision follows the course of the nerve, distally curving forward to cross the soft spot and continuing across the plantar surface just distal to the heel pad. The flexor retinaculum (laciniate ligament) is divided, as is the superficial fascia of the abductor hallucis. Depending on competence of the plantar fascia, the medial one-third of the plantar fascia is divided or a complete fascia release is performed. By working under the abductor hallucis muscle, the deep fascia of the muscle is fully divided. On the anterior side of the interval between the distal edge of the abductor hallucis and the medial edge of the flexor digitorum brevis muscle, the lateral plantar nerve is located and inspected to ensure that a septum is not isolating and constricting the nerve. The nerve is retracted, and the tendinous fibers of the quadratus plantae muscle lying under the nerve are divided.[50-52] At the confluence of the plantar edge of the superficial fascia of the abductor hallucis as it joins its deep fascia, with the medial edge of the plantar fascia lying over the nerve and the quadratus fibers lying under it, the nerve takes a sharp turn from the medial to the plantar foot. Presumably, this is the point at which traction on the nerve produces irritation with weight bearing and pronation of the foot. The histologic evidence of nerve injury at this point is not conclusive, although some evidence of change at this location can be seen on ultrasonography and MRI.

If a septum is isolating the nerve, the entire abductor hallucis is released by unipolar cautery to improve visualization, and the septum is fully divided. To explore a so-called failed release, the abductor is similarly divided. The procedure ends with closure of the subcutaneous tissue and skin, and protection in a short leg plaster splint.

Gastrocnemius recession is performed concomitantly, when indicated, through a posteromedial incision. The incision is centered at the inflection point of the calf musculature, indicative of the myotendinous junction. Careful dissection through the soft tissues is performed, and the fascia is incised longitudinally. The gastrocnemius tendon is identified and isolated with retractors, and soft tissue is cleared to ensure the sural nerve is free. The tendon is then cut under direct visualization using a #15 blade or heavy tissue scissors while a dorsiflexion force is applied to the tendon. A few centimeters of separation are usually identified as well as a clear improvement in dorsiflexion motion.

The patient must avoid weight bearing for 4 weeks to allow the plantar fascia to reconstitute itself in a lengthened position and thereby prevent the development of lateral border and dorsal arch pain. The orthotic device, often custom, is used for an additional 9 to 12 months. At a mean 19.6-month follow-up (range, 3 to 24 months), 93% of 92 patients (104 feet) had complete or significantly improved outcomes with pain relief after release of the plantar fascia and tarsal tunnel, as described.[52]

Lateral Plantar Nerve Involvement

The lateral and medial plantar nerves diverge from the tibial nerve at the upper edge of the abductor hallucis or more proximally. The lateral plantar nerve continues distally and crosses the soft spot entering the foot. The medial plantar nerve runs under the muscle of the abductor, with the medial plantar artery and accompanying vein, and does not cross under the potentially restrictive area of the distal edge of the abductor hallucis fascia and proximal edge of the plantar fascia. The lateral plantar nerve typically is the more affected branch of the tibial nerve in distal tarsal tunnel syndrome. Involvement is managed with the total-contact orthotic shoe insert, and surgical release, if necessary, is the same as for chronic plantar fasciitis. Partial release of the plantar fascia and the tarsal tunnel is not reliably successful.

First Branch of the Lateral Plantar Nerve Involvement (Central Heel Pad Syndrome)

The first branch of the lateral plantar nerve typically emerges from the nerve just distal to the branching of the

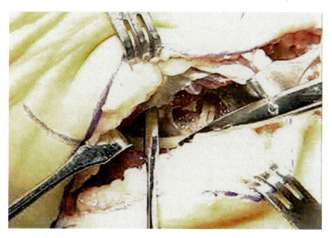

FIGURE 5 Intraoperative photograph showing an extended surgical release of the tarsal tunnel and plantar fascia, in which the lateral plantar nerve is exposed in the interval between the abductor hallucis and flexor digitorum brevis after release of the laciniate ligament, the superficial and deep fascia of the abductor hallucis, the entire plantar fascia, and the tendinous fibers and fascia of the quadratus plantae. (Reprinted from Gould JS: Tarsal tunnel syndrome. *Foot Ankle Clin* 2011;16[2]:275-286. Copyright 2011, with permission from Elsevier.)

lateral from the tibial nerve, but occasionally it emerges from the tibial nerve itself. The branch runs posteriorly under the abductor hallucis, over the quadratus plantae to innervate it, and over the periosteum and the flexor digitorum brevis; the branch sends a sensory branch to the central heel pad and continues into the abductor digiti quinti as a motor branch. The first branch of the lateral plantar nerve has been described as the cause of central heel pad syndrome in runners, for which release of the deep fascia of the abductor hallucis and the medial third of the plantar fascia is the surgical treatment of choice.[53,54] The recommended nonsurgical treatment is to use the total-contact orthotic shoe insert, with widening of the nerve relief channel posteriorly on the medial and plantar surfaces, and to modify the patient's running regimen.[49] If surgical treatment is necessary, a relatively complete release may be needed if significant attenuation of the plantar fascia is noted. This procedure has been successful in football, soccer, baseball, and distance-running athletes.

It is important to differentiate the first branch of the lateral plantar nerve from the calcaneal branches of the tibial nerve, which usually emerge more proximally and end in the subcutaneous tissue and skin of the medial and posteromedial heel. The first branch of the lateral plantar nerve passes under the abductor hallucis, but the calcaneal nerve remains superficial. The distinction between these two nerves is important because they are of similar diameter, and both emerge from the nerve posteriorly and often close together.

A contusion of the central heel with a neuroma of the nerve can be treated by surgical exposure of the first branch through the tarsal tunnel incision, with excision of the branch, insertion into a conduit, and placement of the conduit into the retrocalcaneal space. Improvement of the symptoms can be expected (**Figure 6**).

Other Peripheral Nerve Involvement

Involvement of other peripheral nerves can be a cause of heel pain, but these are less common. Other potentially problematic nerves include the medial plantar, calcaneal, and sural nerves. These are less frequently involved than the tibial and lateral plantar nerves, but with appropriate knowledge of anatomy, can still be managed nonsurgically or released during surgical approached.

The medial plantar nerve can be involved in tarsal tunnel distal or proximal conditions; it also can be involved individually as it leaves the course of the lateral plantar nerve and passes under the abductor hallucis muscle with the medial plantar artery and veins. Slightly more distal, medial plantar nerve meets the flexor digitorum longus and flexor hallucis longus at the master knot of Henry. Here, in the proximal

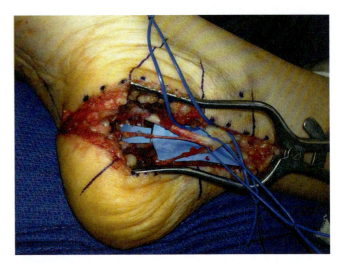

FIGURE 6 Intraoperative photograph showing a neuroma of the first branch of the lateral plantar nerve. (Reproduced with permission from Gould JS, Florence MN: Neuromas of the foot and ankle. *Orthop Knowl Online J* 2014;12[7].

longitudinal arch, medial plantar nerve may be affected by tenosynovitis of these tendons.[55] The pain typically is in the arch and occurs with active or passive movement of the involved tendons, but the nerve may be tender under the abductor hallucis posteromedially Nonsurgical management consists of similar offloading inserts with anterior extension of the nerve relief channel, or stiffer shoes/orthoses to limit tendon excursion. Surgical release uses the same incision as in the release just described for the combined tarsal tunnel and plantar fascia release, but this is extended more distally as necessary once the nerve is identified beneath the abductor hallucis.

The medial plantar heel is innervated by the calcaneal branch or branches of the tibial nerve, which can cause medial plantar heel pain after contusion or surgery in the area.[56] Palpation should allow relatively straightforward identification of the site of the lesion. The history of injury or a surgical incision over the area should be compatible. The treatment can be difficult, with a variable response to nonsurgical desensitization and cushioning, and limited data on surgical treatment.

Branches of the sural nerve innervate the lateral plantar heel, the lateral border of the foot, the plantar aspect of the fifth toe, and the dorsal aspects of the fourth and fifth toes. Lesions of the first branch of the lateral plantar nerve can cause pain in both the central heel pad and lateral heel pad aching through the continuation of the branch to the abductor digiti quinti. A history of trauma to the sural nerve, including a surgical procedure that puts the nerve at risk, may account for injury to the nerve and resulting pain in the lateral heel.[57,58] The pain may be accompanied by loss of sensibility in the area and

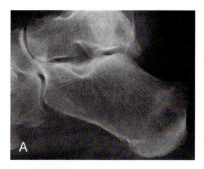 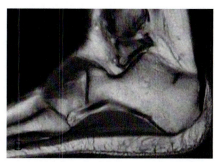 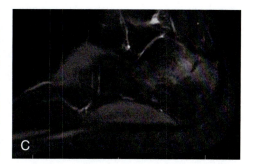

FIGURE 7 Radiographic imaging of calcaneus stress fracture. **A**, Lateral plain radiograph. **B**, T1-weighted magnetic resonance image of stress fracture. **C**, T2-weighted magnetic resonance image demonstrating surrounding bony edema.

tenderness or a positive Tinel sign with palpation over the nerve. Sensory electrical testing may be helpful. A sural nerve block can be a useful adjunctive tool for diagnosis. A backless shoe and manual desensitization with topical medications are the initial treatments of choice. The use of neurolysis is unpredictable, but excision of the nerve can be curative. If a symptomatic neuroma develops at the excision site, a more proximal excision of the entire nerve just below the popliteal space may be needed.

Stress Fractures of the Calcaneus

Stress fracture of the heel can occur in runners, young women who are amenorrheic (female athlete triad), people who have osteoporosis, and otherwise healthy people who have had an increase in stress to the bone.[59] The patient often becomes aware of the pain at the moment the injury occurs or shortly after the inciting activity. The pain initially is constant but becomes worse with activity. Eventually, the pain is present with activity but is relieved by rest, and typically the pain disappears after the requisite 6 weeks of healing. Visual inspection may be normal aside from some soft-tissue swelling and at times bruising. Examination reveals point tenderness with side-to-side calcaneal compression known as a positive squeeze test of the calcaneus. Swelling may be seen on radiographs with good soft-tissue definition, but the fracture may not be apparent until 10 to 14 days after the injury, when resorption is seen at the fracture site. Beyond a few weeks from injury, radiographs will typically show a radiodense band (**Figure 7**), which represents a bony healing response. Patients with a positive calcaneal squeeze test and negative findings on plain radiographs and a history consistent with bone pain often have a calcaneal stress reaction or precursor to a complete stress fracture. Symptomatic treatment is typically used for a stress fracture or stress reaction and includes ice, NSAIDs, and protected weight bearing in a walking boot with soft insert or cast for 2 to 3 weeks. Significant improvement is often seen in this time frame, with a decrease in pain on calcaneal squeeze test on clinical examination. If the diagnosis is unclear or the patient is not responding as anticipated, advanced imaging with MRI or CT would be the next step in management.

Rheumatologic Diagnoses

An important class of diagnoses for the orthopaedic surgeon to consider is systemic or rheumatologic diseases. Although these are less common than mechanical and anatomic causes, heel pain can be a presenting symptom in a young patient and warrant laboratory workup. Patients with recalcitrant unilateral or often bilateral heel pain might suffer from rheumatoid arthritis, systemic lupus erythematosus, psoriasis, inflammatory bowel diseases, ankylosing spondylitis, Reiter syndrome, Behçet syndrome, or others.[60] In patients with nonclassic bilateral plantar heel pain, the physician may consider laboratory studies including complete blood count, C-reactive protein, erythrocyte sedimentation rate, rheumatoid factor, human leukocyte antigen-B27, antinuclear antibodies, cyclic citrullinated protein, and uric acid. Bilateral heel symptoms with atypical response to orthopaedic treatment and/or elevated markers may warrant consultation with rheumatology.

SUMMARY

Plantar heel pain has multiple etiologies, although plantar fasciitis is the most common. In chronic plantar fasciitis with nerve entrapment at either the proximal and/or distal tarsal tunnel, the neurogenic findings may evolve and require modification of the diagnosis and treatment. Management begins with a proper diagnosis based on a careful history and physical examination followed by inductive reasoning. Adjunctive testing may be indicated to clarify and document the diagnosis. An algorithmic treatment plan is developed and followed to the level indicated. Despite recent studies on plantar heel pain, the fundamentals of diagnosis and management remain unchanged.

KEY STUDY POINTS

- Although plantar fasciitis is the most common cause of plantar heel pain, other common disorders that should be included in the differential diagnosis when evaluating each patient include plantar fascia rupture, calcaneal stress fracture, and chronic plantar fasciitis with tarsal tunnel syndrome.
- Nonsurgical treatment is the mainstay of isolated plantar fasciitis and has good evidence-based studies to guide treatment and should be followed. Tissue conditioning and plantar fascia–specific and Achilles tendon stretching, ice, NSAIDs, and over-the-counter soft inserts are preferred treatment approaches.
- When plantar fasciitis becomes chronic, symptoms often evolve with neurogenic component of proximal and/or distal tarsal tunnel syndrome. Patients should be evaluated for associated nerve compression, which often involves the first branch of the lateral plantar nerve.
- Surgical treatment should be reserved for chronic plantar heel symptoms presenting for more than 9 months, and should address both plantar fascia pathology and nerve compression. There is more limited evidence to guide surgical treatment, and surgical outcomes can be unpredictable.

ANNOTATED REFERENCES

1. Gould JS: General workup of the foot and ankle patient, in Gould JS, ed: *The Handbook of Foot and Ankle Surgery: An Intellectual Approach to Complex Problems.* Jaypee Brothers Medical Publishers, 2013, pp 3-4.

2. Lareau CR, Sawyer GA, Wang JH, DiGiovanni CW: Plantar and medial heel pain: Diagnosis and management. *J Am Acad Orthop Surg* 2014;22(6):372-380.

3. Gould JS: Making the diagnosis and the discussion of management with the patient, in Gould JS, ed: *The Handbook of Foot and Ankle Surgery: An Intellectual Approach to Complex Problems.* Jaypee Brothers Medical Publishers, 2013, pp 5-7.

4. Riddle DL, Pulisic M, Pidcoe P, Johnson RE: Risk factors for plantar fasciitis: A matched case-control study. *J Bone Joint Surg Am* 2003;85(5):872-877.

5. Wolgin M, Cook C, Graham C, Mauldin D: Conservative treatment of plantar heel pain: Long-term follow-up. *Foot Ankle Int* 1994;15(3):97-102.

6. DiGiovanni BF, Nawoczenski DA, Lintal ME, et al: Tissue-specific plantar fascia-stretching exercise enhances outcomes in patients with chronic heel pain: A prospective, randomized study. *J Bone Joint Surg Am* 2003;85(7):1270-1277.

7. Nakale NT, Strydom A, Saragas NP, Ferrao PNF: Association between plantar fasciitis and isolated gastrocnemius tightness. *Foot Ankle Int* 2018;39(3):271-277.

8. Pearce CJ, Seow D, Lau BP: Correlation between gastrocnemius tightness and heel pain severity in plantar fasciitis. *Foot Ankle Int* 2021;42(1):76-82.

   A strong correlation was found between gastrocnemius tightness and heel pain in plantar fasciitis. There was evidence of improvement in pain proportional to improvements in tightness. Level of evidence: IV.

9. DiGiovanni BF, Moore AM, Zlotnicki JP, Pinney SJ: Preferred management of recalcitrant plantar fasciitis among orthopaedic foot and ankle surgeons. *Foot Ankle Int* 2012;33(6):507-512.

10. Engkananuwat P, Kanlayanaphotporn R, Purepong N: Effectiveness of the simultaneous stretching of the Achilles tendon and plantar fascia in individuals with plantar fasciitis. *Foot Ankle Int* 2018;39(1):75-82.

11. DiGiovanni BF, Nawoczenski DA, Malay DP, et al: Plantar fascia-specific stretching exercise improves outcomes in patients with chronic plantar fasciitis. A prospective clinical trial with two-year follow-up. *J Bone Joint Surg Am* 2006;88(8):1775-1781.

12. Pfeffer G, Bacchetti P, Deland J, et al: Comparison of custom and prefabricated orthoses in the initial treatment of proximal plantar fasciitis. *Foot Ankle Int* 1999;20(4):214-221.

13. Mahindra P, Yamin M, Selhi HS, Singla S, Soni A: Chronic plantar fasciitis: Effect of platelet-rich plasma, corticosteroid, and placebo. *Orthopedics* 2016;39(2):e285-e289.

14. Monto RR: Platelet-rich plasma efficacy versus corticosteroid injection treatment for chronic severe plantar fasciitis. *Foot Ankle Int* 2014;35(4):313-318.

15. Jain SK, Suprashant K, Kumar S, Yadav A, Kearns SR: Comparison of plantar fasciitis injected with platelet-rich plasma vs corticosteroids. *Foot Ankle Int* 2018;39(7):780-786.

16. Lee HS, Choi YR, Kim SW, Lee JY, Seo JH, Jeong JJ: Risk factors affecting chronic rupture of the plantar fascia. *Foot Ankle Int* 2014;35(3):258-263.

17. Celik D, Kuş G, Sırma SÖ: Joint mobilization and stretching exercise vs steroid injection in the treatment of plantar fasciitis: A randomized controlled study. *Foot Ankle Int* 2016;37(2):150-156.

18. Peerbooms JC, Lodder P, den Oudsten BL, Doorgeest K, Schuller HM, Gosens T: Positive effect of platelet-rich plasma on pain in plantar fasciitis: A double-blind multicenter randomized controlled trial. *Am J Sports Med* 2019;47(13):3238-3246.

   When compared with corticosteroid injection, PRP for plantar fasciitis demonstrated better improvements in pain/function up to 1 year in a group of 115 subjects. Level of evidence: I.

19. Jiménez-Pérez AE, Gonzalez-Arabio D, Diaz AS, Maderuelo JA, Ramos-Pascua LR: Clinical and imaging effects of

corticosteroids and platelet-rich plasma for the treatment of chronic plantar fasciitis: A comparative non randomized prospective study. *Foot Ankle Surg* 2019;25(3):354-360.

In a nonrandomized nonblind trial, PRP led to greater improvement in visual analog scale pain score, American Orthopaedic Foot and Ankle Society score, and ultrasound-measured plantar fascia thickness at 6 months compared with corticosteroid injections. Level of evidence: III.

20. Hohmann E, Tetsworth K, Glatt V: Platelet-rich plasma versus corticosteroids for the treatment of plantar fasciitis: A systematic review and meta-analysis. *Am J Sports Med* 2021;49(5):1381-1393.

A meta-analysis of 15 studies suggests some benefit of PRP over corticosteroid injection lasting at least 1 year. Unfortunately, there is much variability in the studies, limited quality, and a high risk of bias. Level of evidence: III.

21. Kandil MI, Tabl EA, Elhammady AS: Prospective randomized evaluation of local injection of allogeneic growth factors in plantar fasciitis. *Foot Ankle Int* 2020;41(11):1335-1341.

There was some positive effect in visual analog scale pain and Foot Function Index scores with allogeneic growth factors when compared with control saline injection. Satisfaction was 92% in treatment group versus 78% in the control group. Level of evidence: I.

22. Hanselman AE, Tidwell JE, Santrock RD: Cryopreserved human amniotic membrane injection for plantar fasciitis: A randomized, controlled, double-blind pilot study. *Foot Ankle Int* 2015;36(2):151-158.

23. Ahmad J, Ahmad SH, Jones K: Treatment of plantar fasciitis with botulinum toxin. *Foot Ankle Int* 2017;38:1-7.

24. Abbasian M, Baghbani S, Barangi S, et al: Outcomes of ultrasound-guided gastrocnemius injection with botulinum toxin for chronic plantar fasciitis. *Foot Ankle Int* 2020;41(1):63-68.

When compared with placebo saline injection, botulinum toxin injection into the medial head of the gastrocnemius produced significant improvements in pain, function, and patient satisfaction at 12-month follow-up in patients with plantar fasciitis. Level of evidence: I.

25. Elizondo-Rodríguez J, Simental-Mendía M, Peña-Martínez V, Vilchez-Cavazos F, Tamez-Mata Y, Acosta-Olivo C: Comparison of botulinum toxin A, corticosteroid, and anesthetic injection for plantar fasciitis. *Foot Ankle Int* 2021;42(3):305-313.

A randomized, blind trial comparing placebo anesthetic, corticosteroid, and botulinum injections for plantar fascia demonstrates no differences between groups through 6 months of follow-up in pain, function, or plantar fascia thickness. Level of evidence: I.

26. Hoefnagels EM, Weerheijm L, Witteveen AG, Louwerens JWK, Keijsers N: The effect of lengthening the gastrocnemius muscle in chronic therapy resistant plantar fasciitis. *Foot Ankle Surg* 2021;27(5):543-549.

Isolated gastrocnemius recession demonstrates significant improvements in visual analog scale pain score and functional outcomes in chronic plantar fasciitis. Dorsiflexion increases by a mean of 16° and loading shifts toward the medial midfoot while decreasing at the hallux. Level of evidence: II.

27. Busquets R, Sanchez-Raya J, Sallent A, Maled I, Duarri G: Proximal medial gastrocnemius release: Muscle strength evaluation. *Foot Ankle Surg* 2020;26(7):828-832.

Proximal gastrocnemius recession not only avoids weakening the surgical limb, but actually increases the strength on isometric and isokinetic testing at 6 months and 1 year. Level of evidence: II.

28. Kou JX, Balasubramaniam M, Kippe M, Fortin PT: Functional results of posterior tibial tendon reconstruction, calcaneal osteotomy, and gastrocnemius recession. *Foot Ankle Int* 2012;33(7):602-611.

29. MacInnes A, Roberts SC, Kimpton J, Pillai A: Long-term outcome of open plantar fascia release. *Foot Ankle Int* 2016;37(1):17-23.

30. Sammarco GJ, Helfrey RB: Surgical treatment of recalcitrant plantar fasciitis. *Foot Ankle Int* 1996;17(9):520-526.

31. Hogan KA, Webb D, Shereff M: Endoscopic plantar fascia release. *Foot Ankle Int* 2004;25(12):875-881.

32. Karagounis P, Tsironi M, Prionas G, Tsiganos G, Baltopoulos P: Treatment of plantar fasciitis in recreational athletes: Two different therapeutic protocols. *Foot Ankle Spec* 2011;4(4):226-234.

33. Patel A, DiGiovanni BF: Association between plantar fasciitis and isolated contracture of the gastrocnemius. *Foot Ankle Int* 2011;32(1):5-8.

34. Maskill JD, Bohay DR, Anderson JG: Gastrocnemius recession to treat isolated foot pain. *Foot Ankle Int* 2010;31(1):19-23.

35. Abbassian A, Kohls-Gatzoulis J, Solan MC: Proximal medial gastrocnemius release in the treatment of recalcitrant plantar fasciitis. *Foot Ankle Int* 2012;33(1):14-19.

36. Yucel U, Kucuksen S, Cingoz HT, et al: Full-length silicone insoles versus ultrasound-guided corticosteroid injection in the management of plantar fasciitis: A randomized clinical trial. *Prosthet Orthot Int* 2013;37(6):471-476.

37. Gollwitzer H, Saxena A, DiDomenico LA, et al: Clinically relevant effectiveness of focused extracorporeal shock wave therapy in the treatment of chronic plantar fasciitis: A randomized, controlled multicenter study. *J Bone Joint Surg Am* 2015;97(9):701-708.

38. Gerdesmeyer L, Frey C, Vester J, et al: Radial extracorporeal shock wave therapy is safe and effective in the treatment of chronic recalcitrant plantar fasciitis: Results of a confirmatory randomized placebo-controlled multicenter study. *Am J Sports Med* 2008;36(11):2100-2109.

39. Acevedo JI, Beskin JL: Complications of plantar fascia rupture associated with corticosteroid injection. *Foot Ankle Int* 1998;19(2):91-97.

40. Keck C: The tarsal-tunnel syndrome. *J Bone Joint Surg Am* 1962;44(1):180-182.

41. Lam SJ: A tarsal-tunnel syndrome. *Lancet* 1962;2(7270):1354-1355.

42. Lopez-Ben R: Imaging of nerve entrapment in the foot and ankle. *Foot Ankle Clin* 2011;16(2):213-224.

43. Gould JS: Tarsal tunnel syndrome. *Foot Ankle Clin* 2011;16(2):275-286.

44. Heimkes B, Posel P, Stotz S, Wolf K: The proximal and distal tarsal tunnel syndromes: An anatomical study. *Int Orthop* 1987;11(3):193-196.

45. Lau JT, Daniels TR: Effects of tarsal tunnel release and stabilization procedures on tibial nerve tension in a surgically created pes planus foot. *Foot Ankle Int* 1998;19(11):770-777.

46. DiGiovanni BF, Gould JS: Tarsal tunnel syndrome and related entities. *Foot Ankle Clin* 1998;3:405-426.

47. Labib SA, Gould JS, Rodriguez-del-Rio FA, Lyman S: Heel pain triad (HPT): The combination of plantar fasciitis, posterior tibial tendon dysfunction and tarsal tunnel syndrome. *Foot Ankle Int* 2002;23(3):212-220.

48. Roy PC: Electrodiagnostic evaluation of lower extremity neurogenic problems. *Foot Ankle Clin* 2011;16(2):225-242.

49. Gould JS, Ford D: Orthoses and insert management of common foot and ankle problems, in Schon LC, Porter DA, eds: *Baxter's The Foot and Ankle in Sports.* Mosby Elsevier, 2008, pp 595-593.

50. DiGiovanni BF, Abuzzahab FS, Gould JS: Plantar fascia release with proximal and distal tarsal tunnel release: Surgical approach to chronic disabling plantar fasciitis with associated nerve pain. *Tech Foot Ankle Surg* 2003;2:254-261.

51. Gould JS, DiGiovanni BF: Plantar fascia release in combination with proximal and distal tarsal tunnel release, in Weisel SW, ed: *Operative Techniques in Orthopaedic Surgery.* Wolters Kluwer/Lippincott Williams & Wilkins, 2011, vol 4, pp 3911-3919.

52. Gould JS: Entrapment syndromes, in Gould JS, ed: *The Handbook of Foot and Ankle Surgery: An Intellectual Approach to Complex Problems.* Jaypee Brothers Medical Publishers, 2013, pp 247-269.

53. Baxter DE, Thigpen CM: Heel pain: Operative results. *Foot Ankle* 1984;5(1):16-25.

54. Rondhuis JJ, Huson A: The first branch of the lateral plantar nerve and heel pain. *Acta Morphol Neerl Scand* 1986;24(4):269-279.

55. Rask MR: Medial plantar neurapraxia (jogger's foot): Report of 3 cases. *Clin Orthop Relat Res* 1978;134:193-195.

56. Govsa F, Bilge O, Ozer MA: Variations in the origin of the medial and inferior calcaneal nerves. *Arch Orthop Trauma Surg* 2006;126(1):6-14.

57. Pringle RM, Protheroe K, Mukherjee SK: Entrapment neuropathy of the sural nerve. *J Bone Joint Surg Br* 1974;56B(3):465-468.

58. Flanigan RM, DiGiovanni BF: Peripheral nerve entrapments of the lower leg, ankle, and foot. *Foot Ankle Clin* 2011;16(2):255-274.

59. Leabhart JW: Stress fractures of the calcaneus. *J Bone Joint Surg Am* 1959;41-A:1285-1290.

60. Falsetti P, Frediani B, Acciai C, Baldi F, Filippou G, Marcolongo R: Heel fat pad involvement in rheumatoid arthritis and in spondyloarthropathies: An ultrasonographic study. *Scand J Rheumatol* 2004;33(5):327-331.

CHAPTER 16

Foot and Ankle Tumors

YAZAN KADKOY, MS • DANIEL J. GARCIA, BS • JOSEPH BENEVENIA, MD, FAAOS

ABSTRACT

Musculoskeletal tumors of the foot or ankle are rare tumors with varying pathology. Thorough history and physical assessment of the patient can provide insight into differentiating benign and malignant conditions and are essential for guiding this diagnostic workup. Radiographic imaging can assist in delineating types of different lesions and lead to a diagnosis. Plain radiographs can evaluate the soft tissues as well as bone and may indicate aggressiveness of osseous lesions. Further evaluation with CT or MRI may be needed to confirm diagnosis or for surgical planning. In many cases, diagnosis can only be made with tissue sample from biopsy. Tumors of the foot or ankle can range from benign soft-tissue tumors to malignant soft-tissue sarcomas. Benign osseous tumors may be found in the foot or ankle as well as malignant osseous tumors including osteosarcoma, Ewing sarcoma, and chondrosarcoma. Metastatic carcinomas have been known to metastasize to sites in the foot

or ankle. Malignant lesions about the foot or ankle may be more often misdiagnosed as benign conditions, which can delay appropriate treatment. Reconstructive treatments for the foot and ankle include amputation, custom endoprosthetic reconstruction, and osseous grafting techniques.

Keywords: ankle tumor; benign tumor; foot tumor; limb salvage; malignant tumor

INTRODUCTION

The evaluation, diagnosis, treatment, and referral of patients with a tumor of the foot or ankle are important in clinical practice. Orthopaedic surgeons should be vigilant to detect these tumors. A foot or ankle tumor is classified as benign or, less often, malignant and may occur within the soft tissue or bone. A mass can develop in the foot as a result of a posttraumatic or neuropathic condition or because of bone or soft-tissue infection.

Dr. Benevenia or an immediate family member has received royalties from Merete Medical and Rutgers University/Creosso LLC; is a member of a speakers' bureau or has made paid presentations on behalf of Musculoskeletal Transplant Foundation; serves as a paid consultant to or is an employee of Merete and Onkos; serves as an unpaid consultant to Implant Cast and NJOS; has stock or stock options held in Creosso LLC; has received research or institutional support from Creosso, Merete Medical, and Musculoskeletal Transplant Foundation; has received nonincome support (such as equipment or services), commercially derived honoraria, or other non–research-related funding (such as paid travel) from Implantcast, Merete, and Onkos; and serves as a board member, owner, officer, or committee member of American Academy of Orthopaedic Surgeons, Musculoskeletal Transplant Foundation, Musculoskeletal Tumor Society and WAIOT, SICOT, ISOLS. Neither of the following authors nor any immediate family member has received anything of value from or has stock or stock options held in a commercial company or institution related directly or indirectly to the subject of this chapter: Yazan Kadkoy and Daniel Garcia.

This chapter is adapted from Neilson JC, Lelkes VM: Foot and ankle tumors, in Chou LB, ed: *Orthopaedic Knowledge Update®: Foot and Ankle 6*. American Academy of Orthopaedic Surgeons, 2020, pp 253-268.

INCIDENCE

Tumors of the foot or ankle are rare, and their incidence has not been well studied. In a retrospective review of 7,487 musculoskeletal tumors at any anatomic site that were surgically treated at a tertiary center over 18 years, 413 tumors were in the bone or soft tissue of the foot or ankle (5.52%; mean patient age, 36 years).[1] Sixty of the foot and ankle tumors (39.2%) were considered to be malignant, and the remaining 93 were considered to be benign. Eighty patients (52.3%) had a soft-tissue tumor, of which giant cell tumor of the tendon sheath and pigmented villonodular synovitis (PVNS) were the most common. The remaining 73 patients (47.7%) had a bone tumor; giant cell tumor was the most common type.

PATIENT EVALUATION

History

A thorough patient history is key to the differential diagnosis of a mass or lesion of the foot or ankle. The most common initial symptom of a bony lesion is pain, and identifying the onset, duration, location, and character of the pain can be useful in determining the etiology. Any aggravating or alleviating activities may be especially important. In general, an aggressive malignant bone lesion is painful. Many benign bone lesions are found incidentally. NSAIDs can provide significant pain relief in a patient with aggressive tumor or some specific types of tumors, such as osteoid osteoma. A soft-tissue mass, whether malignant or benign, usually is not painful, although discomfort may result from displacement or destruction of adjacent structures or a change in gait pattern. When a mass has been identified, the duration, onset, as well as changes in the size, location, and number of masses can be helpful in determining the best management. Most masses that have been present for years without increasing in size are benign, but some benign masses are at risk for malignant dedifferentiation. A stable tumor that begins to grow may represent malignant progression to a sarcoma and should be evaluated and treated by a musculoskeletal oncologist. Some tumors, such as vascular anomalies, have a distinct pattern of enlarging and shrinking, especially with activity. Some foot masses, such as Morton neuroma and plantar fibroma, have a distinct location. In addition to the history of the tumor itself, the patient history should include a complete discussion of any earlier tumors, whether benign or malignant, as well as any risk factors such as tobacco smoking, chemical exposure, recent or past trauma or infection, or a family history of tumors.

Physical Examination

In addition to the involved foot and ankle, a complete examination should include the contralateral extremity, proximal draining lymph node beds, any masses identified while taking the history, and any skin lesions. This evaluation may lead to identification of primary or metastatic tumor sites or a syndrome such as neurofibromatosis or plantar fascial fibromatosis (Ledderhose disease). The size and depth of the mass should be measured because these are the two factors most useful for determining the likelihood of malignancy. A large subfascial tumor (>5 cm) is most likely to be malignant. Direct palpation of the mass may elicit pain. The mass may be firm or fluctuant, although a mass that usually is fluctuant, such as a ganglion, can appear to be firm because of the tension exerted by the many structures in the foot. The mobility of the mass can help in identifying both its depth and its origin; for example, a schwannoma usually is only mobile perpendicular to the plane of the nerve. Provocative testing with percussion for a Tinel sign can be useful in evaluating neural tumors. Transillumination can help characterize solid, rather than fluid-filled, masses. Auscultation and palpation for bruits can be useful in identifying arteriovascular malformations. Evaluation for other common generators of pain in the foot should be undertaken as suggested by the patient's history.

Imaging

Radiographic analysis is important in the evaluation of both soft-tissue and bone tumors. Radiographs can indicate the aggressiveness of an osseocentric tumor. A permeative pattern suggests an aggressive, often malignant process. A geographic pattern often is characterized by a thin, eggshell-like margin of bone around the tumor and connotes a less aggressive process. This observed difference is explained by the response of the bone to the tumor. The bone is able to respond to and even contain a relatively slow-growing, unaggressive tumor. Some types of tumors are most likely to occur in a diaphyseal, metaphyseal, or epiphyseal area, but because the foot bones are small and irregular, the specific origin of a tumor can be difficult to identify.

Periosteal elevation may be the result of a mass effect from tumor, and subperiosteum elevated off the bone usually indicates a relatively aggressive tumor. The pattern of periosteal elevation is described as a sunburst, onion skinning, or a Codman triangle.

The matrix of any lesion can give important clues to its origin. Cartilage tumors often have a lucent appearance and over time become mineralized in a punctate pattern. Fibrous dysplasia typically has a ground-glass radiographic appearance. In comparison with normal bone, other tumors are more or less lucent or have mixed lucency; this characteristic often is helpful in the differential diagnosis of primary and metastatic tumors of bone. Cortical destruction also can indicate a relatively aggressive tumor. Extraosseous mineralization may appear adjacent to a bone lesion or in some soft-tissue masses. The most commonly seen forms of extraskeletal bone are phleboliths in an arteriovascular malformation or synovial sarcoma, mineralization of the necrotic center of soft-tissue sarcoma, peripheral mineralization of myositis ossificans, or cloud-like mineralization of an extraskeletal osteosarcoma. Radiographs can differentiate soft-tissue masses within different tissue planes by the density of air, fat, water (muscle), and bone.

CT is helpful for evaluating the character of mineralized structures, which have many characteristics in common with those of bone, as seen on plain radiographs. As discussed in a 2020 study, CT of the chest, abdomen, and pelvis is an important part of the workup for a patient with suspected metastatic carcinoma to bone.[2] Although CT angiography is an effective tool for a patient who cannot undergo MRI, usually MRI is superior for precise evaluation of tumors and important surrounding structures in the foot and ankle. Obtaining high-quality MRI results for small structures in areas such as the forefoot requires the use of small coils and a high-Tesla machine. MRI with gadolinium contrast is recommended for all soft-tissue and most bone lesions because this technique shows the amount of blood flow to a mass. By enhancing the rim of a cystic structure such as a ganglion, as well as some arteriovascular malformations and bone cysts, MRI can differentiate between a fluid-filled and a solid mass. Diffusion-weighted MRI sequences are most commonly used to assess the tumor response to radiation, chemotherapy, or ablative treatment. Magnetic resonance angiography has supplanted traditional angiography for most tumor indications, and it is useful for evaluating the blood supply to the foot before resection or reconstruction. As discussed in a 2019 study, the soft-tissue detail provided by a high-quality MRI is critical to the surgical resection of soft-tissue and bone tumors of the foot and ankle.[3] Technetium Tc-99 bone scanning is useful for evaluating a stress fracture or a stress reaction that can masquerade as an osseous lesion of the foot. Whole body scanning is commonly used to identify malignant metastasis to bone, but it must be interpreted with caution because some tumors, such as multiple myeloma, eosinophilic granulomas, and large renal cell cancers, may not show significant uptake.

The use of ultrasonography in the diagnosis and management of soft-tissue tumors is constantly evolving. Ultrasonography is used to differentiate solid and fluid-filled masses, and it is an excellent tool for measuring flow in vascular anomalies. The usefulness of ultrasonography increases with the surgeon's experience with this modality. In the treatment of tumors, ultrasonography most commonly is used for guidance during soft-tissue biopsy or the treatment of a vascular anomaly. Positron emission tomography (PET) is useful in the evaluation of many but not all types of malignancies. Inclusion of the lower extremities is not standard during PET staging of many cancerous conditions, and whole body PET should be specified if PET evaluation is appropriate for the patient's lesion. PET is rarely ordered by a physician other than an oncologist. PET can be useful for evaluation of the lymphatic spread of hidradenocarcinoma, melanoma, or epithelioid sarcoma, usually in conjunction with lymphoscintigraphy and sentinel node resection.[4] Although PET-MRI is a promising tool for identifying tumor metastasis at diagnosis and during subsequent staging, its use has not yet been completely validated according to a 2020 study.[5]

Laboratory Evaluation

Laboratory testing is not necessary for most tumors of the foot and ankle. However, inflammatory markers, white blood cell analysis, and cultures are appropriate if an infectious origin is suspected. Complete blood cell counts are useful for identifying leukemia or lymphoma and may reveal anemia in a patient with multiple myeloma or a widely metastatic cancer. Protein electrophoresis and light chain evaluations can be diagnostic for multiple myeloma. Some other primary cancers have blood markers, such as prostate-specific antigen. Metabolic analysis can reveal kidney or liver damage, malnutrition, or electrolyte abnormalities.[2] Calcium levels should be checked in all patients with metastatic disease to the bone because increased bone turnover can lead to increased serum calcium or to cardiac conditions including fatal arrhythmias.

Biopsy

Pathologic analysis should be performed in all masses. An excision, incision, or needle technique can be used, depending on the size, location, and imaging characteristics of the lesion as well as the experience of the surgeon. Excisional biopsy is appropriate if a cuff of normal tissue can be obtained around the lesion to ensure negative margins. This saves the patient from a wider re-excision if the lesion is determined to be malignant by pathology. Incisional biopsy should be considered for a relatively large mass, which should be presumed to be malignant until histologic analysis proves otherwise. In general, biopsies should be performed or guided by a surgeon trained in treating primary malignant tumors of the extremity. Frozen section should be obtained during an open biopsy to determine whether lesional tissue is obtained and thereby increase the likelihood of a correct diagnosis. A needle biopsy can be done with or without imaging guidance. Ultrasonography or CT can be used to increase the likelihood of obtaining tissue from the lesion by targeting solid, nonnecrotic areas and correlating these findings with those of contrast-enhanced MRI. According to a 2020 study, a thoughtful approach to needle biopsy is essential because bleeding from deep or subcutaneous vessels could allow tumor tissue to spread along uninvolved tissue planes and thereby increase the resection area.[6] Fine-needle aspiration biopsy can be used in many masses, but this technique is operator dependent. Core biopsy allows more tissue to be obtained, but its use is limited to tumors large enough to accommodate the throw of the needle. The small amount of subcutaneous tissue in the foot and ankle often allows relatively early identification of a mass. Usually, a mass smaller than 3 cm is benign. A mass larger than 3 cm is more likely to be malignant. However, a study found that malignant bone tumors in the foot are 5 to 30 times smaller than those in other skeletal areas.[7] Although complications from bone biopsy are rare (0.52%), all biopsies should be done with great care, as an inexpert biopsy can increase the risk of hardware failure, tumor dissemination, and infection, as discussed in a 2022 literature review.[8]

BENIGN SOFT-TISSUE TUMORS

Synovial Tumors

Ganglion

A synovial ganglion is the most common mass of the foot and ankle. A study found that 11% of all synovial ganglia occur at the ankle and foot.[9] Synovial ganglia result from a weakness in the wall of a synovial structure. On MRI, a ganglion most commonly is seen in the tarsal canal and on the dorsum of the foot.[10] The most common site of origin involves the lateral column of the Lisfranc joint. These structures often are painless but can create pain when they compress adjacent structures, and they can become irritating with shoe wear. Ganglia can be diagnosed clinically if they increase and decrease in size, are over a joint and superficial tendon, are subcutaneous, or can be transilluminated (if sufficiently large). In addition, fluid can be aspirated using a large-bore needle. If all of these factors are present, resection without advanced imaging may be appropriate. However, if these factors are not present, high-quality gadolinium-enhanced MRI is needed to consolidate the diagnosis. The mass should be characterized by a homogeneous low signal with T1 weighting, a high signal with T2 weighting, and rim enhancement with gadolinium[3] (**Figure 1**). The use of hand/foot MRI coils decreases the field of view and improves the quality of the image for a small mass. The treatments include observation, corticosteroid injection, and surgical resection. Marginal resection can be undertaken with an attempt to remove the stalk and entire cyst capsule. Arthroscopic internal drainage or resection has been described with recurrence rate of 12%.[11]

Pigmented Villonodular Synovitis

Pigmented villonodular synovitis (PVNS) is an intra-articular process characterized by hemorrhage, hemosiderin deposition, giant cells, histiocytes, and fibrous stroma. The estimated incidence of PVNS is around 1.8 cases per million people in a population.[12] Although the knee is the most commonly affected joint, PVNS sometimes occurs in the ankle. In the earlier stages, patients may have a painful or painless effusion. Patients with long-standing disease may have large masses, poor joint motion, and arthritis. MRI classically shows a low signal with T1 and T2 weighting, with peripheral contrast enhancement. A blooming pattern can be seen in larger

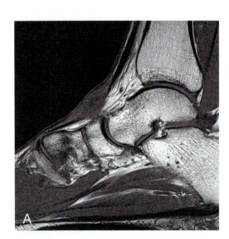
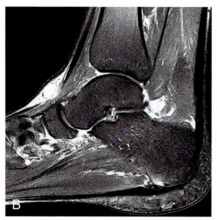
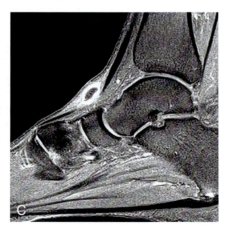

FIGURE 1 Magnetic resonance images showing the characteristics typical of a synovial ganglion on the dorsum of the ankle. **A**, T1-weighted image with homogenous low signal intensity. **B**, T2-weighted image with high signal intensity. **C**, Rim enhancement in a gadolinium-enhanced T1-weighted image.

masses. In the foot or ankle, the tumor may involve more than one adjacent joint as a result of direct extension. PVNS is categorized as localized or diffuse. The localized form more likely occurs in the forefoot[11] and is treated with open or arthroscopic resection of the nodule, and recurrence rates are low. The diffuse form often occurs in the hindfoot[11] and is treated with open and/or arthroscopic surgery but is associated with high recurrence rates up to 14% to 55%[13] because of the difficulty of obtaining a complete resection. Some patients with degenerative disease can benefit from fusion or arthroplasty.

Giant Cell Tumor of Tendon Sheath

Giant cell tumor of tendon sheath is histologically identical to PVNS but is extra-articular and associated with synovial structures such as tendon sheaths. The mass itself is painless, but it may impinge upon or irritate adjacent structures. The MRI signal characteristics are similar to those of PVNS. Marginal resection is the appropriate treatment. Needle or incisional biopsy should be considered for a relatively large and fast-growing tumor because it is possible for such a tumor to degenerate into a malignant giant cell tumor of tendon sheath that, like a sarcoma, should undergo wide resection.

Synovial Chondromatosis

Synovial chondromatosis is much less common than PVNS, but it can be no less debilitating. This abnormality is thought to be a cartilaginous metaplasia of the synovium that breaks off to form loose bodies. This tumor has been associated with an abnormality in chromosome 6. Open or arthroscopic treatment is appropriate, with anterior-posterior arthroscopic approach being proposed as the most effective surgical management.[14] A small 2020 study reported that the recurrence rate within its analysis was low at 5%, while reporting no transformation into chondrosarcoma.[14] Degeneration to chondrosarcoma is difficult to diagnose correctly, and a questionable diagnosis should be reviewed by an experienced musculoskeletal pathologist.

Lipoma Arborescens

Lipoma arborescens is an extremely rare synovial disorder that most likely represents a reactive process made up of intra-articular lipoma-like masses of hypertrophic synovial villi distended by fat. Open or arthroscopic treatment usually is curative.[15]

Other Synovial Proliferations

Significant synovial proliferations similar to those of PVNS can be caused by medical conditions including acute or chronic infection, gout, calcium pyrophosphate disease, amyloidosis, rheumatologic disease, and foreign material in the joint.

Vascular Anomalies

Vascular anomalies are a broad group of tumors that stem from an abnormality in the arteries, veins, capillaries, or lymph tissues. These tumors can occur in any tissue in the body. A superficial vascular anomaly often is seen as a change in skin color and character. Deeper intramuscular growths often change in size with activity. Often the growth infiltrates areas between the muscle fibers, and as a result complete resection is difficult. A deep tumor can become painful or cause cramping as it grows. Well-circumscribed soft-tissue calcifications often are seen on radiographs. Ultrasonography and some MRI sequences can differentiate between high-flow and low-flow lesions. The appearance of the lesion on MRI often is serpiginous and has been described as an axial slice through a bowl of worms. Although surgical resection is an option, many vascular anomalies can be effectively treated with serial percutaneous sclerosing therapy, usually under ultrasonographic guidance. Very few vascular anomalies of the foot require systemic treatment.[16,17]

Nodular Fasciitis

Nodular fasciitis is a rapidly growing, very cellular tumor with a high mitotic rate. It is sometimes misdiagnosed as a sarcoma, and only an experienced pathologist may be able to arrive at the correct diagnosis. Patients age 20 to 40 years are most often affected. Unclear borders can be seen on MRI as the tumor infiltrates the surrounding soft tissue; T1-weighted and T2-weighted signal intensities are mixed, and there is a mixed pattern with gadolinium enhancement. Pain can come from local irritation as the tumor grows to a significant size within weeks. The tumor is self-limiting and often regresses with biopsy.

Fibroma

Benign fibromas primarily occur in the subcutaneous tissues and can be found in any area of the body. Histologically dense, mature fibrocytes are present. T1-weighted and T2-weighted MRI shows low signal intensity, and there is no enhancement with gadolinium. Marginal resection usually is curative, and recurrence is rare.

Plantar Fibroma/Fibromatosis

Plantar fibroma appears as one or more lesions, usually along the medial border of the plantar fascia, most often in adolescents or young adults. The tissue is histologically similar to that of Dupuytren or Peyronie contracture, which is found in older adults. The lesions rarely grow larger than 2 cm and remain static in size. Bilateral masses occur in as many as half of patients. On MRI, there is low T1 signal and low to intermediate T2 signal, with variable enhancement. Most patients are asymptomatic. A patient with pain should be evaluated for the presence of another pain generator and should undergo extensive nonsurgical treatment including physical therapy and the use of night splints, shoe modification, and over-the-counter pain medications. Resection is rarely recommended. The recurrence rate for primary lesions after local excision is between 57% and 100%, whereas the recurrence rate for primary lesions after complete plantar fasciotomy is between zero and 50%.[15] Resection may leave a hypersensitive area on the plantar aspect of the foot. A recent study showed that extracorporeal shockwave therapy in patients with ultrasonography-confirmed plantar fibromatosis was beneficial for pain relief and functional outcomes, while softening the fibroma and reducing its thickness. Patients in the study were given 12 rounds of extracorporeal shockwave therapy over 6 months with statistically significant improvements in pain and functional scores at both long-term and short-term follow-up.[18]

Extra-abdominal Fibromatosis

Extra-abdominal fibromatosis (also known as desmoid tumor) is a locally aggressive, monoclonal proliferative disease that occurs anywhere in the musculoskeletal system. The tumor grows at a variable rate and in some patients is latent for long periods of time. The peak incidence is in patients approximately 30 years old. These tumors are firm and may adhere to underlying structures. MRI classically shows low T1 and T2 signal, but some tumors have a mixed T2 signal; enhancement with gadolinium is low or mixed. Unlike a sarcoma, fibromatosis often infiltrates the surrounding tissues, and planning a wide resection is difficult. As many as 28% of these tumors are associated with previous trauma, including a surgical scar. The treatment is evolving. Medical therapies have included the use of NSAIDs, antiestrogen therapies, and other chemotherapies. Radiation has been used alone and in conjunction with surgical resection for tumor control. Local control rates after surgical resection range from 50% to 80%.[19,20]

Epidermoid Inclusion Cyst

An epidermoid inclusion cyst usually is subungual and occurs as the result of traumatic disruption of the nail matrix beneath the skin, with subsequent collection of keratin in a cyst-like structure that can erode into the distal phalanx. The treatment is with biopsy and intralesional excision and grafting, if necessary. Secondary infection can complicate the treatment.

Glomus Tumor

The vascular glomus tumor appears as a small, painful red to blue discoloration beneath the nail bed. Patients have a triad of symptoms involving paroxysmal pain, point tenderness, and cold hypersensitivity.[21] Other subungual tumors, especially malignant melanoma, should be considered in the differential diagnosis. A glomus tumor usually is smaller than 1 cm. Imaging is difficult, but MRI signal is low with T1 weighting and high with T2 weighting; a low-intensity central nidus is seen with gadolinium enhancement. Tumor pressure on the bone can cause erosion of the phalanx. This tumor usually occurs in early adulthood and is treated with marginal excision with low rates of recurrence, except in cases of incomplete excision.[22]

Morton Interdigital Neuroma

Morton neuroma is a fibrosing process of the plantar digital nerve that causes pain in the plantar aspect of the foot. This disorder most commonly occurs between the heads of the third and fourth metatarsals and less often between the second and third metatarsals. Pain radiates proximally along the innervations and into the toes. A mass may be palpable on physical examination; squeezing the forefoot or palpating the mass aggravates the symptoms. On MRI, a large Morton neuroma has a characteristic low-intensity signal with T1 weighting, an intermediate-intensity signal with T2 weighting, and mild uptake with gadolinium enhancement (**Figure 2**). Nonsurgical treatment including shoe wear modification and the use of an in-shoe orthotic device may alleviate

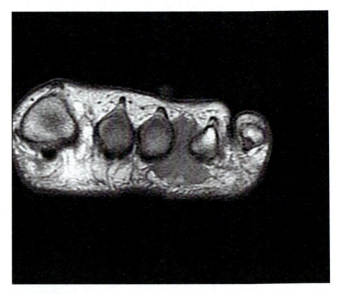

FIGURE 2 T1-weighted MRI showing a large Morton neuroma between the third and fourth metatarsals.

the symptoms. Corticosteroid injections may decrease the symptoms and tumor size. If these measures are unsuccessful, marginal surgical resection leads to pain relief in most patients.

Neurilemmoma or Schwannoma

Neurilemmoma or schwannoma is a benign proliferation of Schwann cells in the nerve sheath. This tumor is most common in patients age 20 to 50 years. Tumors usually occur on the flexor surfaces of the extremities, and 90% are isolated. The tumor often is identifiable on physical examination because of a positive Tinel sign and restriction of the movement of the mass to one plane as a result of nerve tethering. MRI characteristically shows a mass along the tract of a nerve with a central low signal known as a target sign. When left untreated for a long period of time, a tumor can develop atypia; such a tumor is called an ancient schwannoma. This transformation does not necessarily have malignant potential. Most patients have an isolated tumor, but schwannomatosis syndromes do exist. The tumor can be resected by marginal excision, leaving the nerve intact.

Neurofibroma

Neurofibroma is a benign spindle cell tumor of a peripheral nerve that usually is superficial. Like schwannoma, neurofibroma is isolated in 90% of patients. The tumor occurs in patients age 20 to 30 years. Multiple lesions are seen in patients with neurofibromatosis.[1] These patients have a 10% risk of dedifferentiation of one of their many tumors into a neurosarcoma. Resection of these tumors from major nerves is not recommended because no plane exists between the neurofibroma and the nerve.

Lipoma

Lipomas are fatty tumors that can occur in any part of the body. Most lipomas appear in patients age 40 to 60 years. The lipoma itself is painless, but it can compress other structures or painfully herniate out of the fascial covering. A small superficial tumor has a soft, doughy consistency, rarely grows larger than 10 cm, and can be monitored with simple observation. A large subfascial tumor often is excised because of the difficulty of monitoring and the risk of malignant dedifferentiation. MRI can be used to diagnose lipoma without a biopsy. The key is to examine every MRI sequence to ensure that the tumor has the signal characteristics of subcutaneous fat. Further evaluation by an orthopaedic oncologist is advised if any of the sequences differ in even a portion of the tumor because this signal change might represent progression of the tumor to a well-differentiated or dedifferentiated liposarcoma. The many subtypes of lipomas,

including angiolipoma, spindle cell lipoma, lipoblastoma, hibernoma, myolipoma, chondroid lipoma, and myelolipoma, also may have signal characteristics different from those of subcutaneous fat. For a true lipoma, a marginal excision of less than 5 cm is sufficient, and no follow-up is necessary.

MALIGNANT SOFT-TISSUE TUMORS

Soft-Tissue Sarcomas

Most types of soft-tissue sarcomas can occur in the foot or ankle. A low-grade tumor may be slow growing and exist in the foot for a long time, but a high-grade tumor can progress in a short period of time to a large and fungating mass within the thin soft-tissue covering of the ankle (**Figure 3**). Benign or low-grade tumors that have been present for many years can dedifferentiate into a higher grade sarcoma and suddenly begin to grow. Benign pathology is significantly much more common in the foot and ankle compared with soft-tissue sarcomas, and they can often be misdiagnosed and have unplanned excisions.[23] Sarcomas often have an indeterminate profile on MRI, and the diagnosis must be confirmed by biopsy. In general, sarcomas have a low T1 signal intensity and a mixed or high T2 intensity, with significant gadolinium enhancement. A patient with a suspected soft-tissue sarcoma should be referred to a sarcoma center for a wide surgical excision with adjuvant or neoadjuvant radiation therapy and/or chemotherapy. Soft-tissue sarcomas of the ankle have a higher recurrence rate compared with the foot after treatment, and previous unplanned excisions may increase rate of recurrence.

Synovial Sarcoma

Synovial sarcoma is the most common sarcoma of the foot. More than 25% of synovial sarcomas occur below the knee, with 13% in the foot alone.[9] Like other sarcomas, synovial sarcoma often is smaller in the distal extremities than in the rest of the body. Mineralization occurs in many synovial sarcomas.[24] As described in a 2021 study, synovial sarcomas predominantly appear as well-defined heterogeneously enhancing multilobulated tumors.[25] Treatments for synovial sarcoma rely on wide margin surgical resection. Limb salvage should not be attempted at the expense of wide margins. Because of the need for a large resection, amputation is commonly performed at either the ankle or lower leg.[26]

Acral Myxoinflammatory Fibroblastic Sarcoma

Acral myxoinflammatory fibroblastic sarcoma is a poorly defined, slow-growing, painless mass that involves the underlying tendon sheath. Most patients are age 30 to 50 years. Thirty percent of these rare tumors occur in the

Section 5: Special Problems of the Foot and Ankle

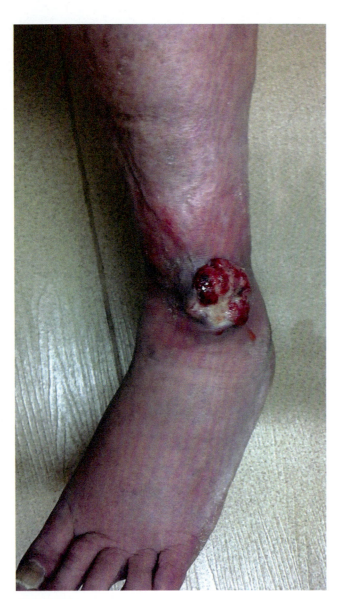

FIGURE 3 Photograph showing a high-grade myxofibrosarcoma. These fungating soft-tissue sarcomas have a poor prognosis.

foot or ankle.[9] On MRI, the tumor is seen as less well encapsulated than most sarcomas (**Figure 4**). Most cases have variable numbers of local recurrences, but metastatic potential is relatively rare with a local recurrence rate between 22% and 67%. Current treatment consists of wide local excision with close observation for local recurrence and metastatic disease.[27]

Epithelioid Sarcoma

Nine percent of epithelioid sarcomas occur in the foot or ankle.[9] Most patients are age 10 to 35 years, and two-thirds of these tumors occur in boys or men. Metastasis occurs through lymphatic chains. PET and sentinel node evaluation should be considered. The use of isolated limb infusion, a relatively new technique for treating regional metastasis, may preclude the need for amputation.[28,29]

Clear Cell Sarcoma

Clear cell sarcoma is rare. Most patients are age 20 to 40 years, with the tumor usually found deep to the fascia and producing melanin. Sometimes clear cell sarcoma is thought to be a deep-tissue variant of malignant melanoma. Because the tumor often is spread throughout the lymphatic system, the sentinel nodes should be evaluated. Isolated limb infusion may be an option for a patient with clear cell sarcoma. The prognosis is poor because of a high incidence of pulmonary metastasis.

Malignant Melanoma

Acral lentiginous melanoma is the most common malignancy of the foot. Most patients are in the fourth decade of life, and more women than men are affected. A patient with a pigmented or otherwise concerning skin lesion should be referred to a melanoma specialist. The acral variant of melanoma has a worse prognosis than all other types of melanoma.[30] In a recent study, metastasis to sentinel lymph nodes was shown to be a significant prognostic factor for melanoma-specific survival and disease-free survival. Sentinel lymph node biopsy was recommended specifically for patients with thick (>1 mm) or ulcerated lesions. Here patients with ulcerated lesions have a 10% greater risk of death at the 5-year time point.[31]

Isolated limb infusion commonly is used to treat patients with in-transit melanoma.

BENIGN OSSEOUS TUMORS

Osteochondroma

Osteochondroma is the most common tumor of bone, and it can occur anywhere in the body. The tumors can be isolated or multiple. Osteochondroma develops during childhood or adolescence, and the tumors grow until the patient reaches skeletal maturity. Although many masses go unnoticed, the thin covering of the foot and ankle often allows detection. The growths are pedunculated (growing from a single stalk) or sessile (having a broad base similar in size to the tumor). Resection of the tumor, with or without subsequent protected weight bearing, may be appropriate for tumors that are unsightly or are irritating surrounding structures. Observation is recommended for asymptomatic tumors. The diagnosis requires the identification of a continuum between the marrow space of the bone and the marrow space of the osteochondroma. Plain radiographs often are sufficient for diagnosis, but advanced imaging sometimes is necessary.

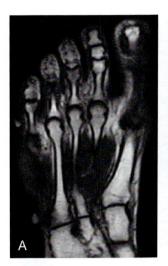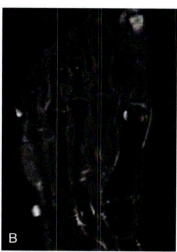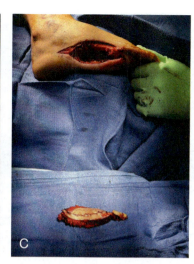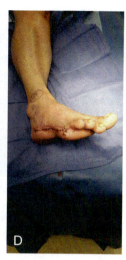

FIGURE 4 T1-weighted (**A**) and T2-weighted (**B**) magnetic resonance images of myxoinflammatory fibroblastic sarcoma. The patient was treated with a ray resection of the fifth ray. Intraoperative photographs show resection (**C**) and closure (**D**).

Biopsies are not necessary for tumors with cartilage caps smaller than 3 cm that have not changed in size. Chondrosarcomatous differentiation should be considered if a tumor enlarges substantially after adolescence. Patients with multiple hereditary exostosis have a loss of function related to one of three known exostosin (EXT) tumor suppressor genes. Whereas previous studies had reported a 25% risk of malignant degeneration, later studies indicate that malignant degeneration involves only 2% to 4% of those with multiple hereditary exostosis.[32]

Subungual Exostosis

Subungual exostosis is a benign osteochondral lesion that does not arise from a physis but rather from the tip of the distal phalanx. This tumor often is painful and causes nail deformity. The treatment involves removing the nail to gain access to the bone below, and usually it is curative.

Enchondroma/Chondroma

Enchondroma is a benign proliferation of hyaline cartilage that occurs when dysplastic embryonal cartilage becomes trapped in a bone. Eight percent of these tumors occur in the bones of the foot, most commonly in the forefoot,[33] with the most commonly involved bones being the proximal phalanges.[34] The lesions usually are centrally located in the bone along the trajectory of an epiphyseal plate. Enchondromas most commonly are incidentally found after they have begun normal mineralization in a specified pattern but may become symptomatic with pain and swelling. MRI shows a low T1 and a high T2 signal with a well-defined popcorn-type margin. Observation is the treatment of choice for lesions with a benign appearance. There is a very low risk of malignant transformation. Malignant presentations are more common in the midfoot and hindfoot.[35] Radiographic features causing concern include cortical thinning, soft-tissue masses, and growth. The most common symptom of malignant degeneration is pain from weakening of the bone. Pathologic fractures are common. Biopsy is appropriate for suspicious lesions; for small foot and ankle lesions, simple curettage may be an appropriate excisional biopsy (**Figure 5**). The risk of local recurrence for lesions excised with simple curettage is very low. Patients with Ollier disease or Maffucci syndrome are at increased risk for malignant transformation and should be observed closely.

Periosteal Chondroma

Periosteal chondroma is a rare benign eccentric tumor of bone that is more common in the long bones of the body than in the foot or ankle. Usually this tumor is found incidentally, and excision biopsy or curettage is the usual treatment.[36]

Chondroblastoma

Chondroblastoma is a rare benign lesion that accounts for fewer than 1% of primary bone tumors and is one of very few epiphyseal or apophyseal tumors. More than 80% of patients are younger than 25 years, and often they have open growth plates.[33] In the foot, chondroblastoma usually occurs in the talus or calcaneus. Despite its benign nature, chondroblastoma carries a small (less than 1%) risk of pulmonary metastasis, and plain radiography of the chest should be part of the initial workup. Radiographs and CT show dystrophic calcification in the epiphysis, with possible enlargement of the bone. MRI often shows low signal with T1 weighting and high

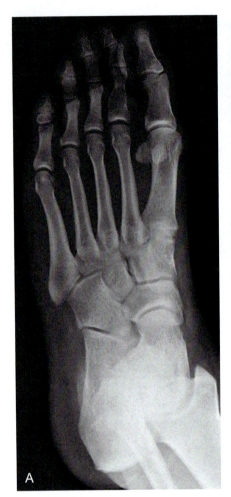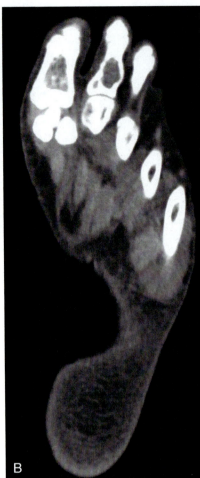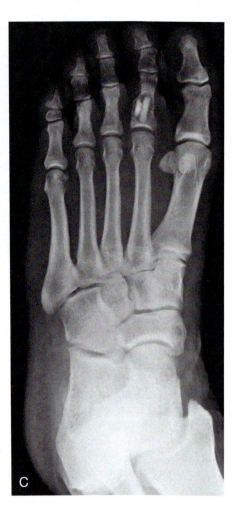

FIGURE 5 Preoperative radiograph (**A**), CT (**B**), and postoperative radiograph (**C**) of enchondroma treated by calcium phosphate and allograft.

signal with T2 weighting. Many lesions are cystic or have secondary aneurysmal bone cysts; this characteristic can make diagnosis difficult because of the small epiphysis of the small bones. Microscopically, these tumors have a characteristic chicken wire appearance between the chondroid cells. Lesions are treated with curettage and high-speed burning. Often adjuvant peroxide, phenol, cryotherapy, or argon beam laser treatment is useful for extending the margin and decreasing the risk of local recurrence.

Giant Cell Tumor of Bone

Giant cell tumor of bone is a locally aggressive epiphyseal neoplasm that accounts for 5% of primary bone tumors with only 6% of these tumors occurring in the foot or ankle.[33] Giant cell tumors of bone most commonly occur in the distal tibia, talus, and the metatarsals. This disease is most common in patients age 20 to 40 years. In contrast to patients with chondroblastoma, patients with giant cell tumor of bone usually have closed growth plates, and there is no significant mineralization within the lesion. The risk of benign metastasis to the lung is approximately 1%, but in patients with metastasis the risk of mortality is 15% to 20%. Malignant giant cell tumors are found in 1% of patients with giant cell tumor of bone.[37] This high-grade sarcoma often represents a recurrence of a tumor treated with radiation. Radiographically, these lesions are purely lytic, and they may enlarge to destroy the metaphysis. MRI shows low signal with T1 weighting and high signal with T2 weighting, often with fluid levels that may represent secondary aneurysmal bone cysts. The pathologic findings classically are described as the nuclei of the giant cells having an appearance similar to that of the nuclei of the surrounding stromal cells. The treatment usually entails biopsy followed by wide curettage, mechanical burring, adjuvant treatment, and cementing and/or bone grafting of the lesion. Completely destructive lesions may require bone replacement with allograft or endoprosthesis. In a review of 31 patients with a distal tibial giant cell tumor of bone who underwent an extended curettage, the recurrence rate was 29%.[38] In another study that compared the recurrence of giant cell tumor of bone of the foot with giant cell tumor of bone of appendicular skeleton after en block excisions, researchers showed that one out of seven patients with giant cell tumor of bone of the foot (14.3%) developed recurrence, whereas just four out of 124 patients with giant cell tumor of bone of appendicular skeleton (4.8%) developed recurrence.[39] These rates are higher than that reported in previous studies. The use of alternative treatments including embolization, diphosphonates, and denosumab is becoming more common in the treatment of giant cell tumors, especially those in difficult locations such as the spine and pelvis.

Unicameral Bone Cyst

Unicameral bone cyst is a destructive tumor that most commonly occurs in the calcaneus of teenagers. The tumor may or may not be symptomatic and often is identified incidentally. Patients most often complain of heel pain. The lesions usually are lateral on the calcaneus and adjacent to the middle facet. MRI shows a fluid-filled lesion with few or no fluid-fluid levels; peripheral rim enhancement is seen with gadolinium enhancement. The risk of fracture is low in patients with these lesions. Observation is appropriate for an asymptomatic patient. A painful cyst usually is treated with percutaneous techniques including the injection of steroids, bone marrow, a sclerosing agent, and/or a bone graft substitute (**Figure 6**). Surgical interventions can lead to 93% healing rate on plain radiographs.[40] Open surgery may be indicated for a displaced fracture.

Aneurysmal Bone Cyst

Approximately 10% of aneurysmal bone cysts are found in the distal tibia or foot.[33] The most common bones affected are the metatarsals. Patients with this lesion commonly report pain during weight bearing or activity. Most patients are in the first or second decades of life. In the long bones, radiographs classically show aggressive, eccentric, expansile lucent lesions with a surrounding thin sclerotic layer of reactive bone. MRI shows multiple fluid-fluid levels throughout the lesion. These lesions classically are treated with extended curettage, with or without adjuvant treatments or bone grafting. Curettage alone may lead to a recurrence rate of 21%.[41] Some patients currently are treated with sclerosing agents, however. This technique often involves multiple fluoroscopic injections of sodium tetradecyl sulfate or a similar agent into the lesions, causing involution of the tumor and mineralization of the bone. A sclerosing agent often is used to treat lesions, including some foot and ankle tumors, that are difficult to reach surgically, are small and carry a low risk of fracture, or have caused too much bone destruction to allow allograft reconstruction. Aneurysmal bone cysts can arise secondary to another type of bone lesion, including but not limited to non-ossifying fibroma, chondromyxoid fibroma, chondroblastoma, or giant cell tumor. Caution is necessary in diagnosing aneurysmal bone cyst because the differential diagnosis includes telangiectatic osteosarcoma, which can have an identical appearance on imaging studies. Biopsy is recommended before treatment is initiated.

Chondromyxoid Fibroma

Chondromyxoid fibroma is a tumor of adolescence that occurs in the foot or ankle in as many as 25% of patients.[33] There may be a delay in treatment from the first visit seeking care because of misdiagnosis, often mistaken for a unicameral bone cyst. In the long bones, chondromyxoid fibroma commonly is an eccentric metaphyseal lesion and has a sclerotic margin with cortical scalloping or expansion. There is little matrix calcification. On MRI, lesions often have a high signal with T2 weighting. The preferred treatment is aggressive curettage with high-speed burring and optional adjuvant treatment or grafting. A zero to 20% recurrence rate recently has been documented in the foot and ankle.[42,43]

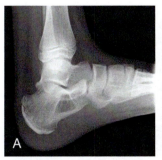 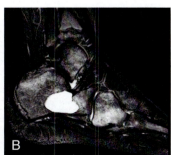 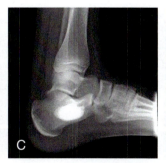 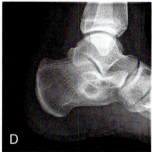

FIGURE 6 A painful unicameral cyst in the calcaneus. **A**, Lateral radiograph with a geographic lesion of the calcaneus. **B**, T2 sagittal MRI demonstrating fluid signal within the calcaneus lesion. **C**, Postoperative radiograph after irrigation and percutaneous injection of calcium sulfate–calcium phosphate. **D**, Radiograph showing near-complete resolution 1 year after surgery.

Nonossifying Fibroma

Approximately 25% of nonossifying fibromas (also called fibroxanthomas) occur in the distal tibia or fibula.[33] but this tumor is rare in the bones of the foot. Patients often are adolescents with an ankle sprain; the tumor is an incidental geographic lesion separate from the area of pain. Observation is the most common treatment. Surgical curettage and grafting are reserved for lesions that are painful or at a high risk for fracture.

Osteoid Osteoma

Osteoid osteoma is a small, cortically based tumor that occurs in the foot or ankle in approximately 10% of patients.[33] The most common bone affected is the talus.[44] Patients classically describe night pain that is relieved by the use of NSAIDs. Sometimes the pain is referred from or perceived as coming from an adjacent joint. Tumors near a joint may cause early arthritis. The lesion is smaller than 2 cm on radiography and has a sclerotic rim around a lucent area with a central, small, dense sclerotic nidus resembling a target. Significant local sclerosis may be present. These lesions may be found within cortical bone, cancellous, or subcortical cancellous locations. Previous studies have suggested CT is preferable to MRI for imaging of these lesions because of potential inaccuracy. However, recent improvements to the spatial resolution of modern equipment and the use of volumetric isotropic sequences could potentially make MRI preferred to CT. According to a 2021 study, this especially true in pediatric populations, where minimizing ionizing radiation is an important consideration.[45] If adequate relief cannot be obtained with NSAID therapy, the treatment of choice is radiofrequency ablation, which has excellent results. Radiofrequency ablation may not be optimal if the nidus is found to be within close proximity of neurovascular structures within the foot. Open treatments include en bloc resection, unroofing and curettage, and curettage with cortical peeling. There is low risk of recurrence of symptoms after treatment.

Osteoblastoma

Osteoblastoma in the foot or ankle is rare. The symptoms are similar to those of osteoid osteoma, but pain is not usually relieved with NSAIDs. Osteoblastomas have a varied appearance, and many have aggressive radiographic characteristics.[33] The tumor is treated with curettage and grafting.

Intraosseous Lipoma

Intraosseous lipoma in the calcaneus is common and often is found incidentally in a patient with plantar fasciitis or Achilles tendinitis. Radiographically, this benign-appearing lesion has well-defined borders and central lucency with occasional areas of mineralized septa. MRI or CT can confirm the presence of adipose tissue. Asymptomatic patients do not require treatment. Patients with corresponding bone edema or fracture are best treated with simple curettage and grafting.

MALIGNANT OSSEOUS TUMORS

Primary malignant bone tumors of the foot or ankle classically have been treated with amputation. Patients can achieve an excellent functional outcome after transtibial amputation. Limb salvage is now offered to most patients as a primary treatment. A patient with a suspicious lesion should be referred to a musculoskeletal oncologist before biopsy to decrease the risk of morbidity. Delay in diagnosis of osteosarcoma, Ewing sarcoma, and chondrosarcoma has been found to be significantly longer in the foot compared with other osseous sites.[7]

Chondrosarcoma

Chondrosarcoma occurs in the foot or ankle in only 3% of patients[31] and is the most common primary malignant tumor of the foot.[46] Sixty percent of high-grade tumors are partially calcified, with cortical destruction.[33] Relatively large lesions may have associated soft-tissue masses. The treatment is primarily based on tumor grade. Grade 1 chondrosarcomas in the lower extremity can be treated with extended curettage using a high-speed burr, with adjuvant treatment using cryotherapy, argon beam, phenol, or cementation grafting. Resection of the lesion may be necessary with allograft or autograft reconstruction. Grade 2 and 3 lesions are treated with wide resection and reconstruction or amputation. For grade 4 (dedifferentiated) lesions, primary amputation should be considered because of the high risk of local recurrence and metastasis.

Osteosarcoma

Approximately 3% of osteosarcomas occur in the foot or ankle[33] with the tarsal bones being most commonly affected site in the foot.[47] Most patients are adolescents. The tumor usually is painful, and patients often report night pain. Aggressive lucent or mixed lesions often have periosteal new bone formation and mineralized soft-tissue masses. Pathologic analysis shows malignant osteoid. The treatment routinely includes neoadjuvant and adjuvant chemotherapy, with surgery for removal of the primary tumor and any metastases.

Ewing Sarcoma

Approximately 8% of Ewing sarcomas occur in the distal tibia, fibula, or foot.[33] Patients report pain with activity and at night. These tumors often have fast-growing soft-tissue masses that expand from the bone. Radiographs show lucency within the bone and often impressive periosteal reactions. The histopathologic funding is of a small round blue cell tumor, with little surrounding stroma. The course of treatment is similar to that of osteosarcoma. Radiation can be substituted for surgical excision, but because of slightly inferior outcomes, radiation usually is reserved for tumors in areas that are extremely difficult to resect, such as the spine.

Metastatic Carcinoma

The incidence of metastatic bone tumors greatly increases with advancing patient age. Metastatic carcinoma is the most common destructive bone lesion in patients older than 40 years, many of whom have no known history of cancer. The initial symptom is pain. Because of their metastatic nature, these tumors are stage IV. With advances in the treatment of carcinomas, many patients live with the disease for years or decades. As patient survival rates improve, so does the need for durable reconstruction of the destroyed bone. If possible, an intervention to stabilize a foot or ankle metastatic site must create a strong construct that will bear the patient's weight soon and for many years to come.

Patients older than 40 years are more likely to have a destructive metastatic carcinoma than a primary bone sarcoma. The primary tumor site and sites of metastasis must be identified. For a patient with newly diagnosed lesions, a thorough history and physical examination are important for identifying risk-increasing behaviors, a family history of cancer, or other relevant factors. A laboratory evaluation should be considered, including a complete blood cell count to identify any blood disorder or anemia, a metabolic panel to identify renal dysfunction in multiple myeloma, and disease-specific markers such as prostate-specific antigen, thyroid-specific hormone, and electrophoresis in multiple myeloma. The most useful means of identifying a primary tumor is contrast CT of the chest, abdomen, and pelvis. A bone scan is recommended for a patient thought to have metastatic carcinoma to identify sites at risk for fracture and possibly to identify a biopsy site that will not increase the risk of fracture.

The most common primary sites of metastatic carcinoma are the breast, kidney, thyroid gland, lung, and prostate gland. Because of its acral metastases, lung cancer most often leads to destructive carcinoma of the foot and ankle. Many lung cancers are radio responsive, and excellent pain relief usually is achieved early in the course of radiation. With a large, painful lesion that is at risk for pathologic fracture, the patient may be able to bear weight soon after biopsy, curettage, adjuvant treatment, and stabilization with plates, screws, and cementation of

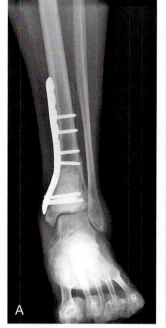
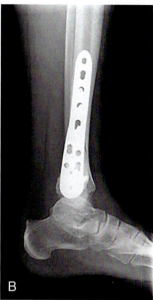

FIGURE 7 AP (**A**) and lateral (**B**) radiographs showing a treated metastatic lesion to the distal tibia. The patient was able to bear weight as tolerated immediately after surgery.

the defect. In treating characteristically vascular tumors, as in kidney or thyroid cancers, embolization should be considered to limit blood loss during surgical stabilization (**Figure 7**). Amputation rarely is necessary.

Multiple Myeloma

Multiple myeloma is the most common primary bone tumor in patients older than 40 years. Many patients have multiple purely radiolucent lesions. Patients who have a lesion, anemia, and renal dysfunction rarely require biopsy; the diagnosis usually can be made with serum protein electrophoresis, urine protein electrophoresis, and serum light chains. Lesions with a low risk of fracture usually can be treated with chemotherapy and/or radiation. Painful lesions with significant structural loss may be quite vascular, and the treatment should be similar to that of metastatic carcinoma.

RECONSTRUCTIVE TREATMENTS

Amputation and Prosthetic Replacement

Some patients choose amputation to treat their malignant tumor. Excellent functional outcomes can be achieved after amputation. Prosthesis design continues to progress and to lead to increases in normal patient function. A German group has pioneered the use of transcutaneous prostheses that are biologically anchored to bone, thus allowing the patient to attach the prosthesis with a mechanical latch and completely eliminating the need for a socket. Prostheses with this design primarily are used after transfemoral amputation. However, some patients with transtibial amputations with fit issues and short residual bone may be candidates for an endo-exo prosthesis. This technique creates a permanent bone prosthesis interface with an endoprosthesis that extends outside of the bone through a chronic fistula. This endo-exo metal shaft connects mechanically to a prosthetic leg, negating the need for a socket.[48]

Osseous Grafting

Masquelet Technique

The Masquelet technique of bone formation, also called the induced membrane technique, most commonly is used in long bones. This technique also is useful for smaller bone defects of the foot and ankle caused by tumor, trauma, or infection. The two-step surgical process is designed to create structural bone from cancellous graft. A block of polymethyl methacrylate is placed to conform to the shape of the bone defect. The wound is closed, the skin is allowed to heal, and a granulation membrane is induced and matures before the polymethyl methacrylate block is removed. In vitro studies have demonstrated improved alkaline phosphatase activity and calcium deposition if the autograft is placed 1 month after the spacer.[49]

Vascularized Autograft

The most common source of vascularized free-osseous transfers is the fibula, but other bones also are used. Because of its native shape, a vascularized portion of the iliac crest can be used to re-create the medial arch of the foot after resection of portions of the midfoot and forefoot. A vascularized portion of the medial femoral condyle has been used to treat osteonecrosis, nonunion, and small bone defects.[50]

Allograft

The use of osteoarticular allograft in a large joint is fraught with complications, but it can be successful in a small segment (less than 3 to 5 cm). Frozen or freeze-dried morcellized allograft is commonly used to fill defects after curettage of a benign tumor.

Synthetic Bone Fillers

The broad group of synthetic bone fillers includes products with a range of material properties that the treating surgeon may consider desirable. Some products can be percutaneously injected into cystic structures and allowed to harden. Other products can be mixed with an antibiotic to create beads that are absorbed into the body and act as a scaffolding for bone formation.

Allograft-Autograft Composite

The treatment of some tumors of the distal tibia creates massive bone loss. Although some patients choose transtibial amputation as a reliable and functionally satisfactory treatment, others prefer to avoid amputation if at all possible. Intercalary bulk allografting has a high failure rate in massive tibial defects as a result of allograft fracture and junctional nonunion. A technique for structural allografting coupled with intramedullary fibular autografting has led to improved rates of union and allograft vascularization, thereby decreasing fracture rates and improving healing after fracture.[51] The use of this technique allows patients to retain the native ankle joint after cryogenic treatment or radiation of autograft (**Figure 8**).

Allograft Prosthetic Reconstruction

The availability of modular tibial components with long stems for ankle arthroplasty has increased the feasibility of allograft prosthetic reconstruction of the ankle.

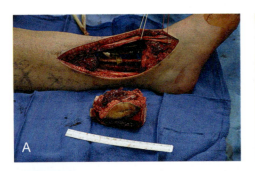
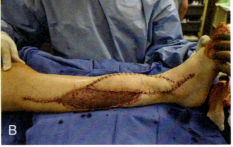
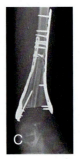
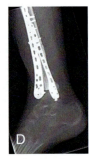

FIGURE 8 Intraoperative photographs and postoperative radiographs showing the surgical treatment of periosteal osteosarcoma of the distal tibia and fibula. The allograft-autograft reconstruction used tissue from the patient's ipsilateral vascularized fibula. **A**, Intraoperative image after resection of the periosteal osteosarcoma. **B**, Intraoperative image after reconstruction of the distal tibia including free fibula osseocutaneous transfer and skin grafting of host site. Six-month postoperative AP (**C**) and lateral (**D**) radiographs with evidence of osseous healing.

Outcomes research is needed to determine whether this technique is superior to allograft fusion or transtibial amputation.

Bone Transport

Ring fixators and rails for bone transport, with or without a rod, can be used for reconstruction of distal tibial bone. The lengthening process can be prolonged depending on the defect size. Patient compliance varies.

Bracing Treatment and Shoe Inserts

Orthotic devices can be used after tumor resection in the foot and ankle. Simple inserts are used for offloading if anatomic changes have led to pain in a portion of the foot after tumor resection. Some orthotic devices are contoured to compensate for the loss of a major portion of the foot.

ISOLATED LIMB INFUSION

In isolated limb infusion, high-dosage chemotherapy is circulated through the extremity in a closed loop after tourniquet inflation proximally to the catheters. Isolation of the leg allows for administration of much higher dosages than is possible systemically without damaging solid organs. Isolated limb infusion is a well-established treatment of in-transit metastatic melanoma of the extremities, and it is now being used for other lymphatically spread diseases, such as Merkel cell carcinoma and epithelioid sarcoma. This technique was found to be useful in shrinking unresectable extremity tumors to allow limb salvage.[28] Isolated limb infusion has great potential for treating foot and ankle tumors, but it should be used with caution because of the risk of severe toxicity to the skin.[29]

NONONCOLOGICALLY EXCISED MALIGNANT TUMORS

Nononcologic excision of malignant tumors continues to be a major concern for orthopaedic oncologists. Patients are referred to oncologists not only by orthopaedic surgeons but also by podiatrists and general surgeons after removal of a small mass that was thought to be benign. Most such masses are soft-tissue sarcomas, and routine re-excision is recommended if negative margins were not obtained during the original surgery. This protocol decreases the risk of recurrence to the same level as in a wide primary excision. Unfortunately, re-excision requires greater flap coverage, and in some patients amputation may be necessary to control the disease.

SUMMARY

A thorough understanding of the common benign and malignant tumors of the foot and ankle is essential to the evaluation, diagnosis, and treatment of masses in the foot. Despite the small size of tumors on presentation, the possibility of malignancy should be considered before any surgical intervention is undertaken.

KEY STUDY POINTS

- Thorough history and physical examination of a patient with a suspected foot or ankle tumor will help guide treatment and need for further imaging studies.
- Benign tumors of the foot and ankle may be symptomatic warranting surgical intervention or may be treated nonsurgically.
- Malignant tumors of the foot and ankle may require chemotherapy or radiation treatment in addition to surgical interventions for limb salvage.
- Reconstruction techniques for treating tumors of the foot and ankle include bone transport, masquelet, vascularized autograft, allografts, and autograft-allograft composites.

ANNOTATED REFERENCES

1. Toepfer A, Harrasser N, Recker M, et al: Distribution patterns of foot and ankle tumors: A University Tumor Institute experience. *BMC Cancer* 2018;18(1):735.

2. Pesapane F, Downey K, Rotili A, Cassano E, Koh DM: Imaging diagnosis of metastatic breast cancer. *Insights Imaging* 2020;11(1):79.

   Imaging modalities that characterize metastases in breast cancer were reviewed to update evidence on comparative imaging accuracy using 40 scientific papers. Level of evidence: IV.

3. Hughes P, Miranda R, Doyle AJ: MRI imaging of soft tissue tumours of the foot and ankle. *Insights Imaging* 2019;10(1):60.

   A systematic literature review provided a comprehensive overview of MRI characteristics of the most common benign and soft-tissue neoplasms, which occur around the foot and ankle. Level of evidence: IV.

4. Gauerke S, Driscoll JJ: Hidradenocarcinomas: A brief review and future directions. *Arch Pathol Lab Med* 2010;134(5):781-785.

5. De Luca F, Bolin M, Blomqvist L, Wassberg C, Martin H, Falk Delgado A: Validation of PET/MRI attenuation correction methodology in the study of brain tumours. *BMC Med Imaging* 2020;20(1):126.

A retrospective cohort of 14 patients with suspected or confirmed brain tumor and 11C-methionine PET/MRI compared proton density–weighted MRI with reference standard CT. Level of evidence: III.

6. Klein A, Birkenmaier C, Fromm J, Knosel T, Di Gioia D, Durr HR: Sarcomas of the extremities and the pelvis: Comparing local recurrence after incisional and after core-needle biopsy. *World J Surg Oncol* 2022;20(1):14.

A retrospective case series of 162 patients with minimum follow-up of 6 months after wide resection of extremity sarcomas evaluated the influence of biopsy type and other clinical factors on the rate of local recurrence and survival. Level of evidence: IV.

7. Brotzmann M, Hefti F, Baumhoer D, Krieg AH: Do malignant bone tumors of the foot have a different biological behavior than sarcomas at other skeletal sites? *Sarcoma* 2013;2013:767960.

8. Masood S, Mallinson PI, Sheikh A, Ouellette H, Munk PL: Percutaneous bone biopsy. *Tech Vasc Interv Radiol* 2022;25(1):100800.

This is a systematic literature review to cover the core concepts of percutaneous bone biopsy including indications, appropriate imaging modalities, common approaches, and complications. Level of evidence: IV.

9. Sakamoto A, Okamoto T, Matsuda S: Persistent symptoms of ganglion cysts in the dorsal foot. *Open Orthop J* 2017;11:1308-1313.

10. Weishaupt D, Schweitzer ME, Morrison WB, Haims AH, Wapner K, Kahn M: MRI of the foot and ankle: Prevalence and distribution of occult and palpable ganglia. *J Magn Reson Imaging* 2001;14(4):464-471.

11. Lui TH: Arthroscopic ganglionectomy of the foot and ankle. *Knee Surg Sports Traumatol Arthrosc* 2014;22(7):1693-1700.

12. Karami M, Soleimani M, Shiari R: Pigmented villonodular synovitis in pediatric population: Review of literature and a case report. *Pediatr Rheumatol Online J* 2018;16(1):6.

13. Staals EL, Ferrari S, Donati DM, Palmerini E: Diffuse-type tenosynovial giant cell tumour: Current treatment concepts and future perspectives. *Eur J Cancer* 2016;63:34-40.

14. Al Farii H, Doyle-Kelly C; Marwan Y; Volesky M; Turcotte R: Arthroscopic management of synovial chondromatosis of the ankle joint: A systematic review of the literature. *JBJS Rev* 2020;8(9):e2000045.

This is a systematic literature review of 22 postoperative patients following arthroscopic management of ankle synovial chondromatosis to better understand recurrence patterns and suggest an alternative approach to open arthrotomy. Level of evidence: IV.

15. Carroll P, Henshaw RM, Garwood C, Raspovic K, Kumar D: Plantar fibromatosis: Pathophysiology, surgical and nonsurgical therapies – An evidence-based review. *Foot Ankle Spec* 2018;11(2):168-176.

16. Behr GG, Johnson C: Vascular anomalies: Hemangiomas and beyond. Part 1: Fast-flow lesions. *AJR Am J Roentgenol* 2013;200(2):414-422.

17. Behr GG, Johnson CM: Vascular anomalies: Hemangiomas and beyond. Part 2: Slow-flow lesions. *AJR Am J Roentgenol* 2013;200(2):423-436.

18. Hwang JT, Yoon KJ, Park CH, et al: Follow-up of clinical and sonographic features after extracorporeal shock wave therapy in painful plantar fibromatosis. *PLoS One* 2020;15(8):e0237447.

A retrospective cohort study of 26 patients with plantar fibromatosis confirmed by ultrasonography evaluated long-term clinical outcome of extracorporeal shockwave therapy in plantar fibromatosis and ultrasonographic changes of plantar fibroma following therapy. Level of evidence: III.

19. Pritchard DJ, Nascimento AG, Petersen IA: Local control of extra-abdominal desmoid tumors. *J Bone Joint Surg Am* 1996;78(6):848-854.

20. Bonvalot S, Desai A, Coppola S, et al: The treatment of desmoid tumors: A stepwise clinical approach. *Ann Oncol* 2012;23(suppl 10):x158-x166.

21. Trehan SK, Soukup DS, Mintz DN, Perino G, Ellis SJ: Glomus tumors in the foot: Case series. *Foot Ankle Spec* 2015;8(6):460-465.

22. Netscher DT, Aburto J, Koepplinger M: Subungual glomus tumor. *J Hand Surg Am* 2012;37(4):821-823.

23. Houdek MT, Beahrs TR, Wyles CC, Rose PS, Sim FH, Turner NS: What factors are predictive of outcome in the treatment of soft tissue sarcomas of the foot and ankle? *Foot Ankle Spec* 2017;10(1):12-19.

24. Wilkerson BW, Crim JR, Hung M, Layfield LJ: Characterization of synovial sarcoma calcification. *AJR Am J Roentgenol* 2012;199(6):W730-W734.

25. Gazendam AM, Popovic S, Munir S, Parasu N, Wilson D, Ghert M: Synovial sarcoma: A clinical review. *Curr Oncol* 2021;28(3):1909-1920.

A systematic literature review of synovial sarcoma included diagnostic options, predictive factors of prognosis, and systemic therapies. Level of evidence: IV.

26. Rammelt S, Fritzsche H, Hofbauer C, Schaser KD: Malignant tumours of the foot and ankle. *Foot Ankle Surg* 2020;26(4):363-370.

27. Ieremia E, Thway K: Myxoinflammatory fibroblastic sarcoma: Morphologic and genetic updates. *Arch Pathol Lab Med* 2014;138(10):1406-1411.

28. Vohra NA, Turaga KK, Gonzalez RJ, et al: The use of isolated limb infusion in limb-threatening extremity sarcomas. *Int J Hyperthermia* 2013;29(1):1-7.

29. Kroon HM, Thompson JF: Isolated limb infusion: A review. *J Surg Oncol* 2009;100(2):169-177.

30. Durbec F, Martin L, Derancourt C, Grange F: Melanoma of the hand and foot: Epidemiological, prognostic and genetic features. A systematic review. *Br J Dermatol* 2012;166(4):727-739.

31. Ito T, Wada M, Nagae K, et al: Acral lentiginous melanoma: Who benefits from sentinel lymph node biopsy? *J Am Acad Dermatol* 2015;72(1):71-77.

32. Porter DE, Lonie L, Fraser M, et al: Severity of disease and risk of malignant change in hereditary multiple exostoses. A genotype phenotype study. *J Bone Joint Surg Br* 2004;86(7):1041-1046.

33. Wold LE, Unni KK, Sim FH, Sundaram M: *Atlas of Orthopaedic Pathology*, ed 3. Saunders, 2008.

34. Chun KA, Stephanie S, Choi JY, Nam JH, Suh JS: Enchondroma of the foot. *J Foot Ankle Surg* 2015;54(5):836-839.

35. Gajewski DA, Burnette JB, Murphey MD, Temple HT: Differentiating clinical and radiographic features of enchondroma and secondary chondrosarcoma in the foot. *Foot Ankle Int* 2006;27(4):240-244.

36. Parodi KK, Farrett W, Paden MH, Stone PA: A report of a rare phalangeal periosteal chondroma of the foot. *J Foot Ankle Surg* 2011;50(1):122-125.

37. Siebenrock KA, Unni KK, Rock MG: Giant-cell tumour of bone metastasising to the lungs. A long-term follow-up. *J Bone Joint Surg Br* 1998;80(1):43-47.

38. Rajani R, Schaefer L, Scarborough MT, Gibbs CP: Giant cell tumors of the foot and ankle bones: High recurrence rates after surgical treatment. *J Foot Ankle Surg* 2015;54(6):1141-1145.

39. Co HL, Wang EH: Giant cell tumor of the small bones of the foot. *J Orthop Surg (Hong Kong)* 2018;26(3):2309499018801168.

40. Levy DM, Gross CE, Garras DN: Treatment of unicameral bone cysts of the calcaneus: A systematic review. *J Foot Ankle Surg* 2015;54(4):652-656.

41. Chowdhry M, Chandrasekar CR, Mohammed R, Grimer RJ: Curettage of aneurysmal bone cysts of the feet. *Foot Ankle Int* 2010;31(2):131-135.

42. Roberts EJ, Meier MJ, Hild G, Masadeh S, Hardy M, Bakotic BW: Chondromyxoid fibroma of the calcaneus: Two case reports and literature review. *J Foot Ankle Surg* 2013;52(5):643-649.

43. Jamshidi K, Mazhar FN, Yahyazadeh H: Chondromyxoid fibroma of calcaneus. *Foot Ankle Surg* 2013;19(1):48-52.

44. Jordan RW, Koc T, Chapman AWP, Taylor HP: Osteoid osteoma of the foot and ankle – A systematic review. *Foot Ankle Surg* 2015;21(4):228-234.

45. Carneiro BC, Da Cruz IAN, Ormond Filho AG, et al: Osteoid osteoma: The great mimicker. *Insights Imaging* 2021;12(1):32.

This is a systematic literature review to understand osteoid osteoma and their imaging findings to increase diagnostic accuracy, enable early treatment, and prevent poor prognosis. Level of evidence: IV.

46. Ozer D, Aycan OE, Er ST, Tanrıtanır R, Arıkan Y, Kabukçuoğlu YS: Primary tumor and tumor-like lesions of bones of the foot: Single-center experience of 166 cases. *J Foot Ankle Surg* 2017;56(6):1180-1187.

47. Schuster AJ, Kager L, Reichardt P, et al: High-grade osteosarcoma of the foot: Presentation, treatment, prognostic factors, and outcome of 23 cooperative osteosarcoma study group COSS patients. *Sarcoma* 2018;2018:1632978.

48. Fröllce JP, van de Meent H: The endo-exo prosthesis for patients with a problematic amputation stump [Dutch]. *Ned Tijdschr Geneeskd* 2010;154:A2010.

49. Aho OM, Lehenkari P, Ristiniemi J, Lehtonen S, Risteli J, Leskelä HV: The mechanism of action of induced membranes in bone repair. *J Bone Joint Surg Am* 2013;95(7):597-604.

50. Haddock NT, Alosh H, Easley ME, Levin LS, Wapner KL: Applications of the medial femoral condyle free flap for foot and ankle reconstruction. *Foot Ankle Int* 2013;34(10):1395-1402.

51. Bakri K, Stans AA, Mardini S, Moran SL: Combined massive allograft and intramedullary vascularized fibula transfer: The Capanna technique for lower-limb reconstruction. *Semin Plast Surg* 2008;22(3):234-241.

CHAPTER 17

Osteonecrosis of the Talus

DANIEL K. MOON, MD, MS, MBA, FAAOS

ABSTRACT

Osteonecrosis of the talus is a challenging entity to treat. Poor outcomes remain all too common. Although most talar osteonecrosis is secondary to trauma, up to 25% of cases are atraumatic and associated with corticosteroid use, alcoholism, hyperlipidemia, irradiation, thrombophilia, or idiopathic etiologies. Treatment strategies for osteonecrosis of the talus can be divided into three categories: nonsurgical, joint-sparing surgery, and joint-sacrificing surgery. Before collapse of the articular surface, nonsurgical treatment designed to protect the joint along with limited weight bearing should be pursued until revascularization. Patients for whom nonsurgical treatment has been unsuccessful or who have articular collapse of the talar dome may undergo surgical options such as core decompression and bone grafting. Joint-sacrificing surgery should be considered as a last resort for recalcitrant osteonecrosis or patients with end-stage arthritic changes.

Keywords: joint-sacrificing surgery; joint-sparing surgery; nonsurgical; osteonecrosis of the talus; talus fracture

---

Dr. Moon or an immediate family member serves as a board member, owner, officer, or committee member of American Academy of Orthopaedic Surgeons, American Orthopaedic Foot and Ankle Society, and Colorado Orthopaedic Society.

INTRODUCTION

Osteonecrosis of the talus is difficult to diagnose and treat because of the anatomic location of the talus and its limited blood supply.[1] Osteonecrosis of the talus is not always clinically symptomatic, and patients should be followed until revascularization and consolidation are complete. As discussed in a 2019 study, the pathophysiology and natural course of the disease likely vary based on etiology.[2] Many treatments and surgical techniques have been attempted, but few long-term outcome reports have been published.

The incidence of talar osteonecrosis is rising, along with an increasing incidence of high-energy trauma.[1] Studies cite an incidence of 0.1% to 2.5% for all fractures, and an estimated 1,000 adult ankle osteonecrosis cases from all causes may present annually in the United States.[2,3] Traumatic fractures of the talus require extreme force, and falls from substantial height as well as motor vehicle collisions are leading mechanisms.[4] Increased use of advanced imaging techniques has led to greater numbers of patients in whom an early talar lesion is diagnosed.

ANATOMY AND VASCULAR SUPPLY

An understanding of the unique anatomy of the talus and its blood supply is crucial for comprehending diagnosis of talar osteonecrosis. The orientation of the talar neck differs from that of the body of the talus in both the horizontal and sagittal planes. In the horizontal plane, the neck deviates medially. In the sagittal plane, the neck deviates downward. This complex shape can lead to difficulty in determining the accuracy of reduction on radiographs. The talus has seven articular surfaces that comprise almost 60% of its surface, and screw fixation

---

Section 5: Special Problems of the Foot and Ankle

This chapter is adapted from Lee YK, Jegal H, Lee KB, Lee TH: Osteonecrosis of the talus, in Chou LB, ed: *Orthopaedic Knowledge Update®: Foot and Ankle 6*. American Academy of Orthopaedic Surgeons, 2020, pp 287-299.

© 2025 American Academy of Orthopaedic Surgeons   Orthopaedic Knowledge Update®: Foot and Ankle 7   267

Section 5: Special Problems of the Foot and Ankle

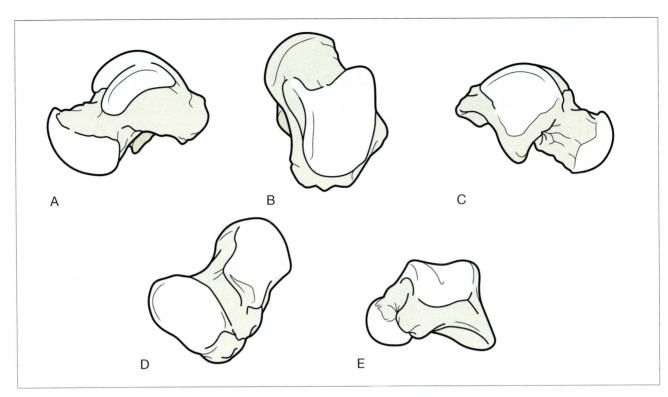

FIGURE 1 Schematic drawings showing the important anatomic features of the talus. **A**, Medial view. **B**, Dorsal view. **C**, Lateral view. **D**, Plantar view. **E**, Posterior view.

using the anteromedial approach is complicated[1] (**Figure 1**). The talus is most stable in the mortise with dorsiflexion because the body is wider anteriorly than posteriorly. The bone is recessed for dorsiflexion at the neck of the talus, which is a common site of talar fracture particularly during hyperdorsiflexion with axial loading.

The talus has no tendinous attachments or muscular origins. The entire blood supply comes from several direct vascular insertions; understanding the contribution of each of these is important to avoid iatrogenic vascular injury. The posterior tibial, dorsalis pedis, and perforating peroneal arteries are the three main extraosseous arteries that supply the talus[5] (**Figure 2**). The posterior tibial artery constitutes the principal blood supply of the talar body through the artery of the tarsal canal and deltoid artery.[6] The artery of the tarsal canal arises from the posterior tibial artery within the deltoid ligament below the medial malleolus and passes between the sheath of the flexor digitorum longus and flexor hallucis longus to enter the tarsal canal. The deltoid artery, which travels between the deep and superficial deltoid ligament and arises near the origin of the artery of the tarsal canal, is an important source of extraosseous circulation to the body of the talus. Preservation of the deltoid artery is therefore critical during stabilization or reduction of the talar neck and body. The artery of the tarsal sinus is formed from the anatomic loop between the dorsalis pedis and perforating peroneal arteries and merges with the artery of the tarsal canal. Together, these arteries feed most of the talar neck and head.[1,5,6]

ETIOLOGY AND INCIDENCE

Osteonecrosis of the talus has three primary causes. Approximately 75% of patients have a history of trauma including talar neck or body fracture. The incidence of osteonecrosis after talar neck fracture increases with greater initial fracture displacement.[7] Fifteen percent of patients have a nontraumatic medical condition as well as a history of steroid use (regardless of dosage or duration of use).[1] Some of these patients have alcoholism, sickle cell disease, dialysis, hemophilia, hyperuricemia, or lymphoma.[6,8-11] The remaining 10% of patients have idiopathic talar necrosis without a determined traumatic or medical cause.[12]

The original Hawkins classification system for talar neck fractures stratified risk of osteonecrosis based on fracture displacement and joint congruency.[13] The risk after type I talar fracture was reported as 10%; 42% after type II fracture; and 86% after type III fracture. Talar body and neck fractures do not differ significantly in terms of the risk of the development of osteonecrosis.[14] The Hawkins type II classification was subdivided into subluxated (type IIA) and dislocated (type IIB)

Chapter 17: Osteonecrosis of the Talus

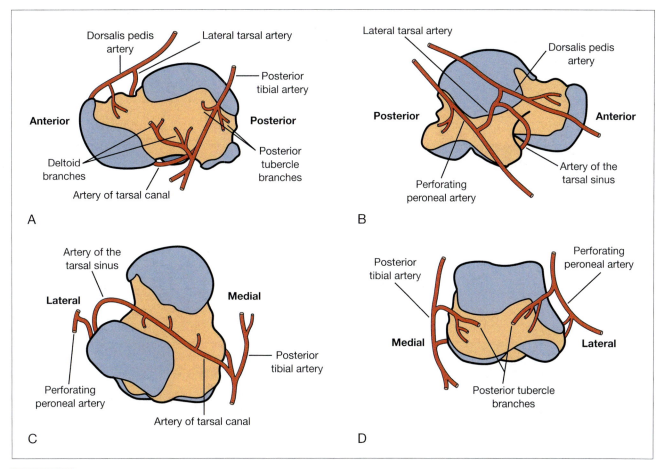

FIGURE 2 Schematic drawings showing the blood supply of the talus. **A**, The medial talar blood supply. The first branches of the posterior tibial artery are the posterior tubercle branches. More distally, the posterior tibial artery comes off the tarsal canal artery with its deltoid branches. This artery courses through the tarsal canal. **B**, The lateral talar blood supply. The lateral tarsal artery connects the dorsalis pedis artery to the perforating peroneal artery and branches to form the tarsal sinus artery. **C**, The inferior talar blood supply. The tarsal sinus artery and the tarsal canal artery form an anastomotic loop within the tarsal canal. **D**, The posterior talar blood supply. The posterior tubercle branches of the posterior tibial artery and perforating peroneal artery supply the medial and lateral tubercles.

subtalar joint in terms of predicting the development of osteonecrosis of the talus, concluding that osteonecrosis risk of the talar body was associated with the degree of initial displacement.[15] Osteonecrosis did not occur when the subtalar joint was not dislocated. In some reports, talar fracture osteonecrosis rates are lower than those reported by Hawkins, with overall osteonecrosis rates of approximately 25% to 30%. This reduction in osteonecrosis rate may be due to advances in treatment and fixation.[7,15,16]

The osteonecrotic progression from initial insult to structural compromise appears to be etiology dependent and may involve varied pathophysiology. For example, traumatic osteonecrosis, which may be ischemic-dominant, likely proceeds differently than atraumatic osteonecrosis where mechanisms may be apoptotic-dominant. Yet, all osteonecrotic pathways converge on a general reparative process where there is new appositional, living bone laid upon dead trabeculae in subchondral bone and where there is resorption of dead trabeculae (**Figure 3**). Bone density decreases as resorption outpaces bone formation, and the affected areas are susceptible to microfractures, which can accumulate to the point of subchondral collapse, macroscopic fracture, and joint incongruity.[2,6]

SYMPTOMS AND DIAGNOSIS

Pain is the most common symptom of talar osteonecrosis and is strongly associated with a loss of articular integrity.[17] Before articular collapse, a patient may be asymptomatic. Because osteonecrosis weakens the trabeculae in subchondral bone, collapse can occur from the pressure of body weight on the articular surface. These subchondral fractures can cause pain as well as mechanical symptoms.[1]

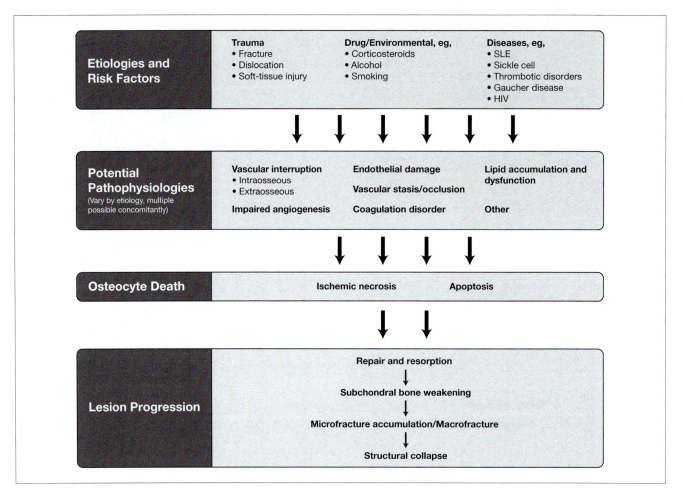

FIGURE 3 Osteonecrosis pathophysiology and lesion progression illustrating convergence of multiple etiologic pathways. SLE = systemic lupus erythematosus. (Reproduced with permission from Moon DK: Epidemiology, cause, and anatomy of osteonecrosis of the foot and ankle. *Foot Ankle Clin* 2019;24[1]:1-16. Copyright 2018, Elsevier.)

Although MRI and bone scanning are useful for early detection of talar osteonecrosis, evaluation should begin with plain radiography of the ankle. Early sclerotic changes, cystic changes, and advanced changes related to subchondral collapse may be seen on plain radiographs. The Hawkins sign may provide evidence of revascularization and is thought to be a reliable early indicator of vascular viability, with few false-negative results[1] (**Figure 4**). The Hawkins sign is a subchondral radiolucent band in the dome of the talus that can be seen on AP radiographs of the ankle at 6 to 8 weeks after fracture, and on lateral radiographs at 10 to 12 weeks. Subchondral collapse often has no symptoms, and it is rare to detect lesions on plain radiographs during the early stage of talar osteonecrosis. MRI is considered a key diagnostic tool during the early stage.[5] It is used to diagnose and quantify the extent of osteonecrosis because of its sensitivity to altered fat cell signals. Bone marrow is predominantly composed of fat components responsible for strong T1-weighted images, and bone marrow necrosis with subsequent edema is an early indication of osteonecrosis.[1] Necrotic regions with increased edema are revealed with high signal intensity on T2-weighted images. The prognostic value of the Hawkins sign and diagnostic value of MRI after talar neck fractures were studied. It was concluded that a positive Hawkins sign has no predictive value regarding ankle function in low-energy fractures and may predict better ankle function in high-energy fractures. It was recommended that MRI be performed in patients with a negative Hawkins sign 12 weeks after fracture, especially with high-energy trauma cases.[18]

MRI can also be useful in examining advanced stages of talar osteonecrosis. Titanium implants may be preferable to stainless steel implants for talar fracture fixation because their nonmagnetic properties minimize signal interference on MRI. Technetium Tc 99m bone scanning is also helpful for diagnosing early-stage talar osteonecrosis; it is usually performed 6 to 12 weeks after internal fixation of the talar fracture and shows decreased uptake

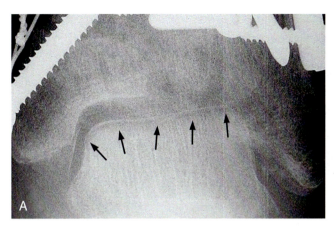 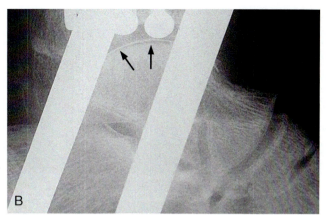

FIGURE 4 The Hawkins sign in a woman who had undergone external and internal fixation of a complex pilon fracture. Mortise view (**A**) and lateral (**B**) radiographs of the ankle reveal striking subchondral radiolucency (arrows), indicating talar viability.

in the talar body. The Ficat and Arlet classification system is frequently applied to radiographs to assess the extent of talar osteonecrosis[17] (**Table 1**).

TREATMENT

Many treatments for talar osteonecrosis have been described, but few long-term or critical-outcome studies have been published, and there is no consensus as to the best form of treatment regardless of stage. Treatment options for talar osteonecrosis can be grouped into three categories: nonsurgical, joint-sparing surgery, and joint-sacrificing treatment.

Nonsurgical treatment includes addressing etiologic factor, immobilization and restricted weight bearing, pharmacologic approaches, and ultrasound modalities. Surgical joint-sparing treatments include internal implantation of a bone stimulator,[19] vascularized autograft, and core decompression. Joint-sacrificing procedures include arthrodesis or talar replacement (partial or total).

Table 1
The Ficat and Arlet Classification of the Radiographic Appearance of Talar Osteonecrosis

Stage	Radiographic Appearance
I	Normal
II	Cystic and sclerotic lesions. Normal talar contour
III	Crescent sign. Subchondral collapse
IV	Narrowing of the joint space. Secondary changes in the tibia

Adapted with permission from Delanois RE, Mont MA, Yoon TR, Mizell M, Hungerford DS: Atraumatic osteonecrosis of the talus. *J Bone Joint Surg Am* 1998;80(4):529-536.

Nonsurgical Treatment

In general, treatment for osteonecrosis should logically start with addressing etiologic factors. For example, addressing modifiable risk factors for osteonecrosis such as chronic use of steroids, excessive consumption of alcohol, and smoking is an important consideration in potentially limiting the progression of the osteonecrosis and perhaps improving chances at recovery.

Nonsurgical treatment is preferred for talar osteonecrosis at Ficat and Arlet stage I, II, or III. Some early studies found benefit in avoiding weight bearing until revascularization was complete.[20-22] A study of 23 patients with posttraumatic osteonecrosis found that patients who were non–weight bearing on crutches for an average of 8 months had a fair-to-excellent result.[9] Those who were partially weight bearing in a patellar tendon brace or short leg brace with limited ankle motion had a poor-to-good result. Most of those who received no treatment (defined as non–weight bearing for less than 3 months) had a poor result. Other investigators reported that protected weight bearing using a patellar tendon brace had a favorable outcome and that delayed weight bearing had no benefit.[23,24] The amount and duration of weight bearing should be determined for each individual patient based on the location of the lesion and its symptoms. There is no need to restrict ambulation if sufficient bony structures remain to support weight bearing.[24] Regardless of the extent of weight bearing, it is important to preserve ankle motion, especially flexion and extension, and to protect the ankle from varus and valgus stress by using a patellar tendon brace or a cam boot walker (**Figure 5**).

Pharmacologic treatment for osteonecrosis of the talus is under investigation. Oral or intravenous diphosphonates have been applied to talar osteonecrosis.[25] Diphosphonates are antiresorptive agents that inhibit the action of mature osteoclasts on bone, thereby changing

Section 5: Special Problems of the Foot and Ankle

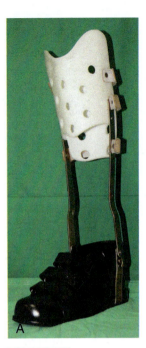
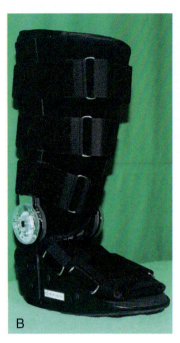

FIGURE 5 Photographs showing a patellar tendon brace (**A**) and a cam boot walker (**B**).

the balance between resorption and deposition of bone to allow greater deposition. Diphosphonates appear to transiently stimulate the proliferation of pro-osteoblast cells, increase their differentiation, increase the production of antiresorptive protein osteoprotegerin by osteoblasts, and decrease edema at the site of osteonecrosis.[26] Although diphosphonates have been used more widely for femoral head osteonecrosis, their use for talar osteonecrosis is off-label and controversial; concerns exist that in rare cases, osteoporotic medication such as diphosphonates and denosumab actually induce osteonecrosis of the jaw.[27]

Ultrasound bone stimulators can also be attempted for bone regeneration.[25] Low-intensity pulsed ultrasound was found to enhance the osteogenic differentiation of mesenchymal stem cells, stimulate the differentiation and proliferation of osteoblasts, inhibit the activities of osteoclasts, improve local blood perfusion and angiogenesis, and accelerate stress fracture healing.[28] Extracorporeal shock wave therapy was found to be an effective treatment for osteonecrosis of the femoral head but remains a controversial off-label treatment for talar osteonecrosis.[29]

Joint-Sparing Treatment
Core Decompression
Core decompression can be used before collapse of the talar dome. Increased pressure in the osteonecrotic areas as a result of marrow response to glucocorticoids or cell death edema is suspected to inhibit intraosseous blood flow, although pressure increases alone may not be sufficient to cause osteonecrosis.[2,30,31] The purpose of core decompression is to decrease core pressure using multiple drilling procedures, thereby enhancing revascularization and potentially decreasing pain. In a rabbit model, the effect of core decompression was enhanced by negative pressure in necrotic areas of the femoral head.[31] Histologic analysis revealed better healing in animals treated with additional negative pressure than in those who underwent core decompression only.

Drills with a diameter of 1.5 to 4 mm are usually used to decompress talar osteonecrotic lesions, using posterolateral, lateral, or medial approaches depending on the location of the lesion.[32] In one study, 32 ankles with stage II talar osteonecrosis that remained severely symptomatic after standard nonsurgical treatment went on to receive core decompression. At a mean 7-year follow-up (range, 2 to 15 years), 29 of the ankles had a fair-to-excellent clinical outcome; the remaining 3 ankles underwent arthrodesis after unsuccessful core decompression.[17] In another case report, a patient with stage I talar osteonecrosis had a satisfactory outcome after percutaneous core decompression using a 3.5-mm cannulated drill through a small stab incision.[33]

Core decompression is a relatively simple procedure that does not preclude subsequent arthrodesis or arthroplasty. However, articular surface collapse decompresses the lesion and necrotic anatomic changes are then too far advanced for treatment with decompression.

Biologic injections are being investigated as adjuncts to decompression. Percutaneous stem cell injections of bone marrow concentrate as well as platelet-rich plasma have been combined with decompression for osteonecrosis.[34,35] A study compared a group of patients who received percutaneous injection of progenitor cells (autologous bone marrow concentrate from the iliac crest) with core decompression and those who received core decompression alone. For the 45 ankles in the autologous bone marrow concentrate grafting group, the treatment revealed a lower prevalence of articular surface collapse and a longer duration before collapse or arthrodesis, compared with the 34 ankles in the control group that underwent core decompression alone.[34] Despite potential for adjuncts to improve the efficacy of core decompression, much remains to be understood about how the adjuncts specifically lead to improved outcome.

Bone Grafting
Autograft or allograft bone grafting treatments attempt to restore an articulating, living joint and can be used before a joint-sacrificing procedure is considered.[32] Nonvascularized autograft from the iliac crest is the most widely used bone graft, followed by allograft. Advantages of autograft over allograft include biocompatibility and rapid union. Disadvantages include donor site pain and limited volume of harvested bone.

Autologous bone grafting is usually performed with resection or curettage of the necrotic area. Tricortical bone block and cancellous bone can be used for filling defects. Favorable outcomes were reported when autologous bone grafting was used after 6 months of unsuccessful nonsurgical treatment in patients with a wide area of talar osteonecrosis. At 2-year follow-up, the patients were almost symptom free with ongoing creeping substitution[32] (**Figure 6**). Patients treated with iliac bone grafting followed by matrix-associated autologous chondrocyte transplantation returned to their former activities of daily living and recreation without restriction and with only a slight deficit in the range of motion.[36] Morphologic and biochemical MRI at 12-month follow-up showed interval bone healing with no intraosseous edema.

If the lesion is large and primarily involves the articular surface, structural talar allograft is a viable option. Osteochondral allograft can be considered for partial joint resurfacing in a young patient with focal lesions[25] (**Figure 7**). Talar allograft has a narrow range of indications because of the difficulty of matching donor talar morphology to the recipient, a limited supply of fresh allograft, and high associated costs. Although successful outcomes are possible, the procedure has modest failure rates, suggesting that patient factors such as age and activity level may be important considerations.[37]

Vascularized autologous bone graft has been used for treating osteonecrosis of the femoral head. Its theoretical advantages are a direct vascular supply to the necrotic area and mechanical support to prevent further collapse. This procedure is technically demanding and requires microsurgical technique and longer surgical times. Free vascularized bone graft is more difficult to use in the talus than in the femoral head because the vessels are smaller around the ankle than the hip.[38] Furthermore, vessel-pedicled bone graft can be used, although this demanding technique requires sacrifice from a donor small bone around the talus, and may require multiple joints around the donor bone to be fused. A cadaver study identified a consistent blood supply to the distal fibula, the cuboid, and the first and second cuneiforms with reliable nutrient arteries.[39] In every cadaver specimen, the transverse pedicle branch of the proximal lateral tarsal artery supplying

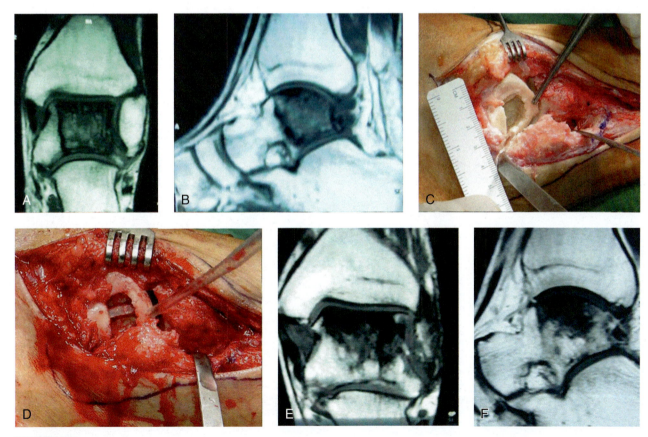

FIGURE 6 **A** and **B**, Preoperative magnetic resonance images showing wide osteonecrosis, which was revealed with low signal intensity. Intraoperative photographs showing removal and curettage of necrotic tissue (**C**) and insertion of autologous tricortical bone block and cancellous bone grafting (**D**). **E** and **F**, magnetic resonance images obtained 2-year follow-up show a well revascularized talus.

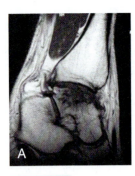 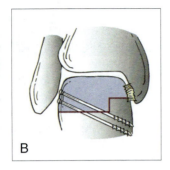 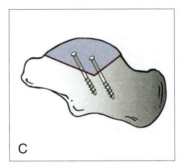 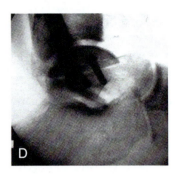

FIGURE 7 Segmental osteochondral allograft resurfacing for an ankle with focal talar osteonecrosis. **A**, Preoperative magnetic resonance image showing large segmental involvement. **B** and **C**, Drawings showing preoperative planning for partial joint arthroplasty. **D**, Lateral radiograph showing placement of prepared allograft with screws from a transmalleolar approach.

the cuboid, approximately 4.1 cm long, could be rotated to reach as far as the medial malleolus (**Figure 8**). The transverse segment of the anterolateral malleolar artery to the lateral malleolus is approximately 4 cm long but is usually quite thin. When 20 patients with talar osteonecrosis were treated with transposition of a vascularized cuneiform bone flap and iliac cancellous bone grafting, clinical symptoms were completely or partially relieved, the necrotic area was filled with newly formed bone, and 18 patients (90%) had a good or excellent result.[40] A study reported 13 patients who underwent vascularized pedicle bone grafting from the cuboid combined with bracing treatment. Two patients experienced treatment failure and subsequently underwent total ankle arthroplasty, one patient underwent arthroscopic débridement for soft-tissue impingement, and no other patient required secondary surgery. The study authors suggested that vascularized pedicle bone grafting from the cuboid combined with bracing treatment for 1 year may be a viable treatment option for osteonecrosis of the talus.[41] A cadaver and clinical study introduced vascularized tibial grafting for revascularization of osteonecrosis of the talus and for arthrodesis of the ankle in patients with osteoarthritis secondary to osteonecrosis of the talus. The procedure was performed in eight patients with isolated osteonecrosis of the talus and 12 patients with osteoarthritis secondary to osteonecrosis of the talus. In all eight revascularizations, bone healing occurred without progression to talar collapse and union was established in 11 of 12 revascularizations of the talus in all patients.[42] Vessel-pedicled bone grafts are technically demanding but promising; further outcome studies are warranted although this procedure may not be practical in many settings.

Joint-Sacrificing Treatment
Talar Body Prostheses

A talar body prosthesis attempts to preserve talar function while avoiding the drawbacks of arthrodesis or total talectomy for large talar osteonecrosis defects.

Partial talus prostheses have had limited success in replacing the osteonecrotic body but retaining the native talar head and neck. One study of a stainless steel partial talar prosthesis reported 14 of 16 patients experienced

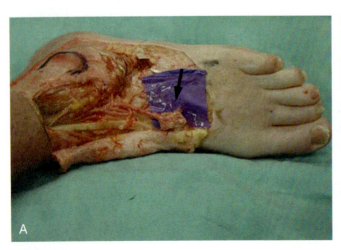 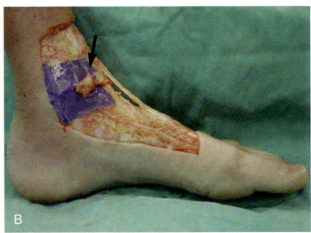

FIGURE 8 Photographs showing the transverse pedicle branch of the proximal lateral tarsal artery with the cuboid pedicle (arrow) (**A**) and its range (arrow) of rotation, which can extend even to the medial malleolus (**B**).

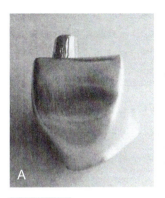 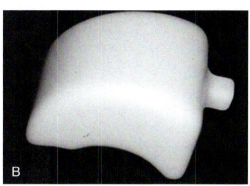 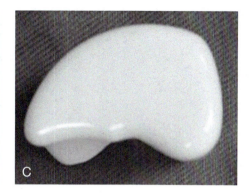

FIGURE 9 Photographs showing a stainless steel talar prosthesis (**A**), a first-generation ceramic talar prosthesis with a peg for an intact talar neck (**B**), and a second-generation implant without the peg (**C**).

favorable outcomes with respect to pain and function. A later study of additional patients with the implant after modifications demonstrated 94% of patients with good results at a minimum 5-year follow-up.[43,44] A different group designed an alumina-ceramic partial talar prosthesis that had limited success but was complicated by loosening of the peg fixation to the talar neck. Despite removing the peg in a subsequent design, additional results led the study authors to abandon their partial talar prosthesis design and instead recommend shifting to total talus prostheses[45,46] (**Figure 9**).

Total talus prostheses replace the entire native talus with an artificial anatomically shaped implant, which acts as a spacer articulating with the tibia, calcaneus, and navicular. In a study, 51 patients (55 ankles) with osteonecrosis of the talus who were treated with total talar replacement (alumina implant) were followed up. The authors of the study suggested that the favorable congruency of the custom-made implant with adjacent joints produced stability and maintained ankle function.[46] These devices are becoming more accessible as three-dimensional printing techniques combined with CT allow for custom, anatomic-matched implant creation. According to a 2020 study, total talus prostheses may best be reserved for talar osteonecrosis where adjacent articular surfaces are relatively intact, yet long-term follow-up including consideration of patient factors such as age and activity is needed.[47]

Total Ankle Arthroplasty

Total ankle arthroplasty for a patient with talar osteonecrosis was first reported more than 35 years ago.[48] A few published studies are available, all of which reported unsatisfactory outcomes as well as some revisions to arthrodesis[49-52] (**Table 2**). Surgeons rarely use total ankle arthroplasty in patients with talar osteonecrosis because of poor bone ingrowth and the lack of supporting bony structures.

In cases of talar osteonecrosis with concomitant arthritic changes, combining total talar prostheses with a tibial arthroplasty implant shows some preliminary

Table 2

Studies of Noncemented Total Ankle Arthroplasty for Talar Osteonecrosis

Study (Year)	Number of Patients	Follow-Up (Years)	Implant (Manufacturer)	Results
Newton (1982)	3	3	Scandinavian Total Ankle Replacement (small bone innovations)	Collapse in two patients; conversion to fusion in one. Persistent pain in one patient
Buechel et al (1988)	2	2	Buechel-Pappas (Endotec)	Complex regional pain syndrome in one patient
Buechel et al (2003)	2	5	Buechel-Pappas	Collapse in one patient; complex regional pain syndrome in one patient
Takakura et al (2004)	2	2	TNK ankle (Japan medical materials)	Collapse in both patients; conversion to fusion

Adapted with permission from Lee KB, Cho SG, Jung ST, Kim MS: Total ankle arthroplasty following revascularization of osteonecrosis of the talar body: Two case reports and literature review. *Foot Ankle Int* 2008;29:852-858.

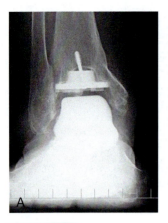 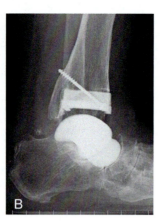

FIGURE 10 Radiographs demonstrating a total talar prosthesis combined with total ankle arthroplasty. **A**, AP radiograph. **B**, Lateral radiograph. (Reproduced from Yamamoto T, Nagai K, Kanzaki N, et al: Comparison of clinical outcomes between ceramic-based total ankle arthroplasty with ceramic total talar prosthesis and ceramic-based total ankle arthroplasty. Foot Ankle Int 2022;43[4]:529-539.)

promise by precluding the risk of traditional talar component failure due to osteonecrotic bone stock (**Figure 10**). A 2022 study compared the results of ceramic total talar prostheses combined with total ankle arthroplasty with those of conventional total ankle arthroplasty and found that clinical outcomes were similar, and fewer revisions were needed in the total talar prosthesis group.[53]

Arthrodesis

Arthrodesis is an option when other treatments have been unsuccessful or impractical, or in patients with stage IV talar osteonecrosis. A critical analysis of arthrodesis for the management of ankle arthrosis and talar body osteonecrosis found that the osteonecrotic talus was retained, thereby preserving ankle biomechanics and leg length.[54] Fusion was obtained in 16 out of 19 ankles, perhaps disproving the belief that fusion cannot be achieved in an osteonecrotic talus.

Subtalar arthrodesis has been attempted to hasten ingrowth of blood vessels to the talus and avoid osteonecrosis and subsequent arthrosis, but subsequent reports indicate potentially poor results.[1,55,56]

Ankle fusions for talar osteonecrosis can be attained with a variety of implants. Large cannulated screws, blade plates, locking plates, locked intramedullary rods, or multiplane thin-wire external fixators have been extensively studied.[25,57] Resection of a necrotic talar body and bulk autograft placement with tibiotalocalcaneal arthrodesis using an intramedullary nail was a reasonable option for the management of type IV posttraumatic talar deformity.[58]

Arthroscopic ankle arthrodesis is possible when there is little or no malalignment of the ankle joint.[59] The anterolateral, anteromedial, and posterolateral portals are used to denude the entire cartilage while maintaining the contour of the bony surfaces. Fixation is accomplished using two or three percutaneous, cancellous, cannulated, or noncannulated screws placed parallel or convergent. In one study, a series of 16 patients underwent arthroscopic ankle arthrodesis for noncollapsed talar osteonecrosis, with results demonstrating arthrodesis in all 15 available patients.[60] Advantages of an arthroscopic procedure include minimal blood loss, a relatively short time to union, and minimal interruption of the surrounding soft tissue. The subsequent blood supply leads to a better union rate than that after an open procedure. A multicenter comparative study found that arthroscopic arthrodesis required a shorter hospital stay and led to better outcomes than an open procedure at 1- and 2-year follow-up.[61]

The mini-open technique, similar to the arthroscopic technique, uses an extended small incision at the same locations as arthroscopic portals. Advantages and disadvantages are similar to those of the arthroscopic technique, but the mini-open technique allows additional iliac crest grafting.[32] Nine patients treated using the mini-open technique had a satisfactory clinical and radiographic outcome at a mean 55-month follow-up.[62]

Curettage or resection of the necrotic area during ankle arthrodesis can cause shortening. The risk is minimal during the early stages of osteonecrosis if the necrotic area is small and shallow. However, most patients who undergo ankle arthrodesis have stage III or IV talar osteonecrosis, and shortening from resection is an important consideration.

In severe cases of osteonecrosis with an unsalvageable talus, a study reported a salvage procedure combining ankle and hindfoot arthrodesis without structural bone graft. The authors of the study enrolled 14 patients with ankle and hindfoot arthrodesis who underwent retrograde intramedullary nailing and analyzed the clinical and radiographic outcomes. The study concluded that tibiocalcaneal arthrodesis without structural allograft was possible in cases of complete loss of the talar body and significantly improved clinical and radiographic outcomes.[63]

Arthrodesis between the tibia and talar neck and head can also be used for patients with fracture and collapse of the talar body.[64] The procedure involves removing the fragments of the talar body and inserting a sliding tibial graft into the talar neck. Modified procedures have had favorable outcomes.[65-67]

TREATMENT ALGORITHM

The treatment of talar osteonecrosis has been marked by controversy, but there is growing consensus on optimum

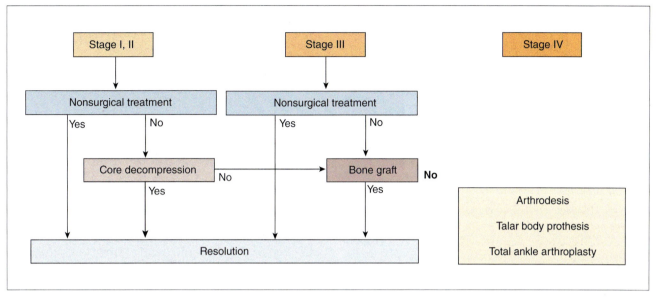

FIGURE 11 Treatment algorithm for osteonecrosis of the talus.

treatment modalities. A recommended algorithm uses the Ficat and Arlet classification (**Figure 11**). Treatment success is defined as the relief of pain or cessation of articular collapse. A widened necrotic area on MRI or a widened sclerotic margin on plain radiographs does not necessarily mean failure of treatment. If articular collapse has been halted, even with progression of necrosis, the surgeon can wait for revascularization and resolution of the lesion. Initial nonsurgical treatment is recommended for patients with stage I or II talar osteonecrosis. If there is no effect, core decompression or bone grafting can be considered. A patient with stage III talar osteonecrosis with collapse of the articular surface will not benefit from core decompression; bone grafting is therefore the only possible procedure. A salvage procedure such as arthrodesis can be performed if there are arthritic changes.

SUMMARY

Osteonecrosis of the talus is an uncommon disease, which if left untreated can lead to collapse of the talus and progressive pain with arthritic changes. As many as 90% of patients may be at risk for talar osteonecrosis after a displaced talar neck fracture, depending on the fracture and dislocation pattern, because of the vulnerable vascular structures around the talus. Osteonecrosis of the talus can lead to end-stage arthritis requiring arthrodesis or arthroplasty. Only a few comparative outcome studies on the treatment of osteonecrosis of the talus have been published. Appropriate treatment selection requires careful evaluation. Radiographs should be used in conjunction with CT, bone scans, or MRI, with MRI serving as the most useful imaging modality for the disease. Identification of revascularization using bone scans or MRI is essential in deciding the best treatment plan. Before articular surface collapse, nonsurgical treatment with limited weight bearing can be used to protect the joint until revascularization. For a patient who has undergone unsuccessful nonsurgical treatment or has articular collapse of the talar dome, treatment options may include core decompression and bone grafting. Salvage procedures should be considered as a last resort or for a patient with end-stage arthritic changes or widespread structural collapse.

KEY STUDY POINTS

- An understanding of the unique anatomy of the talus and its blood supply is crucial for comprehending talar osteonecrosis.
- Osteonecrosis of the talus has multiple etiologies broadly grouped as trauma, nontraumatic medical conditions, and idiopathic.
- Treatment strategies for osteonecrosis of the talus can be divided into three categories: nonsurgical, joint-sparing surgery, and joint-sacrificing surgery.
- Careful evaluation and treatment decision making are of the utmost importance for the prognosis.

ANNOTATED REFERENCES

1. Adelaar RS, Madrian JR: Avascular necrosis of the talus. *Orthop Clin North Am* 2004;35(3):383-395, xi.

2. Moon DK: Epidemiology, cause, and anatomy of osteonecrosis of the foot and ankle. *Foot Ankle Clin* 2019;24:1-16.

   The actual incidence of osteonecrosis of the ankle in the United States is unknown. Applying epidemiologic data, approximately 1,000 adult ankle osteonecrosis cases are estimated to present annually. Level of evidence: V.

3. Vallier HA: Fractures of the talus: State of the art. *J Orthop Trauma* 2015;29(9):385-392.

4. Zwipp H: *Severe Foot Trauma in Combination With Talar Injuries*. Springer-Verlag, 1993, pp 123-135.

5. Pearce DH, Mongiardi CN, Fornasier VL, Daniels TR: Avascular necrosis of the talus: A pictorial essay. *Radiographics* 2005;25(2):399-410.

6. DiGiovanni CW, Patel A, Calfee R, Nickisch F: Osteonecrosis in the foot. *J Am Acad Orthop Surg* 2007;15(4):208-217.

7. Dodd A, Lefaivre KA: Outcomes of talar neck fractures: A systematic review and meta-analysis. *J Orthop Trauma* 2015;29(5):210-215.

8. Langevitz P, Buskila D, Stewart J, Sherrard DJ, Hercz G: Osteonecrosis in patients receiving dialysis: Report of two cases and review of the literature. *J Rheumatol* 1990;17(3):402-406.

9. Kemnitz S, Moens P, Peerlinck K, Fabry G: Avascular necrosis of the talus in children with haemophilia. *J Pediatr Orthop B* 2002;11(1):73-78.

10. Miskew DB, Goldflies ML: Atraumatic avascular necrosis of the talus associated with hyperuricemia. *Clin Orthop Relat Res* 1980;148:156-159.

11. David R: *Sports Injuries of the Ankle*. Mosby, 2013, p 4234.

12. Ando Y, Yasui T, Isawa K, Tanaka S, Tanaka Y, Takakura Y: Total talar replacement for idiopathic necrosis of the talus: A case report. *J Foot Ankle Surg* 2016;55(6):1292-1296.

13. Hawkins LG: Fractures of the neck of the talus. *J Bone Joint Surg Am* 1970;52(5):991-1002.

14. Lindvall E, Haidukewych G, DiPasquale T, Herscovici D Jr, Sanders R: Open reduction and stable fixation of isolated, displaced talar neck and body fractures. *J Bone Joint Surg Am* 2004;86(10):2229-2234.

15. Vallier HA, Reichard SG, Boyd AJ, Moore TA: A new look at the Hawkins classification for talar neck fractures: Which features of injury and treatment are predictive of osteonecrosis? *J Bone Joint Surg Am* 2014;96(3):192-197.

16. Jordan RK, Bafna KR, Liu J, Ebraheim NA: Complication of talar neck fractures by Hawkins classification- a systemic review. *J Foot Ankle Surg* 2017;56:817-821.

17. Delanois RE, Mont MA, Yoon TR, Mizell M, Hungerford DS: Atraumatic osteonecrosis of the talus. *J Bone Joint Surg Am* 1998;80(4):529-536.

18. Chen H, Liu W, Deng L, Song W: The prognostic value of the Hawkins sign and diagnostic value of MRI after talar neck fractures. *Foot Ankle Int* 2014;35(12):1255-1261.

19. Holmes GB Jr, Wydra F, Hellman M, Gross CE: A unique treatment for talar osteonecrosis: Placement of an internal bone stimulator. A case report. *JBJS Case Connect* 2015;5(1):e4-e5.

20. Adelaar RS: The treatment of complex fractures of the talus. *Orthop Clin North Am* 1989;20(4):691-707.

21. Canale ST: Fractures of the neck of the talus. *Orthopedics* 1990;13(10):1105-1115.

22. Kenwright J, Taylor RG: Major injuries of the talus. *J Bone Joint Surg Br* 1970;52(1):36-48.

23. Penny JN, Davis LA: Fractures and fracture-dislocations of the neck of the talus. *J Trauma* 1980;20(12):1029-1037.

24. Comfort TH, Behrens F, Gaither DW, Denis F, Sigmond M: Long-term results of displaced talar neck fractures. *Clin Orthop Relat Res* 1985;199:81-87.

25. Saltzmann C: *Talar Avascular Necrosis*, ed 8. Mosby, 2007, pp 952-960.

26. Agarwala S, Jain D, Joshi VR, Sule A: Efficacy of alendronate, a bisphosphonate, in the treatment of AVN of the hip. A prospective open-label study. *Rheumatology (Oxford)* 2005;44(3):352-359.

27. Beth-Tasdogan NH, Mayer B, Hussein H, Zolk O, Peter JU: Interventions for managing medication-related osteonecrosis of the jaw. *Cochrane Database Syst Rev* 2022;7(7):CD012432.

    Medication-related osteonecrosis of the jaw is a severe adverse reaction to certain medications commonly used in the treatment of osteoporosis, including diphosphonates, denosumab, and antiangiogenic agents. Level of evidence: V.

28. Yan SG, Huang LY, Cai XZ: Low-intensity pulsed ultrasound: A potential non-invasive therapy for femoral head osteonecrosis. *Med Hypotheses* 2011;76(1):4-7.

29. Wang CJ, Wang FS, Yang KD, et al: Treatment of osteonecrosis of the hip: Comparison of extracorporeal shockwave with shockwave and alendronate. *Arch Orthop Trauma Surg* 2008;128(9):901-908.

30. Urbaniak JR, Harvey EJ: Revascularization of the femoral head in osteonecrosis. *J Am Acad Orthop Surg* 1998;6(1):44-54.

31. Zhang YG, Wang X, Yang Z, et al: The therapeutic effect of negative pressure in treating femoral head necrosis in rabbits. *PLoS One* 2013;8(1):e55745.

32. Horst F, Gilbert BJ, Nunley JA: Avascular necrosis of the talus: Current treatment options. *Foot Ankle Clin* 2004;9(4):757-773.

33. Grice J, Cannon L: Percutaneous core decompression: A successful method of treatment of stage I avascular necrosis of the talus. *Foot Ankle Surg* 2011;17(4):317-318.

34. Hernigou P, Dubory A, Flouzat Lachaniette CH, Khaled I, Chevallier N, Rouard H: Stem cell therapy

in early post-traumatic talus osteonecrosis. *Int Orthop* 2018;42(12):2949-2956.

35. Houdek MT, Wyles CC, Collins MS, et al: Stem cells combined with platelet-rich plasma effectively treat corticosteroid-induced osteonecrosis of the hip: A prospective study. *Clin Orthop Relat Res* 2018;476(2):388-397.

36. Dickschas J, Welsch G, Strecker W, Schoffl V: Matrix-associated autologous chondrocyte transplantation combined with iliac crest bone graft for reconstruction of talus necrosis due to villonodular synovitis. *J Foot Ankle Surg* 2012;51(1):87-90.

37. El-Rashidy H, Villacis D, Omar I, Kelikian AS: Fresh osteochondral allograft for the treatment of cartilage defects of the talus- a retrospective review. *J Bone Joint Surg Am* 2011;93(17):1634-1640.

38. Hussl H, Sailer R, Daniaux H, Pechlaner S: Revascularization of a partially necrotic talus with a vascularized bone graft from the iliac crest. *Arch Orthop Trauma Surg* 1989;108(1):27-29.

39. Gilbert BJ, Horst F, Nunley JA: Potential donor rotational bone grafts using vascular territories in the foot and ankle. *J Bone Joint Surg Am* 2004;86(9):1857-1873.

40. Yu XG, Zhao DW, Sun Q, et al: Treatment of non-traumatic avascular talar necrosis by transposition of vascularized cuneiform bone flap plus iliac cancellous bone grafting. *Zhonghua Yi Xue Za Zhi* 2010;90(15):1035-1038.

41. Nunley JA, Hamid KS: Vascularized pedicle bone-grafting from the cuboid for talar osteonecrosis: Results of a novel salvage procedure. *J Bone Joint Surg Am* 2017;99(10):848-854.

42. Kodama N, Takemura Y, Ueba H, Imai S, Matsusue Y: A new form of surgical treatment for patients with avascular necrosis of the talus and secondary osteoarthritis of the ankle. *Bone Joint J* 2015;97-B(6):802-808.

43. Harnroongroj T, Vanadurongwan V: The talar body prosthesis. *J Bone Joint Surg Am* 1997;79(9):1313-1322.

44. Harnroongroj T, Harnroongroj T: The talar body prosthesis: Results at ten to thirty-six years of follow-up. *J Bone Joint Surg Am* 2014;96(14):1211-1218.

45. Taniguchi A, Takakura Y, Sugimoto K, et al: The use of a ceramic talar body prosthesis in patients with aseptic necrosis of the talus. *J Bone Joint Surg Br* 2012;94(11):1529-1533.

46. Taniguchi A, Takakura Y, Tanaka Y, et al: An alumina ceramic total talar prosthesis for osteonecrosis of the talus. *J Bone Joint Surg Am* 2015;97(16):1348-1353.

47. Kadakia RJ, Akoh CC, Chen J, Sharma A, Parekh SG: 3D printed total talus replacement for avascular necrosis of the talus. *Foot Ankle Int* 2020;41(12):1529-1536.

Twenty-seven patients underwent total talar replacement for talar osteonecrosis with a mean follow-up of 22.2 months. Ankle range of motion was unchanged. Significant improvements were noted in visual analog scale pain score, Foot and Ankle Outcome Score, general symptoms, quality of life, and activities of daily living. Three complications requiring reoperation occurred. Level of evidence: IV.

48. Manes HR, Alvarez E, Llevine LS: Preliminary report of total ankle arthroplasty for osteonecrosis of the talus. *Clin Orthop Relat Res* 1977;127:200-202.

49. Buechel FF, Pappas MJ, Iorio LJ: New Jersey low contact stress total ankle replacement: Biomechanical rationale and review of 23 cementless cases. *Foot Ankle* 1988;8(6):279-290.

50. Buechel FF Sr, Buechel FF Jr, Pappas MJ: Ten-year evaluation of cementless Buechel-Pappas meniscal bearing total ankle replacement. *Foot Ankle Int* 2003;24(6):462-472.

51. Newton SE III: Total ankle arthroplasty. Clinical study of fifty cases. *J Bone Joint Surg Am* 1982;64(1):104-111.

52. Takakura Y, Tanaka Y, Kumai T, Sugimoto K, Ohgushi H: Ankle arthroplasty using three generations of metal and ceramic prostheses. *Clin Orthop Relat Res* 2004;424:130-136.

53. Yamamoto T, Nagai K, Kanzaki N, et al: Comparison of clinical outcomes between ceramic-based total ankle arthroplasty with ceramic total talar prosthesis and ceramic-based total ankle arthroplasty. *Foot Ankle Int* 2022;43(4):529-539.

Forty-six ankles undergoing conventional total ankle arthroplasty (mean 42-month follow-up) were compared with 26 ankles undergoing combined total ankle arthroplasty with total talar prosthesis (mean 46-month follow-up). Although preoperative range of motion was worse for patients with combined total ankle arthroplasty/prosthesis, postoperatively there were no significant differences. No significant differences were noted for the Japanese Society for Surgery of the Foot ankle-hindfoot scale and Self-Administered Foot Evaluation Questionnaires. Revision rate was 10.9% in conventional total ankle arthroplasty and zero in combined total ankle arthroplasty. Level of evidence: III.

54. Kitaoka HB, Patzer GL: Arthrodesis for the treatment of arthrosis of the ankle and osteonecrosis of the talus. *J Bone Joint Surg Am* 1998;80(3):370-379.

55. McKeever FM: Treatment of complications of fractures and dislocations of the talus. *Clin Orthop Relat Res* 1963;30:45-52.

56. Pennal GF: Fractures of the talus. *Clin Orthop Relat Res* 1963;30:53-63.

57. Devries JG, Philbin TM, Hyer CF: Retrograde intramedullary nail arthrodesis for avascular necrosis of the talus. *Foot Ankle Int* 2010;31(11):965-972.

58. Abd-Ella MM, Galhoum A, Abdelrahman AF, Walther M: Management of nonunited talar fractures with avascular necrosis by resection of necrotic bone, bone grafting, and fusion with an intramedullary nail. *Foot Ankle Int* 2017;38(8):879-884.

59. Myerson MS, Quill G: Ankle arthrodesis. A comparison of an arthroscopic and an open method of treatment. *Clin Orthop Relat Res* 1991;268:84-95.

60. Kendal AR, Cooke P, Sharp R: Arthroscopic ankle fusion for avascular necrosis of the talus. *Foot Ankle Int* 2015;36(5):591-597.

61. Townshend D, Di Silvestro M, Krause F, et al: Arthroscopic versus open ankle arthrodesis: A multicenter comparative case series. *J Bone Joint Surg Am* 2013;95(2):98-102.

Section 5: Special Problems of the Foot and Ankle

62. Wrotslavsky P, Giorgini R, Japour C, Emmanuel J: The miniarthrotomy ankle arthrodesis: A review of nine cases. *J Foot Ankle Surg* 2006;45(6):424-430.

63. Tenenbaum S, Stockton KG, Bariteau JT, Brodsky JW: Salvage of avascular necrosis of the talus by combined ankle and hindfoot arthrodesis without structural bone graft. *Foot Ankle Int* 2015;36(3):282-287.

64. Blair HC: Comminuted fractures and fracture dislocations of the body of the astragalus: Operative treatment. *Am J Surg* 1943;59(1):37-43.

65. Lionberger DR, Bishop JO, Tullos HS: The modified Blair fusion. *Foot Ankle* 1982;3(1):60-62.

66. Lin SY, Cheng YM, Huang PJ, Tien YC, Yap WK: Modified Blair method for ankle arthrodesis. *Kaohsiung J Med Sci* 1998;14(4):217-220.

67. Hantira H, Al Sayed H, Barghash I: Primary ankle fusion using Blair technique for severely comminuted fracture of the talus. *Med Princ Pract* 2003;12(1):47-50.

SECTION 6

Foot and Ankle Trauma

Section Editor:
Andrew Haskell, MD, FAAOS

CHAPTER 18

Ankle and Pilon Fractures

BRIAN C. LAU, MD • MALCOLM R. DEBAUN, MD
MICHAEL J. GARDNER, MD, FAAOS

ABSTRACT

The treatment of ankle and pilon fractures continues to evolve, as understanding of optimal surgical indications, timing, and reduction and fixation techniques improves. Rotational ankle fractures are extremely common injuries and present with a wide spectrum of bony and soft-tissue injuries. The first and most important decision point is determining whether the ankle mortise is stable. Recently, emphasis has been on direct fixation of all disrupted structures around the unstable ankle, including the bony and ligamentous structures. Controversy persists regarding syndesmosis reduction assessment and fixation techniques. Pilon fractures are high-energy, axial-loading injuries that involve disruption of the distal tibial articular surface. Traditionally, staged treatment with open reduction and internal fixation following external fixation and soft-tissue rest was common, although select injuries may be appropriate for early open reduction. Anterior approaches are the mainstay for accessing the bony injury, and predictable fracture fragment, surgical fixation sequences, and precontoured periarticular plates provide the highest likelihood for a good outcome.

Keywords: ankle fracture; mortise; pilon fractures; syndesmosis

Dr. Lau or an immediate family member serves as a paid consultant to or is an employee of DePuy, a Johnson & Johnson Company; has received research or institutional support from Arthrex, Inc. and Wright Medical Technology, Inc.; and serves as a board member, owner, officer, or committee member of American Orthopaedic Society for Sports Medicine and Arthroscopy Association of North America. Dr. DeBaun or an immediate family member has received royalties from Metalogix; serves as a paid consultant to or is an employee of Metalogix, Next Science, Reselute, Shukla, SI Bone, and Synthes; has stock or stock options held in NSite; and has received research or institutional support from DePuy, a Johnson & Johnson Company. Dr. Gardner or an immediate family member has received royalties from Conventus, Globus Medical, SI-Bone, and Synthes; is a member of a speakers' bureau or has made paid presentations on behalf of KCI; serves as a paid consultant to or is an employee of Conventus, Globus Medical, KCI, OsteoCentric, SI-Bone, StabilizOrtho, and Synthes; has stock or stock options held in Conventus, Genesis Innovations Group, Imagen Technologies, Intelligent Implants, and N'Site Medical; and serves as a board member, owner, officer, or committee member of American Academy of Orthopaedic Surgeons and Orthopaedic Trauma Association.

ANKLE FRACTURES

Introduction

The ankle is the most frequently injured weight-bearing joint. Ankle fractures are among the most common of all fractures; the annual incidence was found to be 71 to

---

This chapter is adapted from Spiguel AR, Jo MJ: Ankle and pilon fractures, in Chou LB, ed: *Orthopaedic Knowledge Update®: Foot and Ankle 6.* American Academy of Orthopaedic Surgeons, 2020, pp 303-317.

© 2025 American Academy of Orthopaedic Surgeons

187 fractures per 100,000 people.[1-3] Fractures about the ankle range in severity from a minor malleolar avulsion fracture to a comminuted fracture of the articular surface, with a resulting spectrum of stability and congruity of the mortise. Although an ankle fracture often is considered to be appropriate for introductory surgical training, the evaluation, diagnosis, and decision making required to achieve an optimum outcome can prove to be difficult.

A small incongruity in the ankle leads to dramatic changes in the pressure distribution of the joint surface and subsequently leads to arthritis.[4,5] Even a 1-mm shift of the talus can result in a 40% loss of contact area with the plafond. The goal of treatment of a patient with an ankle fracture is to restore congruity and stability to the ankle and to maintain them through the healing process. Whether this goal is best achieved by surgical or nonsurgical means is best decided by weighing the risks and benefits of the treatment options while taking patient-specific factors into account.

Evaluation

Patient History

A thorough patient history should give particular attention to any medical comorbidities. The presence of diabetes, peripheral neuropathy, or peripheral vascular disease is important for risk stratification and decision making.[6,7] The patient's age, preinjury activity level, occupation, and recreational activities also can be important in decision making. Patients should be asked if osteoporosis has been diagnosed or if they have had a fragility fracture, such as a compression fracture of the spine, a hip fracture, or a distal radius fracture.[8] The presence of a medical comorbidity can increase the risk of infection, nonunion, malunion, or soft-tissue complications.[7,9] A patient with obesity is at increased risk for soft-tissue complications.[10] A patient who uses tobacco or abuses alcohol should be counseled about the associated fracture and wound-healing risks as well as the potential benefits of cessation.[7,11]

The details of the injury should be noted because an understanding of the mechanism and energy of the injury can be helpful for evaluation, initial reduction, and treatment planning.

Physical Examination

A thorough, circumferential examination of the ankle should be performed to evaluate the soft tissue of the entire ankle region. Evaluation of the soft-tissue envelope around an ankle fracture is paramount because its condition can be the determining factor while making treatment decisions. The ankle has little soft-tissue coverage, and substantial edema, fracture blisters, and soft-tissue compromise can occur even with a low-energy ankle fracture. An ankle fracture–dislocation may require urgent reduction to minimize the comorbidity associated with inside-out pressure on the soft tissue. Open fractures typically cause a transverse medial wound over the medial malleolus. Findings such as venous stasis skin changes, chronic skin discoloration, and ulceration may be signs of diabetes or peripheral vascular disease.

Tenderness in the medial and lateral malleoli and the collateral ligaments should be noted, regardless of the presence of a fracture. Tenderness to palpation in the absence of a fracture may indicate ligamentous injury, although the accuracy of this finding has been challenged.[12,13] Evaluation of a syndesmotic injury can be difficult. Tenderness over the anterior tibiofibular joint or a positive squeeze test (performed 5 cm above the distal tibiofibular joint) may indicate the presence of a syndesmotic injury. The entire tibia and fibula should be palpated up to the knee joint. Tenderness to palpation about the proximal fibula may indicate a Maisonneuve fracture variant with injury to the syndesmosis.

A thorough neurovascular examination and contralateral-side comparison should be done. Decreased sensation in a stocking distribution indicates advanced peripheral neuropathy. A size 5.07 Semmes-Weinstein monofilament should be used to test sensation if there is a question about peripheral neuropathy.[9] The ankle-brachial index can be measured to detect a vascular injury or peripheral vascular disease, and a vascular consultation may be warranted.

Radiographic Studies

Urgent intervention may be required for an ankle dislocation, open fracture, or acutely evolving neurovascular injury. An ankle dislocation with skin tenting or neurovascular compromise may need immediate reduction after only the most pertinent history and physical examination are obtained. Imaging studies done with the ankle in an almost reduced position may provide more detail about the fracture pattern than studies with the joint in a grossly deformed state.

Imaging of an ankle fracture should begin with AP, lateral, and mortise radiographic views. A full-length tibiofibular series is helpful for diagnosing a proximal fibula fracture. The radiographs should be used to understand the fracture pattern and detect signs of instability. Any incongruity of the talus and the plafond is a sign of instability. Displacement of the medial or lateral malleolus or a talar shift of less than 2 mm historically was associated with a satisfactory result and was used as a criterion for fracture fixation.[14] On the AP radiograph, tibiofibular overlap of less than 10 mm or a clear space of more than 5 mm suggests a syndesmotic injury.[15] On the mortise radiographic view, a medial clear space that

Chapter 18: Ankle and Pilon Fractures

is larger than 5 mm or unequal to the superior clear space suggests a medial-side ligament injury. Tibiofibular overlap of less than 10 mm on the mortise view also may indicate a syndesmotic injury. The lateral radiograph may show a posterior malleolus fracture, malpositioning of the fibula relative to the tibia, and/or talar subluxation. The positioning of the ankle during the radiographic procedure is important; the medial clear space was found to become wider with increasing plantar flexion of the ankle, possibly leading to an incorrect diagnosis of deep deltoid injury.[16] Comparison views of the contralateral side may be helpful for detecting asymmetry or associated instability.

Stress radiographs may be indicated to assess stability if the talus and syndesmosis appear reduced, but the injury mechanism or pattern suggests an unstable ankle. A manual external rotation or gravity stress mortise view radiograph can be used to assess deltoid ligament integrity and talus stability in an isolated lateral malleolus fracture.[12,13,17] With instability, this fracture pattern commonly is called a bimalleolar-equivalent fracture. Similarly, a stress view can be used to assess for syndesmotic injury, as in a proximal fibula fracture with a well-reduced ankle. Widening of the tibiofibular joint with an associated lateral shift of the talus is positive for syndesmotic instability. Evaluation of the syndesmosis may be more sensitive in the sagittal plane than in the coronal plane.[18]

CT is essential for evaluating the fracture pattern and planning treatment of an axial-loading injury or a suspected plafond or pilon-type fracture. CT is also beneficial for a complex fracture or a fracture with posterior malleolus fragments.

MRI is useful for detecting ligamentous injury. Although MRI may not be economically feasible for every ankle fracture, it can be beneficial if the diagnosis is difficult. MRI was found to be useful for distinguishing partial and complete tears of the deltoid ligament as well as evaluation of the syndesmotic ligament complex.[19,20]

Classification

An ideal classification system is reliable, reproducible, useful for treatment decision making, and able to provide prognostic information. Although no system for classifying ankle fractures meets all of these goals, the Lauge-Hansen, Danis-Weber, and AO/Orthopaedic Trauma Association (OTA) systems are most commonly used.

The Lauge-Hansen classification uses the position of the foot at the time of injury as well as the direction of the force causing the injury to define four types of injuries: supination–external rotation, supination-adduction, pronation–external rotation, and pronation-abduction.

Each of these types has four subtypes (I through IV) denoting injury severity. The Lauge-Hansen system is popular but difficult to reproduce. A cadaver study found that a short oblique fracture of the distal fibula can occur with the foot in the pronated position, and a high fibular fracture can occur with abduction of the ankle.[21] A novel study compared online videotape clips showing the mechanism of ankle fractures with postinjury radiographs showing the same injuries.[22] The Lauge-Hansen classification was correctly correlated with supination-adduction–type injuries but had only a 29% correlation with injuries of pronation–external rotation type. The Lauge-Hansen classification system is not ideal for guiding treatment decisions or providing prognostic information. However, because this system correlates the mechanism of injury with the fracture pattern, it may be useful for communicating patterns of injury and guiding closed reduction techniques. Countering the injuring force with a splint, cast, or external fixator may improve the reduction.

The Danis-Weber classification is based on the level of a lateral malleolus fracture. A type A fracture is below the level of the plafond; a type B fracture, at the level of the plafond; and a type C fracture, above the plafond. A type A fracture without a medial fracture probably is an avulsion-type fracture that does not lead to lateral instability of the talus and can be treated nonsurgically. A type C fracture is inherently unstable and may involve the syndesmosis. The stability of a type B fracture is more difficult to assess because it may combine a syndesmotic injury with a deltoid ligament injury or may be a stable injury.[23] A stress radiograph can be helpful in type B fractures.

The combined AO/OTA system uses alphanumeric labels to systematically classify fractures.[24] This classification system is reproducible and can be used to describe a wide range of injury types as well as specific fracture patterns. Although the AO/OTA system is useful in data collection and research endeavors, it is cumbersome to use clinically and lacks specific diagnostic and prognostic components.

Initial Management

Reduction and splinting of an ankle fracture should be done in a timely manner. The health of the soft tissue is paramount. Reduction of any dislocation or subluxation will help to alleviate pressure on the skin and subcutaneous tissues, and proper reduction can alleviate any pressure, tethering, or kinking of the neurovascular structures. Reduction helps to alleviate atypical joint contact pressure that can contribute to posttraumatic arthritis. A successful reduction typically depends on recognizing the fracture pattern and reversing the deforming force.

Section 6: Foot and Ankle Trauma

© 2025 American Academy of Orthopaedic Surgeons

Orthopaedic Knowledge Update®: Foot and Ankle 7

285

For example, the commonly used Quigley maneuver for laterally translated or externally rotated ankle fractures applies a varus and internal rotation force through the first toe.[25] The Quigley maneuver consists of rolling the patient onto the affected side and suspending the limb by the great toe to allow the talus to internally rotate and translate medially. An unsuccessful reduction may result from the use of an incorrect technique, inadequate anesthesia, or the interposition of structures such as surrounding tendons or fracture fragments. An open reduction may be needed if reduction with closed methods is unsuccessful.

Timely splinting also is beneficial for soft-tissue preservation. The splint helps hold the reduction, which decreases shear forces on surrounding soft-tissue injury. Incorrect splinting technique can cause serious damage, however. The combination of insufficient padding and the pressures added during molding can create pressure points and lead to ulceration. Excess padding can cause the splint to be too loose, increase the shear forces, and even lead to loss of reduction. A study of plaster splints showed that dipping the plaster in water hotter than 24°C can lead to thermal injury.[26] The use of multiple plaster layers, as when excess plaster is folded over at its end or layers are added to create a stirrup or strut, also was found to increase the temperature. The recommended method is to cut the plaster to the exact length needed. Placing the curing splint on a pillow or overwrapping it with fiberglass also can increase the temperature to a dangerous level.[26,27]

Routine postsplinting radiography of a minimally or nondisplaced fracture that was not unnecessarily manipulated exposes patients to radiation, increases clinical waiting times, increases health care costs, and does not provide meaningful information.[28]

Definitive Management

The treatment goal for a rotational ankle fracture is healing with the mortise in an anatomic position. Attaining this goal may or may not require anatomic positioning of the fibular fracture. Nonsurgical treatment is appropriate if there is no medial malleolar fracture, the deep deltoid remains competent, and the mortise is stable, as can be confirmed using an external rotation or gravity stress mortise radiograph. A positive stress test results in lateral translation of the talus and is demonstrated by the medial clear space being larger than the superior clear space. The larger the medial clear space is on a stress radiograph, the greater the likelihood of syndesmotic injury.[29] If the mortise stress radiograph is negative, nonsurgical management typically consists of early functional treatment, with weight bearing as tolerated. A soft orthosis, walking boot, or walking cast initially can provide comfort and

protection from further injury. Its use can be discontinued as symptoms allow.

Ankle fracture–dislocations are inherently unstable and, after initial closed reduction, typically require open reduction and internal fixation (ORIF) of the malleoli to ensure anatomic healing. A Weber type B ankle fracture with a positive stress radiograph that remains well reduced within the mortise without stress can be considered for nonsurgical treatment. A prospective randomized study found that nonsurgically and surgically treated unstable fibula fractures had similar outcomes at 1-year follow-up, although 20% of the patients who were nonsurgically treated had medial clear space widening, and 20% had a delayed union or nonunion suggesting longer follow-up is necessary before concluding reduction and fixation is not beneficial.[30]

Arthroscopy

Arthroscopy at the time of ORIF may be a useful adjuvant to evaluate for intra-articular fractures, loose bodies, associated osteochondral lesions, syndesmosis, and deltoid injuries.[31] Osteochondral lesions at the time of ankle fracture can affect subsequent outcomes, and early identification is key for management.[32] In addition, the washout effect of the catabolic environment within the acute phase after an ankle fracture may decrease the risk of posttraumatic arthritis.[33,34]

Lateral Malleolus

If surgical treatment is indicated, attention to the fibular fracture is the key to restoring ankle reduction and stability. Care must be taken to accurately re-create fibular length, alignment, and rotation. The most common fracture pattern is a Weber type B with a spiral configuration at the level of the distal tibiofibular joint that exits posterolaterally. Effective fixation methods include the use of multiple lag screws, one or more lag screws with neutralization plating, or antiglide plating. Common plating surfaces are directly lateral or posterolateral. Laterally based plates tend to be more prominent because of their subcutaneous location, and posterolateral plates can cause peroneal irritation theoretically if placed inappropriately distal. Recent clinical evidence suggests posterolateral antiglide plating is biomechanically favorable, leads to less reoperation for implant removal, and does not increase peroneal tendon irritation or preoperative time compared with lateral plating[35-37] (**Figure 1**).

Novel interlocking lateral malleolar nailing systems have recently become available. In the absence of soft-tissue concern precluding a direct approach, comparative advantage over traditional plating techniques has yet to be supported.[38,39]

Chapter 18: Ankle and Pilon Fractures

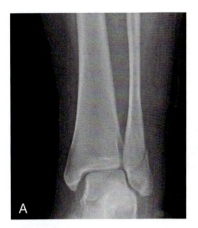
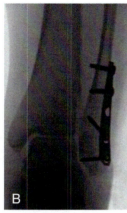

FIGURE 1 Mortise radiographic views demonstrating unstable Weber B (**A**) affixed with an antiglide posterolateral one-third tubular plate and lag screw through the plate (**B**). (Courtesy of Malcolm R. DeBaun, MD, Durham, NC.)

Medial Malleolus

The medial side of the ankle can fail through the medial malleolus or the medial ligamentous structures. The medial malleolus consists of the anterior malleolus, to which the superficial deltoid attaches, and the posterior malleolus, to which the deep deltoid attaches. The clinical significance is that when the anterior malleolus is reduced and stabilized, the deep deltoid, and thus the ankle mortise, may remain incompetent.[31] Medial malleolar fixation typically consists of two lag screws directed from the tip of the malleolus into the distal tibia after open reduction. Depending on the size of the fragment, one screw, a screw and pin, or a tension band technique can be used. Biomechanical and clinical data indicate that cortical lag screws engaged in the far lateral cortex of the distal tibia provide greater fixation strength than screws ending in the distal tibial metaphysis.[32] Although most medial malleolus fractures are transverse after failing in tension, a medially directed traumatic force may create a vertical shear fracture as in supination-adduction patterns, often with marginal impaction of the distal tibia joint surface at the fracture edge. This fracture pattern requires disimpaction and possibly grafting of any joint irregularity, typically followed by a buttress plate and screw fixation with screws directed from medial to lateral rather than from the tip of the malleolus (**Figure 2**). Anatomic reduction of impaction remains critical to mitigate risk of posttraumatic arthritis. In supination–external rotational injuries, clinical outcomes are equivalent whether the medial-side injury was ligamentous or bony.[40,41]

Posterior Malleolus

Treatment of the posterior malleolus component has received increased attention. The decision to fix the posterior malleolus historically was based on the percentage of the articular surface involved, as measured on a lateral radiograph. A fracture involving more than one-quarter to one-third of the articular surface area or a fracture in which the talus is subluxated posteriorly with the posterior malleolar fragment typically requires reduction and fixation (**Figure 3**). It is now recognized that a posterior malleolus fracture involving the posterolateral corner of the distal tibia represents avulsion of the posterior tibiofibular ligaments, which are a component of the syndesmosis complex. Thus, reduction and fixation of the posterior malleolar component restores the tension and competence of the syndesmosis in this fracture type, and it may provide better stability than a syndesmotic screw.[42] The posterior malleolus contributes to the

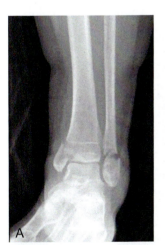
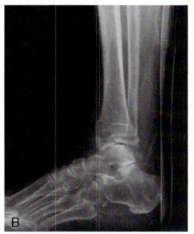
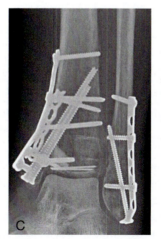
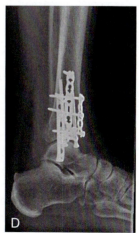

FIGURE 2 **A**, AP mortise radiographic view from a patient who sustained a supination-adduction ankle fracture with significant marginal impaction. **B**, Lateral radiograph demonstrating a tension band plate that was used for the Weber A fibula. Mortise and lateral radiographic views demonstrating the marginal impaction on the medial column that was anatomically reduced directly and stabilized with intraosseous threaded wires (**C**), calcium phosphate cement, and a high density of fixation to include a buttress plate (**D**). (Courtesy of Malcolm R. DeBaun, MD, Durham, NC.)

© 2025 American Academy of Orthopaedic Surgeons — Orthopaedic Knowledge Update®: Foot and Ankle 7

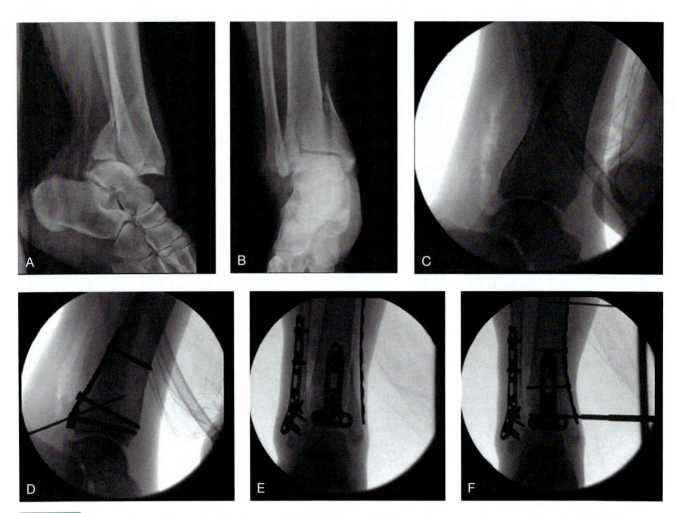

FIGURE 3 Preoperative radiographs showing mortise (**A**) and lateral (**B**) views demonstrating a complex trimalleolar fracture-dislocation of the ankle. **A**, Note the vertical fracture pattern of the medial malleolus but with no evidence of articular impaction in this case. **B**, The posterior dislocation of the talus is placing pressure on the anterior soft tissues. This will necessitate prompt reduction to protect the articular surfaces and soft tissues. Preoperative planning should include whether the posterior malleolus fracture needs to be addressed surgically as well as consideration of the planned approach (anterior or posterior) and positioning of the patient. **C** and **D**, Intraoperative fluoroscopic images showing lateral views. **C**, After appropriate reduction of the talus, there is concomitant reduction of the posterior malleolus fragment. **D**, The posterior malleolus fragment was initially secured using a Kirschner wire. The plate was then placed using a buttress technique with the initial screw placed through the plate just proximal to the apex of the fracture. The construct was then finalized using lag screws through the fragment. **E** and **F**, Intraoperative fluoroscopic images showing mortise views. **E**, After appropriate reduction of the posterior malleolus and fibula, that medial malleolus has a near-anatomic reduction. A low-profile plate was placed in the appropriate position using a percutaneous technique. The plate was undercontoured to achieve the desired buttress effect. **F**, The initial screw was placed at the apex of the fracture, and with tightening of the screw, anatomic reduction was achieved with the plate. The construct was then completed using horizontal screws placed with a lag technique. For both the posterior and medial malleolus fragment, a lag screw was placed in the subchondral bone to provide compression close to the articular surface.

posterior lip of the tibial incisura, and reduction and fixation may improve syndesmotic reduction accuracy. The less common transverse-type posterior malleolus fracture typically involves a greater percentage of the articular surface and may extend to the medial malleolus. This fracture typically requires ORIF, either percutaneously or through a direct posterior approach. CT can be used to improve the characterization of the transverse-type posterior malleolus fracture.

The method of internal fixation has also been studied. Anterior to posterior directed screws and direct posterior plating are two common options. Anterior to posterior lag screws have the advantages to be able to be done in the supine position with minimal soft-tissue disruptions and may be technically less challenging. However, these may lead to hardware prominence in the posterior soft tissues, damage to the neurovascular and tendinous structures anteriorly, and malreduction and may be biomechanically inferior to buttress plating.[43] Direct visualization and reduction as well as posterior buttress plating may be a superior mode of fixation for clinically significant posterior malleolus fractures. This technique may be technically more challenging and cause a larger soft-tissue insult during dissection, but recent studies have shown that there may be clinical benefits to this method.[44]

Syndesmosis

Reduction and fixation of the syndesmosis has been a source of controversy (**Figure 4**). Two key points have been established: syndesmosis malreduction is common, and it has a substantial effect on functional outcomes.[45,46]

Instability of the syndesmosis can be diagnosed intraoperatively with an external rotation stress test after fixation of the malleolar fracture, although the accuracy of this test has been questioned.[47] Evidence of syndesmosis injury should be sought in all ankle fractures requiring surgical treatment; its incidence is as high as 40% in Weber type B fractures and is even higher in Weber type C fractures.[48]

The risk of anterior or posterior translation of the syndesmosis can be minimized by reduction of the posterior malleolus fragment, meticulous clamp placement, direct visualization, and comparing the true talar dome lateral fluoroscopic views of the injured ankle with those of the contralateral ankle.[49,50] It has been shown that positioning of the medial tine of the reduction clamp can greatly affect the reduction and that direct visualization and manual reduction using direct pressure with a finger may actually result in a more accurate reduction.[51,52]

Overcompression of the syndesmosis previously was thought to be impossible, regardless of the position of the ankle during reduction.[52] Evidence suggests that overcompression is possible, however, and can affect the functional outcome.[49,53]

There continues to be various options for fixation of the syndesmosis. Flexible (suture) rather than rigid fixation has become increasingly popular, but the long-term outcomes and effectiveness require more investigation.[54] When using screws to fix the syndesmosis, the number of screws, number of cortices, and postoperative breakage of screws do not seem to affect the long-term outcome.[55]

Postoperative Management

A splint is used to keep patients from bearing weight immediately after surgery. Elevation can be used to reduce swelling. The splint and sutures are removed 2 weeks after surgery. If the fracture fixation is thought to be stable, the patient begins to use a removable boot, and range of motion may begin. For patients with surgically fixed unstable fibula, bimalleolar, and trimalleolar ankle fractures with less than 25% involvement of the posterior malleolus, immediate weight bearing and range of motion has not been shown to increase complications and does improve short-term outcomes compared with those treated in casts for 6 weeks after surgery.[56]

To minimize the risk of neuroarthropathic (Charcot) collapse, immobilization and protection from weight bearing should be continued for a longer period in patients who have neuropathy from any source or diabetes-related nephropathy or retinopathy. For patients older than 70 years, with unstable surgical ankle fractures, poor bone quality, and difficulty adhering to restrictions on bearing weight, a novel construct using Kirschner wires and cement augmentation was found to permit safe early weight bearing.[57]

Complications

Nonunion is a rare complication usually related to nonsurgical treatment of the medial malleolus. This is often a fibrous nonunion and not painful. Malunion is most common in fractures treated nonsurgically. In surgically treated fractures, care must be taken to obtain anatomic reduction of the mortise and syndesmosis to avoid posttraumatic arthrosis and recurrent instability.[58] Wound-healing complications are uncommon, particularly with 2 weeks of splint immobilization to prevent tissue shearing. Tobacco smoking substantially increases the risk of all complications, including impaired wound healing.[59]

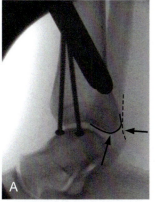 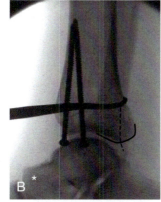

FIGURE 4 **A**, True talar dome lateral fluoroscopic image showing syndesmotic malreduction after clamp placement, indicated by the relative posterior position of the posterior border of the fibula (dashed line) in relation to the posterior edge of the plafond (solid line). **B**, Fluoroscopic image showing reduction of the fibular anterior translation using a hook after clamp removal. Note the intersection of the posterior border of the fibular at the posterior corner of the plafond. (Courtesy of Michael J. Gardner, MD, Stanford, CA.)

PILON FRACTURES

Introduction

Fractures of the articular surface of the distal tibia are commonly referred to as pilon fractures. A pilon fracture occurs when the talus is forced cranially into the distal tibia. The force is transmitted through the articular surface (tibial plafond) into the metaphysis leading to extensive injury. Frequently the resulting injury involves a high degree of comminution and articular impaction. These injuries can be high or low energy, with high-energy injuries leading to a compromised soft-tissue envelope. The soft-tissue envelope must be considered when planning surgical incisions. The fracture pattern and articular impaction are determined by the direction of the force and position of the foot at the time of injury.[60] There is no consensus on the optimal treatment of these fractures. Surgical treatment is technically demanding, requires careful planning, and can be very challenging. The outcomes tend to be unpredictable and often lead to residual disability.

Clinical and Radiographic Evaluation

As in any initial patient evaluation, a history and physical examination are essential. A thorough medical history helps to determine whether the patient is at increased risk for a poor outcome (soft-tissue complications, poor fracture healing, or fixation failure). Patients at increased risk include those who smoke tobacco; abuse alcohol; are long-term users of steroids; or have diabetes, neuropathy, malnutrition, osteoporosis, or peripheral vascular disease.

The mechanism of injury is directly related to the amount of force sustained by the limb and is the key to understanding the potential soft-tissue injury, which acutely is more important than the fracture itself. Perfusion, swelling, tissue necrosis, and fracture blisters must be carefully assessed and will influence the treatment algorithm. Early intervention, including limb realignment with closed reduction, is imperative to minimize impending skin compromise from fracture fragments and to restore circulation and nerve function.

The radiographic evaluation of the ankle should begin with standard AP, lateral, and mortise radiographic views as well as full-length tibiofibular radiographic views. For a complex pilon fracture, radiographs of the contralateral limb can be helpful to understand unique morphologic variations of the distal tibia and provide a preoperative planning template. CT should always be obtained after restoration of limb length and alignment. CT is useful for understanding the fracture pattern and determining the extent of articular involvement for preoperative planning as well as determination of the appropriate surgical approach and fixation strategies.[61,62]

Classification

Fracture classification systems are tools for describing the fracture pattern and understanding factors related to prognosis and treatment. Several classification systems for tibial pilon fractures have been proposed; however, the Rüedi-Allgöwer classification and the AO/OTA classification are the two most commonly used. The Rüedi-Allgöwer classification types, described in 1968, are based on articular displacement and degree of comminution. They increase in severity from low-energy to high-energy injuries. Type I is an intra-articular fracture with a nondisplaced articular surface, type II is a fracture-dislocation with an incongruous joint without comminution, and type III fractures have associated articular comminution and impaction of the metaphysis.

The AO/OTA system is much more detailed than the Rüedi-Allgöwer classification. All fractures of the distal tibia, including extra-articular metaphyseal fractures, are classified in a manner similar to that of other periarticular fractures, with differentiation between partial and complete articular injuries. Type A is an extra-articular fracture, type B is a partial articular fracture, and type C is a complete articular fracture (**Figure 5**).

Initial Management

The timing of definitive surgery for pilon fractures is critical to minimize complication risks. In early clinical series, the use of immediate ORIF with large exposures and bulky implants resulted in unacceptably high rates of complications primarily in regard to the soft-tissue envelope. This led to contemporary treatment principles and a staged protocol to minimize this risk. The initial focus should be on treating the soft-tissue envelope and the swelling, restoring the length and alignment of the tibia, and decompressing the joint surface. Premature definitive ORIF can lead to skin necrosis, dehiscence, and infection. Performing surgery after the soft-tissue injury is allowed to recover has considerably reduced all wound complications as well as deep osteomyelitis and infected nonunions.[63,64] In the staged protocol, most surgeons currently use external fixation with or without limited internal fixation to achieve the goal of length and alignment.[63,64] Studies evaluating high-energy open pilon fractures using a staged treatment protocol with external fixation followed by definitive ORIF found acceptable outcomes and a low rate of soft-tissue complications.[63-67]

Limited internal fixation with external fixation can be used in a pilon fracture with a long oblique or spiral fracture extending into the diaphysis. The soft tissues along the diaphysis are typically outside the area of greatest injury and can be treated with minimal exposure and reduction using an antiglide-type plate application. This method can help reestablish limb length, rotation,

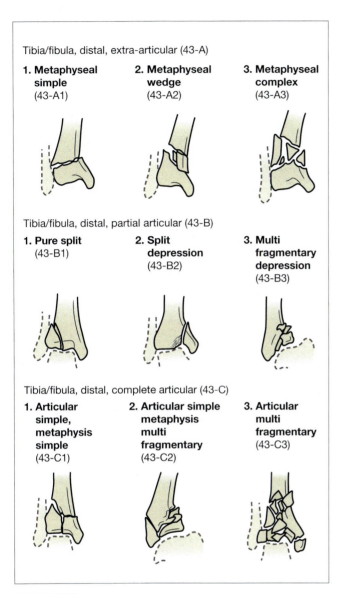

FIGURE 5 Schematic drawings showing the AO/OTA classification of pilon fractures. (Adapted with permission from TIBIA/FIBULA. *J Orthop Trauma* 2007;21[10]:S43-S58.)

and alignment and can provide early intimate contact of fracture fragments at the diaphysis to encourage early union and minimize the need for secondary procedures. However, limited internal fixation with external fixation should be used only in specific situations in which the articular block is spanned, and the limited internal fixation will assist in obtaining the final reduction.[66]

A staged protocol has been described for surgical fixation of a high-energy pilon fracture (AO/OTA type 43C) in which the articular fracture has a displaced posterior component. The researchers thought that it was difficult to obtain an accurate reduction through an anterior approach alone, with an indirect reduction of the posterior fragment, and the result would be less than optimal. Their staged approach involved application of an initial external fixator followed by a limited ORIF through a posterolateral approach. When the soft tissues were amenable, an anterior approach was used to reduce the anterior and medial fragments to a stable posterior fragment. On the basis of CT, the researchers concluded that the use of this protocol improved their ability to obtain an anatomic articular reduction in comparison with the use of an anterior approach only and an indirect posterior reduction. They were unable to demonstrate between-group difference in postoperative complications, and the functional outcomes were significantly improved in the patients treated with posterior plating[67] (**Figure 6**).

Despite the known benefits of provisional external fixation, soft-tissue rest, and future definitive management, some surgeons still prefer early surgical fixation. A study found similar complication rates and overall functional scores regardless of whether a staged protocol or single-stage ORIF was used to treat high-energy pilon fractures during the acute period. This study was performed by experienced surgeons who were able to evaluate and expedite the treatment of these injuries. This may be impractical for most centers and therefore not generalizable.[68] Pilon fractures that are largely rotational or torsional injuries with minimal axial load tend to be lower energy in nature and tolerate surgical incisions much sooner. Errors in timing of surgery can be costly with severe consequences for the patient.

There are some important indicators that can be helpful in decision making regarding timing of surgical intervention. Fracture blisters are quite common and are the result of delamination of the dermis from the epidermis or subcutaneous tissue from the fascia. They are an indicator of deep tissue injury, which can contribute to wound-healing issues, and should give pause to thoughts of early surgical intervention. The wrinkle sign is also another reliable examination finding that indicates it is safer to proceed with surgical intervention. When wrinkles are present, edema has usually decreased to a point that skin can be mobilized for surgery without too much tension during closure.

Surgical Treatment

Surgical Approaches

The surgical approach for a pilon fracture must be chosen carefully and is dictated by the location of the articular injury, the mechanically appropriate fixation needed, and the soft-tissue injuries that are present. Classically the anteromedial, anterolateral, posterolateral, posteromedial, and direct medial incisions have

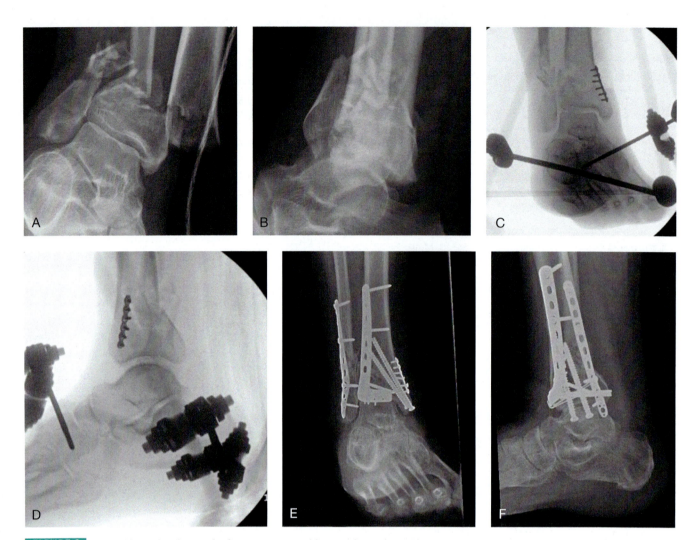

FIGURE 6 AP and lateral radiographs from a 69-year-old man who sustained a type III open pilon fracture (43C) with a transverse medial wound (**A** and **B**). Mortise and lateral radiographic views demonstrate irrigation and débridement with limited internal fixation and ankle spanning external fixation that was applied at the first stage (**C** and **D**). Given the tenuous medial soft tissue envelope, anterolateral and posterolateral approaches were used for the definitive reduction and fixation to the plafond and fibula, respectively. Mortise and lateral radiographic views show percutaneous large frag screws that provided medial column support (**E** and **F**). (Courtesy of Malcolm R. DeBaun, MD, Durham, NC.)

been described (**Figure 7**). The anteromedial approach was popularized by the AO. Traditionally used for ORIF of pilon fractures where the medial column is involved, it is the most extensile approach, providing access to the entire distal tibial articular surface and offering the ability to place a plate medially, laterally, or anteriorly. The anteromedial approach is also associated with more difficulty in reaching the lateral Chaput fragment. In addition, wound complications are a concern with this approach, given it is necessary to rely on the survival of full-thickness skin flaps that have undergone significant trauma. When an extensile version of the anteromedial approach was used to treat 21 patients after provisional stabilization with a spanning external fixator, all wounds healed, there were no nonunions, and one superficial infection occurred.[69] Another retrospective review found a statistically significant correlation between skin necrosis and this approach, which they attributed to potential poor vascularization to the medial aspect of the tibia.[70]

The anterolateral approach is useful for most complete articular fractures. This approach is indicated for pilon fractures that involve the lateral column, usually allows adequate visualization of the medial shoulder, avoids dissection over the anteromedial surface of the distal tibia, and may lead to fewer wound complications. The muscles of the anterior compartment provide good soft-tissue coverage over an implant, but the anterior tibial artery and vein as well as the superficial and deep peroneal nerves are at risk of injury or impingement. Impaction of the medial articular surface is difficult to reduce when this exposure is used, and the proximal

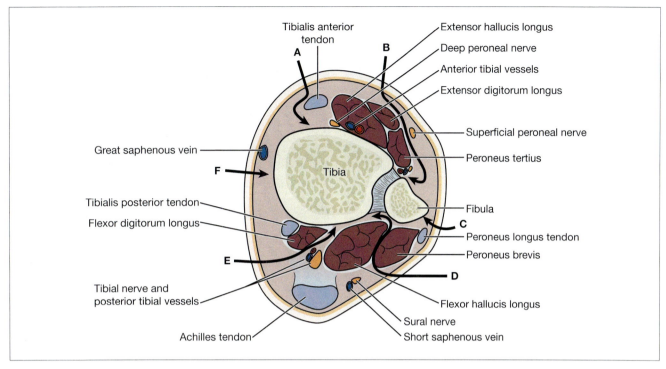

FIGURE 7 Drawing showing the axial view of the anteromedial (**A**), anterolateral (**B**), posterolateral (fibula) (**C**), posterolateral (tibia) (**D**), posteromedial (**E**), and medial (**F**) approaches used for treatment of tibial plafond and associated fibula fractures.

extent of the exposure is limited because of the muscle origins of the anterior compartment on the fibula and the intraosseous membrane distally.[71]

Posterior approaches can also be used for exposure and fixation of the posterior component of a pilon fracture. The posterolateral approach is useful primarily in posterior partial articular fractures (AO/OTA type 43B). It also has the advantage that the surgeon can approach the fibula through the same incision. Articular visualization is almost impossible; the articular reduction usually is done indirectly with cortical reductions of the metaphysis and diaphysis. The posteromedial approach is not commonly used and rarely required for fixation of a pilon fracture. As in the posterolateral approach, it is difficult to see the articular surface, and reduction is done indirectly with an extra-articular cortical reduction. These posterior approaches sometimes are used as an adjunct to an anterior approach for the purpose of treating a complex pilon fracture.[72] A cadaver study proposes a modified posteromedial approach for more complex fractures that involve both the medial and lateral parts of the posterior plafond, providing a greater degree of exposure. Classically the posteromedial approach is between the flexor digitorum longus and the flexor hallucis longus, which provides limited visualization to the lateral one-third of the posterior malleolus, including the syndesmosis and the fibula. To gain better access, instead of retracting the neurovascular bundle laterally with the flexor hallucis longus, it should be retracted with the flexor digitorum longus medially, which allows for better visualization of the posterior malleolus. In this study, 64% of the posterior malleolus could be visualized with the standard posteromedial approach and 91% could be visualized with the modified posteromedial approach.[73]

Dual approaches to the plafond are often required to adequately reduce and stabilize all components of the injury. If performed with meticulous attention to soft-tissue handling and adequate skin bridge (>5 to 6 cm), dual approaches are safe and effective.[74,75]

Internal Fixation

Pilon fractures in the distant past typically were treated nonsurgically, given their overall poor results. A comparison of nonsurgical treatment with ORIF found better results in surgically treated patients.[76] The researchers recommended four principles to guide the surgical treatment of a pilon fracture: restoration of fibular length, reconstruction of the articular surface and metaphysis, bone grafting, and medial buttressing to stabilize the metaphysis and assist the diaphyseal reduction. The results of this study were difficult to reproduce, however, probably because the patients in the study had a relatively low-energy mechanism of injury (eg, from a skiing accident) in contrast to the high-energy mechanisms (eg, from a motor vehicle crash) that have become increasingly common.

Section 6: Foot and Ankle Trauma

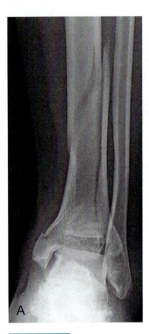
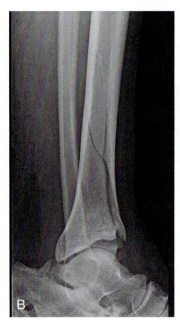
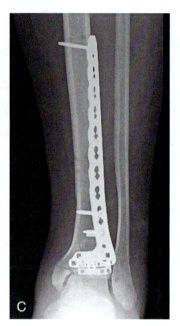
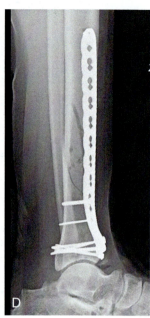

FIGURE 8 Preoperative radiographs showing AP (**A**) and lateral (**B**) views of a complex pilon fracture with extension into the diaphysis. Postoperative radiographs showing mortise (**C**) and lateral (**D**) views. An anterolateral approach to treat a pilon fracture allows excellent access to the anterior distal tibial articular surface. After the impaction was reduced and stabilized, the metaphysis was fixed with an anterolateral plate. (Courtesy of Michael J. Gardner, MD, Stanford, CA.)

The decision for where to place the implant is determined by the injury radiographs and which column needs to be supported. Plate fixation should be on the compression side of the fracture, or on the concave side of the deformity to act as a buttress to support the column that has failed. Assessing the fibula can also help make this decision; comminuted fibula fractures usually signify that the lateral column failed because of a valgus force and the lateral side needs to be buttressed (**Figure 8**). Conversely, transverse tension fractures of the fibula are typically seen with varus angulation and deformity on the injury radiographs requiring medial column buttress and support. Ultimately, tibial plates should be applied to resist the original deforming forces sustained.[73] High-energy OTA 43C fractures with extensive metaphyseal comminution sometimes require both medial and lateral column support to adequately reduce, buttress, and maintain alignment of the distal tibia. Most modern precontoured tibial plates lack the ability to adequately capture all fracture fragments of type C fractures in high-energy pilon injuries when a single plate is used without additional fixation.[77] According to a 2019 study, failure to establish balanced fixation especially with medial column implants increases complications, especially nonunion, even for valgus fracture patterns.[78] As described in a 2021 study, when tenuous medial soft tissues preclude plate fixation, large frag screws can provide adequate medial column stability.[79]

As discussed in a 2020 study, despite advances in implant technology and surgical approaches, the four principles from 1979 still guide surgeons treating pilon fractures.[80] Precontoured locked distal tibia and fibula plates are available for use in osteoporotic bone and/or fractures with significant metaphyseal comminution. Attention to soft-tissue devitalization has led to minimally invasive plate osteosynthesis using small incisions and indirect or percutaneous reduction techniques. This technique may minimize soft-tissue complications, but the surgeon should balance this with the ability to achieve articular reduction and restoration of the mechanical axis.

External Fixation

Definitive external fixation with hybrid external fixators usually is reserved for a fracture with large articular fragments, a contaminated open fracture, or soft-tissue injury that compromises standard surgical exposures. A limited open reduction of the articular surface sometimes can be done in addition to hybrid external or percutaneous fixation.

SUMMARY

Ankle fracture treatment centers around mortise stability. In isolated lateral malleolar fractures, mortise stability can be assessed by radiographic stress views. Posterior malleolar fixation may improve mortise stability, syndesmotic reduction, and syndesmotic stability. Syndesmotic malreduction is common and significantly affect outcomes. Reduction should be performed by direct visualization or careful comparison with contralateral radiographic views.

Surgical intervention for pilon fractures historically has led to high complication rates and poor outcomes. To minimize the risk of complications, definitive surgical treatment should be delayed until the soft-tissue envelope is optimal. There is still no consensus on the surgical management of these difficult fractures, and it is important that patients understand that pilon fracture is a life-altering injury.

KEY STUDY POINTS

- In rotational ankle fractures, carefully assess for anatomic mortise position, or stability on stress testing, to determine surgical indications.
- Syndesmotic reduction is difficult and is a main determinant of functional outcome.
- Pilon fractures carry a high risk of soft-tissue problems, and definitive surgery should be delayed after closed reduction and external fixation if there is any question or doubt.

ANNOTATED REFERENCES

1. Phillips WA, Schwartz HS, Keller CS, et al: A prospective, randomized study of the management of severe ankle fractures. *J Bone Joint Surg Am* 1985;67(1):67-78.

2. Daly PJ, Fitzgerald RH Jr, Melton LJ, Ilstrup DM: Epidemiology of ankle fractures in Rochester, Minnesota. *Acta Orthop Scand* 1987;58(5):539-544.

3. Thur CK, Edgren G, Jansson KA, Wretenberg P: Epidemiology of adult ankle fractures in Sweden between 1987 and 2004: A population-based study of 91,410 Swedish inpatients. *Acta Orthop* 2012;83(3):276-281.

4. Ramsey PL, Hamilton W: Changes in tibiotalar area of contact caused by lateral talar shift. *J Bone Joint Surg Am* 1976;58(3):356-357.

5. Lloyd J, Elsayed S, Hariharan K, Tanaka H: Revisiting the concept of talar shift in ankle fractures. *Foot Ankle Int* 2006;27(10):793-796.

6. Olsen JR, Hunter J, Baumhauer JF: Osteoporotic ankle fractures. *Orthop Clin North Am* 2013;44(2):225-241.

7. Miller AG, Margules A, Raikin SM: Risk factors for wound complications after ankle fracture surgery. *J Bone Joint Surg Am* 2012;94(22):2047-2052.

8. Cummings SR, Melton LJ: Epidemiology and outcomes of osteoporotic fractures. *Lancet* 2002;359(9319):1761-1767.

9. Wukich DK, Kline AJ: The management of ankle fractures in patients with diabetes. *J Bone Joint Surg Am* 2008;90(7):1570-1578.

10. Chaudhry S, Egol KA: Ankle injuries and fractures in the obese patient. *Orthop Clin North Am* 2011;42(1):45-53, vi.

11. Ovaska MT, Makinen TJ, Madanat R, et al: Risk factors for deep surgical site infection following operative treatment of ankle fractures. *J Bone Joint Surg Am* 2013;95(4):348-353.

12. Egol KA, Amirtharajah M, Tejwani NC, Capla EL, Koval KJ: Ankle stress test for predicting the need for surgical fixation of isolated fibular fractures. *J Bone Joint Surg Am* 2004;86(11):2393-2398.

13. McConnell T, Creevy W, Tornetta P III: Stress examination of supination external rotation-type fibular fractures. *J Bone Joint Surg Am* 2004;86(10):2171-2178.

14. de Souza LJ, Gustilo RB, Meyer TJ: Results of operative treatment of displaced external rotation-abduction fractures of the ankle. *J Bone Joint Surg Am* 1985;67(7):1066-1074.

15. Joy G, Patzakis MJ, Harvey JP Jr: Precise evaluation of the reduction of severe ankle fractures. *J Bone Joint Surg Am* 1974;56(5):979-993.

16. Saldua NS, Harris JF, LeClere LE, Girard PJ, Carney JR: Plantar flexion influences radiographic measurements of the ankle mortise. *J Bone Joint Surg Am* 2010;92(4):911-915.

17. Michelson JD, Varner KE, Checcone M: Diagnosing deltoid injury in ankle fractures: The gravity stress view. *Clin Orthop Relat Res* 2001;387:178-182.

18. Candal-Couto JJ, Burrow D, Bromage S, Briggs PJ: Instability of the tibio-fibular syndesmosis: Have we been pulling in the wrong direction? *Injury* 2004;35(8):814-818.

19. Koval KJ, Egol KA, Cheung Y, Goodwin DW, Spratt KF: Does a positive ankle stress test indicate the need for operative treatment after lateral malleolus fracture? A preliminary report. *J Orthop Trauma* 2007;21(7):449-455.

20. Cheung Y, Perrich KD, Gui J, Koval KJ, Goodwin DW: MRI of isolated distal fibular fractures with widened medial clear space on stressed radiographs: Which ligaments are interrupted? *AJR Am J Roentgenol* 2009;192(1):W7-W12.

21. Haraguchi N, Armiger RS: A new interpretation of the mechanism of ankle fracture. *J Bone Joint Surg Am* 2009;91(4):821-829.

22. Kwon JY, Chacko AT, Kadzielski JJ, Appleton PT, Rodriguez EK: A novel methodology for the study of injury mechanism: Ankle fracture analysis using injury videos posted on YouTube.com. *J Orthop Trauma* 2010;24(8):477-482.

23. Ebraheim NA, Elgafy H, Padanilam T: Syndesmotic disruption in low fibular fractures associated with deltoid ligament injury. *Clin Orthop Relat Res* 2003;409:260-267.

24. Marsh JL, Slongo TF, Agel J, et al: Fracture and dislocation classification compendium – 2007: Orthopaedic Trauma Association classification, database and outcomes committee. *J Orthop Trauma* 2007;21(10 suppl):S1-S133.

25. Quigley TB: A simple aid to the reduction of abduction-external rotation fractures of the ankle. *Am J Surg* 1959;97(4):488-493.

26. Halanski MA, Halanski AD, Oza A, Vanderby R, Munoz A, Noonan KJ: Thermal injury with contemporary cast-application techniques and methods to circumvent morbidity. *J Bone Joint Surg Am* 2007;89(11):2369-2377.

27. Deignan BJ, Iaquinto JM, Eskildsen SM, et al: Effect of pressure applied during casting on temperatures beneath casts. *J Pediatr Orthop* 2011;31(7):791-797.

28. Chaudhry S, DelSole EM, Egol KA: Post-splinting radiographs of minimally displaced fractures: Good medicine or medicolegal protection? *J Bone Joint Surg Am* 2012;94(17):e128.

29. Tornetta P III, Axelrad TW, Sibai TA, Creevy WR: Treatment of the stress positive ligamentous SE4 ankle fracture: Incidence of syndesmotic injury and clinical decision making. *J Orthop Trauma* 2012;26(11):659-661.

30. Sanders DW, Tieszer C, Corbett B, Canadian Orthopedic Trauma Society: Operative versus nonoperative treatment of unstable lateral malleolar fractures: A randomized multicenter trial. *J Orthop Trauma* 2012;26(3):129-134.

31. Chan KB, Lui TH: Role of ankle arthroscopy in management of acute ankle fracture. *Arthroscopy* 2016;32(11):2373-2380.

32. Stufkens SA, Knupp M, Horisberger M, Lampert C, Hintermann B: Cartilage lesions and the development of osteoarthritis after internal fixation of ankle fractures: A prospective study. *J Bone Joint Surg Am* 2010;92(2):279-286.

33. Adams SB, Reilly RM, Huebner JL, Kraus VB, Nettles DL: Time-dependent effects on synovial fluid composition during the acute phase of human intra-articular ankle fracture. *Foot Ankle Int* 2017;38(10):1055-1063.

34. Adams SB, Setton LA, Bell RD, et al: Inflammatory cytokines and matix metalloproteinases in the synovial fluid after intra-articular ankle fracture. *Foot Ankle Int* 2015;36(11):1264-1271.

35. Deng Y, Staniforth TL, Zafar MS, Lau YJ: Posterior antiglide plating vs lateral neutralization plating for Weber B distal fibular fractures: A systematic review and meta-analysis of clinical and biomechanical studies. *Foot Ankle Int* 2022;43(6):850-859.

    A systematic review with meta-analysis of 1,122 patients with Weber B ankle fractures demonstrated twofold greater odds of requiring removal of hardware in lateral plating compared with posterior plating. Level of evidence: IV.

36. DeKeyser GJ, Campbell ML, Kellam PJ, et al: True antiglide fixation of Danis-Weber B fibula fractures has lower rates of removal of hardware. *Injury* 2022;53(3):1289-1293.

    A retrospective review of 96 patients with Weber B fractures showed a lower risk of reoperation of antiglide plate compared with lateral neutralization plate. Level of evidence: III.

37. Minihane KP, Lee C, Ahn C, Zhang LQ, Merk BR: Comparison of lateral locking plate and antiglide plate for fixation of distal fibular fractures in osteoporotic bone: A biomechanical study. *J Orthop Trauma* 2006;20(8):562-566.

38. White TO, Bugler KE, Olsen L, et al: A prospective, randomized, controlled, two-center, international trial comparing the fibular nail with open reduction and internal fixation for unstable ankle fractures in younger patients. *J Orthop Trauma* 2022;36(1):36-42.

    One hundred twenty-five patients were randomized to fibular nail or plate fixation. In patients younger than 65 years, a fibular nail demonstrated no difference with plate fixation of ankle fractures with patient-reported outcomes, complications, and reintervention. Level of evidence: I.

39. Weinfeld SB: Fibular nailing did not differ from standard open reduction and internal fixation for unstable ankle fractures in elderly patients. *J Bone Joint Surg Am* 2017;99(10):885-885.

40. Githens MF, DeBaun MR, Jacobsen KA, Ross H, Firoozabadi R, Haller J: Plafond malreduction and talar dome impaction accelerates arthrosis after supination-adduction ankle fracture. *Foot Ankle Int* 2021;42(10):1245-1253.

    A retrospective review of 79 patients showed that articular malreduction gap or step-off >2 mm was associated with development of arthrosis. Level of evidence: IV.

41. Tornetta P III: Competence of the deltoid ligament in bimalleolar ankle fractures after medial malleolar fixation. *J Bone Joint Surg Am* 2000;82(6):843-848.

42. Ricci WM, Tornetta P, Borrelli J Jr: Lag screw fixation of medial malleolar fractures: A biomechanical, radiographic, and clinical comparison of unicortical partially threaded lag screws and bicortical fully threaded lag screws. *J Orthop Trauma* 2012;26(10):602-606.

43. Berkes MB, Little MTM, Lazaro LE, et al: Malleolar fractures and their ligamentous injury equivalents have similar outcomes in supination-external rotation type IV fractures of the ankle treated by anatomical internal fixation. *J Bone Joint Surg Br* 2012;94(11):1567-1572.

44. Gardner MJ, Brodsky A, Briggs SM, Nielson JH, Lorich DG: Fixation of posterior malleolar fractures provides greater syndesmotic stability. *Clin Orthop Relat Res* 2006;447:165-171.

45. Bennett C, Behn A, Daoud A, et al: Buttress plating versus anterior-to-posterior lag screws for fixation of the posterior malleolus: A biomechanical study. *J Orthop Trauma* 2016;30(12):664-669.

46. O'Connor TJ, Mueller B, Ly TV, Jacobson AR, Nelson ER, Cole PA: "A to P" screw versus posterolateral plate for posterior malleolus fixation in trimalleolar ankle fractures. *J Orthop Trauma* 2015;29(4):e151-e156.

47. Gardner MJ, Demetrakopoulos D, Briggs SM, Helfet DL, Lorich DG: Malreduction of the tibiofibular syndesmosis in ankle fractures. *Foot Ankle Int* 2006;27(10):788-792.

48. Sagi HC, Shah AR, Sanders RW: The functional consequence of syndesmotic joint malreduction at a minimum 2-year follow-up. *J Orthop Trauma* 2012;26(7):439-443.

49. Pakarinen H, Flinkkila T, Ohtonen P, et al: Intraoperative assessment of the stability of the distal tibiofibular joint in supination-external rotation injuries of the ankle: Sensitivity, specificity, and reliability of two clinical tests. *J Bone Joint Surg Am* 2011;93(22):2057-2061.

50. Stark E, Tornetta P III, Creevy WR: Syndesmotic instability in Weber B ankle fractures: A clinical evaluation. *J Orthop Trauma* 2007;21(9):643-646.

51. Miller AN, Barei DP, Iaquinto JM, Ledoux WR, Beingessner DM: Iatrogenic syndesmosis malreduction via clamp and screw placement. *J Orthop Trauma* 2013;27(2):100-106.

52. Miller AN, Carroll EA, Parker RJ, Boraiah S, Helfet DL, Lorich DG: Direct visualization for syndesmotic stabilization of ankle fractures. *Foot Ankle Int* 2009;30(5):419-426.

53. Summers HD, Sinclair MK, Stover MD: A reliable method for intraoperative evaluation of syndesmotic reduction. *J Orthop Trauma* 2013;27(4):196-200.

54. Cosgrove CT, Putnam SM, Cherney SM, et al: Medial clamp tine positioning affects ankle syndesmosis malreduction. *J Orthop Trauma* 2017;31(8):440-446.

55. Cosgrove CT, Spraggs-Hughes AG, Putnam SM, et al: A novel indirect reduction technique in ankle syndesmotic injuries: A cadaveric study. *J Orthop Trauma* 2018;32(7):361-367.

56. Phisitkul P, Ebinger T, Goetz J, Vaseenon T, Marsh JL: Forceps reduction of the syndesmosis in rotational ankle fractures: A cadaveric study. *J Bone Joint Surg Am* 2012;94(24):2256-2261.

57. Michelson JD, Wright M, Blankstein M: Syndesmotic ankle fractures. *J Orthop Trauma* 2018;32(1):10-14.

58. Wikerøy AKB, Hoiness PR, Andreassen GS, Hellund JC, Madsen JE: No difference in functional and radiographic results 8.4 years after quadricortical compared with tricortical syndesmosis fixation in ankle fractures. *J Orthop Trauma* 2010;24(1):17-23.

59. Dehghan N, McKee MD, Jenkinson RJ, et al: Early weight-bearing and range of motion versus non-weightbearing and immobilization after open reduction and internal fixation of unstable ankle fractures: A randomized controlled trial. *J Orthop Trauma* 2016;30(7):345-352.

60. Assal M, Christofilopoulos P, Lubbeke A, Stern R: Augmented osteosynthesis of OTA 44-B fractures in older patients: A technique allowing early weightbearing. *J Orthop Trauma* 2011;25(12):742-747.

61. Lubbeke A, Salvo D, Stern R, Hoffmeyer P, Holzer N, Assal M: Risk factors for post-traumatic osteoarthritis of the ankle: An eighteen year follow-up study. *Int Orthop* 2012;36(7):1403-1410.

62. Nasell H, Ottosson C, Tornqvist H, Linde J, Ponzer S: The impact of smoking on complications after operatively treated ankle fractures—A follow-up study of 906 patients. *J Orthop Trauma* 2011;25(12):748-755.

63. Jacob N, Amin A, Giotakis N, Narayan B, Nayagam S, Trompeter AJ: Management of high-energy tibial pilon fractures. *Strategies Trauma Limb Reconstr* 2015;10(3):137-147.

64. Liporace FA, Yoon RS: Decisions and staging leading to definitive open management of pilon fractures: Where have we come from and where are we now? *J Orthop Trauma* 2012;26(8):488-498.

65. Crist BD, Khazzam M, Murtha YM, Della Rocca GJ: Pilon fractures: Advances in surgical management. *J Am Acad Orthop Surg* 2011;19(10):612-622.

66. Sirkin M, Sanders R, DiPasquale T, Herscovici D Jr: A staged protocol for soft tissue management in the treatment of complex pilon fractures. *J Orthop Trauma* 1999;13(2):78-84.

67. Patterson MJ, Cole JD: Two-staged delayed open reduction and internal fixation of severe pilon fractures. *J Orthop Trauma* 1999;13(2):85-91.

68. Boraiah S, Kemp TJ, Erwteman A, Lucas PA, Asprinio DE: Outcome following open reduction and internal fixation of open pilon fractures. *J Bone Joint Surg Am* 2010;92(2):346-352.

69. Dunbar RP, Barei DP, Kubiak EN, Nork SE, Henley MB: Early limited internal fixation of diaphyseal extensions in select pilon fractures: Upgrading AO/OTA type C fractures to AO/OTA type B. *J Orthop Trauma* 2008;22(6):426-429.

70. Ketz J, Sanders R: Staged posterior tibial plating for the treatment of Orthopaedic Trauma Association 43C2 and 43C3 tibial pilon fractures. *J Orthop Trauma* 2012;26(6):341-347.

71. White TO, Guy P, Cooke CJ, et al: The results of early primary open reduction and internal fixation for treatment of OTA 43.C-type tibial pilon fractures: A cohort study. *J Orthop Trauma* 2010;24(12):757-763.

72. Assal M, Ray A, Stern R: The extensile approach for the operative treatment of high-energy pilon fractures: Surgical technique and soft-tissue healing. *J Orthop Trauma* 2007;21(3):198-206.

73. Carbonell-Escobar R, Rubio-Suarez JC, Ibarzabal-Gil A, Rodriguez-Merchan EC: Analysis of the variables affecting outcome in fractures of the tibial pilon treated by open reduction and internal fixation. *J Clin Orthop Trauma* 2017;8(4):332-338.

74. Howard JL, Agel J, Barei DP, Benirschke SK, Nork SE: A prospective study evaluating incision placement and wound healing for tibial plafond fractures. *J Orthop Trauma* 2008;22(5):299-305.

75. Campbell ST, DeBaun MR, Kleweno CP, Nork SE: Simultaneous posterolateral and posteromedial approaches for fractures of the entire posterior tibial plafond: A safe technique for effective reduction and fixation. *J Orthop Trauma* 2022;36(1):49-53.

    A retrospective review of 35 patients with posterior pilon fractures demonstrated a low rate of wound problems (6%) when combined posterolateral and posteromedial approaches were used. Level of evidence: IV.

76. Mehta S, Gardner MJ, Barei DP, Benirschke SK, Nork SE: Reduction strategies through the anterolateral exposure for fixation of type B and C pilon fractures. *J Orthop Trauma* 2011;25(2):116-122.

77. Stannard JP, Schmidt AH, Kregor PJ: *Surgical Treatment of Orthopaedic Trauma*. Thieme, 2007.

78. Haller JM, Githens M, Rothberg D, Higgins T, Nork S, Barei D: Risk factors for tibial plafond nonunion: Medial column fixation may reduce nonunion rates. *J Orthop Trauma* 2019;33(9):443-449.

    A retrospective review of 740 tibial plafond fractures identified failure to treat the medial column as a risk factor for failure and nonunion. Level of evidence: IV.

79. Goodnough LH, Tigchelaar SS, Van Rysselberghe NL, et al: Medial column support in pilon fractures using percutaneous intramedullary large fragment fixation. *J Orthop Trauma* 2021;35(12):e502-e506.

A narrative review of technique and indications for medial column support in pilon fractures using percutaneous large fragment fixation and a case series of seven patients demonstrated well-healed fractures and maintained alignment. Level of evidence: V.

80. Hebert-Davies J, Kleweno CP, Nork SE: Contemporary strategies in pilon fixation. *J Orthop Trauma* 2020;34(suppl 1):S14-S20.

This study provides a narrative review and technique guide for treatment strategies in pilon fixation. Level of evidence: V.

CHAPTER 19

Talar Fractures

SAMUEL B. ADAMS, MD, FAAOS, FAOA

ABSTRACT

Talar fractures are relatively uncommon injuries and can be challenging to treat. The unique blood supply and complex surrounding articulations of the talus are critical to understand in terms of injury prognosis and surgical planning. Talar neck and body fractures most commonly are encountered following high-energy trauma and can result in complications such as talus osteonecrosis and posttraumatic arthritis of one or more surrounding joints, which can be difficult to treat. Fractures of the lateral and posterior processes were once ignored but have garnered more appreciation with recent data supporting surgical fixation.

Keywords: osteonecrosis; posttraumatic arthritis; talar body fracture; talar neck fracture; talar process fracture

INTRODUCTION

Talar fractures are uncommon injuries representing less than 1% of all fractures and only 3% to 6% of all foot fractures. Injuries to the talus can be devastating as the

---

Dr. Adams or an immediate family member serves as a paid consultant to or is an employee of Conventus/Flower, DJO, Exactech, Inc., Orthofix, Inc., Regeneration Technologies, Inc., and Stryker; has stock or stock options held in Medshape; and serves as a board member, owner, officer, or committee member of American Orthopaedic Foot and Ankle Society.

talus is the link between the ankle and the foot including the subtalar, transverse tarsal, and ankle joints. When a talar fracture occurs and peritalar arthritis ensues, the universal combined motion of the foot and ankle becomes compromised, and severe disability can result.

ANATOMY

To better understand talar fractures and their treatment, the unique anatomy of the talus must be understood. The talus is considered the universal joint of the foot because of its multiple joint articulations allowing motion in all planes. The variety of coupled actions occurring from the motion of this bone and surrounding articulations permit the flexibility of the hindfoot and midfoot. The talus articulates with the tibia, fibula, calcaneus, and navicular. Therefore, approximately two-thirds of the talar surface is covered with articular cartilage, and neither tendons nor muscles insert or originate from this bone. The talus is held in position by the articulating bony constraints and by constraining ligaments of the ankle joint. For the purposes of understanding fractures, the talus can be divided into the following parts: head, neck, body, lateral process, posterior medial process, and posterolateral process.

The blood supply to the talus is complex and has been extensively documented because of the incidence of osteonecrosis after fractures and dislocations. Areas for vessel entry into the talus are limited because of the majority cartilage surface. The extraosseous arteries to the talus include branches from the posterior tibial, dorsal pedis/anterior tibial, and peroneal arteries. The posterior tibial artery supplies the talus through two branches. The first branch is the artery of the tarsal canal. The artery of the tarsal canal then gives rise to the deltoid branch

---

This chapter is adapted from Hak DJ, Martin MP III: Talus fractures, in Chou LB, ed: *Orthopaedic Knowledge Update®: Foot and Ankle 6*. American Academy of Orthopaedic Surgeons, 2020, pp 303-317.

that supplies the medial and posterior talar body. The second branch derived from the posterior tibial artery forms a vascular plexus over the posterior medial tubercle of the talus with branches from the peroneal artery. The anterior tibial (dorsalis pedis) artery provides blood to the superior surface of the talar neck. The anterior tibial artery also gives rise to the anterolateral malleolar artery, which can anastomose with the perforating peroneal artery that becomes the artery of the tarsal sinus. The peroneal artery also forms a plexus with the posterior tibial artery to form the vascular plexus over the posterior tubercle of the talus. The peroneal artery also anastomoses with other vessels to form the artery of the tarsal sinus. The arteries of the tarsal sinus and tarsal canal further anastomose.

TALAR NECK FRACTURES

Mechanism of Injury

Talar neck fractures are usually caused by high-energy trauma such as motor vehicle collisions. The smallest cross-sectional area of the talus is in the region of the talar neck, which is covered with a relatively weak cortex, making it more susceptible to fracture. The high-energy trauma that produces displaced talar neck fractures frequently damages the limited blood supply to the talus and often causes varying degrees of articular cartilage damage.

Classification

The Hawkins classification is the most widely accepted classification system for talar neck fractures[1] (**Figure 1**). It is based on displacement and dislocation and therefore correlates with the presumed talar blood supply damage. The Hawkins classification was expanded by Canale and Kelly, who added the type IV group.[2] A Hawkins type I fracture is nondisplaced, without subluxation or dislocation of the surrounding joints. Hawkins type II is a displaced vertical talar neck fracture, with a subluxation or dislocation of the subtalar joint. Hawkins type III is a displaced fracture extending through the talar neck with dislocation at both the subtalar and tibiotalar joints. The type IV category consists of a dislocation of the ankle and subtalar joint, along with a dislocation or subluxation of the head of the talus at the talonavicular joint. The degree of displacement and dislocation is thought to be the primary determinant of blood supply damage and therefore of the risk for the development of osteonecrosis.

The type II classification has been subdivided into two subtypes: type IIA, those with a subluxated subtalar joint, and type IIB, those with a dislocated subtalar joint.[3] In a series of 81 talar neck fractures, osteonecrosis did not develop in any of the 19 Hawkins type IIA (subluxated subtalar joint) fracture, but osteonecrosis developed in 4 of 16 Hawkins type IIB fractures (25%).

Radiologic Evaluation

Routine ankle radiographs (AP, mortise, and lateral views) are used to identify talar fractures. The Canale oblique view of the talar neck provides the best evaluation of talar neck angulation and shortening[2] (**Figure 2**). This view is obtained with the ankle in maximum equinus and the foot pronated 15° while the x-ray tube is angled 75° from the horizontal plane. Although this view can be obtained preoperatively, it is most beneficial at the time of surgery to assess talar neck reduction. In addition to plain radiographs, talar fractures should be assessed with CT. CT is useful for assessing comminution and displacement of the fractures as well as providing accurate images of the ankle, subtalar, and transverse tarsal joints.

An association between talar fractures and peroneal tendon subluxation has been reported. Evaluation of preoperative CT scans in 30 patients who underwent talar fracture internal fixation identified dislocation of the peroneal tendon in 8 patients, but in only 1 of the patients was it diagnosed and treated at the time

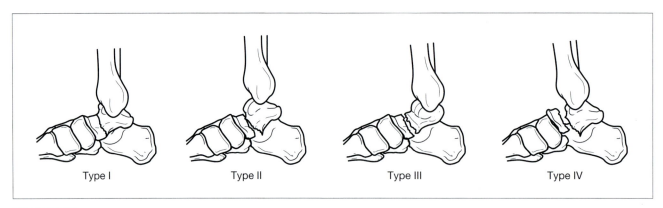

FIGURE 1 Illustration showing modified Hawkins classification of talar neck fractures.

Chapter 19: Talar Fractures

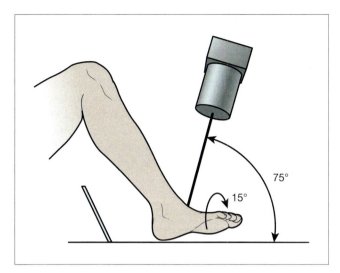

FIGURE 2 Illustration showing Canale view to evaluate the talar neck.

of fracture surgery.[4] The presence of peroneal tendon dislocation was associated with the presence of a fleck sign of the distal fibula, which represents an avulsion fracture at the insertion of the superior peroneal retinaculum. Dislocation was found at the time of a second surgery in another patient, in whom preoperative CT images did not show peroneal tendon dislocation, leading to an overall incidence of peroneal tendon dislocation of 30% (9 of 30 patients). The clinical diagnosis of peroneal tendon dislocation in these cases is obviously difficult, requiring clinicians to have a high index of suspicion for the possibility of associated peroneal tendon dislocations when treating both talar and calcaneal fractures.

Emergency Treatment and Timing of Surgical Fixation

Historically, talar neck fractures were considered surgical emergencies requiring immediate reduction and fixation to minimize the risk of osteonecrosis. Recent studies, however, have found no correlation between surgical timing and the development of osteonecrosis.

In a retrospective review of 102 talar neck fractures, the study authors were unable to find a correlation between surgical delay and the development of osteonecrosis. The mean time to fixation was 3.4 days for patients in whom osteonecrosis developed compared with 5 days for patients in whom osteonecrosis did not develop. Instead, the authors found that osteonecrosis was associated with talar neck comminution and open fracture.[5]

In another retrospective review of 106 surgically treated talar fractures (76 neck fractures, 25 body fractures, and five process fractures), the study authors reported that surgical timing did not affect the development of osteonecrosis or posttraumatic osteoarthritis.[6] Open fractures were found to be associated with the development of osteonecrosis or posttraumatic osteoarthritis. Thirty-five percent of the patients (15 of 43) in whom osteonecrosis or posttraumatic osteoarthritis developed had open injuries, but in the patients in whom osteonecrosis or posttraumatic osteoarthritis did not develop, only 16% (10 of 63) had open injuries. The study authors indicated that urgent surgical treatment is necessary for threatened soft-tissue or neurovascular compromise, but that the reduction quality is likely more important than the reduction timing.

A survey[7] found that most expert orthopaedic trauma surgeons do not think that immediate surgical treatment is necessary for displaced talar neck fractures. Most stated that talar neck fracture surgery can wait more than 8 hours, with a significant proportion stating that even a delay of more than 24 hours is acceptable. Because of the high-energy mechanism and limited soft-tissue envelope around the foot and ankle, 21% of talar neck fractures are open fractures,[1] requiring antibiotic therapy and urgent surgical débridement and irrigation to reduce the risk of infection.

Although delayed fixation of displaced talar neck fractures is acceptable, an initial closed reduction of any associated dislocation is recommended with a goal to achieve near-anatomic alignment of the talar neck. If a closed reduction attempt in the emergency department fails and there is skin or vascular compromise, then surgical closed or open reduction should be performed. Once reduced, the dislocated joint typically stabilizes because of the shape and fit of the articular surfaces and surrounding structures, but the use of both provisional Kirschner wire fixation and spanning external fixation has been described if there is instability.[8] Some studies have advocated the use of an external fixator to provide distraction of the ankle joint to unload the talus with hopes to reduce the incidence of osteonecrosis.[9] However, a study concluded that external fixation has no effect on the prevention of osteonecrosis following talar neck fractures.[10]

OPEN REDUCTION AND INTERNAL FIXATION

Surgical treatment is indicated for Hawkins type II, III, and IV talar neck fractures. Although completely nondisplaced fractures can be managed nonsurgically, fractures must be carefully followed with serial radiographs to ensure that the fracture does not displace during treatment. Caution must be exercised during nonsurgical treatment to avoid subsequent displacement and deformity, leading some authors to recommend internal fixation for even nondisplaced talar neck fractures.[8] In addition, internal fixation will permit early ankle and subtalar motion.

Anatomic reduction of both the talar neck and subtalar joint is the goal of talar neck fracture treatment because even minimal residual displacement can adversely affect subtalar joint mechanics.[11] It is important to avoid reducing the fracture in supination, pronation, or axial malalignment. Because rotational alignment is very difficult to judge, most surgeons recommend the use of dual surgical approaches, anteromedial and anterolateral, to allow accurate visualization and anatomic reduction of talar neck fractures. The anteromedial approach begins at the medial malleolus anterior border and extends toward the navicular tuberosity running between the anterior tibial and posterior tibial tendons. The lateral incision begins at the Chaput tubercle on the tibia and extends toward the bases of the third and fourth metatarsals. If the fracture progresses posteriorly into the body of the talus, a medial malleolar osteotomy may be necessary. An alternative two-incision approach is the direct anterior incision of the ankle and the sinus tarsi incision. The talar neck can be visualized through the anterior incision and the posterior body can be reduced, and any small fracture fragments can be removed from the subtalar joint using the sinus tarsi incision.

Kirschner wires placed in the talar head and body fragments can be used as joysticks to manipulate the reduction and correct the displacement and deformity. To achieve stable internal fixation and decrease the risk for malunion, at least two screws are required.

Anterior-to-posterior screw placement is used frequently because the entrance site is routinely exposed during the anterior approach (**Figure 3**). However, posterior-to-anterior screw fixation has been shown to be biomechanically stronger in a transverse noncomminuted talar neck fracture model.[12] Another biomechanical study compared three anterior-posterior screws, two cannulated posteroanterior screws, and one screw from anterior to posterior and a medially applied blade plate in a comminuted talar neck fracture model. In this study, researchers found a trend toward the anterior-posterior screws having approximately 20% lower yield point and stiffness compared with the posteroanterior screws or blade plate techniques, but this difference was not statistically significant.[13] Posterior-to-anterior screw fixation may be placed percutaneously or through a small posterolateral incision. A retrospective review of 24 consecutive talar neck fractures treated by posterior-to-anterior screw fixation reported favorable clinical, functional, and radiographic outcomes.[14,15] Complications included six patients with complaints of numbness or paresthesias in the sural nerve distribution (five transient, one permanent), one nonunion with hardware failure, one superficial wound infection, one patient with flexor hallucis longus muscle stiffness, and one revision surgery to exchange a screw impinging on the talonavicular joint. However, the study authors noted no cases of posterior impingement.

Lag or compression screws should be used cautiously for fixation of the medial talar neck. Compression in the setting of comminution will cause varus deformity. When there is comminution, fully threaded, nonlagging screws can be used to maintain the correct neck length. Bone grafting may be needed occasionally to replace impaction defects and restore the neck length. A 2022 study demonstrated the use of tibia autograft for the management of medial bone defects in 12 talar neck fractures.[16] Union was achieved in 11 patients (92%) and there was only 1 malunion (8%) with no complications associated with the use of the autograft.

Plate fixation with or without neutralization screw fixation is also a valid means of fixation for comminuted

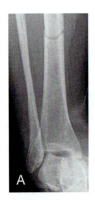
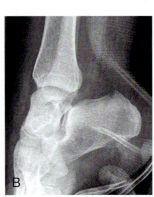
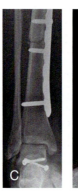
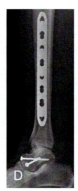
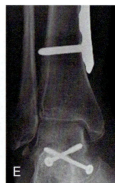
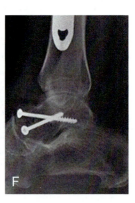

FIGURE 3 Radiographs from a 37-year-old woman who sustained multiple injuries in an automobile versus train accident including a minimally displaced talar neck fracture with subluxation/dislocation of the ankle and subtalar joints. **A** and **B**, AP and lateral plain radiographic views of the injury. **C** and **D**, The patient was initially treated with closed reduction and ankle spanning external fixation, followed by open reduction and internal fixation of the talar neck fracture using dual surgical approaches on postinjury day 5 (AP and lateral radiographs). **E** and **F**, AP and lateral radiographs 20 months postoperatively show no evidence of osteonecrosis, but some narrowing of the joint space is present.

Chapter 19: Talar Fractures

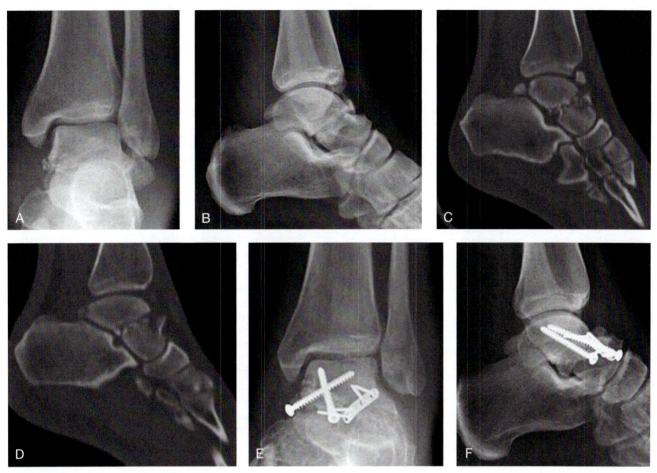

FIGURE 4 Radiographs from a 24-year-old man who sustained a comminuted Hawkins type II talar neck fracture while riding his bicycle with a fixed cleat pedal. **A** and **B**, AP and lateral plain radiograph injury views. **C** and **D**, CT showing the extensive comminution of the talar neck fracture. **E** and **F**, AP and lateral plain radiographs 7 months after open reduction and internal fixation. Because of the comminution, a 2.0-mm plate was used laterally and a fully threaded screw was used medially to prevent compression and shortening of the talar neck.

talar neck fractures.[8] Plates, sizes typically ranging from 2.0 to 2.7 mm, can be placed on the most comminuted column of the talus, either medially, laterally, or bilaterally (**Figure 4**). In addition to providing longitudinal structural support, they also resist supination or pronation of the distal fragment. The use of lateral minifragment plate fixation to augment medially placed sagittal plane position screws was shown to provide length-stable fixation, preventing talar neck shortening and malunion in a series of 26 patients with displaced and comminuted talar neck fractures.[17] In this series, posttraumatic arthritis was the most common complication, occurring in 38% of cases. Other complications included osteonecrosis (27% of cases) and nonunion (11.5% of cases). No patients required hardware removal.

Proximal talar neck fractures with extension into the body can be treated with medial malleolar osteotomies for fracture visualization and reduction. Surgical treatment through a medial malleolar osteotomy approach with miniplate fixation has been reported in 22 Hawkins type III talar neck fractures.[18] The sutdy authors reported that this approach resulted in decreased soft-tissue trauma, adequate talar neck exposure, and restoration of the talar anatomy; however, long-term complications of osteonecrosis and arthritis were still commonly seen. At an average 29.6 months follow-up, complications included 8 cases of partial osteonecrosis, 5 cases of complete osteonecrosis, 4 cases requiring secondary surgery, and 1 malunion. Subtalar arthritis was noted in 14 cases, talocrural arthritis is 13 cases, and talonavicular arthritis in 3 cases.

The use of intraoperative fluoroscopy is imperative to assess reduction accuracy and implant position. A Canale view must be obtained to assess the talar neck reduction. In addition, arthroscopic evaluation may be performed to provide better visualization of the articular surface, which may enhance reduction accuracy and allow débridement of any loose intra-articular debris.

COMPLICATIONS

Osteonecrosis

Osteonecrosis of the talar body caused by interruption of the precarious blood supply to the talus is the most feared complication following talar neck fracture. The risk of osteonecrosis is almost completely determined by the injury severity; however, surgical management techniques, including prompt and accurate reduction and meticulous surgical dissection that avoids further vascular damage, may decrease its likelihood. The osteonecrosis risk in Hawkins type I fractures is only zero to 15%, because only the blood supply entering through the neck is disrupted. Hawkins type II fractures have a 20% to 50% risk of osteonecrosis, with both the artery of the tarsal canal and the dorsal blood supply from the neck being disrupted. Type III and IV fractures have a 69% to 100% risk of osteonecrosis, with all three main sources of blood supply damaged.[1,2] With partial or full collapse of the talar dome, the subsequent degenerative changes lead to pain and disability in both the ankle and subtalar joints, along with shortening of the affected leg.

The Hawkins sign was described as a prognostic indicator of talar body vascularity. It can appear between 6 and 8 weeks after talar neck fractures and can be seen on the AP or mortise view radiographs. When a patient is non–weight bearing, the preserved blood supply permits resorption of the subchondral bone of the talar dome that appears as a radiolucency of the talar dome.[1,2] In clinical practice, the presence of the Hawkins sign is strongly predictive of the absence of osteonecrosis, although the absence of subchondral radiolucency does not universally predict osteonecrosis, and additional testing may be required.[2,19]

On plain radiographs, osteonecrosis will appear as sclerosis of the talar body when compared with the surrounding bone; however, the presence of this relative sclerosis may not become apparent until as late as 4 to 6 months after injury. MRI is the most sensitive test for evaluating the presence and extent of osteonecrosis and can help direct appropriate treatment.[20] For this reason, some surgeons advocate the use of titanium screws to minimize hardware artifact.

Treatment of talar osteonecrosis is extremely challenging. Long periods of non–weight bearing have been proposed to prevent talar dome collapse and allow time for creeping substitution and revascularization. However, non–weight bearing is of questionable value and there is no consensus on either the duration or degree of restricted weight bearing, or on the utility of bracing treatment or immobilization, in minimizing the sequelae of osteonecrosis.[21] Arthrodesis of either the ankle or the subtalar joint, which can be difficult to achieve in the presence of osteonecrotic bone, should be a last resort although subtalar fusion has been shown in a 2019 study to be successful in the setting of osteonecrosis.[22] Core decompression has been reported successful in select cases of talar osteonecrosis without collapse.[23] Talectomy and tibiocalcaneal arthrodesis yields poor outcomes, resulting in frequent pain, a short limb, and significant loss of ankle and subtalar motion.

Replacing the entire talus in the setting of osteonecrosis has been described in many ways. First, a stainless steel talar body prosthesis has been described for use in treating osteonecrosis or severe crush injuries of the talus.[24] In a review of 33 cases, 8 were performed because of a comminuted talar fracture, 2 for a talar body tumor, and 23 for idiopathic osteonecrosis. Implant failure before 6 years occurred in 5 cases, whereas 28 implants were still in place at the time of final follow-up ranging from 10 to 36 years. Early prosthesis failure occurred as a result of size mismatch in two patients, tumor recurrence in one patient, infection in one patient, and osteonecrosis of the talar head and neck in one patient.

The use of an alumina ceramic total talar prosthesis was reported in 55 ankles with talar osteonecrosis; however, only four of these were as a result of a talar neck fracture and the remainder were idiopathic.[25] These implants were custom designed based on the normal contralateral talus. The favorable congruency of the custom-made implant with the adjacent joints provides stability and maintains ankle function. No revisions were required at an average follow-up of 52.8 months (range, 24 to 96 months). Outcomes for these patients were assessed using the Japanese Society for Surgery of the Foot ankle-hindfoot score, which has a maximum score of 100 points (40 points for pain, 50 points for function, and 10 points for alignment). The patients' mean pain score improved from 15 to 34 points, mean function scores improved from 21.2 to 45.1 points, and mean alignment scores improved from 6.0 to 9.8 points, and their total scores improved from 43.1 to 89.4 points.

Additive manufacturing, or three-dimensional printing, has recently been used to treat osteonecrosis of the talus. The so-called total talus arthroplasty has come into favor. Three-dimensional printing allows for an exact replica of the patient's talus to be printed out of titanium or cobalt-chromium by using CT data from the contralateral talus. In addition, the dome of the three-dimensional printed talus can be changed to be congruent with the polyethylene of an ankle replacement if the patient has associated ankle arthritis.[15] The inferior aspect of the implant can be printed to be porous for bony ingrowth if a subtalar arthrodesis is performed. However, there are limited data on the use of these implants.

Vascularized pedicle bone grafting from the cuboid to the talus as a novel salvage procedure for patients with talar osteonecrosis has been described.[26] In a retrospective review of 13 patients whose MRI showed osteonecrosis involving less than 60% of the talus volume, good pain relief and improved physical function were reported in most patients at a mean follow-up of 6 years (range, 2 to 12 years). Three patients required a secondary surgical procedure. In two patients, the treatment failed and they underwent total ankle arthroplasty, and one patient had arthroscopic débridement for soft-tissue impingement.

Promising results of early posttraumatic talus osteonecrosis treatment by the percutaneous injection of autologous bone marrow concentrate have been reported.[27] Forty-five patients with early osteonecrosis without collapse treated with autologous bone marrow concentrate were compared with 34 patients treated with only core decompression. Outcomes studied were the progression in radiographic stages to collapse, the need for arthrodesis, and, in patients who required arthrodesis, the time to successfully achieve fusion. Radiographic collapse frequency was significantly lower in patients treated with autologous concentrate bone marrow grafting (27%, 12 of 45) compared with those treated by core decompression (71%, 24 of 34). There were significantly fewer arthrodesis procedures in patients treated with autologous concentrate bone marrow grafting (20%, 9 of 45) compared with those treated by core decompression (71%, 24 of 34). Patients treated with autologous concentrate bone marrow grafting also showed longer duration of survival before collapse or arthrodesis. For patients requiring arthrodesis, 100% of patients treated with autologous concentrate bone marrow grafting achieved successful fusion, compared with 75% of patients treated by core decompression. The time to successfully achieve fusion was also significantly shorter in patients treated with autologous concentrate bone marrow grafting (mean, 5 months, range, 3 to 7 months in nine patients undergoing arthrodesis) compared with those treated by core decompression (mean, 11 months, range, 6 to 18 months in 24 patients undergoing arthrodesis).

Malunion and Nonunion

The incidence of malunion following talar neck fracture has been reported to be approximately 30%.[2] The typical malunion findings include varus malalignment of the talar neck and associated medial column deformity.

Varus malunion can result in subalar arthritis and lateral column overload. Malalignment of only 2 mm results in significant changes in the subtalar contact characteristics that could lead to the progressive development of posttraumatic arthritis.[11] It is difficult to accurately evaluate residual step-offs and alignment on plain radiographs. CT is the most accurate method to measure malunion and can be helpful in preoperative planning.[28]

Talar neck osteotomy to reconstruct the normal anatomic shape of the talus is recommended for the management of malunions but is dependent on the status of the soft tissues, the joint cartilage, and the presence of osteonecrosis.[29] This salvage procedure corrects the foot malposition by an osteotomy through the malunited fracture, restoring the medial neck length using additional bone grafting if necessary.

Nonunion is rare following talar neck fracture, with an incidence of approximately 2.5%.[5]

Posttraumatic Arthritis

Long-term follow-up studies after talar neck fractures have shown that posttraumatic arthritis is more common than osteonecrosis, with an incidence ranging from 50% to 100%.[30,31] The causes of posttraumatic arthritis are multifactorial and include articular cartilage damage at the time of injury, progressive cartilage degeneration from fracture malunion or nonunion causing malalignment and incongruence, and from osteonecrosis. Posttraumatic arthritis primarily involves the subtalar joint but may also affect the ankle and talonavicular joints. In a study of 39 patients with talar neck fracture, osteonecrosis was seen in 19 patients (49%).[5] Osteonecrosis was associated with comminution of the talar neck ($P < 0.03$) and open fracture ($P < 0.05$). Posttraumatic arthritis developed in 21 of 39 patients (54%), which was more common after comminuted fractures ($P < 0.07$) and open fractures ($P = 0.09$).

TALAR BODY FRACTURES

Fractures of the talar body are uncommon injuries, accounting for only 7% to 38% of talar fractures.[32] A wide spectrum of fractures can occur in the talar body, ranging from small osteochondral shear injuries to severe crush injuries involving the entire talar body. These fractures commonly occur because of a high-energy axial loading injury such as a fall from height.

Small osteochondral injuries may not be apparent and should be at the top of the differential diagnosis in patients with persistent ankle pain 6 to 8 weeks following an apparent simple ankle sprain. Osteochondral injuries are commonly located in the anterolateral and posteromedial talar dome.

The literature on isolated talar body fractures is sparse. Complications frequently were reported in a series of 38 patients who had sustained a talar body fracture evaluated at an average of 33 months following injury. Of the 26 patients with full radiographs, 10 showed evidence of osteonecrosis, 17 showed evidence of posttraumatic tibiotalar arthritis, and 9 showed evidence of posttraumatic subtalar arthritis. In total, 88% of patients showed either evidence of osteonecrosis and/or posttraumatic osteoarthritis. Osteonecrosis and posttraumatic osteoarthritis were more commonly seen in open injuries and in patients with associated talar neck fractures.[32]

In a series of 19 patients having sustained a talar body fracture with an average follow-up of 26 months (range, 18 to 43 months), investigators reported 7 cases of osteonecrosis, 1 delayed union, and 1 malunion. Clinical outcome using American Orthopaedic Foot and Ankle Society Ankle/Hindfoot Scale scoring was rated as excellent in four patients, good in six, fair in four, and poor in five.[33]

LATERAL PROCESS FRACTURES

The lateral process of the talus is a wedge-shaped prominence that has two articular facets. One articular facet articulates with the distal fibula and the other larger facet forms the anterolateral portion of the subtalar joint. The prevalence of this injury in snowboarders has led to its eponymic naming as snowboarder's fracture. There is debate regarding the exact mechanism that produces a fracture of the lateral process. Some theorize that this fracture is caused by axial loading, ankle dorsiflexion, and inversion, whereas others indicate the necessity of an external rotation or eversion force.[34] In one series of 20 patients who sustained a lateral process fracture from snowboarding, the injury mechanism included axial impact (100%), dorsiflexion (95%), external rotation (80%), and eversion (45%).[35] Fractures of the lateral process of the talus are often missed on plain radiographs, with these patients usually being diagnosed as having sustained an ankle sprain. CT best identifies the size and position of the lateral process fracture (**Figure 5**).

Nondisplaced fractures are generally managed nonsurgically with 6 weeks of immobilization, and then advanced to partial weight bearing until radiographic evidence of healing. Larger noncomminuted displaced fractures require open reduction and internal fixation with lag screw fixation, often using either 2.0- or 2.7-mm screws. The surgical approach is a 5- to 8-cm gently curved incision over the sinus tarsi to expose the subtalar joint. Primary surgical treatment for displaced lateral process fractures has been shown to improve outcomes and lower the risk of subtalar arthritis.[35] Displaced comminuted fractures may not be amenable to internal fixation and instead may be treated by excision.

In a 2020 retrospective review of eight patients with talar process fractures, the most common mechanism of injury was dorsiflexion, supination, and external rotation under axial load.[36] Arthritis developed in two patients (ankle arthritis in one and subtalar arthritis in the other). Moreover, in a 2019 study of 22 patients with lateral process fractures, subtalar arthritis developed in 50% of patients.[37] Subtalar arthritis was the independent factor associated with a poor patient-rated outcome regarding pain and patient-reported outcomes.

POSTERIOR PROCESS FRACTURES

The posterior process of the talus commonly makes up approximately 25% of the posterior subtalar articulation. It consists of a medial and a lateral tubercle that are separated by a groove for the flexor hallucis longus tendon.

Posterior process fractures of the talus are infrequent injuries that usually involve an isolated fracture of either the medial or lateral tubercle. An unfused os trigonum may also be confused with a fracture of the posterior process.

Fractures of the entire posterior talar process are most likely caused by forceful maximal plantar flexion of the ankle, which produces a nutcracker-like compression of the posterior talus process between the posterior malleolus and the calcaneus.[38] Fracture of the medial tubercle of the posterior process may occur when the foot is suddenly forced into combined dorsiflexion and pronation, placing the posterior talotibial portion of the deltoid ligament under tension, and resulting in avulsion of the

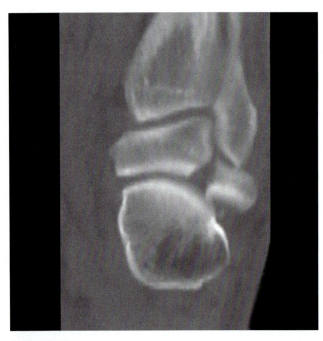

FIGURE 5 Coronal reconstruction CT scan that shows a lateral talar process fracture.

tubercle.[39] The lateral tubercle of the posterior process may be fractured because of repetitive plantar flexion, similar to a stress fracture.[38]

Fracture of the entire posterior talar process is usually treated by open reduction and internal fixation because they comprise a significant portion of the subtalar joint. The surgical approach for fixation is selected based on the direction of major displacement.

A posteromedial approach between the flexor digitorum longus tendon and the neurovascular bundle is used when the fragment is displaced posteromedially, whereas a posterolateral approach between the peroneal tendons and the Achilles tendon is used when the fragment is displaced posterolaterally.

There is sparse literature describing the outcomes of posterior process fractures. A 2019 study evaluated the functional outcome and quality of life of 29 patients with posterior process fractures.[40] The study authors found that surgical management of posterior process fractures provided good functional outcome, quality of life, and patient satisfaction. Patients who were treated nonsurgically were found to have worse outcomes.

SUMMARY

Fractures of the talus are uncommon but often serious injuries. The high-energy injury required to produce a displaced talar neck fracture may also cause severe associated soft-tissue damage, including damage to the precarious talar blood supply. Anatomic reduction and stable internal fixation of displaced talar neck fractures may minimize complication rates; however, the sequelae of posttraumatic complications may be inevitable. The risk of osteonecrosis is almost completely determined by the injury severity and not surgical timing; however, surgical management techniques including prompt and accurate reduction, and meticulous surgical dissection that avoids further vascular damage, may decrease its likelihood. Both osteonecrosis and posttraumatic arthritis are challenging complications to treat. Talar body fractures are also associated with a high rate of complications. Lateral process fractures of the talus can be overlooked and may also lead to posttraumatic sequelae.

KEY STUDY POINTS

- The goals of surgical management of talar fractures are to obtain an anatomic reduction and minimize additional vascular damage.
- Timing of surgical management of talar neck fractures is less important than quality of reduction, although soft-tissue compromise and neurovascular injury should prompt early surgical management.

Fracture-dislocations should be treated with closed reduction on initial evaluation.
- The risk of development of osteonecrosis after talar neck fractures is increased with fracture displacement and associated dislocations, in open injuries, and when there is significant comminution. Osteonecrosis is less common than posttraumatic arthritis.
- Outcomes of displaced lateral and posterior process fractures are better after surgical management.

ANNOTATED REFERENCES

1. Hawkins LG: Fractures of the neck of the talus. *J Bone Joint Surg Am* 1970;52(5):991-1002.

2. Canale ST, Kelly FB Jr: Fractures of the neck of the talus. Long-term evaluation of seventy-one cases. *J Bone Joint Surg Am* 1978;60(2):143-156.

3. Vallier HA, Reichard SG, Boyd AJ, Moore TA: A new look at the Hawkins classification for talar neck fractures: Which features of injury and treatment are predictive of osteonecrosis? *J Bone Joint Surg Am* 2014;96(3):192-197.

4. Sadamasu A, Yamaguchi S, Nakagawa R, et al: The recognition and incidence of peroneal tendon dislocation associated with a fracture of the talus. *Bone Joint J* 2017;99-B(4):489-493.

5. Vallier HA, Nork SE, Barei DP, Benirschke SK, Sangeorzan BJ: Talar neck fractures: Results and outcomes. *J Bone Joint Surg Am* 2004;86(8):1616-1624.

6. Buckwalter VJA, Westermann R, Mooers B, Karam M, Wolf B: Timing of surgical reduction and stabilization of talus fracture-dislocations. *Am J Orthop (Belle Mead NJ)* 2017;46(6):E408-E413.

7. Patel R, Van Bergeyk A, Pinney S: Are displaced talar neck fractures surgical emergencies? A survey of orthopaedic trauma experts. *Foot Ankle Int* 2005;26(5):378-381.

8. Rammelt S, Zwipp H: Talar neck and body fractures. *Injury* 2009;40(2):120-135.

9. Milenkovic S, Radenkovic M, Mitkovic M: Open subtalar dislocation treated by distractional external fixation. *J Orthop Trauma* 2004;18(9):638-640.

10. Besch L, Drost J, Egbers HJ: Treatment of rare talus dislocation fractures. An analysis of 23 injuries [German]. *Unfallchirurg* 2002;105(7):595-601.

11. Sangeorzan BJ, Wagner UA, Harrington RM, Tencer AF: Contact characteristics of the subtalar joint: The effect of talar neck misalignment. *J Orthop Res* 1992;10(4):544-551.

12. Swanson TV, Bray TJ, Holmes GB Jr: Fractures of the talar neck. A mechanical study of fixation. *J Bone Joint Surg Am* 1992;74(4):544-551.

13. Attiah M, Sanders DW, Valdivia G, et al: Comminuted talar neck fractures: A mechanical comparison of fixation techniques. *J Orthop Trauma* 2007;21(1):47-51.

14. Beltran MJ, Mitchell PM, Collinge CA: Posterior to anteriorly directed screws for management of talar neck fractures. *Foot Ankle Int* 2016;37(10):1130-1136.

15. Akoh CC, Chen J, Adams SB: Total ankle total talus replacement using a 3D printed talus component: A case report. *J Foot Ankle Surg* 2020;59(6):1306-1312.

    The three-dimensional custom total talus replacement is a novel treatment for osteonecrosis of the talus. However, patients who require a total talus replacement often have concomitant degenerative changes to the tibiotalar, subtalar, or talonavicular joints. The combined three-dimensional custom total ankle–total talus replacement is used for patients with an unreconstructable talus and adjacent tibial plafond involvement. The goal of performing a total ankle–total talus replacement is to provide pain relief, retain motion at the tibiotalar joint, maintain or improve the patient's functional status, and minimize limb shortening. Total ankle–total talus replacement is made possible by three-dimensional printing. The advent of three-dimensional printing has allowed for the accurate re-creation of the native talar anatomy with a talar dome that can be matched to a total ankle replacement polyethylene bearing. In this article, a case of talar osteonecrosis treated with a combined total ankle–total talus replacement is discussed and the current literature for total ankle–total talus replacement is reviewed. Level of evidence: V.

16. McMurtrie JT, Patch DA, Frazier MB, et al: Union rates of talar neck fractures with substantial bone defects treated with autograft. *Foot Ankle Int* 2022;43(3):343-352.

    Tibial autograft was used in 12 patients with talar neck fractures for primary osteosynthesis of comminuted talar neck fractures with substantial bone defects. In this series the autograft application to the talar neck was associated with excellent union rates and low malunion rates. Despite high union rates, secondary outcomes of osteonecrosis with or without collapse, ankle and subtalar posttraumatic arthritis, and relatively low patient-reported outcomes were common. Level of evidence: IV.

17. Maceroli MA, Wong C, Sanders RW, Ketz JP: Treatment of comminuted talar neck fractures with use of minifragment plating. *J Orthop Trauma* 2016;30(10):572-578.

18. Liu H, Chen Z, Zeng W, et al: Surgical management of Hawkins type III talar neck fracture through the approach of medial malleolar osteotomy and mini-plate for fixation. *J Orthop Surg Res* 2017;12(1):111.

19. Tezval M, Dumont C, Sturmer KM: Prognostic reliability of the Hawkins sign in fractures of the talus. *J Orthop Trauma* 2007;21(8):538-543.

20. Thordarson DB, Triffon MJ, Terk MR: Magnetic resonance imaging to detect avascular necrosis after open reduction and internal fixation of talar neck fractures. *Foot Ankle Int* 1996;17(12):742-747.

21. DiGiovanni CW, Patel A, Calfee R, Nickisch F: Osteonecrosis in the foot. *J Am Acad Orthop Surg* 2007;15(4):208-217.

22. Dekker TJ, Pellegrini MJ, Schiff AP, et al: Isolated subtalar arthrodesis for avascular necrosis of the talus. *J Surg Orthop Adv* 2019;28(2):132-136.

    A retrospective review of subtalar arthrodeses was performed on a cohort of 12 patients with talar osteonecrosis who underwent subtalar arthrodesis. The primary outcome was radiographic fusion with secondary outcomes of subsequent procedures, recurrent pain, and perioperative complications. Radiographic fusion of the subtalar arthrodesis occurred in all 12 patients. Five of six patients with traumatic etiology went on to have secondary procedures. One of six patients with atraumatic etiology underwent a secondary procedure for advancement of tibiotalar arthritis. In the setting of atraumatic talar osteonecrosis, this small cohort demonstrates that isolated subtalar arthrodesis is a safe and reliable procedure with high fusion rates and low need for secondary procedures. Level of evidence: IV.

23. Grice J, Cannon L: Percutaneous core decompression: A successful method of treatment of stage I avascular necrosis of the talus. *Foot Ankle Surg* 2011;17(4):317-318.

24. Harnroongroj T, Harnroongroj T: The talar body prosthesis: Results at ten to thirty-six years of follow-up. *J Bone Joint Surg Am* 2014;96(14):1211-1218.

25. Taniguchi A, Takakura Y, Tanaka Y, et al: An alumina ceramic total talar prosthesis for osteonecrosis of the talus. *J Bone Joint Surg Am* 2015;97(16):1348-1353.

26. Nunley JA, Hamid KS: Vascularized pedicle bone-grafting from the cuboid for talar osteonecrosis: Results of a novel salvage procedure. *J Bone Joint Surg Am* 2017;99(10): 848-854.

27. Hernigou P, Dubory A, Flouzat Lachaniette CH, Khaled I, Chevallier N, Rouard H: Stem cell therapy in early post-traumatic talus osteonecrosis. *Int Orthop* 2018;42(12):2949-2956.

28. Chan G, Sanders DW, Yuan X, Jenkinson RJ, Willits K: Clinical accuracy of imaging techniques for talar neck malunion. *J Orthop Trauma* 2008;22(6):415-418.

29. Rammelt S, Winkler J, Heineck J, Zwipp H: Anatomical reconstruction of malunited talus fractures: A prospective study of 10 patients followed for 4 years. *Acta Orthop* 2005;76(4):588-596.

30. Frawley PA, Hart JA, Young DA: Treatment outcome of major fractures of the talus. *Foot Ankle Int* 1995;16(6):339-345.

31. Lindvall E, Haidukewych G, DiPasquale T, Herscovici D Jr, Sanders R: Open reduction and stable fixation of isolated, displaced talar neck and body fractures. *J Bone Joint Surg Am* 2004;86(10):2229-2234.

32. Vallier HA, Nork SE, Benirschke SK, Sangeorzan BJ: Surgical treatment of talar body fractures. *J Bone Joint Surg Am* 2003;85(9):1716-1724.

33. Ebraheim NA, Patil V, Owens C, Kandimalla Y: Clinical outcome of fractures of the talar body. *Int Orthop* 2008;32(6):773-777.

34. Funk JR, Srinivasan SC, Crandall JR: Snowboarder's talus fractures experimentally produced by eversion and dorsiflexion. *Am J Sports Med* 2003;31(6):921-928.

35. Valderrabano V, Perren T, Ryf C, Rillmann P, Hintermann B: Snowboarder's talus fracture: Treatment outcome of 20 cases after 3.5 years. *Am J Sports Med* 2005;33(6):871-880.

36. von Winning D, Lippisch R, Pliske G, Adolf D, Walcher F, Piatek S: Surgical treatment of lateral and posterior process fractures of the talus: Mid-term results of 15 cases after 7 years. *Foot Ankle Surg* 2020;26(1):71-77.

    Fifteen patients who underwent internal fixation for lateral or posterior process fractures were examined for radiologic and clinical functional outcomes. The independent parameters evaluated were age, sex, extent of general injury, soft-tissue damage, surgical latency, and fracture type. All fractures healed completely. Osteoarthritis developed in three patients. The American Orthopaedic Foot and Ankle Society Ankle/Hindfoot Scale score was 79.5 ± 18.6, the Functional Foot Index score was 31.1 ± 31.4, and the physical and mental component summary scores of the Short Form 36, version 2, were 46.6 ± 11.8 and 50.3 ± 9.1, respectively. The clinical outcomes of internal fixation of talar process fractures were good. Delayed surgical treatment (≥14 days) did not significantly lead to poorer outcomes. Level of evidence: IV.

37. Horterer H, Baumbach SF, Lemperle S, et al: Clinical outcome and concomitant injuries in operatively treated fractures of the lateral process of the talus. *BMC Musculoskelet Disord* 2019;20(1):219.

    This was a retrospective review of 23 lateral talar process fractures. After a follow-up of over 3.5 years, surgically treated fractures resulted in only moderate results. Fifty percent had posttraumatic symptomatic subtalar osteoarthritis, which was the primary independent parameter for a poor outcome following lateral process fractures. Level of evidence: III.

38. Berkowitz MJ, Kim DH: Process and tubercle fractures of the hindfoot. *J Am Acad Orthop Surg* 2005;13(8):492-502.

39. Kim DH, Berkowitz MJ, Pressman DN: Avulsion fractures of the medial tubercle of the posterior process of the talus. *Foot Ankle Int* 2003;24(2):172-175.

40. Wijers O, Engelmann EWM, Posthuma JJ, Halm JA, Schepers T: Functional outcome and quality of life after nonoperative treatment of posterior process fractures of the talus. *Foot Ankle Int* 2019;40(12):1403-1407.

    This study was a retrospective review of 29 patients with posterior process fractures. Patients were treated nonsurgically or surgically. Surgical management of extended posterior talar fractures was found to provide good functional outcome, quality of life, and patient satisfaction. Although the patients treated nonsurgically were found to have less severe injuries, they demonstrated worse overall outcome, which is supportive of surgical management. Nonsurgical treatment is therefore only justified in selected patients. Level of evidence: IV.

CHAPTER 20

Calcaneal Fractures

JESSE F. DOTY, MD, FAAOS

ABSTRACT

Calcaneal fractures can be low-energy or high-energy injuries, affecting patients of all ages. Both early morbidity and long-term sequelae can be expected. Although nondisplaced fractures are treated nonsurgically, displaced fractures present a treatment dilemma. Radiographic classifications are based on the morphology of the primary fracture line, and CT classifications are based on the degree of subtalar facet comminution. Studies reveal high complication rates and wound healing issues with the extensile lateral approach. Minimally invasive approaches decrease wound complications and may provide similar radiographic and clinical results. Percutaneous methods may further decrease wound complications, deep infection, and stiffness. The optimal treatment for displaced, intra-articular fractures is largely based on the amount of gross morphologic displacement, the degree of articular involvement, and patient factors.

Keywords: calcaneal fracture; extensile lateral approach; sinus tarsi approach; subtalar arthritis

INTRODUCTION

Calcaneal fractures are debilitating injuries often associated with long-term pain, posttraumatic arthritis, and the need for further surgical intervention. Management of patient expectations is imperative, and the best treatment approach is largely based on patient factors in addition to fracture patterns. The increasing popularity of minimally invasive and percutaneous surgical approaches minimizes the risk of complications and may provide more predictable outcomes.

PATHOANATOMY AND EPIDEMIOLOGY

Calcaneal fractures are often intra-articular injuries from a high-energy mechanism, such as a motor vehicle crash or a high fall. Commonly these are young, active individuals in industrial settings with a long-term significant socioeconomic impact. Calcaneal fracture impairment is more severe than other fractures and can rival a serious medical event such as an organ transplant or myocardial infarction.[1,2] Polytrauma, alcohol abuse, psychiatric illness, nonworking status, and posttraumatic arthritis have been associated with worse functional outcomes.[3] Typically, an axial load drives the talus into the calcaneus.

Dr. Doty or an immediate family member has received royalties from Arthrex, Inc., Globus Medical, and Wright Medical Technology, Inc.; is a member of a speakers' bureau or has made paid presentations on behalf of Arthrex, Inc., BoneSupport AB, Globus Medical, Immersive Tech, Inc., International Life Sciences, Novastep Inc., and Wright Medical Technology, Inc.; serves as a paid consultant to or is an employee of Arthrex, Inc., BoneSupport AB, Depuy/Synthes, Globus Medical, Immersive Tech, Inc., International Life Sciences, Novastep Inc., and Wright Medical Technology, Inc.; has stock or stock options held in Globus Medical; has received research or institutional support from Arthrex, Inc. and Wright Medical Technology, Inc.; and serves as a board member, owner, officer, or committee member of American Orthopaedic Foot and Ankle Society.

This chapter is adapted from Kim TS: Fractures of the calcaneus, in Chou LB, ed: *Orthopaedic Knowledge Update®: Foot and Ankle 6*. American Academy of Orthopaedic Surgeons, 2020, pp 331-348.

The foot position, bone quality, and the amount of energy determine the fracture pattern.[4] Severe swelling with blisters and compartment syndrome can occur, and the heel is often shortened, widened, and displaced into varus. Although a documented association with lumbar spine fractures exists, a multitude of associated injuries may be present in up to 75% of patients, and the most common concomitant fractures are in close proximity to the calcaneus.[5] Soft-tissue injuries, especially to the peroneal tendons and their retinacular sheath, are also common. A systematic review including 1,050 calcaneal fractures revealed injury to the peroneal tendons in approximately 30% of patients.[6] The treatment algorithm is largely determined by the extent of bony dysmorphism and the degree of involvement of the subtalar joint where articular impaction universally leads to the development of posttraumatic arthritis.

INTRA-ARTICULAR FRACTURES

Classification and Imaging

Plain radiographs should include AP and lateral foot views and a Harris axial heel view. On the lateral view, a decreased Böhler angle, an increased angle of Gissane, and an inferior displacement of the posterior facet can be seen (**Figure 1**). If only the lateral portion of the joint is displaced, a double density sign (when two portions of the posterior facet articular surface are visible on the lateral radiograph) can be seen. The AP foot view may show extension of the fracture into the anterior process. The axial view may show varus displacement and shortening of the tuberosity. The AP calcaneal profile view was recently described to be equally as accurate and more easy to obtain for evaluating the axial varus alignment of the fracture displacement[7] (**Figure 2**). CT is recommended to evaluate the extent of joint involvement and the degree of displacement.[8]

A displaced intra-articular calcaneal fracture is identified as a joint-depression fracture or a tongue-type fracture, based on the Essex-Lopresti[9] classification. A posterior directed force may cause the fracture line to extend into the posterior facet to produce a joint-depression fracture. An inferiorly directed force may produce a fracture line extending inferior to the posterior facet with a tongue-type fracture pattern. A tongue-type fracture may be more associated with disruption of the gastrocnemius-soleus complex insertion and plantar-medial fragment avulsion at the plantar fascia origin. A joint-depression fracture may have increased articular fragmentation and subtalar dislocation.[10]

Sanders[8] expanded Soeur and Remy's[11] classification to define a system based on articular involvement of the posterior facet, as seen on coronal CT. Type I fractures are nondisplaced. Type II fractures are two parts with subtypes based on fracture line location. Type III fractures are three parts, often with a centrally depressed

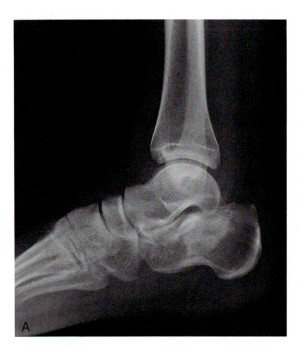
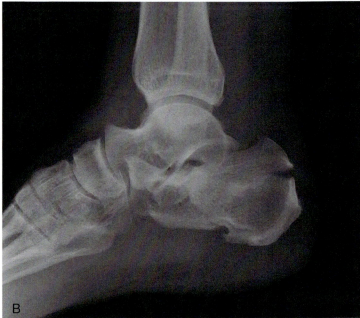

FIGURE 1 Lateral radiographs of displaced intra-articular calcaneal fractures with loss of calcaneal height, depressed articular fragments, decreased Böhler angle, and increased angle of Gissane. Radiographically these can be classified as a joint-depression (**A**) and a tongue-type (**B**) fracture pattern.

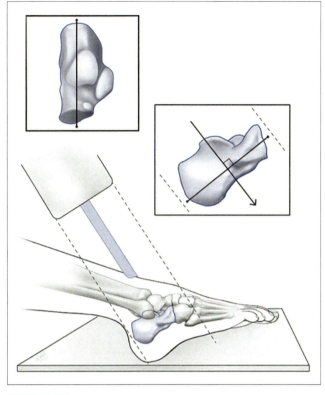

FIGURE 2 Demonstration of the AP calcaneal profile view. (Reprinted with permission from Kwon JY, Moura B, Gonzalez T, et al: Anterior-posterior (AP) calcaneal profile view: A novel radiographic image to assess varus malalignment. *Foot Ankle Int* 2020;41[10]:1249-1255.)

fragment. Type IV fractures are four or more articular fragments. Historically, the medial sustentacular constant fragment was thought to remain nondisplaced because of ligamentous attachments. However, CT suggests the fragment is actually displaced or angulated in more than 20% of fractures.[12]

Nonsurgical Treatment

A nondisplaced fracture is generally treated with non–weight bearing and early range of motion.

Displaced fractures are also sometimes treated nonsurgically, particularly in patients with diabetes, patients with neuropathy, and those with multiple medical comorbidities. Chronologic age may be considered, but improved results with surgical treatment have been reported in a patient cohort older than 60 years.[13]

Surgical Versus Nonsurgical Treatment of a Displaced Fracture

The definitive treatment of patients with displaced intra-articular calcaneal fracture largely depends on patient factors. Improved understanding and management of the associated soft-tissue injury and lower profile implants have led to the development of surgical techniques with lower complication rates. The first randomized prospective study on surgical treatment included 30 patients and was published in 1996 with improved outcomes at 1.5 years in the surgically treated group.[14] Since then, there have been multiple multicenter randomized controlled trials evaluating surgical versus nonsurgical treatment for displaced fractures, but benefits of surgical intervention have been difficult to demonstrate based on high wound complication rates with utilization of the extensile lateral approach (**Figure 3**).

In a large multicenter randomized study, validated outcome measures revealed no overall difference when including all surgical and nonsurgical patients.[15] However, further analysis revealed women, younger patients, non–workers' compensation patients, and those with the most significant displacement benefited the most from surgery. Nonsurgically treated patients were more likely to require subsequent subtalar arthrodesis for post-traumatic arthritis.

Another randomized controlled multicenter study looked at surgical versus nonsurgical treatment in 82 patients with displaced fractures.[16] Pain and functional outcome measures showed no difference between the groups acutely, but at 10-year follow-up, there was a trend toward improved functional outcomes, and also less subtalar arthritis, in the surgically treated group.

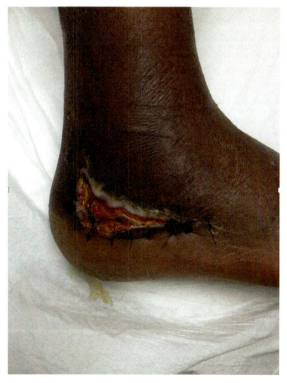

FIGURE 3 Clinical photograph of an extended lateral incision with early skin edge necrosis and wound dehiscence.

A third large randomized controlled study evaluated 151 patients at 22 centers.[17] Complications were higher in the surgical group (23% versus 4%), and there were no differences in pain or function at 2-year follow-up. Given the complexity of calcaneal fractures and the ongoing evolution of treatment, many experts have cautioned against broad and definitive conclusions on surgical versus nonsurgical treatment based on single studies.[18] Meta-analyses report higher complication rates, but also improved anatomic recovery, higher rate of return to work, and decreased rate of late subtalar arthrodesis with surgical treatment.[6,19-21]

Open Reduction and Internal Fixation of a Displaced Fracture

In recent decades, open reduction and internal fixation has frequently been recommended for surgical candidates with a Sanders type II or III intra-articular fractures.[4] Outcomes are poor if these injuries are treated nonsurgically. Historically, most studies reported open reduction and internal fixation through an extensile lateral approach.[22-24] A study presented long-term follow-up (average 15.2 years) on 108 of 208 fractures that underwent open reduction and internal fixation with the extensile lateral approach.[25] Postoperative CT indicated 95% of patients had an anatomic articular reduction. Sanders classification was predictive of late subtalar fusion and clinical and functional results were maintained and acceptable if fusion was not needed (77 of 108 fractures).

Delayed wound healing and infection lead some surgeons to recommend delaying surgical treatment for weeks after the injury as the initial injury swelling subsided.[26,27] However, one study revealed no benefit with regard to wound complications and surgical delay.[28] This evolved to early aggressive soft-tissue management to shorten the surgical delay as fracture reductions are more difficult to obtain weeks after injury. With the use of less invasive approaches and indirect reduction techniques, earlier surgical intervention may be performed in a safer manner.[28,29]

Surgical Treatment of a Tongue-Type Fracture

A displaced tongue-type fracture may require urgent surgical treatment as the tuberosity fragment places the posterior skin under tension and can lead to skin necrosis. A 21% incidence of posterior soft-tissue compromise was found in a study of 139 tongue-type fractures.[30] Six soft-tissue coverage procedures and one amputation resulted. The patients treated with urgent percutaneous reduction avoided soft-tissue complications. Simple or extra-articular tongue-type fractures are treated with percutaneous fixation. Guidewires placed percutaneously on either side of the Achilles tendon and advanced into

the displaced tuberosity can help with fracture reduction.[31] Definitive fixation can be achieved with cannulated screws placed over the guidewires or small fragment screws placed percutaneously (**Figure 4**).

Complex intra-articular fractures with a tongue-type component may not be amenable to anatomic reduction using the percutaneous Essex-Lopresti technique. In young active patients, the articular surface can be visualized with open reduction and internal fixation through an open extensile lateral or sinus tarsi approach.

Primary Arthrodesis for a Type IV Fracture

Comminuted Sanders type IV fracture pattern progression to posttraumatic arthritis is often inevitable. For this reason, primary arthrodesis may be the surgical treatment of choice.[32,33] In this technique, the extra-articular calcaneal anatomy is restored with open reduction and internal fixation, the cartilage is denuded, and bone graft is added to obtain subtalar fusion. High union rates, quicker return to work, and acceptable clinical outcomes have been reported.[34]

Minimally Invasive Techniques for a Displaced Fracture

These alternate approaches have lower rates of wound complications. In addition, the extensive soft-tissue stripping required for the extensile lateral approach may compromise calcaneal vascularization, contribute to peroneal tendon pathology, and lead to stiffness of the subtalar joint.[35] Less invasive procedures include limited open reduction, percutaneous fixation, and external fixation. Goals include restoration of the height and rotation of the tuberosity, stable fixation to allow early mobilization, and reduction of the articular surface. Because percutaneous and indirect reduction techniques are used, surgical treatment is most effective in the first several days following the injury before fracture consolidation begins, but can be used successfully even 2 weeks after injury.

Multiple studies have compared surgical treatment with minimally invasive techniques to the extensile lateral approach. Similar radiographic and clinical outcomes with decreased surgical time, decreased delay to surgery, shorter hospital stay, and lower wound complications have been reported.[36-40]

Percutaneous Reduction and Fixation

Fixation is most commonly performed with percutaneously placed screws. Of 54 consecutive displaced calcaneal fractures treated with percutaneous reduction and external fixation, 49 (90.7%) had an excellent or good clinical and radiographic result.[20] There were no deep infections and only three superficial pin site infections.

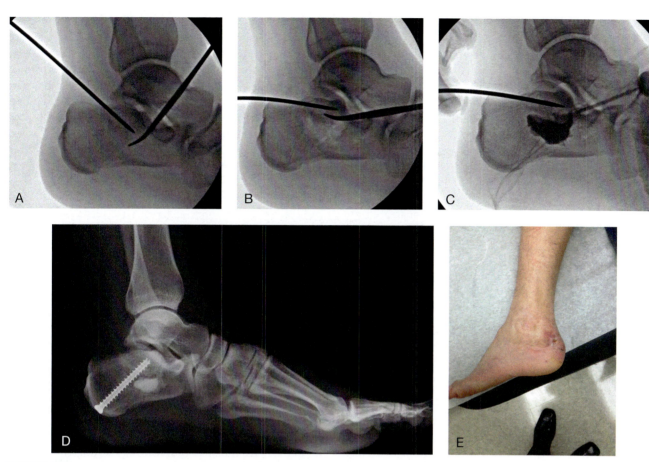

FIGURE 4 Intraoperative lateral fluoroscopic images and radiograph demonstrating Essex-Lopresti maneuver Kirschner wire positioning combined with mini-open approach (**A**) to prepare for elevation, derotation, and reduction of the joint to more optimal alignment (**B**). Percutaneous calcaneoplasty with injection of tricalcium phosphate cement (**C**) is followed by strut screw placement (**D**). Clinical photograph of the healed mini-open approach (**E**).

In 37 displaced calcaneal fractures treated with prone positioning and a temporary external fixator as a reduction aid, followed by percutaneous screw fixation, five wound infections occurred.[41] At 5 years, 2 patients had required subtalar arthrodesis, and 17 (46%) had undergone hardware removal. In a study of 153 consecutive patients with 182 calcaneal fractures treated with percutaneous screw fixation, the deep infection rate was 0.9% and conversion to subtalar fusion was 5.5% at 1 year.[42]

A retrospective study compared 83 fractures treated with percutaneous reduction and fixation with 42 fractures treated with traditional open reduction and internal fixation.[36] The outcomes were similar in terms of the Böhler angle, maintenance of reduction, and rates of late fusion. No deep infections occurred in the patients treated percutaneously, but six deep infections occurred in those treated with open surgical treatment.

A randomized controlled trial of 64 patients compared percutaneous osteosynthesis with the extensile lateral approach.[38] There was no difference in terms of clinical score or radiographic data, but the minimally invasive group demonstrated decreased wound healing problems and infections as well as decreased surgical time and hospital stay.

Limited Open Reduction Using the Sinus Tarsi Approach

The use of the sinus tarsi approach for displaced calcaneal fracture allows open reduction and fixation of the articular fragments through a relatively small and safe incision. This approach can be combined with percutaneous screw or screw and plate fixation of the calcaneal tuberosity. Some surgeons were hesitant to adopt these approaches based on comfort level with articular surface visualization, and much of the research has centered on adequacy of posterior facet reduction. In addition, the use of subtalar joint arthroscopy has been reported to aid in articular reduction with low complication rates.[43]

Research Findings

A 2020 meta-analysis comparing extensile lateral approach with minimally invasive approach for intra-articular calcaneal fractures included 17 randomized controlled studies and 10 retrospective studies with a total of 2,274 fractures. Statistically significant differences all favoring minimally invasive incision were seen with wounds, infection, sural nerve injury, time to surgery, length of surgery, American Orthopaedic Foot and Ankle Society and visual analog scale scores, calcaneal height, and Böhler angle.[44]

A prospective study of displaced fractures treated using a mini-open sinus tarsi approach and percutaneous fixation found a good to excellent clinical result in 16 of 19 patients available for follow-up.[35] Reduction of the posterior facet was graded as good to excellent on CT in 14 of 22 fractures. A single-surgeon series of 39 fractures treated with the sinus tarsi approach demonstrated an articular reduction within 2 mm of anatomic in 91% of cases based on postoperative CT.[45]

In a study comparing the sinus tarsi approach with the extensile lateral approach, no statistical differences in patient satisfaction or outcomes were found between the 33 fractures treated with a sinus tarsi approach and the 79 fractures treated with an extensile approach.[37] Twenty-nine percent of those treated using the extensile lateral approach had a wound complication, compared with only 6% of patients treated using the minimally invasive approach.

A retrospective study of displaced articular fractures in 65 patients treated with the sinus tarsi approach and 60 patients treated with the extensile lateral approach demonstrated decreased wound complications (0 versus 11) and decreased surgical time but equivalent anatomy restoration in the less-invasive group.[39] A similar prospective study of 38 patients at 2-year follow-up reported no differences in radiographic or clinical outcomes between surgical approaches, but the sinus tarsi approach group had less wound complications, decreased surgical time, and decreased delay to surgical treatment.[40]

Two randomized prospective trials have compared the sinus tarsi approach with alternate minimally invasive approaches. A limited posterior longitudinal approach was compared with the sinus tarsi approach in a randomized study of 167 patients.[46] Results were similar for Sanders type II and III fractures. However, the sinus tarsi approach demonstrated better clinical outcomes for Sanders type IV fractures.

A randomized trial of 80 patients compared percutaneous screw fixation with calcium sulfate cement, with the sinus tarsi approach with plate fixation. The percutaneous screw fixation group showed lower complications and lower surgical time. Clinical results were similar for two-part articular fractures, but with increasing articular fragmentation the sinus tarsi approach demonstrated improved clinical outcomes.[26]

A recent meta-analysis of five randomized controlled trials including 707 displaced intra-articular calcaneal fractures revealed similar fixation effectiveness and functional outcomes between cannulated screws only versus plate osteosynthesis. Surgical duration and complications were less in the cannulated screw group.[47] A 2019 study included 51 patients treated with a sinus tarsi approach; the study reported that plates or cannulated screws alone both restored and maintained reduction angles with similar results[48] (**Figure 5**).

Surgical Technique

The lateral decubitus position is used for the sinus tarsi approach. The hip can externally rotate or the C-arm can roll under for an axial view. An external fixator can be used as an intraoperative reduction tool, and when placed medially, it may aid in reduction of tuberosity varus angulation and restoration of calcaneal height. Alternatively, an external Steinmann pin in the tuberosity or a laminar spreader in the primary fracture line may facilitate tuberosity manipulation and reduction.

A longitudinal incision is made from the distal tip of the fibula toward the base of the fourth metatarsal. Joint distractors with fixation in the talus and the distal calcaneus can be helpful for visualization and reduction of the articular fragments. The ability to reduce the tuberosity in relation to the sustentaculum tali at the medial cortex should be confirmed on axial view before final fixation of the posterior facet. Direct reduction maneuvers of the sustentaculum and tuberosity while working inside the primary fracture from the lateral incision are sometimes beneficial before reduction and fixation of the posterior facet, which will further preclude visualization.

Once adequate exposure of the posterior facet is established, direct reduction maneuvers can be used to achieve reduction of the articular surface. Initial fixation of the articular reduction can be done with a Kirschner wire or small screw placed from the lateral articular fragment toward the sustentaculum. Additional screws or a periarticular plate will provide more fixation depending on the fracture pattern. The approach can be extended distally to address the anterior process or proximally to address the peroneal tendons, as long as the blood supply to the lateral skin flap is preserved with protection of the lateral calcaneal artery.[49]

Reduction of the tuberosity and the anterior process can be confirmed fluoroscopically. Percutaneous screws can be placed in the tuberosity and the anterior process. In an unstable or comminuted fracture with poor bone quality, the external fixator can be left in place until early fracture consolidation occurs. Patients are kept non–weight bearing for 6 to 12 weeks, although early joint mobilization is encouraged once the wounds have healed.

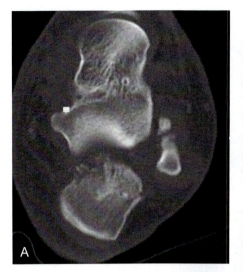 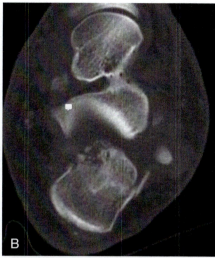 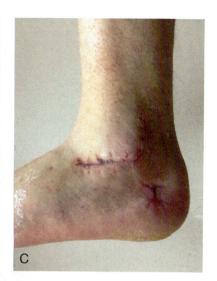
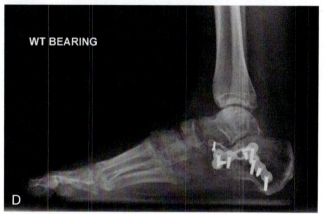

FIGURE 5 **A** and **B**, CT images revealing dislocation of the peroneal tendons to the lateral aspect of the fibula. Photograph (**C**) and radiograph (**D**) showing that extension of the sinus tarsi approach proximally (**C**) allows relocation of the tendons and repair of the superior peroneal retinaculum simultaneously to plate fixation of the fracture.

EXTRA-ARTICULAR FRACTURES

Up to one-third of calcaneal fractures are considered extra-articular because they do not extend into the posterior facet. They are often lower energy mechanisms, commonly seen in children, and many can be treated nonsurgically.[50] Surgical treatment may be indicated to prevent a problematic malunion with shortening of the gastrocnemius-soleus complex, or with widening, which could affect the peroneal tendons or shoe wear. Displaced body fractures with more than 30° of angulation or more than 1 cm of translation are more likely to benefit from surgical treatment.[4]

Tuberosity fractures result from forced dorsiflexion and can involve a portion of the Achilles tendon insertion, which can put the posterior skin at risk.[51] Simple extra-articular avulsion fractures are the most common type. This fracture generally occurred with a low-energy mechanism in older patients.[52] A true nondisplaced fracture can be treated nonsurgically with immobilization in plantar flexion. Because of the inherent risk to the strength of the gastrocnemius-soleus complex, in active patients, a displaced fracture can be treated surgically. Depending on the size of the fracture fragment and the bone quality, fixation can be achieved with percutaneous lag screw fixation. With posterior avulsion fractures, the smaller fragments can be excised and the Achilles tendon reapproximated to the tuberosity with suture anchors.

Isolated fractures of the sustentaculum tali are rare and CT provides accurate delineation of the fracture pattern. Fractures that involve the posterior facet or are displaced more than 2 mm may benefit from surgical treatment. A study of 15 patients who underwent open reduction and internal fixation through a medial approach to the sustentaculum tali found that all fractures healed with maintained reduction.[53]

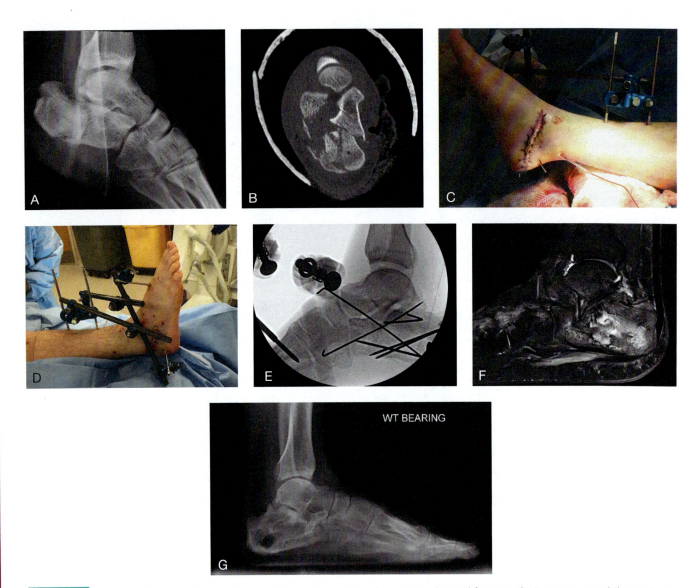

FIGURE 6 Lateral radiograph from a 14-year-old boy who sustained an open calcaneal fracture during an automobile accident (**A**), which can be seen to be severely comminuted on CT (**B**). Photograph showing emergently performed irrigation and débridement of the fracture with primary closure of the open wound (**C**). A sinus tarsi approach was used for provisional Kirschner (K-wire) reduction of the articular facet (**D**) with the assistance of an external fixator (**E**). After K-wire and external fixator removal, the patient presented 8 months later with a draining medial wound and evidence of osteomyelitis on MRI (**F**). The infection was irradiated via a lateral window corticotomy for burr and curet access to thoroughly débride and irrigate the entire inner body of the tuberosity and anterior process, followed by resorbable antibiotic cement implantation. A lateral radiograph 2 years later reveals posttraumatic arthritis (**G**).

Many anterior process fractures can be treated nonsurgically, and historically, surgical treatment has been reserved for displaced fractures that involve 25% of the calcaneocuboid joint.[4] If the fracture fragments are small or comminuted, they can be excised. Delayed excision sometimes is necessary to treat chronically painful avulsion fractures.

COMPLICATIONS

Wound Complications

The most common early complications of surgical treatment of calcaneal fracture are delayed wound healing and infection, occurring in up to 25% of patients undergoing surgery via an extensile approach.[24,26,27,54] Despite surgical

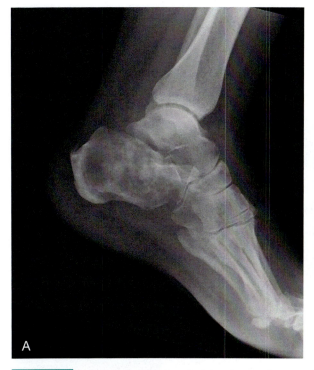
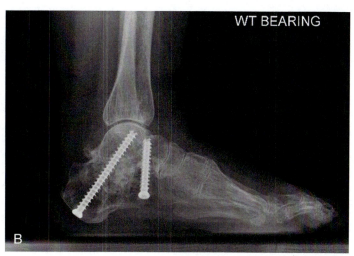

FIGURE 7 Lateral radiographs of a joint-depression type fracture (**A**) undergoing primary arthrodesis with fully threaded screws to maintain position (**B**).

delay, careful retraction of the flap, and meticulous closure, delayed healing and skin necrosis can occur. Treatment using local wound care, antibiotics, or surgical débridement may be necessary. The most common infectious pathogens are Enterobacteriaceae and *Staphylococcus aureus*.[55]

A study of 490 calcaneal fractures treated with open reduction and internal fixation found a wound complication rate of 17.8%.[27] Risk factors such as smoking, diabetes, severity of intra-articular fracture, duration of procedure, amount of blood loss, 10 or more people in the operating room, or the presence of residents or fellows were identified. Use of a tourniquet was associated with a lower risk of wound complications. Other reported risk factors include high body mass index, increased time from injury to surgery, and a single-layer closure.[54]

Open calcaneal fractures have a much higher complication rate than closed calcaneal fractures. A study of 115 surgically treated open fractures found superficial wound infection in 9.6%, deep infection in 12.2%, and culture-positive osteomyelitis in 5.2%.[56] Six patients (5.2%) underwent amputation. In a separate series of 64 open calcaneal fractures, 8% of patients eventually underwent amputations[57] (**Figure 6**).

Posttraumatic Arthritis

Posttraumatic arthritis of the subtalar joint is a common complication of calcaneal fracture. The energy on impact often causes direct and irreversible articular cartilage injury that can be identified at the time of procedure.[58-61] Further joint destruction will occur if the articular surface is not anatomically reduced. Fractures treated nonsurgically and fractures treated surgically with a suboptimal reduction can progress quickly to subtalar arthrosis with a reported 10% rate of late subtalar fusion, which most strongly correlated with the severity of initial injury.[62] Nonsurgical treatment and the existence of a workers' compensation claim also predicted a poor outcome and the need for late subtalar fusion. A large study of patients who underwent subtalar fusion for posttraumatic arthritis found that the patients who had undergone initial surgical treatment for the fracture had better outcomes with fusion than those who had been treated nonsurgically.[63] The initial open reduction and internal fixation restored the calcaneal shape, alignment, and height, even if subtalar fusion later was required (**Figures 7 and 8**).

Section 6: Foot and Ankle Trauma

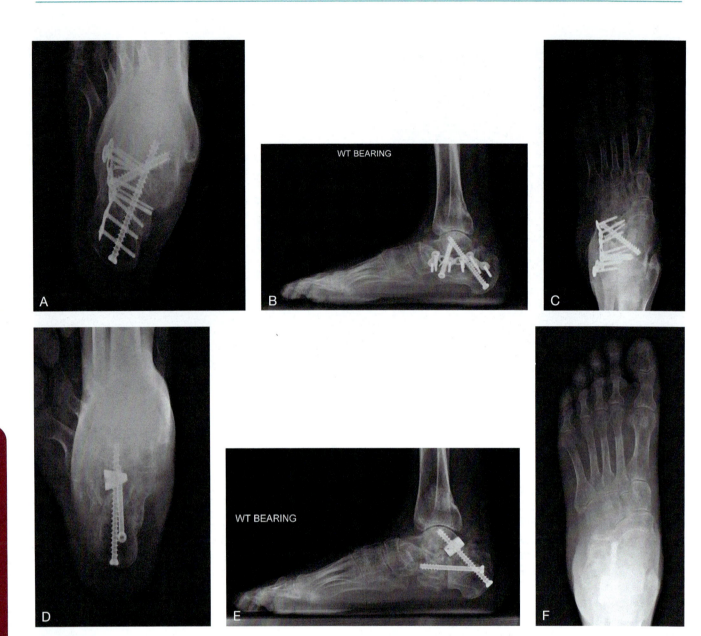

FIGURE 8 Valgus axial, collapsed lateral, and abducted AP radiographs (**A** through **C**, respectively) of a nonplantigrade subtalar fusion malunion for calcaneal fracture requiring revision fusion with medial tuberosity shift (**D**), distraction through the subtalar joint (**E**), and lateral column lengthening to restore talonavicular joint alignment (**F**).

Calcaneal Malunion

If anatomy is not restored, a displaced calcaneal fracture often leads to a problematic malunion. Loss of calcaneal height results in shortening of the gastrocnemius-soleus complex and can affect ankle dorsiflexion with anterior impingement. Varus malalignment of the tuberosity negatively affects gait, ankle stability, and shoe wear. Widening of the calcaneus causes subfibular impingement and peroneal tendon dysfunction (**Figure 9**).

The classification of calcaneal malunion is based on the presence of a lateral wall exostosis, subtalar joint arthrosis, and varus malunion.[64] Fusion with an attempt to restore calcaneal height can provide pain relief. A 93% union rate was reported in a study of 40

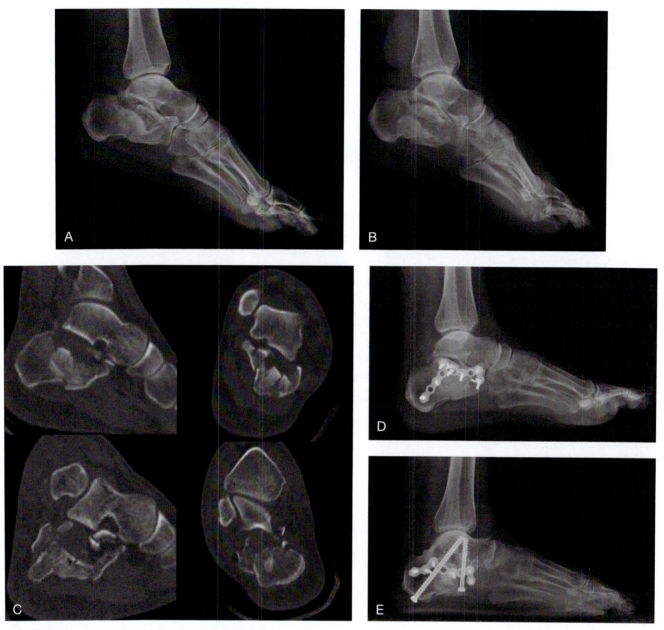

FIGURE 9 Lateral views of the left (**A**) and right (**B**) bilateral calcaneal fractures in a 44-year-old patient who worked as a laborer. CT images (**C**) reveal bilateral Sanders type IV fractures (top row = left calcaneus, bottom row = right calcaneus). The fractures on the left underwent open reduction and internal fixation (ORIF) (**D**) and the fractures on the right underwent ORIF combined with primary subtalar fusion (**E**).

subtalar arthrodesis procedures to correct malunion.[65] The functional results were acceptable, but there was difficulty in restoring calcaneal height, and therefore, the authors recommended surgical treatment of acute fractures to prevent malunion. Corrective osteotomy with preservation of the subtalar joint is another option possibly providing functional improvement after calcaneal malunion.[66] Only one conversion to a subtalar fusion had been required at 3-year follow-up in a series of 26 patients.

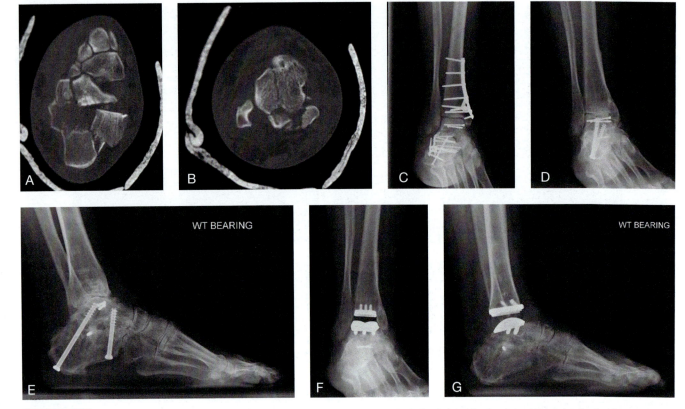

FIGURE 10 CT images and radiographs of an open calcaneal fracture with dislocated subtalar joint (**A**) and talar body comminuted fracture (**B**) requiring soft-tissue flap reconstruction with open reduction and internal fixation using a medial malleolus osteotomy (**C**). Posttraumatic degenerative arthritis subsequently developed 4 years later (**D**), which was managed with staged subtalar fusion (**E**) and ankle arthroplasty (**F** and **G**).

SUMMARY

Chronic pain and disability often ensue regardless of treatment type for calcaneal fractures. No single treatment method is suitable for all calcaneal fractures.[67] Percutaneous and minimally invasive approaches decrease the risk of wound complications, length of surgery, and length of hospital stay, and afford improved clinical results for extra-articular and less comminuted intra-articular fractures.[68] The extensile lateral approach allows excellent visualization and lateral buttressing for severely comminuted fractures. Rare fracture variants such as sustentacular fractures and tuberosity avulsions are treated through more direct medial or posterior approaches. Fracture patterns and patient characteristics are highly variable and therefore best practice treatment algorithms vary depending on multiple factors (**Figure 10**).

KEY STUDY POINTS

- Calcaneal fractures are often high-energy injuries resulting in long-term pain and disability.
- Classification is based on posterior facet articular involvement and can predict progression to posttraumatic arthritis.
- Fracture severity and the ability to surgically restore alignment predict the future necessity and success of subtalar arthrodesis.
- Nonsurgical treatment of displaced fractures frequently results in poor outcomes.
- Surgical treatment is associated with high rates of wound complications and may not be superior to nonsurgical treatment in certain patient groups.
- Minimally invasive surgical approaches have lower complication rates with promising early clinical results.

ANNOTATED REFERENCES

1. van Tetering EA, Buckley RE: Functional outcome (SF-36) of patients with displaced calcaneal fractures compared to SF-36 normative data. *Foot Ankle Int* 2004;25(10):733-738.

2. Potter MQ, Nunley JA: Long-term functional outcomes after operative treatment for intra-articular fractures of the calcaneus. *J Bone Joint Surg Am* 2009;91(8):1854-1860.

3. Simske NM, Hermelin MJ, Vallier HA: Impact of psychosocial and economic factors on functional outcomes after operative calcaneus fractures. *J Orthop Trauma* 2021;35(11):e423-e428.

    Seventy-two patients completed functional outcome scores, which were evaluated to stratify psychosocial and economic risk factors. Level of evidence: III.

4. Sanders R, Clare MP: Fractures of the calcaneus, in Coughlin MJ, Mann RA, Saltzman CL, eds: *Surgery of the Foot and Ankle*, ed 8. Mosby Elsevier, 2007, pp 2017-2073.

5. Bohl DD, Ondeck NT, Samuel AM, et al: Demographics, mechanisms of injury, and concurrent injuries associated with calcaneus fractures: A study of 14 516 patients in the American College of Surgeons National Trauma Data Bank. *Foot Ankle Spec* 2017;10(5):402-410.

6. Mahmoud K, Mekhaimar MM, Alhammoud A: Prevalence of peroneal tendon instability in calcaneus fractures: A systematic review and meta-analysis. *J Foot Ankle Surg* 2018;57(3):572-578.

7. Kwon JY, Gonzalez T: Response to "letter regarding: Anterior-posterior (AP) calcaneal profile view – A novel radiographic image to assess varus malalignment". *Foot Ankle Int* 2020;41(11):1444-1445.

    The AP calcaneal profile view is a novel radiographic technique to evaluate hindfoot alignment in calcaneal fracture treatment. Level of evidence: V.

8. Sanders R: Displaced intra-articular fractures of the calcaneus. *J Bone Joint Surg Am* 2000;82(2):225-250.

9. Essex-Lopresti P: The mechanism, reduction technique, and results in fractures of the OS calcis. *Br J Surg* 1952;39(157):395-419.

10. Adams MR, Koury KL, Mistry JB, Braaksma W, Hwang JS, Firoozabadi R: Plantar medial avulsion fragment associated with tongue-type calcaneus fractures. *Foot Ankle Int* 2019;40(6):634-640.

    This case report and technique tip evaluated plantar medial avulsion fragment reduction. Level of evidence: V.

11. Soeur R, Remy R: Fractures of the calcaneus with displacement of the thalamic portion. *J Bone Joint Surg Br* 1975;57(4):413-421.

12. Berberian W, Sood A, Karanfilian B, Najarian R, Lin S, Liporace F: Displacement of the sustentacular fragment in intra-articular calcaneal fractures. *J Bone Joint Surg Am* 2013;95(11):995-1000.

13. Su J, Cao X: Can operations achieve good outcomes in elderly patients with Sanders II-III calcaneal fractures? *Medicine (Baltimore)* 2017;96(29):e7553.

14. Thordarson DB, Krieger LE: Operative vs. Nonoperative treatment of intra-articular fractures of the calcaneus: A prospective randomized trial. *Foot Ankle Int* 1996;17(1):2-9.

15. Buckley R, Tough S, Mccormack R, et al: Operative compared with nonoperative treatment of displaced intra-articular calcaneal fractures: A prospective, randomized, controlled multicenter trial. *J Bone Joint Surg Am* 2002;84(10):1733-1744.

16. Ågren PH, Wretenberg P, Sayed-Noor AS: Operative versus nonoperative treatment of displaced intra-articular calcaneal fractures: A prospective, randomized, controlled multicenter trial. *J Bone Joint Surg Am* 2013;95(15):1351-1357.

17. Griffin D, Parsons N, Shaw E, et al: Operative versus non-operative treatment for closed, displaced, intra-articular fractures of the calcaneus: Randomised controlled trial. *BMJ* 2014;349:g4483.

18. Buckley R: Operative care did not benefit closed, displaced, intra-articular calcaneal fractures. *J Bone Joint Surg Am* 2015;97(4):341.

19. Luo X, Li Q, He S, He S: Operative versus nonoperative treatment for displaced intra-articular calcaneal fractures: A meta-analysis of randomized controlled trials. *J Foot Ankle Surg* 2016;55(4):821-828.

20. Magnan B, Bortolazzi R, Marangon A, Marino M, Dall'Oca C, Bartolozzi P: External fixation for displaced intra-articular fractures of the calcaneum. *J Bone Joint Surg Br* 2006;88(11):1474-1479.

21. Meena S, Gangary SK, Sharma P: Review article: Operative versus non-operative treatment for displaced intra-articular calcaneal fracture – A meta-analysis of randomised controlled trials. *J Orthop Surg (Hong Kong)* 2016;24(3):411-416.

22. Benirschke SK, Sangeorzan BJ: Extensive intraarticular fractures of the foot. Surgical management of calcaneal fractures. *Clin Orthop Relat Res* 1993;292:128-134.

23. Gould N, Seligson D: *Technique tips: Footings*: Lateral approach to the Os calcis. *Foot Ankle* 1984;4(4):218-220.

24. Sanders R, Fortin P, Dipasquale T, Walling A: Operative treatment in 120 displaced intraarticular calcaneal fractures. Results using a prognostic computed tomography scan classification. *Clin Orthop Relat Res* 1993;290:87-95.

25. Sanders R, Vaupel ZM, Erdogan M, Downes K: Operative treatment of displaced intraarticular calcaneal fractures: Long-term (10-20 years) results in 108 fractures using a prognostic CT classification. *J Orthop Trauma* 2014;28(10):551-563.

26. Folk JW, Starr AJ, Early JS: Early wound complications of operative treatment of calcaneus fractures: Analysis of 190 fractures. *J Orthop Trauma* 1999;13(5):369-372.

27. Ding L, He Z, Xiao H, Chai L, Xue F: Risk factors for postoperative wound complications of calcaneal fractures following plate fixation. *Foot Ankle Int* 2013;34(9):1238-1244.

28. Kwon JY, Guss D, Lin DE, et al: Effect of delay to definitive surgical fixation on wound complications in the treatment of closed, intra-articular calcaneus fractures. *Foot Ankle Int* 2015;36(5):508-517.

29. Bergin PF, Psaradellis T, Krosin MT, et al: Inpatient soft tissue protocol and wound complications in calcaneus fractures. *Foot Ankle Int* 2012;33(6):492-497.

30. Gardner MJ, Nork SE, Barei DP, Kramer PA, Sangeorzan BJ, Benirschke SK: Secondary soft tissue compromise in tongue-type calcaneus fractures. *J Orthop Trauma* 2008;22(7):439-445.

31. Tornetta P: The essex-lopresti reduction for calcaneal fractures revisited. *J Orthop Trauma* 1998;12(7):469-473.

32. Buch BD, Myerson MS, Miller SD: Primary subtaler arthrodesis for the treatment of comminuted calcaneal fractures. *Foot Ankle Int* 1996;17(2):61-70.

33. Huefner T, Thermann H, Geerling J, Pape HC, Pohlemann T: Primary subtalar arthrodesis of calcaneal fractures. *Foot Ankle Int* 2001;22(1):9-14.

34. Schepers T: The primary arthrodesis for severely comminuted intra-articular fractures of the calcaneus: A systematic review. *Foot Ankle Surg* 2012;18(2):84-88.

35. Nosewicz T, Knupp M, Barg A, et al: Mini-open sinus tarsi approach with percutaneous screw fixation of displaced calcaneal fractures: A prospective computed tomography–based study. *Foot Ankle Int* 2012;33(11):925-933.

36. DeWall M, Henderson CE, McKinley TO, Phelps T, Dolan L, Marsh JL: Percutaneous reduction and fixation of displaced intra-articular calcaneus fractures. *J Orthop Trauma* 2010;24(8):466-472.

37. Kline AJ, Anderson RB, Davis WH, Jones CP, Cohen BE: Minimally invasive technique versus an extensile lateral approach for intra-articular calcaneal fractures. *Foot Ankle Int* 2013;34(6):773-780.

38. Jin C, Weng D, Yang W, He W, Liang W, Qian Y: Minimally invasive percutaneous osteosynthesis versus ORIF for sanders type II and III calcaneal fractures: A prospective, randomized intervention trial. *J Orthop Surg Res* 2017;12(1):10.

39. Schepers T, Backes M, Dingemans SA, de Jong VM, Luitse JSK: Similar anatomical reduction and lower complication rates with the sinus tarsi approach compared with the extended lateral approach in displaced intra-articular calcaneal fractures. *J Orthop Trauma* 2017;31(6):293-298.

40. Basile A, Albo F, Via AG: Comparison between sinus tarsi approach and extensile lateral approach for treatment of closed displaced intra-articular calcaneal fractures: A multicenter prospective study. *J Foot Ankle Surg* 2016;55(3):513-521.

41. Tomesen T, Biert J, Frölke JP: Treatment of displaced intra-articular calcaneal fractures with closed reduction and percutaneous screw fixation. *J Bone Joint Surg Am* 2011;93(10):920-928.

42. Tantavisut S, Phisitkul P, Westerlind BO, Gao Y, Karam MD, Marsh JL: Percutaneous reduction and screw fixation of displaced intra-articular fractures of the calcaneus. *Foot Ankle Int* 2017;38(4):367-374.

43. Grün W, Molund M, Nilsen F, Stødle AH: Results after percutaneous and arthroscopically assisted osteosynthesis of calcaneal fractures. *Foot Ankle Int* 2020;41(6):689-697.

This is a retrospective case series of 25 patients with 1-year follow-up of radiographic alignment, clinical scores, and complication rates. Level of evidence: IV.

44. Seat A, Seat C: Lateral extensile approach versus minimal incision approach for open reduction and internal fixation of displaced intra-articular calcaneal fractures: A meta-analysis. *J Foot Ankle Surg* 2020;59(2):356-366.

A randomized trial of 30 patients evaluated pain and radiographic scores. Level of evidence: II.

45. Scott AT, Pacholke DA, Hamid KS: Radiographic and CT assessment of reduction of calcaneus fractures using a limited sinus tarsi incision. *Foot Ankle Int* 2016;37(9):950-957.

46. Zhang T, Su Y, Chen W, Zhang Q, Wu Z, Zhang Y: Displaced intra-articular calcaneal fractures treated in a minimally invasive fashion: Longitudinal approach versus sinus tarsi approach. *J Bone Joint Surg Am* 2014;96(4):302-309.

47. Fan B, Zhou X, Wei Z, et al: Cannulated screw fixation and plate fixation for displaced intra-articular calcaneus fracture: A meta-analysis of randomized controlled trials. *Int J Surg* 2016;34:64-72.

48. Pitts CC, Almaguer A, Wilson JT, Quade JH, Johnson MD: Radiographic and postoperative outcomes of plate versus screw constructs in open reduction and internal fixation of calcaneus fractures via the sinus tarsi. *Foot Ankle Int* 2019;40(8):929-935.

In this study, 33 patients underwent a modified two-incision sinus tarsi approach for calcaneal fracture, with 2-year follow-up of radiographic, clinical scores, and complications. Level of evidence: III.

49. Femino JE, Vaseenon T, Levin DA, Yian EH: Modification of the sinus tarsi approach for open reduction and plate fixation of intra-articular calcaneus fractures: The limits of proximal extension based upon the vascular anatomy of the lateral calcaneal artery. *Iowa Orthop J* 2010;30:161-167.

50. Schepers T, Ginai AZ, van Lieshout EM, Patka P: Demographics of extra-articular calcaneal fractures: Including a review of the literature on treatment and outcome. *Arch Orthop Trauma Surg* 2008;128(10):1099-1106.

51. Hess M, Booth B, Laughlin RT: Calcaneal avulsion fractures: Complications from delayed treatment. *Am J Emerg Med* 2008;26(2):254.e1-254.e4.

52. Lee SM, Huh SW, Chung JW, Kim DW, Kim YJ, Rhee SK: Avulsion fracture of the calcaneal tuberosity: Classification and its characteristics. *Clin Orthop Surg* 2012;4(2):134-138.

53. della Rocca GJ, Nork SE, Barei DP, Taitsman LA, Benirschke SK: Fractures of the sustentaculum tali: Injury characteristics and surgical technique for reduction. *Foot Ankle Int* 2009;30(11):1037-1041.

54. Abidi NA, Dhawan S, Gruen GS, Vogt MT, Conti SF: Wound-healing risk factors after open reduction and internal fixation of calcaneal fractures. *Foot Ankle Int* 1998;19(12):856-861.

55. Backes M, Spijkerman IJ, de Muinck-Keizer RO, Goslings JC, Schepers T: Determination of pathogens in postoperative wound infection after surgically reduced calcaneal fractures and implications for prophylaxis and treatment. *J Foot Ankle Surg* 2018;57(1):100-103.

56. Wiersema B, Brokaw D, Weber T, et al: Complications associated with open calcaneus fractures. *Foot Ankle Int* 2011;32(11):1052-1057.

57. Worsham JR, Elliott MR, Harris AM: Open calcaneus fractures and associated injuries. *J Foot Ankle Surg* 2016;55(1):68-71.

58. Borrelli J, Silva MJ, Zaegel MA, Franz C, Sandell LJ: Single high-energy impact load causes posttraumatic OA in young rabbits via a decrease in cellular metabolism. *J Orthop Res* 2009;27(3):347-352.

59. Borrelli J, Tinsley K, Ricci WM, Burns M, Karl IE, Hotchkiss R: Induction of chondrocyte apoptosis following impact load. *J Orthop Trauma* 2003;17(9):635-641.

60. Borrelli J, Torzilli PA, Grigiene R, Helfet DL: Effect of impact load on articular cartilage: Development of an intra-articular fracture model. *J Orthop Trauma* 1997;11(5):319-326.

61. Torzilli PA, Grigiene R, Borrelli J Jr, Helfet DL: Effect of impact load on articular cartilage: Cell metabolism and viability, and matrix water content. *J Biomech Eng* 1999;121(5):433-441.

62. Csizy M, Buckley R, Tough S, et al: Displaced intra-articular calcaneal fractures: Variables predicting late subtalar fusion. *J Orthop Trauma* 2003;17(2):106-112.

63. Radnay CS, Clare MP, Sanders RW: Subtalar fusion after displaced intra-articular calcaneal fractures: Does initial operative treatment matter? *J Bone Joint Surg Am* 2010;92(suppl 1 pt 1):32-43.

64. Stephens HM, Sanders R: Calcaneal malunions: Results of a prognostic computed tomography classification system. *Foot Ankle Int* 1996;17(7):395-401.

65. Clare MP, Lee WE, Sanders RW: Intermediate to long-term results of a treatment protocol for calcaneal fracture malunions. *J Bone Joint Surg Am* 2005;87(5):963-973.

66. Yu GR, Hu SJ, Yang YF, Zhao HM, Zhang SM: Reconstruction of calcaneal fracture malunion with osteotomy and subtalar joint salvage: Technique and outcomes. *Foot Ankle Int* 2013;34(5):726-733.

67. Rammelt S, Swords MP: Calcaneal fractures – Which approach for which fracture? *Orthop Clin North Am* 2021;52(4):433-450.

    A descriptive technical tip article evaluated various surgical anatomic approaches and their most appropriate application to calcaneal fracture surgical treatment. Level of evidence: V.

68. Zeng Z, Yuan L, Zheng S, Sun Y, Huang F: Minimally invasive versus extensile lateral approach for sanders type II and III calcaneal fractures: A meta-analysis of randomized controlled trials. *Int J Surg* 2018;50:146-153.

CHAPTER 21

Midfoot and Forefoot Trauma

JOSEPH T. O'NEIL, MD • DAVID I. PEDOWITZ, MD, MS, FAAOS

ABSTRACT

Trauma to the midfoot and forefoot encompasses a wide spectrum of pathology, ranging from subtle sprains to massive crush injuries. Therefore, treatment is wide ranging. A comprehensive history and physical examination in conjunction with a thorough diagnostic workup is paramount to optimizing clinical outcomes. Although uncommon, there is a risk of compartment syndrome, which can be particularly pertinent in the setting of a midfoot crush injury. With regard to the optimal treatment of Lisfranc injuries, controversy still exists. Many fractures in the forefoot can be managed nonsurgically with some notable exceptions.

Keywords: forefoot; Lisfranc; midfoot; trauma

INTRODUCTION

The foot is a complex and durable biomechanical structure composed of 28 bones and their articulations. It is

---

Dr. Pedowitz or an immediate family member has received royalties from Smith & Nephew and Zimmer; is a member of a speakers' bureau or has made paid presentations on behalf of Arthrex, Inc., Ossio, Smith & Nephew, and Zimmer; and serves as a paid consultant to or is an employee of Arthrex, Inc., MiRus, Ossio, Smith & Nephew, and Zimmer. Neither Dr. O'Neil nor any immediate family member has received anything of value from or has stock or stock options held in a commercial company or institution related directly or indirectly to the subject of this chapter.

of integral importance to gait, and fractures of the foot can have a substantial effect on normal function. The area of midfoot and forefoot injury extends from the navicular proximally to the toes distally. Midfoot and forefoot injuries encompass a wide spectrum of pathology, from a subtle sprain incurred on an athletic field to a massive crush injury after a motor vehicle accident. Recent advances may improve the success and efficiency of treatment techniques and implants designed to restore function to patients with traumatic foot injury.

NAVICULAR FRACTURES

Although navicular fractures are not common, they are particularly important to understand. The navicular articulates with four bones in the foot, serves as the major attachment site for the posterior tibial tendon, and is responsible for significant hindfoot motion. The navicular is named for its boat-like shape, which is concave from medial to lateral as well as dorsal to plantar at the talonavicular joint, and convex at the naviculocuneiform joints. The navicular represents a transition zone from the mobile talonavicular joint, which allows the entire foot to pivot on the talus, to the stiff naviculocuneiform joints. Navicular fractures range from simple dorsal and medial avulsion fractures to stress fractures and complex body fractures. Any of these fractures, if missed, can lead to significant morbidity in the midfoot.

AVULSION FRACTURES

Dorsal capsular avulsion fracture, the most common type of navicular fracture, often is caused by an acute plantar flexion injury or ankle sprain. Typically, trauma to a portion of the strong dorsal talonavicular ligament

---

This chapter is adapted from Raikin SM, Palanca A, Gross CE: Midfoot injuries; forefoot, sesamoid, and turf toe injuries, in Chou LB, ed: *Orthopaedic Knowledge Update®: Foot and Ankle 6.* American Academy of Orthopaedic Surgeons, 2020, pp 349-373.

© 2025 American Academy of Orthopaedic Surgeons

causes avulsion of a small piece of the bone. This fracture is relatively benign and can be treated with immobilization in a walking boot for 6 to 8 weeks or until the patient is asymptomatic. Traditionally, treatment with a short period of immobilization has been recommended as leading to minimal disability, with fragment excision recommended if pain persists after immobilization. If the avulsed fragment is a significant portion of the articular surface of the navicular, open reduction and internal fixation (ORIF) is indicated to minimize the risk of posttraumatic arthritis and the likelihood of subsequent midtarsal subluxation. Unfortunately, no clear criteria define the percentage of dorsal navicular involvement, indicating that surgical intervention is necessary.

Avulsion fracture of the navicular tuberosity is the result of forceful eversion of the midfoot. Eversion tensions the posterior tibial tendon insertion, the tibionavicular ligament (the most anterior portion of the deltoid ligament), and the plantar calcaneonavicular (spring) ligament. Because of the broad insertion of the posterior tibial tendon throughout the plantar aspect of the midfoot, usually the tendon is not completely pulled off, and significant tuberosity displacement is rare. These fractures typically cause pain and ecchymosis medially and are easily seen on routine foot radiographs. Immobilization in a walking boot is used for 4 to 6 weeks. If a symptomatic nonunion develops, excision (a Kidner-type procedure) may be undertaken rather than internal fixation. Some experts recommend internal fixation for a fracture displaced more than 5 mm because of the risk of nonunion.[1]

An acute fracture should be distinguished from a type II accessory navicular. The accessory bone and the corresponding medial navicular body have more rounded edges than the fracture. These entities typically are treated in a similar manner but treatment is largely based on the severity of the patient's symptoms.

NAVICULAR BODY FRACTURES

Fractures of the navicular body are uncommon because of the stability imparted by the position of the navicular between numerous bones. Such a fracture often is caused by a high-energy mechanism, as in a fall from a height or an axial load. The classification is based on fracture morphology: a type I fracture is in the coronal plane and has no malalignment of the midfoot; a type II fracture, the most common type, has a dorsolateral to plantarmedial fracture line with the lateral fragment displaced dorsally; and a type III fracture is comminuted centrally or laterally within the navicular body (**Figure 1**). The foot collapses into abduction through the comminution. Many researchers suggest that displaced, comminuted fractures (all type II and III fractures) and larger fracture fragments benefit from internal fixation. As in all foot and ankle trauma, the integrity and suitability of the soft tissues for surgical intervention must be respected,

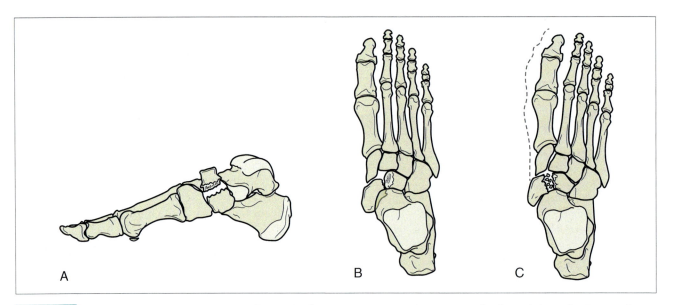

FIGURE 1 Drawing showing the three types of navicular fractures. **A**, Type I is best seen with a lateral view. The fracture line is in the coronal plane, there is no midfoot instability, and dorsal displacement is variable. **B**, Type II is best seen with an AP or oblique view. The fracture line is in the dorsolateral to plantarmedial plane, with medial displacement from the posterior tibial tendon. **C**, Type III is best seen with an AP view and is characterized by midbody comminution and valgus foot angulation as can be seen by comparing the medial column with its normal alignment demonstrated by the dashed line. (Redrawn from Ficke JR: Fractures and dislocation of the midfoot, in Pinzur MS, ed: *Orthopaedic Knowledge Update®: Foot and Ankle 4*. American Academy of Orthopaedic Surgeons, 2008, pp 107-114.)

and for this reason, surgical treatment may need to be delayed 1 to 2 weeks. Temporary spanning external fixation may be necessary if there is gross instability. CT is particularly useful during surgical planning to fully appreciate the anatomy of the fracture fragments, especially in the presence of additional transverse tarsal and tarsometatarsal (TMT) injuries.

Surgical treatment is done through a dorsal approach between the course of the anterior and posterior tibial tendons to facilitate visualization and evaluation. The saphenous vein and nerve must be avoided during the superficial dissection. Because the lateral aspect of the navicular is challenging to fully appreciate, usually it is beneficial to place the incision just over the anterior tibial tendon rather than more medially and closer to the posterior tibial tendon. With this exposure, surgical windows on either side of the tibialis anterior allow both the medial and lateral navicular to be seen fully. Care must be taken to elevate the neuromuscular bundle, which lies lateral to the tibialis anterior and medial to the extensor hallucis longus tendon.

Simple fractures are fixed with lag screws. Screws may be placed medial to lateral or lateral to medial, depending on which placement will provide better fixation. If there is significant comminution, locked or mini-fragment plating of the navicular itself or temporary bridge plating of the medial column may be necessary. Manipulation of fracture fragments may require the use of a small external fixator or Kirschner wire (K-wire) distractor, which eliminates the deforming forces on the navicular and improve visualization.

Late osteonecrosis may occur following these injuries and, in advanced stages, may lead to medial column collapse. Symptoms of posttraumatic arthrosis of the talonavicular joint can be treated with shoe wear modification, a stiff custom insert, or a rigid or rocker-bottom-soled shoe. Some patients require delayed talonavicular, naviculocuneiform, or talonaviculocuneiform (medial column) arthrodesis.

STRESS FRACTURES

The navicular bone historically was thought to be particularly susceptible to stress fracture because of the relatively avascular zone in the central third of the bone. Arterial anatomic studies suggest that biomechanical and other clinical factors play a more significant role in the development of stress fractures than previously thought.[2] With explosive activity, this area undergoes considerable compression, which can cause stress responses including bone bruise, stress reaction, stress fracture, and complete fracture of the navicular. The diagnosis often is delayed because the symptoms are vague in location, insidious,

and sometimes similar to those of a sprain. The fracture may be evaluated only after weeks or months of continued activity. Patients have poorly localized pain in the midfoot and usually are unable to perform the hop test, which requires jumping up and down on the involved forefoot. Radiographs of the foot should be carefully scrutinized for evidence of a fracture. Often the radiographs are normal, however, and a high index of suspicion and MRI confirmation are required. MRI is preferable to CT because CT can only document fractures with cortical disruption, which often does not occur until the later stages of a stress fracture that is evolving into a complete fracture.

The treatment ranges from avoidance of weight bearing to early surgical intervention. The results of any treatment involving partial weight bearing appear to be inferior to those of complete avoidance of weight bearing or early surgical treatment, and therefore partial weight bearing should be discouraged. Although surgical treatment may be the preferred initial treatment for a competitive athlete, avoidance of weight bearing and early surgical treatment appear to have similar results in the general population.[3,4]

CUBOID AND CUNEIFORM FRACTURES

Cuboid Fractures

Through its articulation with the fourth and fifth metatarsal bases and the anterior process of the calcaneus, the cuboid forms an intercalary link from the lateral forefoot to the hindfoot. As in the hand, the medial column is relatively rigid. Conversely, the lateral column of the foot is quite mobile to accommodate ground reactive forces and the geometry of uneven surfaces. Fractures of the cuboid are thought to be rare because its bony surroundings offer some protection. Patients report lateral foot pain and difficulty in weight bearing. Lateral and plantar midfoot and hindfoot ecchymosis is common. Plain radiographs often are sufficient, but CT or MRI is recommended for surgical planning or evaluation to detect additional midfoot pathology. Aside from avulsion injuries, cuboid fractures rarely occur in isolation, so a high index of suspicion should be present for additional injuries.

Avulsion fractures and compression fractures are the two primary types of cuboid fractures. Avulsion fractures, which are more common, can occur even with mild to moderate foot and ankle sprains. These are capsular avulsions and can be treated nonsurgically with weight bearing as tolerated in a fracture boot. Minimally displaced or nondisplaced cuboid fractures also can be treated nonsurgically and may benefit from a 4- to 6-week period of non–weight bearing.

Although displaced fractures do not always require surgical intervention, they often accompany more severe bony and soft-tissue midfoot injuries. Displaced fractures result from a direct crush or from an axial load in plantar flexion accompanied by eversion. In the second scenario, a so-called nutcracker fracture is produced when the cuboid is caught between the fourth and fifth metatarsal bases and the anterior process of the calcaneus, and it is cracked like a nut. In these compression injuries, the lateral column is crushed and becomes shorter because it is no longer held out to length (**Figure 2**). These fractures carry a significant risk of collapse and painful malunion, and therefore surgical treatment to restore length and intra-articular anatomy is thought to be beneficial. No recommendations, however, have been published as to the amount of lateral column shortening required to warrant surgical fixation.

The surgical options range from bone grafting with definitive internal fixation to temporary bridge plating or external fixation. Arthrodesis rarely is required but may be necessary if articular surfaces cannot be reconstructed. Although large studies of surgical treatment of compression injuries with lengthy follow-up are lacking, the importance of timely surgical intervention was underscored by midterm results, suggesting that persistent symptoms often are caused by associated midfoot injuries.[5]

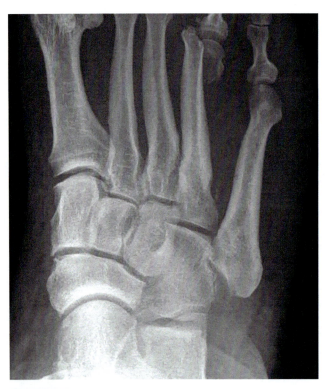

FIGURE 2 Oblique radiograph of the foot showing lateral dislocation of the fifth tarsometatarsal joint with a compression fracture of the cuboid.

Cuneiform Fractures

The cuneiforms are a relatively stable complex of bones between the navicular and the medial three metatarsal bases. The strong intertarsal ligaments allow the cuneiforms only a small amount of motion. Accordingly, displaced fractures are rare and suggest the presence of a more sinister midfoot injury elsewhere. The mechanism usually is direct trauma, and patients have pain over the central to medial midfoot. Plain radiographs should be obtained, but MRI or CT often is needed to evaluate subtle fracture patterns because there is bony overlap on plain radiographs. A nondisplaced fracture is treated with a walking boot and modified weight bearing, as symptoms allow. A displaced fracture occasionally requires internal fixation and, when associated with a TMT injury, primary arthrodesis becomes an option.

TARSOMETATARSAL FRACTURES

TMT injury can be ligamentous, bony, or both. Jacques Lisfranc de St. Martin in 1815 described a fracture-dislocation at the TMT joints that occurred when a soldier caught his foot in a stirrup while dismounting his horse. Such injuries often were managed by amputation, and there is little similarity between classic descriptions and current understanding. Nonetheless, the TMT joints often are called Lisfranc joints, and the terms tarsometatarsal injury and Lisfranc injury are used interchangeably.

Anatomy

The TMT complex spans parts of the transverse and longitudinal arches of the foot and is stabilized by strong plantar ligaments and weaker dorsal ligaments. In the coronal plane, intrinsic stability is provided by the unique position of the second metatarsal base, which is recessed proximally between the medial and lateral cuneiforms. In the axial plane, the unique wedge shape of the bases of the metatarsals and their corresponding cuneiforms provide a bony congruity that maintains the transverse arch and confers tremendous stability.

The ligaments stabilizing the TMT joints are dorsal, plantar, and interosseous. The interosseous ligaments are the strongest; they extend between each of the lateral four metatarsal bases but are conspicuously absent between the first and second metatarsals. The first ray is connected to the second TMT complex by the Lisfranc ligament, which extends from the medial cuneiform to the medial base of the second and third metatarsals, the plantar portion of which is the strongest and most important for midfoot stability.[6]

Little motion occurs at these articulations, but the bones of the TMT joints provide sturdy attachment sites for the anterior and posterior tibial tendons.

The dorsal neurovascular bundle, containing the dorsalis pedis artery and vein and the deep peroneal nerve, runs dorsally over the second TMT joint, just lateral to the extensor hallucis longus tendon.

Patient History and Physical Examination

Patients who have a nonneuropathic Lisfranc injury report swelling and midfoot pain and typically are incapable of weight bearing secondary to pain. The injury can result from low-energy or high-energy trauma that causes direct or indirect force to the midfoot. High-energy injuries often occur during a motor vehicle crash in which the midfoot sustains violent trauma or is crushed under great load. Lower energy sports injuries, commonly seen in American football and rugby, have a twisting mechanism combined with an axial load and midfoot hyperdorsiflexion. To simplify the understanding of Lisfranc injuries, generally they are categorized as direct or indirect. Direct injury results from the application of load precisely over the TMT complex, usually dorsally. Because the soft-tissue envelope overlying the TMT complex is thin, it is important to be aware of concomitant soft-tissue and vascular injury, which can lead to compartment syndrome of the foot. Indirect injury is more common than direct injury and results from an axial load combined with twisting of the midfoot in plantar flexion. Indirect injury often occurs during athletic activities, although occasionally can occur as the result of a misstep off a stair or sidewalk.

Because of the numerous mechanisms and tremendous variability in the forces causing the spectrum of TMT injuries, it is necessary to maintain a high index of suspicion in patients with posttraumatic midfoot pain. More severe injury is easily diagnosed by the severity of swelling and gross displacement. Plantar ecchymosis, a cardinal feature of midfoot injury, should always suggest the need for further workup. On occasion, subtle injury causes only mild swelling and pain. A patient whose history and physical examination suggest a Lisfranc injury should receive prompt radiographic evaluation.

Diagnostic Studies

Plain weight-bearing radiographs of the injured and contralateral extremities should be obtained. Weight bearing often is difficult because of pain but is necessary because diastasis between the medial cuneiform and base of the second metatarsal may not be evident on non–weight-bearing radiographs (**Figure 3**). If the radiographs are equivocal or nondiagnostic, an examination under anesthesia may be warranted to detect instability. CT is used to define bony injury and detect associated fractures. Three-dimensional CT reconstruction can be helpful for appreciating the geometry of the injury.

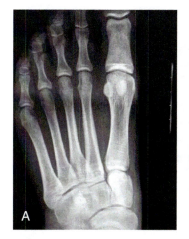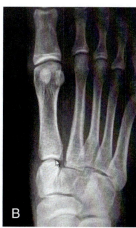

FIGURE 3 Weight-bearing AP radiograph showing widening of the space between the medial cuneiform and second metatarsal base (**A**), which indicates a disruption of the Lisfranc ligament, along with a weight-bearing AP radiograph of the contralateral uninjured foot (**B**).

MRI is useful for diagnosing a more subtle ligamentous injury, such as a Lisfranc tear or sprain, a bony contusion, or an occult fracture. MRI has high predictive value for midfoot instability[7] (**Figure 4**).

On weight-bearing AP radiographs, the medial border of the second metatarsal base should align with the corresponding medial border of the middle cuneiform. Failure to maintain this specific relationship indicates rupture of the strong plantar Lisfranc ligament. On an

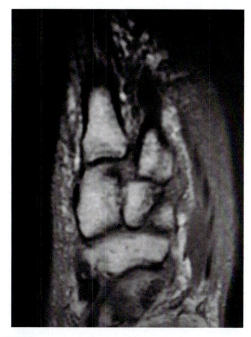

FIGURE 4 MRI showing a Lisfranc injury with lateral deviation of the second metatarsal base.

oblique foot radiograph, the medial border of the fourth metatarsal should align with the medial border of the cuboid. On a lateral radiograph, there should be no dorsal or plantar subluxation of the metatarsals relative to their corresponding cuneiforms or cuboid bone. Any dorsal displacement of the metatarsal bases is abnormal and must be distinguished from posttraumatic or degenerative bossing of the TMT complex. A so-called fleck sign seen on radiographs or CT is indicative of a bony avulsion of the insertion of the Lisfranc ligament on the medial base of the second metatarsal (Figure 5). Because bone-to-bone healing is more reliable than ligament-to-bone healing, the fleck sign is thought to suggest a good prognosis.

Classification

Organizing Lisfranc injuries into specific groups with treatment algorithms is difficult because of tremendous variability in the severity of injury and the contribution of soft-tissue pathology. No single classification scheme appropriately balances ease of use and reproducibility with treatment recommendations and prognosis. A classification system first reported on in 1909,[8] and expanded in later studies[9,10] is predicated on the concept of the three columns of the foot (Figure 6). The medial column includes the first metatarsal, medial cuneiform, and corresponding navicular facet; the middle column includes the second and third metatarsals, middle and lateral cuneiforms, and corresponding navicular facets; and the lateral column includes the fourth and fifth metatarsals and cuboid. A type A injury has total incongruity with a homolateral dislocation. A type B injury has partial incongruity with an incomplete homolateral dislocation. A type C injury is divergent, with partial or total displacement. Although some clinicians find this classification system cumbersome to use, it provides a useful standard terminology for describing these injuries. A review of 54 Lisfranc injuries found those with involvement of all three columns had worse outcomes compared with fewer column involvement.[11]

As discussed in a 2019 study, classifications of low-energy sports–related Lisfranc injuries highlight their more subtle nature as well as the high likelihood of concomitant extension of injury to the intercuneiform joints.[12] Sports-related Lisfranc sprains were classified as stage I injuries when nondisplaced, stage II when there was diastasis with no arch height loss, and stage III when diastasis was associated with arch height loss.[13]

Treatment

The primary objective of the treatment of any Lisfranc injury is to achieve a pain-free, durable, and stable plantigrade foot. This objective is achieved by anatomic reduction and adequate immobilization to ensure stability.

A patient with point tenderness over the Lisfranc articulation, normal plain weight-bearing radiographs, and MRI showing an abnormal Lisfranc ligament may have injured only the dorsal ligaments. With an intact plantar ligament, the appropriate treatment is rest and immobilization in a walking cast or boot, with weight bearing allowed as symptoms decrease, typically at 4 to 6 weeks. A course of physical therapy is useful for strengthening and gait training. After using a walking boot, many patients prefer to use a stiff insole or a carbon fiber insert, which somewhat restricts midfoot motion, as they transition into their preinjury shoe wear. However, imaging studies must be scrutinized because even slight displacement carries a high risk of instability.

Inability to obtain or maintain an anatomically reduced and stabilized Lisfranc complex leads to premature midfoot arch collapse and degenerative arthritis.[10,14] Surgical stabilization is usually required for an injury causing midfoot instability, such as a displaced fracture or disruption of the ligamentous structures connecting the plantarmedial cuneiform to the second and third metatarsal bases. Debate exists as to the optimal primary surgical treatment of Lisfranc injuries. The options include ORIF with transarticular screws and/or pins, ORIF with bridge plate(s), ORIF with suture button techniques, and primary midfoot arthrodesis (Figure 7). Closed reduction with pinning or spanning external fixation is only reserved for injury with severe soft-tissue

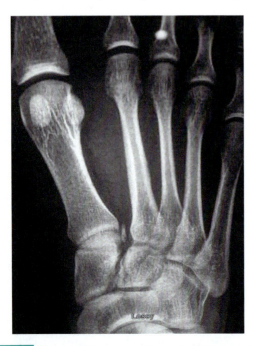

FIGURE 5 AP weight-bearing radiograph of the foot showing the fleck sign, which indicates avulsion of the origin of the Lisfranc ligament.

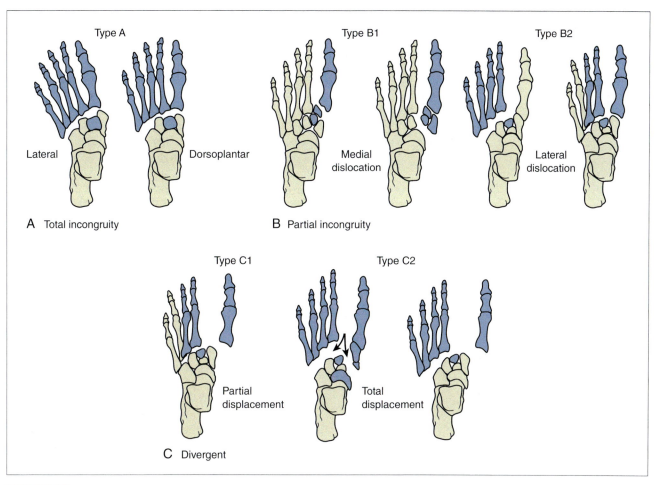

FIGURE 6 Schematic drawing showing the classification of tarsometatarsal joint injury. Shading represents injured or displaced areas of the foot. **A**, In type A, total incongruity, all five metatarsals are displaced, with or without fracture at the base of the second metatarsal. The usual displacement is lateral or dorsolateral, and the metatarsals move as a unit. Type A injury is homolateral. **B**, In type B, one or more articulations remain intact. Type B1 represents partial incongruity with medial dislocation, and type B2 represents partial incongruity with lateral dislocation. The first metatarsal cuneiform joint may be involved. **C**, Type C is divergent, with partial (type C1) or total (type C2) displacement. The arrows in C2 represent the forces through the foot leading to a divergent pattern. (Redrawn from Watson TS, Shurnas PS, Denker J: Treatment of Lisfranc joint injury: Current concepts. *J Am Acad Orthop Surg* 2010;18[12]:718-728. Copyright 2010, by American Academy of Orthopaedic Surgeons.)

compromise because of the difficulty of obtaining anatomic reduction without opening the dislocation site.

Surgical Results and Prognosis

Proponents of ORIF think that maintaining midfoot joint motion is essential for optimal long-term function and prevention of adjacent-segment degeneration. One study found that 28 of 30 patients with anatomic reduction of a Lisfranc injury had a good to excellent functional result.[15] However, none of the 11 patients who underwent gait analysis had a normal gait pattern after anatomic reduction of a displaced Lisfranc injury.[16] As to the type and specific placement of hardware, no universal agreement exists. Advocates of transarticular screw fixation suggest that joint compression and alignment are easily achieved and, when necessary, screw removal is easily facilitated through percutaneous techniques. These surgeons argue that the removal of a dorsal plate is difficult and adds unnecessary morbidity to hardware removal, especially because of the difficulty in differentiating small cutaneous nerves from postsurgical scar. Those who favor dorsal plating mainly do so because transarticular screw fixation without arthrodesis causes significant articular chondral damage that may lead to premature posttraumatic midfoot arthritis. Of note, cadaver research has demonstrated that transarticular screw fixation and bridge plate fixation have similar biomechanical strength for maintaining reduction.[17,18] However, a 2019 simulated limited weight-bearing cadaver study showed increased plantar diastasis with dorsal plating techniques compared with transarticular screws, but it was not statistically significant.[19] Clinical studies have compared

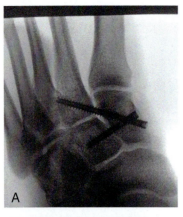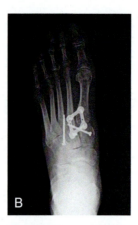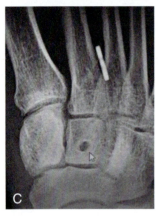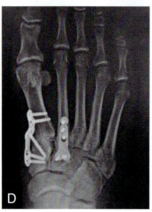

FIGURE 7 Radiographs showing examples of Lisfranc injury fixation. **A**, Open reduction and internal fixation (ORIF) with transarticular screws. **B**, ORIF with bridge plate. **C**, ORIF with suture button technique with additional suture anchor in the middle cuneiform. **D**, Primary arthrodesis.

transarticular screw constructs with dorsal bridge plate constructs. They have corroborated previous findings on the surgical treatment of Lisfranc injuries by showing that an anatomic reduction is the best predictor of functional outcome. Results of these studies have been mixed. One study did not find a significant difference in functional outcomes based on fixation method but did find a higher rate of soft-tissue complications in the dorsal bridge plate group.[20] A second study found better functional outcomes in the bridge plate group, which could be attributed to a trend for better anatomic reduction with a bridge plate construct.[21] A 2021 systematic review looking at various fixation techniques found no significant differences between use of screws versus plating.[22] A small number of the included studies showed superior outcomes with plating. One study using suture button fixation was included and showed superior American Orthopaedic Foot and Ankle Society scores.

Suture button fixation has emerged as an alternative to transarticular screws and dorsal bridge plating. The primary benefit of this technique is the lack of need for hardware removal. Clinical studies have shown promising outcomes for this technique.[23,24] A 2021 study compared suture button fixation with conventional transarticular screw fixation for purely ligamentous Lisfranc injuries and found better outcome scores 6 months postoperatively, but this was before removal of the transarticular screw(s). No differences were seen at 1 year. There was also no difference in radiographic outcomes.[25] In addition, a 2021 biomechanical study looked at the use of flexible suture fixation for Lisfranc injuries.[26] The study did not directly compare this method with screw or plate fixation but did find that adding a supplementary limb of suture across the intercuneiform joint provided mechanical benefit, particularly at higher loads.

Proponents of primary midfoot fusion note that the medial column of the midfoot is inherently more stable and less mobile than the lateral column, and therefore, little motion is lost through arthrodesis. A prospective, randomized study of 41 subacute, purely ligamentous Lisfranc injuries found that patients who underwent primary arthrodesis had significantly better outcome scores than those who underwent ORIF.[27] At an average 46-month follow-up, patients who underwent arthrodesis rated their function at 92% of their preinjury level, compared with 65% for patients who underwent ORIF. Five patients who had ORIF later underwent arthrodesis secondary to persistent pain and deformity or osteoarthrosis. A similar randomized prospective study of 40 patients who underwent ORIF or fusion for treatment of Lisfranc fractures and/or ligamentous injuries reported no significant between-group differences at follow-up intervals extending 2 years after surgical treatment.[28] A telephone survey of these patients at an average 53-month follow-up also found no between-group difference in satisfaction rates. However, 78.6% of patients who underwent ORIF required an additional surgical procedure (including planned removal of transarticular screws), compared with 16.7% of those who underwent fusion.

A number of more recent studies have looked to compare primary arthrodesis with ORIF. A study on low-energy Lisfranc injuries in members of the US military found no differences in Foot and Ankle Ability Measure outcome scores at 35 months between those who underwent primary arthrodesis and those who underwent ORIF. However, those who underwent primary arthrodesis had a quicker return to full duty than the ORIF group (4.5 months versus 6.7 months). Additionally, those who underwent primary arthrodesis had less of a decline in their fitness test running times than those who underwent ORIF (9 seconds slower per mile compared with 39 seconds slower per mile) at the 1-year mark.[29] A study from China demonstrated better American Orthopaedic Foot and Ankle Society scores in patients who underwent primary arthrodesis compared with ORIF.[30] However, other studies, one of which was a systematic review and meta-analysis, have not been able to show significant differences in terms of functional outcomes between patients undergoing primary arthrodesis versus ORIF.[31,32] As mentioned previously, the need for eventual hardware removal has been shown to be lower in patients undergoing primary arthrodesis. A study demonstrated that when hardware removal is excluded, there are no significant differences in revision surgical treatment rates (29.5% in the ORIF group versus 29.6% in the primary arthrodesis group).[33] A database study looked at cost comparison as well as complication rate for primary arthrodesis and ORIF. Primary arthrodesis was found to be significantly more expensive along with having a higher complication rate, likely because of implant costs. However, the highest cost of care was found in patients who had to be converted to a primary arthrodesis, having initially undergone ORIF.[34]

COMPARTMENT SYNDROME OF THE FOOT

Although compartment syndrome of the foot is not common, severe trauma to the foot can lead to elevated intracompartmental pressures that, if unrecognized, can cause soft-tissue injury beyond the injury from the initial trauma. Foot compartment syndrome has been found to be most likely to occur when a crush mechanism was combined with a forefoot injury. One study found Lisfranc injuries to be responsible for two-thirds of the incidences of compartment syndrome of the foot.[35]

Compartment syndrome results from raised pressure within a closed fascial space that exceeds tissue capillary pressure and causes tissue hypoperfusion. The foot is most commonly thought to consist of nine compartments.[36] On the plantar surface, medial, lateral, and central compartments exist. There are four interosseous compartments between the metatarsal shafts and an adductor compartment in the proximal forefoot. A septum divides the central compartment into superficial and deep compartments, although the distinction between these two compartments was called into question.[37] The superficial compartment contains the flexor digitorum brevis muscle, and the deep compartment contains the quadratus plantae muscle and lateral plantar nerve. A calcaneal compartment has been described, which is an extension of the deep central compartment into the hindfoot. The deep calcaneal compartment communicates directly with the deep posterior compartment of the leg.

Severe direct trauma or crush injury is responsible for many incidences of compartment syndrome. The classic signs and symptoms, consisting of pain out of proportion to the injury and pain with passive digital motion, are of little use in the setting of severe foot trauma because it is impossible to determine whether the pain is attributable to the injury or increased intracompartmental pressure.

The diagnosis can be made by direct measurement of compartment pressures higher than 30 mm Hg or within 10 to 30 mm Hg of the patient's diastolic blood pressure. Decompression can be achieved through two dorsal incisions: a medial incision between the first and second metatarsals and a second incision between the fourth and fifth metatarsals. A medial incision may be needed to relieve pressure in the medial, lateral, superficial, and deep central compartments. The use of a piecrust skin incision technique may be adequate if the compartment syndrome is the result of a massive subcutaneous hematoma. Repeat irrigation and débridement with secondary closure or skin grafting may be necessary if soft-tissue swelling precludes primary closure. Missed compartment syndrome can cause ischemic contracture, complex regional pain syndrome, and permanent loss of function. Therefore, a high index of suspicion for compartment syndrome is necessary in a patient with a severe crush and/or traumatic midfoot injury accompanied by profound swelling. A prospective study of surgical outcomes and quality of life in severe foot trauma and associated compartment syndrome after fasciotomy found shorter interval to fasciotomy correlated with less pain and better outcome scores.[38] In contrast, a case-control study of high-energy, combat-related lower extremity trauma found greater incidence of hammertoes (50% versus 17%) in the group that underwent fasciotomy compared with control patients who did not have fasciotomy.[39] The study was unable to demonstrate differences in the development of neuropathic pain, sensory deficits, motor deficits, chronic pain, stiffness, or infection.

FOREFOOT FRACTURES

Most if not all fractures of the forefoot can be successfully managed without surgical treatment. Standard trauma principles include anatomic reduction of the fracture and any involved joints, with sufficiently rigid internal or external fixation. It is important to evaluate the associated soft tissues to avoid incisions in areas at high risk for skin necrosis, dehiscence, or other complications. A surgical procedure should be delayed until resolution of the soft-tissue injury is sufficient to minimize the risk of complications (**Figure 8**).

METATARSAL FRACTURES

Metatarsal fractures are relatively common. Each of the five metatarsals functions in a different manner, and optimal fracture healing requires a different approach to the treatment of each metatarsal. With the exception of the proximal fifth metatarsal, only limited published studies are available on the indications for treating patients with metatarsal fractures and the long-term results.

Section 6: Foot and Ankle Trauma

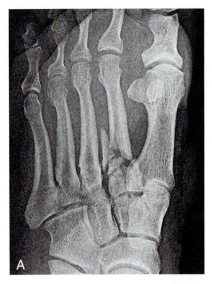
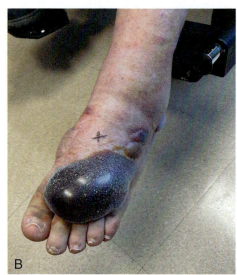
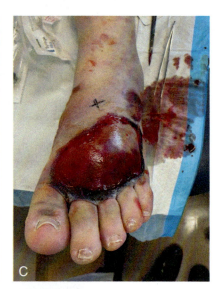
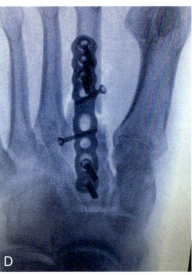
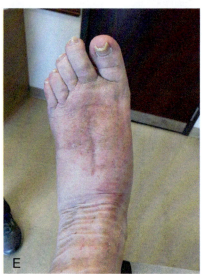

FIGURE 8 **A,** Radiograph showing complex crush injury with second metatarsal fracture. Clinical photographs showing significant soft-tissue injury with fracture blister (**B**) and subsequent unroofing (**C**). **D,** Postoperative AP radiograph demonstrating open reduction and internal fixation of fracture and spanning fixation to include fusion of second tarsometatarsal joint. **E,** Clinical photograph taken 8 weeks after surgical intervention. Treatment needed to be delayed 5 weeks to allow soft tissue to be appropriate for an incision.

Most metatarsal fractures are the result of trauma, whether acute or chronic, and are effectively managed nonsurgically. There does not appear to be an association with the development of metatarsal fractures and long-term diphosphonate therapy.[40] The frequency of metatarsal fractures decreases with increasing age and has a seasonal peak during the summer months.[41] Surgical treatment typically is indicated for severe displacement, multiple fractures, intra-articular injury, an open wound, compartment syndrome, displaced fracture fragments creating risk to the skin, significant sagittal displacement in any ray, or significant transverse displacement in the first or fifth metatarsal. It is considerably less problematic to initially reduce and stabilize a fracture than to do so after malunion, nonunion, or after a skin complication has developed. This can be accomplished with percutaneous pinning, external fixation, and/or ORIF.

First Metatarsal Fractures

The first metatarsal is wider, shorter, and stronger than the lesser metatarsals. It is more mobile because the ligaments and articulation at its base allow more motion. Unlike the lesser metatarsals, the first metatarsal does not have a stout transverse intermetatarsal ligament distally between the adjacent second metatarsal neck. The first metatarsal bears almost half of the body's weight through the forefoot.[42] Displacement of the first metatarsal head in any direction disturbs the tripod-like weight-bearing

Chapter 21: Midfoot and Forefoot Trauma

complex of the anterior portion of the foot and impairs forefoot function. Because even a small malalignment can affect the distribution of weight during ambulation, it is important to tolerate almost no displacement in the coronal or sagittal plane. The primary goal of treatment of a fracture of the first metatarsal is to maintain the normal distribution of weight under all of the metatarsal heads.

Nonsurgical Treatment

A minimally displaced or nondisplaced fracture of the first metatarsal can almost always be successfully treated nonsurgically. A short leg cast or a controlled ankle movement (CAM) walker boot allows protected weight bearing. A boot has the advantages of allowing adjustment, skin assessment, and direct application of ice and anti-inflammatory medications. The disadvantages of the boot include possible difficulty with fit or compliance. For an unstable injury, it is preferable to use a cast and avoid weight bearing for 4 to 6 weeks, until there is evidence of healing. Displacement or nonunion is rare, however, and more aggressive mobilization may enhance healing and recovery.[43] Early displacement of such a fracture can be detected by close follow-up. The patient should begin to use a comfortable, well-cushioned regular shoe as soon as the symptoms and soft tissues permit and bony healing is appropriate on radiographs. Passive motion exercises of the toes should be initiated as soon as tolerable if the fracture is stable.

Surgical Treatment

The first ray should be carefully evaluated for displacement, particularly in the transverse and sagittal planes because malunion can lead to painful weight bearing, early posttraumatic arthritis, transfer metatarsalgia, and difficulty in shoe fitting. Percutaneous or open reduction of the fracture should be followed by internal or external fixation. Internal fixation can be achieved using K-wires, lag screws, or a low-profile, small-caliber plate. The location and position of the plate are determined by the fracture extent and pattern as well as the placement of the incision.

A proximal first metatarsal fracture can be fixed using a bridge plate across the TMT joint. External fixation can allow proper healing if there is significant comminution, particularly near the TMT joint. Primary arthrodesis of the first TMT joint is an option for a severe injury or comminution and has little effect on foot function.[27-30]

After surgical treatment, a well-padded short leg splint should be used initially. The toes should be left uncovered so that swelling and perfusion can be assessed and toe range-of-motion exercises can be initiated to avoid stiffness. When the wounds have healed (generally at 2 to

3 weeks), a short leg walking cast or CAM walker boot gradually can be used with progressive weight bearing. Generally, patients are allowed to increase the amount of weight put onto the foot over 3 to 4 weeks, until it is possible to bear weight without pain. Fusion of the first TMT joint may require a longer period of limited weight bearing. When there is clinical and radiographic healing of the fracture, the transition to a comfortable accommodative shoe can begin, with increasingly aggressive range-of-motion and resistance exercises. Most injuries heal within 2 to 3 months and leave little functional impairment. Dorsal plate fixation in metatarsal fractures occasionally leads to symptomatic hardware with shoe wear, which can easily be solved with delayed hardware removal once full consolidation of a bony union has been achieved.

Middle Metatarsal Fractures

Fracture of a middle (second, third, or fourth) metatarsal is common. The injury can occur in isolation or with other injuries from vehicular or other high-energy trauma. Often a middle metatarsal fracture has a direct mechanism such as a crush injury, a puncture wound, or axial loading of a plantarflexed foot. Heightened suspicion is necessary to identify the fracture in a patient with multiple injuries and to evaluate for open fracture, which is most common with a crush injury. A metatarsal fracture is classified by its location as a neck, shaft, or base fracture.

Metatarsal Neck Fractures

A metatarsal neck fracture is inherently less stable than a shaft or base fracture. Often, more than one metatarsal is affected, further decreasing fracture stability and the ability to maintain adequate alignment by closed means. In particular, sagittal plane deformity can lead to painful plantar callosities, dorsal exostoses, and corns. A nondisplaced or minimally displaced fracture can be managed with a hard-soled shoe with weight bearing as tolerated. A more displaced fracture initially should be managed with closed reduction under sedation, using finger traps and direct manipulation with pressure over the metatarsal heads. An unstable fracture or a fracture with persistent sagittal plane deformity should be treated with closed reduction and retrograde pinning with K-wires (from the plantar surface), open reduction and antegrade-retrograde pinning, or internal fixation with a small-caliber plate (if the head fragment is sufficiently large). A longitudinal skin incision that allows simultaneous access to adjacent metatarsals is used. As an alternative, fixation after closed reduction can be done by driving K-wires from the intact fifth metatarsal neck into the adjacent fractured middle metatarsal necks.[44]

Section 6: Foot and Ankle Trauma

© 2025 American Academy of Orthopaedic Surgeons

Orthopaedic Knowledge Update®: Foot and Ankle 7

337

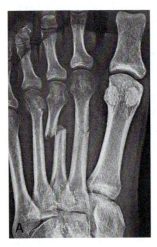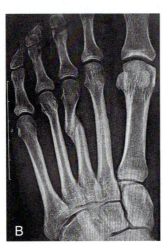

FIGURE 9 **A**, AP radiograph showing significantly displaced fracture of the third metatarsal shaft with coronal plane deformity. Concomitant nondisplaced fractures of the second metatarsal and fourth metatarsal head are seen. **B**, Radiograph shows complete healing and remodeling of all fractures at 6 months with asymptomatic malunion of the third metatarsal shaft.

Metatarsal Shaft Fractures

As with a metatarsal neck fracture, a minimally displaced or nondisplaced metatarsal shaft fracture can be treated with a hard-soled shoe and weight bearing as tolerated. Moderate frontal plane deformity does not typically lead to functional complications, but sagittal plane deformity is more problematic. Although significant displacement may have more predictable results with surgical intervention, malunions, particularly in the coronal plane, are well tolerated (**Figure 9**). A malunited fracture with significant sagittal plane deformity can lead to painful plantar callosities and dorsal exostoses and corns. The typical apex dorsal deformity in a shaft fracture results from plantar flexion of the distal fragment produced by the strong flexor tendons. In general, the more distal the fracture, the greater the apex dorsal deformity, and the higher probability is that open reduction will be required. As for every foot injury, the radiographic evaluation should include AP, lateral, and oblique views. Oblique views are particularly useful because the metatarsals are seen as superimposed on the lateral view.

Most diaphyseal fractures can be managed nonsurgically. The surgical indications generally are limited to metatarsal shortening, significant displacement or angulation, and multiple displaced metatarsal fractures. The methods of fixation include intramedullary K-wires, small plates and screws, and external fixation. K-wires are suitable for many fracture patterns except comminuted length-unstable fractures, for which plates and screws may be more appropriate. K-wires and external fixation are particularly useful for fractures with significant soft-tissue injury. Although plate fixation requires a larger incision, when possible, its use may be favored, especially when there are multiple metatarsals involved, because it allows for earlier weight bearing, tendon mobilization, and better functional outcomes without significant risk of displacement[45] (**Figure 10**).

After surgical treatment, a well-padded short leg splint should be applied and the patient should not bear weight for 1 to 2 weeks, until acute swelling resolves. A walking short leg cast then can be applied if plantar pins are present. If no pins are present, the patient can gradually begin

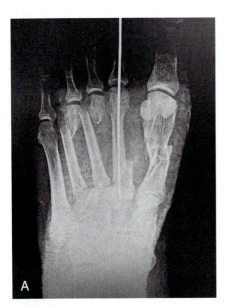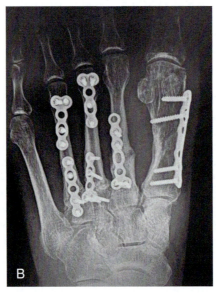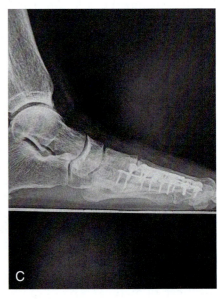

FIGURE 10 AP radiographs of forefoot injury. **A**, Fractures of metatarsals 1 to 4 with initial Kirschner wire stabilization are shown. **B** and **C**, Subsequent AP and lateral radiographs, respectively, show plating and eventual anatomic healing.

to use a CAM walker boot. After the initial 1 to 2 weeks, the patient is allowed to bear weight only through the heel. Pins are removed at the 4- to 6-week mark, based on evidence of fracture healing. In general, a relatively young patient will have radiographic healing earlier than an older patient. Weight bearing following plate fixation may commence at 2 weeks, provided that the incisions are healing appropriately. Compression socks are recommended to help decrease postoperative and dependent edema such that eventual difficulties with shoe wear are minimized.

Metatarsal Base Fractures

A metatarsal base fracture inherently is more stable than a shaft or neck fracture because of the shorter lever arm of the deforming flexor forces and the surrounding interosseous ligaments and capsular attachments. Most base fractures are managed by closed means with a hard-soled shoe and weight bearing as tolerated. Care should be taken to rule out a Lisfranc variant injury before proceeding with closed treatment. Weight-bearing radiographs, if possible, or cross-sectional advanced imaging (MRI and/or CT) should be obtained to rule out such an injury. ORIF should be considered if there is significant displacement, an open injury, or an unstable pattern. Fixation can be achieved with plates, screws, or percutaneous K-wires. Plates spanning the TMT joints can be considered when interfragmentary screw fixation is not an option or when there is insufficient bone in the metatarsal proximal to the fracture to allow for adequate fixation. Primary fusion may be desirable for a comminuted intra-articular injury.

Fifth Metatarsal Fractures

Fifth metatarsal fractures account for approximately one-fourth of all metatarsal injuries. Fractures of the fifth metatarsal differ from those of the other lesser metatarsals in several respects. The fifth metatarsal is the only one with extrinsic tendon attachments; both the peroneus brevis and the peroneus tertius insert at the base of the fifth metatarsal. The fifth metatarsal has very little soft-tissue coverage on the lateral and plantar foot. There is a very strong ligamentous attachment to the plantar aponeurosis. The proximal fifth metatarsal has a vascular watershed area that creates a biomechanical and biologic environment in which fractures are common, often are difficult to treat, and can have problematic healing.

A fifth metatarsal fracture can be classified as a proximal (base) fracture or a diaphyseal fracture. Each of these types has a unique etiology, treatment, and prognosis. The management of a diaphyseal fracture is similar for all metatarsals. Most can be managed nonsurgically; however, stress fractures of the diaphysis have a tendency to prolonged union and refracture, particularly in patients

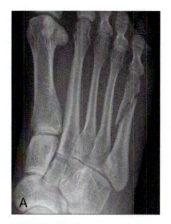 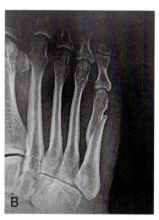

FIGURE 11 **A** and **B**, Oblique radiographs showing an example of a dancer's fracture, a displaced oblique fracture of the fifth metatarsal shaft with early consolidation at 3 months. The patient was made to bear weight as tolerated in a hard-soled shoe for 6 weeks.

with obesity or in the setting of a large fourth-fifth intermetatarsal angle.[46] Despite significant displacement, long oblique fractures of the fifth metatarsal shaft, commonly known as dancer's fractures, heal well without surgery with early weight bearing in a hard-soled shoe with a very high union rate. The surgical indications generally are limited to shortening, sagittal malangulation, significant displacement (>1 cm), and multiple metatarsal fractures (**Figure 11**).

The proximal half of the fifth metatarsal often is classified according to the Lawrence and Botte system into three distinct fracture zones. Zone I includes the styloid process and can extend into the fourth/fifth TMT articulation; zone II, the metadiaphyseal region involving the fourth/fifth intermetatarsal articulation; and zone III, the proximal diaphyseal region where the fracture is typically transverse. Zones I, II, and III are subject to an avulsion fracture, a Jones fracture, and (usually) a stress fracture, respectively (**Figure 12**).

Avulsion Fractures

Almost all fifth metatarsal fractures are avulsion fractures at the base. This injury is thought to occur secondary to the forces exerted on the base by the strong attachment of the peroneus brevis and the lateral plantar aponeurosis. These fracture lines do not extend distally to the fourth/fifth intermetatarsal articulation and are sometimes referred to as pseudo-Jones fractures. The plantar aponeurosis probably has a key role in these fractures because they are rarely displaced, and some fibers of the peroneus brevis remain intact. The mechanism of injury usually is an acute inversion moment, as occurs when stepping off a curb. Many patients describe hearing a popping sound and have acute swelling, ecchymosis, and difficulty in ambulation. The location of tenderness

Section 6: Foot and Ankle Trauma

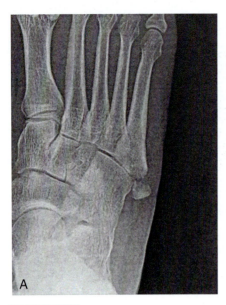 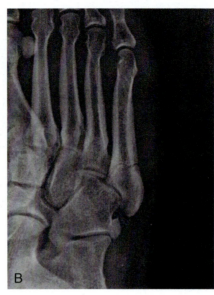 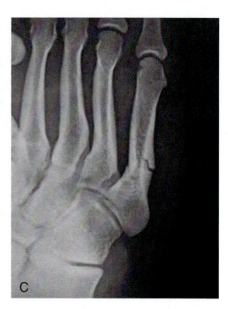

FIGURE 12 Oblique radiographs showing fifth metatarsal base fractures. **A**, Zone I, avulsion, or pseudo-Jones fractures. **B**, Zone II, metadiaphyseal or Jones fracture. **C**, Zone III, diaphyseal fractures.

and swelling determines whether a foot or ankle radiograph should be obtained to look for a fifth metatarsal avulsion fracture or another injury that can occur with the same mechanism, such as a fracture on the anterior process of the calcaneus or distal fibula.

Fifth metatarsal avulsion fractures typically are successfully managed without surgery. Patients can be made weight bearing as tolerated in a cast or boot, or even a well-cushioned shoe with a stiff sole, for 4 to 8 weeks. The progression of treatment often is based on clinical symptoms; radiographs are not correlated with outcome, and radiographic healing can be prolonged or not occur. Most of these injuries clinically heal within 6 to 8 weeks. Painful nonunions are uncommon and are treated by excision of the fragment and repair of the peroneus brevis or, for larger fragments, by fixation and grafting. Primary internal fixation is typically reserved for fractures that include a large fragment entering the metatarsal-cuboid joint with more than 2 mm of displacement. Fixation usually is with a narrow tension band wire or a small-caliber lag screw (Figure 13). Primary surgical fixation may lead to lower rates of malunion and earlier return to weight bearing and work, although patient outcome scores were not significantly improved at 1 year postoperatively compared with patients treated nonsurgically.[47]

Jones (Metadiaphyseal) Fractures

A fracture of the proximal metadiaphyseal junction of the fifth metatarsal, called a Jones fracture,[48] occurs acutely with an adduction moment and axial loading causing an upward force on a plantarflexed foot. The pattern is different from that of an avulsion fracture, in that a Jones fracture exits the intermetatarsal facet rather than the cuboid–fifth metatarsal articulation. Although a Jones fracture often can be successfully managed without surgery, nonunion and refracture are common and can be problematic, especially for athletes. It is thought that the location of the fracture and the high incidence of nonunion are secondary to a vascular watershed area at the metaphyseal/diaphyseal junction.

Successful nonsurgical treatment generally requires cast immobilization and avoidance of weight bearing over a prolonged (6-week) period. For this reason, Jones

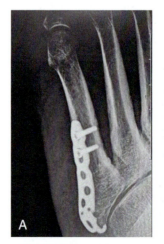 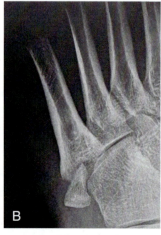

FIGURE 13 **A**, Oblique radiograph showing displaced zone I fracture in a patient who plays professional baseball. **B**, Oblique radiograph obtained after the patient underwent open reduction and internal fixation with plate fixation.

Chapter 21: Midfoot and Forefoot Trauma

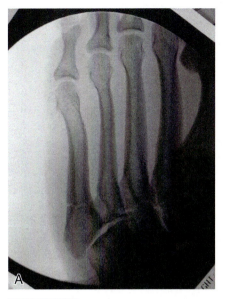 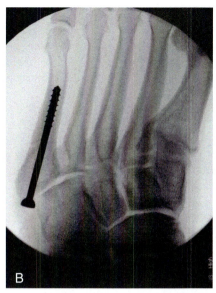 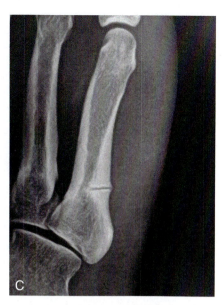

FIGURE 14 **A**, Oblique radiograph showing an acute zone II, Jones fracture. **B**, Oblique radiograph showing subsequent open reduction and internal fixation (ORIF) with intramedullary screw fixation. **C**, Oblique radiograph showing an example of acute on chronic fracture with lateral cortical beaking and endosteal hypertrophy, which required ORIF and bone grafting.

fractures often are treated surgically in young, active individuals. The treatment decision also is affected by whether the fracture represents an acute or a stress injury, as can be accurately determined by the chronicity of symptoms, injury mechanism, radiographic evidence of sclerosis or nonunion at the fracture margins, and the presence of factors predisposing to stress fracture, such as cavovarus alignment (**Figure 14**).

Nonsurgical Treatment
Nonsurgical treatment is reserved for a nondisplaced fracture in a patient who is not an athlete and who chooses this treatment after discussing the risks and benefits of surgical treatment. A well-padded, non–weight-bearing cast or boot should be used. If healing is evident after 6 weeks, the patient begins to bear weight gradually during the next 2 to 3 weeks. Surgical treatment should be considered if the symptoms persist and radiographic union is not seen at 10 weeks, or if there is a refracture.

Surgical Treatment
Percutaneous intramedullary screw fixation is commonly used for an acute displaced fracture or a fracture in a high-performance athlete. Plating also leads to good results and low rates of hardware removal.[49] Surgical treatment leads to a significantly shorter time to bone healing and return to sport than nonsurgical treatment.[49] Bone graft or other biologic supplementation can promote union in a chronic fracture, a nonunion, or a refracture, and is often used in the treatment of the elite athlete with a Jones fracture.[50] Tension band techniques have been described but generally require a larger incision and more soft-tissue dissection than percutaneous screw fixation. The risks of surgical intervention include sural nerve injury, local wound problems including infection and delayed healing, iatrogenic fracture, and pain from the screw head. There is also risk of refracture, particularly in the presence of other mechanical or biologic risk factors. In the competitive athlete, in whom fifth metatarsal fractures commonly occur, a large systematic review of the literature suggests that the average return to play is 11 weeks.[51]

Metatarsal Stress Fractures
A stress fracture is an overuse injury that occurs when activity repetition leads to a mismatch between bone microtrauma and bone repair. Such injuries are common among active patients such as military recruits, athletes, and dancers. It is often related to a sudden increase in activity level. The forefoot is especially vulnerable to stress fracture, and the metatarsals are commonly involved, with the second and third being the most common.[50,52]

Both intrinsic and extrinsic factors can contribute to the development of stress fracture. The intrinsic factors include level of fitness, anatomic alignment, bone morphology, vitamin D levels, menstrual pattern, and bone vascularity. The extrinsic factors include training regimen, shoe wear, and playing surface.[50,53] The fifth metatarsal is especially susceptible to stress fracture because of the poor blood supply to the metadiaphyseal junction, but all metatarsals are at risk. The lateral column is

Section 6: Foot and Ankle Trauma

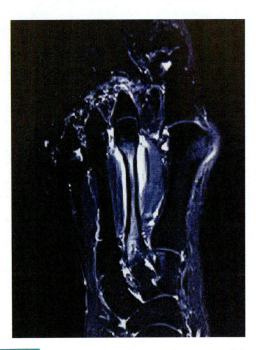

FIGURE 15 Axial T2 image of a second metatarsal shaft stress-fracture with intramedullary and periosteal edema in a 42-year-old woman who is a runner and who has had swelling and pain for 3 weeks.

especially susceptible to stress fracture in those with significant hindfoot varus.

Diagnosis of a metatarsal stress fracture is based on a characteristic history, physical examination, and imaging findings. The key historical feature is insidious pain and swelling, often correlated with new high-impact exercise routines, or a change in activity level, equipment, or training surface. The patient's nutritional, endocrinologic, rheumatologic, and menstrual history should be obtained. Localized tenderness and soft-tissue swelling may be present on physical examination. Imaging should begin with AP, lateral, and oblique foot radiographs. Early in the disease process, radiographs may not show any pathology, although past cortical densities of metatarsals may suggest prior stress fractures. The characteristic radiographic findings include cortical radiolucent lines, periosteal reaction, callus formation, and focal sclerosis. The radiographic evidence of stress fracture may lag several weeks behind the clinical symptoms, and the diagnosis may need to be confirmed by repeating the plain radiographs weeks later. Advanced imaging studies also can confirm the diagnosis. CT, a technetium Tc-99m bone scan, and MRI are useful. For an expeditious diagnosis and implementation of a treatment plan, MRI is the most sensitive test[54,55] (**Figure 15**). Although ultrasonography is user dependent, it has been found to have a high specificity and sensitivity and has the benefit of being able to be used in the office setting.[56]

Nonsurgical Treatment

The cornerstone of nonsurgical treatment is rest from the inciting activity. A postoperative shoe or CAM walker boot can be used for immobilization, but a short leg cast is preferred for a high-risk stress fracture such as a proximal fifth metatarsal stress fracture. Patients should have protected weight bearing for 6 to 8 weeks, depending on the severity of symptoms. Protective modalities can range anywhere from a stiff shank in the shoe to a stiff-soled surgical shoe, CAM boot, or a non–weight-bearing cast—whatever achieves symptomatic resolution for the aforementioned time period. A nutritional assessment should be done, and supplementation with calcium and vitamin D should be considered if deficient. If healing is delayed, extracorporeal shock wave therapy and teriparatide can be considered.[57,58] If appropriate, the patient can be referred to a metabolic bone disease specialist for a diagnostic workup and treatment of any identified disorder.

Surgical Treatment

Surgical treatment should be reserved for a high-level athlete, a patient with an established pseudarthrosis, or a patient with refracture. A preexisting foot deformity that creates a predisposition to metatarsal stress fracture, such as cavovarus foot or metatarsus adductus, should be managed concomitantly, as necessary.[59,60] In general, rigid fixation with compression plating of the first through fourth metatarsals and intramedullary screw fixation of the fifth metatarsal is recommended. Autologous bone grafting can be used in the index surgery, but there is no evidence to support the superiority of bone graft plus internal fixation over internal fixation alone for an acute stress fracture.

The initial postoperative immobilization is in a well-padded non–weight-bearing short leg splint with the toes uncovered. After 2 weeks, the splint can be removed, and the patient can begin partial weight bearing in a CAM walker boot. Low-impact and no-impact rehabilitation exercise to restore motion, strength, and fitness (such as cycling and swimming) can begin. At 6 weeks after surgical treatment, the patient can return to full weight bearing and activity, provided there is clinical and radiographic evidence of fracture healing.

TOE FRACTURES

Fractures of the lesser toes are the most common fractures of the forefoot and account for 3.6% of all fractures in adults.[61,62] Almost all patients with such a fracture can be treated nonsurgically with no long-term pain or functional deficits. Nonetheless, a thorough evaluation and radiographic workup should be done to evaluate for concomitant fractures, open fracture, nail bed injury, or other soft-tissue injury.

The most frequent mechanisms of lesser toe fractures are stubbing and crushing injuries, which account for 75% of the fractures, but penetrating trauma can also cause the injury.[62,63] The fifth toe accounts for half of all fractures of the lesser toes. A fracture of the fifth toe, sometimes called a night walker fracture, is produced by a direct abduction force and often is sustained while walking barefoot in the dark. Almost all phalangeal fractures are nondisplaced or minimally displaced. Extra-articular injuries are far more common than intra-articular injuries.

The treatment of lesser toe fracture is nonsurgical for almost all patients. A toe with mild or no fracture displacement or angulation can be treated with buddy taping, in which gauze sponges are placed between the affected toe and the adjacent toes, and the toes are strapped together with adhesive tape. Some patients find wearing a snug sock is preferable to buddy taping, as the act of donning and taking the tape off is irritating both to the skin and the toe that has been injured. The patient should wear a stiff-soled shoe with an open toe box and is allowed to ambulate as tolerated. If there is deformity of the toe, closed reduction under local anesthesia can be accomplished with longitudinal traction (manual or with finger traps) and angular correction, with an object in the web space serving as a fulcrum.

Surgical treatment is reserved for a patient with an open fracture, an unsuccessful closed reduction, or a grossly displaced, unstable fracture. The risks and benefits of surgical treatment should be carefully weighed because a malunited phalangeal fracture is associated with minimal morbidity. As an alternative to surgical fixation, the patient can be offered exostectomy if the malunion becomes symptomatic. Displaced fractures of the proximal phalanx of the great toe in the sagittal plane can result in a poorly tolerated clawing of the hallux because of the extension and flexion moments, which occur through the fracture site and the distal interphalangeal joint, respectively, by the long flexor and extensor tendons. In these cases, ORIF is recommended (**Figure 16**).

A pediatric injury worth mentioning is an open fracture of the hallux distal phalanx involving the nail bed, otherwise known as a Seymour fracture. In this entity, the proximity of the open nail bed injury communicates with the physis of distal phalanx. Appearing relatively innocuous, nonsurgical management can lead to osteomyelitis, and high index of suspicion for these injuries should be maintained when evaluating the skeletally immature patient with a fracture of the distal phalanx of the great toe.

FIRST METATARSOPHALANGEAL JOINT COMPLEX INJURIES

The first (hallux) metatarsophalangeal (MTP) joint is significantly larger than the lesser MTP joints. Several strong muscles (the abductor hallucis, the extensor hallucis brevis, the adductor hallucis, and the two flexor hallucis brevis tendons) attach to the base of the first proximal phalanx, and a robust plantar plate provides plantar stabilization of the joint. The plantar plate attaches to the base of the proximal phalanx and the metatarsal neck and is reinforced by a lateral transverse metatarsal ligament. The two slips of the flexor hallucis brevis tendon contain the sesamoid bones, which help support weight beneath the first metatarsal head during gait.

Injury to the first MTP joint usually is the result of severe dorsiflexion with an axial-loading component and can range from a mild sprain to a turf toe injury (a severe sprain) or overt dislocation. Normal motion in the hallux MTP joint is from 90° of dorsiflexion to 45° of plantar flexion. The first MTP joint is subject to compression injuries, fractures, sprains, and hyperextension injuries (turf toe injuries). Cartilage damage is common in the first MTP joint and can lead to hallux rigidus and ultimately to osteoarthritis. Traumatic hallux valgus has

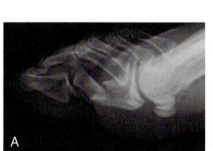
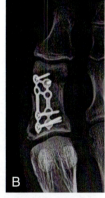
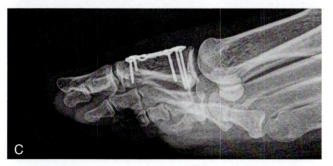

FIGURE 16 **A**, Lateral radiograph of a displaced fracture of the proximal phalanx of the great toe with clawing. **B** and **C**, Subsequent AP and lateral radiographs, respectively, after open reduction and internal fixation.

Section 6: Foot and Ankle Trauma

also been reported. Even seemingly minor injuries can lead to substantial disability.[64] Patients typically report significant plantar pain, swelling, and stiffness in the toe. Routine standing AP, lateral, and oblique foot radiographs are necessary to detect injury to bones, joints, and sesamoid positioning.

Turf Toe Injuries

Turf toe injuries are relatively common in field athletes such as football, soccer, and lacrosse players. The typical mechanism of injury is hyperdorsiflexion with axial loading with the foot fixed in equinus. The plantar structures are avulsed from the plantar metatarsal neck or base of the proximal phalanx as the hallux is dorsally translated. Further stress causes capsule disruption and a plantar plate tear. Although most patients recover with appropriate symptomatic care, some injuries are sufficiently debilitating to keep an athlete out of play for a season and may require surgical repair. It has not yet been proved whether an aggressive open repair has results superior to those of nonsurgical management, particularly because the postoperative rehabilitation can be quite prolonged.[64]

There are several classification systems. It has been proposed that a stretch of the capsuloligamentous complex with mild swelling and plantarmedial tenderness is classified as a grade I injury; partial soft-tissue disruption with moderate swelling and diffuse tenderness is a grade II injury; and severe ligament injury with dorsal impaction of the first MTP articular surface, severe swelling, tenderness, and stiffness about the first MTP joint is a grade III injury.[65] Cartilage injury and bony impaction portend a relatively poor prognosis (**Table 1**).

Contralateral comparison radiographs and stress dorsiflexion radiographs can be helpful for classifying the injury and for detecting any retraction or injury of the sesamoids. A measurement of more than 10.4 mm from base of the proximal phalanx to the distal tibial sesamoid and more than 13.3 mm for the fibular sesamoid is 99.7% sensitive for a plantar plate rupture. Unfortunately, bipartite sesamoids can confound a diagnosis.[64] MRI can be helpful for determining the extent of capsuloligamentous disruption. Sprains and small capsular avulsions can be managed using hard-soled shoes or a carbon fiber orthotic device to limit dorsiflexion until symptoms are resolved. The recovery period typically is 2 to 4 weeks. A grade I or II injury is managed with a short CAM walker boot or postoperative shoe, with 3 to 4 weeks of physical therapy to improve range of motion and reduce swelling, followed by a return to sports using a protective steel or carbon fiber insole (a turf toe plate), as symptoms allow. Taping of the hallux in plantar flexion can be useful. A custom-made total-contact insole also can prevent further injury. A grade III injury may require significantly longer time for recovery than a grade I or II injury. Surgical treatment is indicated if there is a large or incarcerated intra-articular fragment, joint incongruity, complete disruption of the plantar structures, gross instability, or retraction of the sesamoids. These injuries have been associated with late arthrosis and stiffness.

Surgical treatment of a turf toe injury generally entails open repair of the plantar plate to restore congruity to the hallux MTP joint complex. A medial approach is used if the tibial sesamoid is affected and a plantar approach is used for the fibular sesamoid. It is vital to identify and protect the sensory nerves. An injury through the sesamoid bones (a displaced fracture) should be repaired at the time of surgical treatment. Flexor hallucis brevis tendon avulsion from the proximal phalanx can be repaired to the proximal phalanx with suture anchors. The abductor hallucis tendon can be used to augment the plantar plate repair if there is significant loss of healthy collagen. Regardless of repair technique, this is a severe

Table 1

Summary of Turf Toe Grading and Treatment

Grade	Pathology	Clinical	Treatment	Return to Play
I	Stretching of plantar capsule ligament complex	Mild swelling and plantar-medial tenderness	Symptomatic	As tolerated
II	Partial soft-tissue disruption	Moderate swelling and diffuse tenderness	CAM boot ± crutches	2 wk, taping may be needed
III	Severe ligament injury with dorsal impaction of the first MTP articular surface	Severe swelling, tenderness, and stiffness about the first MTP joint; positive vertical Lachman test	Surgical repair or long-term immobilization	6-10 wk, depending on sport/position; taping needed on return to play

CAM = controlled ankle movement, MTP = metatarsophalangeal

Data from Anderson RB, Shawen SB: Great-toe disorders, in Porter DA, Schon LC, eds: *Baxter's the Foot and Ankle in Sport*, ed 2. Elsevier Health Sciences, 2007, pp 411-433.

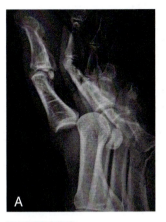 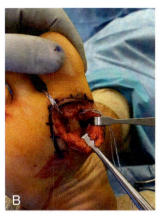

FIGURE 17 **A**, Lateral radiograph of complete first metatarsophalangeal dislocation and turf toe injury in a 20-year-old patient who plays college lacrosse. **B**, Surgical photograph of the complete plantar soft-tissue disruption. Repair was performed with suture anchors proximally in the sesamoids on either side of the flexor hallucis longus tendon.

injury, and time to return to play in competitive athletes requiring a turf toe repair is lengthy and averages 14 weeks postoperatively.[66]

First MTP Joint Dislocations

First MTP joint dislocation is rare and most often occurs in a dorsal direction as a result of a high-energy hyperextension mechanism. Plain radiographs usually are sufficient for diagnosing a first MTP joint dislocation and associated injuries. The plantar plate typically is disrupted at its proximal attachment beneath the metatarsal and then retracts distally. Reduction can be blocked by the intact collateral ligaments and the abductor and adductor tendons. Prompt closed reduction can be attempted with digital block anesthesia: the interphalangeal joint is extended, longitudinal traction is applied, and plantar translation reduces the joint. However, the injury often requires open reduction.

Open reduction usually is successful and can be followed by restricted dorsiflexion in a stiff-soled shoe or a short CAM walker boot for 3 to 4 weeks, with early range-of-motion exercises. Open reduction is required if the joint is unstable or incongruent as a result of bony or soft-tissue interposition after attempted reduction. K-wire fixation should be added. The wire(s) can be removed at 3 to 4 weeks, and range-of-motion exercises can be initiated. Postreduction radiographs and a range-of-motion examination should be done to confirm stability, congruity, and clearance of soft-tissue interposition. Repair of acute ruptured plantar structures can be performed concomitantly with open reduction if performed through a plantar approach (**Figure 17**).

SESAMOID INJURIES

The sesamoids are an important part of the great toe flexor mechanism and have a function similar to that of the patella in the quadriceps mechanism of the knee. The sesamoids support the first metatarsal head and the first MTP joint from pressure during weight bearing and provide a lever arm to the flexor hallucis brevis tendons to plantarflex the proximal phalanx. Each sesamoid is approximately 7 to 10 mm long and slightly oblong. The dorsal surfaces of the sesamoids articulate with the plantar aspect of the first metatarsal head. The strong intersesamoid ligament connects the two sesamoids and extends to the deep transverse intermetatarsal ligament. The flexor hallucis longus tendon runs between the two sesamoid bones, ultimately attaching to the distal phalanx. Typically, the medial (tibial) sesamoid is more centrally located beneath the first metatarsal head than the lateral (fibular) sesamoid, and it probably bears more weight, making it more prone to injury such as sesamoiditis or stress fracture.

Sesamoid injury can cause tremendous pain and disability. Dancers and runners are particularly susceptible to stress fracture in the sesamoids from repeated impact and tension. Dancers and runners who train and perform in thin-soled shoes are vulnerable to these injuries because they land on a hard surface with the toes dorsiflexed. Patients who have pes cavus, equinus, or hindfoot varus are particularly susceptible to overuse injury.

Sesamoid injuries are evaluated with a routine set of AP, lateral, and axial sesamoid radiographs of the foot, which allow assessment of the congruity of each metatarsal-sesamoid articulation, the status of the cartilage surfaces, and any fracture displacement. The patient typically has mild swelling, stiffness of the MTP joint, and point tenderness over the involved sesamoid. Passive or active hyperextension exacerbates the pain by stretching the entire sesamoid apparatus. Resisted plantar flexion also can be painful. It is important to evaluate the patient for signs of a subtle cavus foot deformity.

Sesamoiditis is characterized by pain, tenderness, inflammation, and possible cartilage injury at the metatarsal head–sesamoid articulation. This syndrome typically is caused by repetitive stress on the sesamoids and MTP joint apparatus. Sesamoiditis is aggravated by improper tracking of the sesamoids under the metatarsal head or by progressive metatarsus varus. A plantarflexed first ray and overactivity of the peroneus longus tendon (peroneal overdrive) can overload the sesamoids and produce pain similar to that of sesamoiditis. Such underlying conditions must be identified and treated.

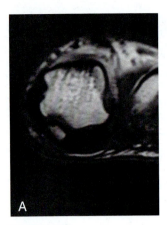 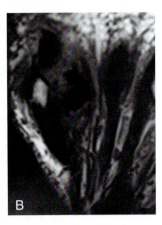

FIGURE 18 Axial (**A**) and coronal (**B**) T1-weighted images of suspected fibular sesamoid osteonecrosis with fragmentation.

SESAMOID OSTEONECROSIS

Patients with sesamoid osteonecrosis are more often women in the second decade of life with pain during toe-off during gait. As with sesamoid stress fractures, the medial sesamoid is more commonly involved. Radiographs can reveal increased sclerosis of the bone and fragmentation, although MRI is more sensitive. Typical patterns of early osteonecrosis include low intensity on T1-weighted images and hyperintensity on T2 images (**Figure 18**). As the osteonecrosis progresses and the sclerosis of the bone occurs, the T2 images will become hypointense.

Sesamoid Fractures

Fracture of a sesamoid can result from tension force on the sesamoid apparatus or from a direct acute or repetitive impact force on the sesamoid itself. Most sesamoid fractures have a simple transverse pattern with minimal displacement and sharp fracture edges. Most often, the medial sesamoid is affected. An acute fracture should be differentiated from a symptomatic bipartite sesamoid although sometimes the treatment is not very different. Unlike a fractured sesamoid, bipartite sesamoids on plain radiographs have smooth edges, are larger in size, and are lacking in callus, and the radiolucent line is oblique, rather than transverse, in fractures. Thirty-four percent of patients have bilateral bipartite sesamoids.

Treatment of Sesamoid Injuries

Acute or suspected stress fracture of a sesamoid is usually managed by immobilizing the hallux in a spica cast for 3 to 6 weeks, ideally with the toe in plantar flexion. Alternatively, a removable great toe spica splint may be fashioned for comfort and ease of use. The patient should avoid weight bearing for at least the first 3 weeks. The cast should be followed by protection in a short CAM walker boot and initiation of range-of-motion exercises. If a sesamoid fracture does not heal with casting and/or if pain persists beyond 6 months, sesamoidectomy is indicated and has historically led to satisfactory outcomes. Sesamoiditis and osteonecrosis usually are successfully treated in a similar fashion. Subsequent use of an orthotic device that offloads the affected sesamoid with a metatarsal pad and a recess for the sesamoid can help prevent reinjury (dancer's pad). With osteonecrosis, a carbon fiber foot plate added to the patient's shoe will help with symptoms but does little for the underlying pathology. There is scant literature regarding ORIF and bone grafting of a sesamoid nonunion. Bone grafting and fixation of a sesamoid fracture is as likely to lead to union as splinting alone. A standard approach is used, a small hole is drilled into the center of the fracture site with a burr, and the fracture site is filled with cancellous autograft. Interfragmentary compression can be obtained with a 1.5-mm screw if the fragments are sufficiently large. This procedure is technically challenging, and the opportunity to gain experience in this technique is limited. Postoperatively, the great toe and ankle are splinted in a plantarflexed position. Protected weight bearing can begin after 6 weeks.

A sesamoidectomy is used only if the patient has severe and painful osteonecrosis or a nonhealing or comminuted fracture. Sesamoidectomy requires a meticulous approach because the surgeon has to carefully remove the bone from its capsule without disrupting the tendon. Although data are limited, it is for this reason that some surgeons have used burrs to remove bone only and maintain the soft-tissue sling, which provides toe stability. If the fracture is small and at one of the poles, partial excision of the smaller sesamoid fragment can be done. For a lateral (fibular) sesamoid excision, a plantar approach between the first and second metatarsal heads is recommended to minimize painful scar formation. Care must be taken to avoid and protect the digital nerve, which traverses the MTP joint immediately adjacent to the sesamoid, because injury to this nerve can be quite debilitating. In cases of moderate to severe hallux valgus with fibular sesamoiditis, a dorsal approach can be used as the sesamoid has typically subluxated into the intermetatarsal space, lateral to the metatarsal head. A direct medial approach is used for a medial (tibial) sesamoid excision, again avoiding the dorsal and plantar digital sensory nerve branches. The incision is typically at the normal glabrous skin interface. After the bone is removed, the tendon is repaired or imbricated with the capsule before wound closure. The toe is splinted in a protected position for 4 to 6 weeks and once wounds have healed, weight bearing as tolerated is permitted in a protective shoe or boot. For tibial sesamoid excisions, a toe spacer is used to prevent residual valgus and to take tension off the medial repair. For fibular sesamoid excisions, preventing the toe from a varus moment is facilitated by a snugly-fitting sock or ACE bandage for 6 weeks.

Disability may result after sesamoidectomy, and although a rare occurrence, pain-free function is not always restored. Excision of the lateral sesamoid can cause medial drift and a cock-up deformity (hallux varus). Removal of the medial sesamoid can create hallux valgus. Careful repair of the flexor hallucis brevis tendon can help prevent these complications. Although rare, a transfer lesion may develop if the remaining sesamoid becomes painful from the extra weight it must support, despite an intact flexor mechanism. In a study of 26 tibial or fibular sesamoidectomies (mean follow-up of 86 months), there was a 19% complication rate, with one hallux varus case, two hallux valgus cases, and two cases of postoperative scarring with neuroma-type symptoms.[67] Often, there is a slight radiographic increase of hallux varus or valgus, but this is rarely clinically symptomatic. Sesamoid excision in the athletic population is found to have a predictable return to desired play with low complication rates.[68] Despite not having a clear biomechanical explanation, pain in the remaining sesamoid following sesamoidectomy for fracture or for osteonecrosis is not frequently encountered and high patient satisfaction rates can be expected with this procedure.[68-70]

SUMMARY

There are myriad injuries that can be seen in the midfoot and forefoot. They range from subtle sprains and stress fractures, to high-energy fracture-dislocations and compartment syndrome. Because of the great range in presentation and severity, the evaluating surgeon must have a high index of suspicion for these injuries to minimize the morbidity of missed pathology. A careful history and physical examination with appropriate radiographic studies can lead to an accurate and complete diagnosis. With an understanding of their mechanisms and natural history, patients with these injuries can be successfully treated, and function usually can be restored. Only after the injury is recognized can the optimal treatment strategy be selected based on the best available data and clinical science.

KEY STUDY POINTS

- The navicular is particularly susceptible to stress fracture, given its relatively avascular zone centrally. Suspicion should be high as the clinical and radiographic presentation can be subtle. MRI is the diagnostic study of choice.
- Controversy exists with regard to the appropriate surgical treatment method for a Lisfranc injury, with some recent studies demonstrating a trend toward slightly improved outcomes in patients treated with a primary arthrodesis. However, further studies are needed before definitive recommendations can be made.

- Patients with turf toe injuries and sesamoid pathology should be treated with a long nonsurgical course because results with surgical intervention are mixed.
- In the forefoot, displaced fractures, multiple metatarsal fractures, irreducible dislocations, and Jones fractures may require surgical management.
- Although rare, patients with compartment syndrome of the foot can experience debilitating long-term consequences if the condition is not diagnosed and treated in a timely manner. It is most common following a crush injury.

ANNOTATED REFERENCES

1. Jackson JB, Ellington JK, Anderson RB: Fractures of the midfoot and forefoot, in Coughlin MJ, Saltzman CL, Anderson RB, eds: *Mann's Surgery of the Foot and Ankle*, ed 9. Mosby-Elsevier, 2014, pp 2154-2186.

2. McKeon KE, McCormick JJ, Johnson JE, Klein SE: Intraosseous and extraosseous arterial anatomy of the adult navicular. *Foot Ankle Int* 2012;33(10):857-861.

3. Mann JA, Pedowitz DI: Evaluation and treatment of navicular stress fractures, including nonunions, revision surgery, and persistent pain after treatment. *Foot Ankle Clin* 2009;14(2):187-204.

4. Torg JS, Moyer J, Gaughan JP, Boden BP: Management of tarsal navicular stress fractures: Conservative versus surgical treatment. A meta-analysis. *Am J Sports Med* 2010;38(5):1048-1053.

5. Weber M, Locher S: Reconstruction of the cuboid in compression fractures: Short to midterm results in 12 patients. *Foot Ankle Int* 2002;23(11):1008-1013.

6. Kaar S, Femino J, Morag Y: Lisfranc joint displacement following sequential ligament sectioning. *J Bone Joint Surg Am* 2007;89(10):2225-2232.

7. Raikin SM, Elias I, Dheer S, Besser MP, Morrison WB, Zoga AC: Prediction of midfoot instability in the subtle Lisfranc injury: Comparison of magnetic resonance imaging with intraoperative findings. *J Bone Joint Surg Am* 2009;91(4):892-899.

8. Quenu E, Kuss G: Etude sur les luxations du metatarse (luxations metatarsotarsiennes) du diastasis entre le 1er et le 2e metatarsien. *Rev Chir* 1909;39:281-336, 720-791, 1093-1134.

9. Hardcastle PH, Reschauer R, Kutscha-Lissberg E, Schoffmann W: Injuries to the tarsometatarsal joint. Incidence, classification and treatment. *J Bone Joint Surg Br* 1982;64(3):349-356.

10. Myerson MS, Fisher RT, Burgess AR, Kenzora JE: Fracture dislocations of the tarsometatarsal joints: End results correlated with pathology and treatment. *Foot Ankle* 1986;6(5):225-242.

11. Lau SC, Guest C, Hall M, Tacey M, Joseph S, Oppy A: Do columns or sagittal displacement matter in the assessment and management of lisfranc fracture dislocation? An alternate approach to classification of the lisfranc injury. *Injury* 2017;48(7):1689-1695.

12. Porter DA, Barnes AF, Rund A, Walrod MT: Injury pattern in ligamentous lisfranc injuries in competitive athletes. *Foot Ankle Int* 2019;40(2):185-194.

    This retrospective study looked at the prevalence of proximal extension to the medial intercuneiform joint in purely ligamentous Lisfranc injuries in competitive athletes. The authors found a 50% rate of proximal extension into the medial intercuneiform joint, suggesting it may be more prevalent than previously thought. Level of evidence: IV.

13. Nunley JA, Vertullo CJ: Classification, investigation, and management of midfoot sprains: Lisfranc injuries in the athlete. *Am J Sports Med* 2002;30(6):871-878.

14. Garriguez-Perez D, Puerto-Vazquez M, Tomé Delgado JL, Galeote E, Marco F: Impact of the subtle Lisfranc injury on foot structure and function. *Foot Ankle Int* 2021;42(10):1303-1310.

    This retrospective study looked at ligamentous Lisfranc injuries and found loss of arch height in 42.9% of patients, chronic pain in 71.4% of patients, and a 16.6% rate of conversion to arthrodesis, demonstrating the long-term implications that even subtle Lisfranc injuries can cause. Level of evidence: IV.

15. Arntz CT, Veith RG, Hansen ST Jr: Fractures and fracture-dislocations of the tarsometatarsal joint. *J Bone Joint Surg Am* 1988;70(2):173-181.

16. Wiss DA, Kull DM, Perry J: Lisfranc fracture-dislocations of the foot: A clinical-kinesiological study. *J Orthop Trauma* 1987;1(4):267-274.

17. Alberta FG, Aronow MS, Barrero M, Diaz-Doran V, Sullivan RJ, Adams DJ: Ligamentous lisfranc joint injuries: A biomechanical comparison of dorsal plate and transarticular screw fixation. *Foot Ankle Int* 2005;26(6):462-473.

18. Ho NC, Sangiorgio SN, Cassinelli S, et al: Biomechanical comparison of fixation stability using a Lisfranc plate versus transarticular screws. *Foot Ankle Surg* 2019;25(1):71-78.

    This is a biomechanical study that compared a dorsal Lisfranc plate with transarticular screws across the Lisfranc joint as well as first and second TMT joint articulations. No significant differences were seen between the two constructs. Level of evidence: IV.

19. Bansal A, Carlson DA, Owen JR, et al: Ligamentous lisfranc injury: A biomechanical comparison of dorsal plate fixation and transarticular screws. *J Orthop Trauma* 2019;33(7):e270-e275.

    This is a biomechanical study comparing use of a dorsal plate to transarticular screws for Lisfranc joint injuries. The authors simulated partial weight bearing only, at a cyclic load of 343 N. Increased plantar diastasis approaching statistical significance was seen in specimens treated with dorsal plating compared with transarticular screws. Level of evidence: IV.

20. Lau S, Guest C, Hall M, Tacey M, Joseph S, Oppy A: Functional outcomes post Lisfranc injury – Transarticular screws, dorsal bridge plating or combination treatment? *J Orthop Trauma* 2017;31(8):447-452.

21. Kirzner N, Zotov P, Goldbloom D, Curry H, Bedi H: Dorsal bridge plating or transarticular screws for lisfranc fracture dislocations: A retrospective study comparing functional and radiological outcomes. *Bone Joint J* 2018;100-B(4):468-474.

22. Philpott A, Epstein DJ, Lau SC, Mnatzaganian G, Pang J: Lisfranc fixation techniques and postoperative functional outcomes: A systematic review. *J Foot Ankle Surg* 2021;60(1):102-108.

    This is a systematic review of all studies reporting functional outcomes in patients who underwent ORIF of acute Lisfranc joint injuries. Numerous fixation methods were included, including bridge plating and transarticular screws, as well as one study reporting on outcomes following suture button fixation. Better outcomes were seen in the suture button group, but this represented only one study. Although a small number of studies showed superior outcomes with plating, overall no significant differences were seen between those fixed with screws versus plates. Level of evidence: III.

23. Yongfei F, Chaoyu L, Wenqiang X, Xiulin M, Jian X, Wei W: Clinical outcomes of Tightrope system in the treatment of purely ligamentous Lisfranc injuries. *BMC Surg* 2021;21(1):395.

    This study reported on the outcomes of 11 patients treated with a suture button device for a Lisfranc joint injury over a 3-year period with average follow-up of 20 months. Good outcomes were shown, without any cases of loss of reduction or need for hardware removal. Level of evidence: IV.

24. Cottom JM, Graney CT, Sisovsky C: Treatment of lisfranc injuries using interosseous suture button: A retrospective review of 84 cases with a minimum 3-year follow-up. *J Foot Ankle Surg* 2020;59(6):1139-1143.

    This study looked at 84 patients treated over a 3-year period with a suture button device for a purely ligamentous Lisfranc joint injury. The authors did augment the suture button across the Lisfranc articulation with a screw across the medial intercuneiform joint. Satisfactory outcomes were shown without any need for conversion to arthrodesis or removal of hardware at minimum of 3-year follow-up. Level of evidence: IV.

25. Cho J, Kim J, Min TH, et al: Suture button vs conventional screw fixation for isolated Lisfranc ligament injuries. *Foot Ankle Int* 2021;42(5):598-608.

    This study was a nonrandomized, retrospective comparison of patients who underwent suture button versus transarticular screw fixation for a ligamentous Lisfranc injury. At 6 months, better American Orthopaedic Foot and Ankle Society and visual analog scale pain scores were observed in the suture button group. However, at 12 months, there were no differences in outcome scores or radiographic outcomes. Level of evidence: III.

26. Koroneos Z, Vannatta E, Kim M, et al: Biomechanical comparison of Fibertape device repair techniques of ligamentous Lisfranc injury in a cadaveric model. *Injury* 2021;52(4):692-698.

    This was a biomechanical cadaver study examining two different constructs using a nonabsorbable suture device (Arthrex InternalBrace). The first construct used the InternalBrace across the Lisfranc articulation, whereas the second construct used a supplementary limb of suture across the medial intercuneiform articulation. The supplementary limb across the intercuneiform joint showed mechanical benefits at higher loads. Level of evidence: IV.

27. Ly TV, Coetzee JC: Treatment of primarily ligamentous Lisfranc joint injuries: Primary arthrodesis compared with open reduction and internal fixation. A prospective, randomized study. *J Bone Joint Surg Am* 2006;88(3): 514-520.

28. Henning JA, Jones CB, Sietsema DL, Bohay DR, Anderson JG: Open reduction internal fixation versus primary arthrodesis for lisfranc injuries: A prospective randomized study. *Foot Ankle Int* 2009;30(10):913-922.

29. Cochran G, Renninger C, Tompane T, Bellamy J, Kuhn K: Primary arthrodesis versus open reduction and internal fixation for low-energy lisfranc injuries in a young athletic population. *Foot Ankle Int* 2017;38(9):957-963.

30. Qiao YS, Li JK, Shen H, et al: Comparison of arthrodesis and non-fusion to treat Lisfranc injuries. *Orthop Surg* 2017;9(1):62-68.

31. Smith N, Stone C, Furey A: Does open reduction and internal fixation versus primary arthrodesis improve patient outcomes for lisfranc trauma? A systematic review and meta-analysis. *Clin Orthop Relat Res* 2016;474(6):1445-1452.

32. Hawkinson MP, Tennent DJ, Belisle J, Osborn P: Outcomes of Lisfranc injuries in an active duty military population. *Foot Ankle Int* 2017;38(10):1115-1119.

33. Buda M, Kink S, Stavenuiter R, et al: Reoperation rate differences between open reduction internal fixation and primary arthrodesis of Lisfranc injuries. *Foot Ankle Int* 2018;39(9):1089-1096.

34. Barnds B, Tucker W, Morris B, et al: Cost comparison and complication rate of Lisfranc injuries treated with open reduction internal fixation versus primary arthrodesis. *Injury* 2018;49(12):2318-2321.

35. Myerson MS: Management of compartment syndromes of the foot. *Clin Orthop Relat Res* 1991;271:239-248.

36. Manoli A II, Weber TG: Fasciotomy of the foot: An anatomical study with special reference to release of the calcaneal compartment. *Foot Ankle* 1990;10(5):267-275.

37. Guyton GP, Shearman CM, Saltzman CL: The compartments of the foot revisited: Rethinking the validity of cadaver infusion experiments. *J Bone Joint Surg Br* 2001;83(2):245-249.

38. Han F, Daruwalla ZJ, Shen L, Kumar VP: A prospective study of surgical outcomes and quality of life in severe foot trauma and associated compartment syndrome after fasciotomy. *J Foot Ankle Surg* 2015;54(3):417-423.

39. Bedigrew KM, Stinner DJ, Kragh JF Jr, Potter BK, Shawen SB, Hsu JR: Effectiveness of foot fasciotomies in foot and ankle trauma. *J R Army Med Corps* 2017;163(5):324-328.

40. West TA, Pollard JD, Chandra M, et al: The epidemiology of metatarsal fractures among older females with bisphosphonate exposure. *J Foot Ankle Surg* 2020;59(2):269-273.

This study examined the epidemiology of metatarsal fractures among females on diphosphonates. Although the authors found an increased relative rate if metatarsal fractures with diphosphonate use, this did not correlate with duration of diphosphonate use. Level of evidence: III.

41. Herterich V, Hofmann L, Böcker W, Polzer H, Baumbach SF: Acute, isolated fractures of the metatarsal bones: An epidemiologic study. *Arch Orthop Trauma Surg* 2022; March 2 [Epub ahead of print].

This study looked at the epidemiology of isolated metatarsal fractures in an adult population. Most of these fractures (81.3%) involved the fifth metatarsal and frequency diminished with increasing age. Increased age and female sex were associated with increased risk for multiple metatarsal fractures. Level of evidence: III.

42. Cavanagh PR, Rodgers MM, Iiboshi A: Pressure distribution under symptom-free feet during barefoot standing. *Foot Ankle* 1987;7(5):262-276.

43. Digiovanni CW, Benirschke SK, Hansen ST: Foot injuries, in Browner BD, Jupiter JB, Levine AM, Trafton PG, eds: *Skeletal Trauma: Basic Science, Management, and Reconstruction*, ed 3. WB Saunders, 2003, pp 2375-2492.

44. Sisk TD: Fractures, in Edmonson AS, Crenshaw AH, eds: *Campbell's Operative Orthopaedics*, ed 6. Mosby, 1980.

45. Egrise F, Bernard E, Galliot F, Pidhorz L, Mainard D: Treatment of two or more metatarsal fractures. *Orthop Traumatol Surg Res* 2022; April 22 [Epub ahead of print].

This study compared the outcomes of multiple metatarsal fractures fixed with either K-wires or plate/screw fixation. Better functional outcomes were found in patients treated with plates/screws as opposed to K-wires. Level of evidence : IV.

46. Dameron TB Jr: Fractures and anatomical variations of the proximal portion of the fifth metatarsal. *J Bone Joint Surg Am* 1975;57(6):788-792.

47. Jones R: I: Fracture of the base of the fifth metatarsal bone by indirect violence. *Ann Surg* 1902;35(6):697-700.2.

48. Hunt KJ, Anderson RB: Treatment of Jones fracture nonunions and refractures in the elite athlete: Outcomes of intramedullary screw fixation with bone grafting. *Am J Sports Med* 2011;39(9):1948-1954.

49. Polzer H, Polzer S, Mutschler W, Prall WC: Acute fractures to the proximal fifth metatarsal bone: Development of classification and treatment recommendations based on the current evidence. *Injury* 2012;43(10):1626-1632.

50. Cosman F, Ruffing J, Zion M, et al: Determinants of stress fracture risk in United States Military Academy cadets. *Bone* 2013;55(2):359-366.

51. Goodloe JB, Cregar WM, Caughman A, Bailey EP, Barfield WR, Gross CE: Surgical management of proximal fifth metatarsal fractures in elite athletes: A systematic review. *Orthop J Sports Med* 2021;9(9):23259671211037647.

This was a systematic review of studies evaluating outcomes of surgical treatment of fifth metatarsal fractures in elite-level athletes. Evaluation of 12 studies showed high union and return-to-play rates, regardless of surgical construct. Recommendations for optimal surgical management of fifth metatarsal fractures could not be made. Level of evidence: IV.

52. Jones BH, Thacker SB, Gilchrist J, Kimsey CD Jr, Sosin DM: Prevention of lower extremity stress fractures in

athletes and soldiers: A systematic review. *Epidemiol Rev* 2002;24(2):228-247.

53. Shindle MK, Endo Y, Warren RF, et al: Stress fractures about the tibia, foot, and ankle. *J Am Acad Orthop Surg* 2012;20(3):167-176.

54. Gaeta M, Minutoli F, Scribano E, et al: CT and MR imaging findings in athletes with early tibial stress injuries: Comparison with bone scintigraphy findings and emphasis on cortical abnormalities. *Radiology* 2005;235(2):553-561.

55. Boden BP, Osbahr DC: High-risk stress fractures: Evaluation and treatment. *J Am Acad Orthop Surg* 2000;8(6):344-353.

56. Syrop I, Fukushima Y, Mullins K, et al: Comparison of ultrasonography to MRI in the diagnosis of lower extremity bone stress injuries: A prospective cohort study. *J Ultrasound Med* 2022;41(11):2885-2896.

    This study evaluated the sensitivity and specificity of ultrasonography in diagnosing stress fractures in the lower extremity. The authors found it comparable to but less sensitive and specific than MRI. Level of evidence: IV.

57. Alvarez RG, Cincere B, Channappa C, et al: Extracorporeal shock wave treatment of non- or delayed union of proximal metatarsal fractures. *Foot Ankle Int* 2011;32(8):746-754.

58. Raghavan P, Christofides E: Role of teriparatide in accelerating metatarsal stress fracture healing: A case series and review of literature. *Clin Med Insights Endocrinol Diabetes* 2012;5:39-45.

59. Carreira DS, Sandilands SM: Radiographic factors and effect of fifth metatarsal Jones and diaphyseal stress fractures on participation in the NFL. *Foot Ankle Int* 2013;34(4):518-522.

60. Rongstad KM, Tueting J, Rongstad M, Garrels K, Meis R: Fourth metatarsal base stress fractures in athletes: A case series. *Foot Ankle Int* 2013;34(7):962-968.

61. Court-Brown CM, Caesar B: Epidemiology of adult fractures: A review. *Injury* 2006;37(8):691-697.

62. Van Vliet-Koppert ST, Cakir H, Van Lieshout EM, De Vries MR, Van Der Elst M, Schepers T: Demographics and functional outcome of toe fractures. *J Foot Ankle Surg* 2011;50(3):307-310.

63. Mittlmeier T, Haar P: Sesamoid and toe fractures. *Injury* 2004;35(suppl 2):SB87-SB97.

64. Frimenko RE, Lievers W, Coughlin MJ, Anderson RB, Crandall JR, Kent RW: Etiology and biomechanics of first metatarsophalangeal joint sprains (turf toe) in athletes. *Crit Rev Biomed Eng* 2012;40(1):43-61.

65. McCormick JJ, Anderson RB: Turf toe: Anatomy, diagnosis, and treatment. *Sports Health* 2010;2(6):487-494.

66. Vopat ML, Hassan M, Poppe T, et al: Return to sport 0after turf toe injuries: A systematic review and meta-analysis. *Orthop J Sports Med* 2019;7(10):2325967119875133.

    A systematic review of 12 studies determined return to play following turf toe injury based on treatment modality as well as compared nonsurgical and surgical treatment outcomes. Return to play is most significantly related to severity of injury and level of competition. Professional athletes return to play sooner than collegiate and high school athletes. No recommendations could be made on ideal treatment and return-to-play protocols. Level of evidence: IV.

67. Crain JM, Phancao JP, Stidham K: MR imaging of turf toe. *Magn Reson Imaging Clin N Am* 2008;16(1):93-103, vi.

68. Saxena A, Krisdakumtorn T: Return to activity after sesamoidectomy in athletically active individuals. *Foot Ankle Int* 2003;24(5):415-419.

69. Saxena A, Fournier M, Patel P, Maffulli N: Sesamoidectomy in athletes: Outcomes from 2-centers. *J Foot Ankle Surg* 2022;61(1):139-142.

    This study evaluated outcomes of sesamoidectomy in an athletic population. Sesamoidectomy was found to be safe and predictably allowed for return to sport in patients in whom nonsurgical management for sesamoid pathology failed. Level of evidence: IV.

70. Kane JM, Brodsky JW, Daoud Y: Radiographic results and return to activity after sesamoidectomy for fracture. *Foot Ankle Int* 2017;38(10):1100-1106.

CHAPTER 22

Amputations of the Foot and Ankle

MICHAEL S. PINZUR, MD, FAAOS

ABSTRACT

Amputations of the foot and ankle are performed for infection, ischemic gangrene, trauma, neoplastic disease, and congenital deformity. Antecedent diabetes and peripheral vascular disease are responsible for most lower extremity amputations. High-energy trauma, both civilian and military, contributes to approximately 10% of lower extremity amputations, and congenital deformity and neoplastic disease comprise a very small proportion of foot and ankle amputations. The goal of amputation surgery is to remove all nonviable or nonfunctional tissue, followed by functionally oriented reconstruction that will optimize the ambulatory potential of the individual patient. The most favorable clinical outcomes are achieved when care is multidisciplinary.

Keywords: amputation; foot infections; peripheral vascular disease

INTRODUCTION

Much as the AO principles of orthopaedics teach surgeons to appreciate the personality of a fracture, the mechanism and magnitude of injury and/or the associated medical comorbidities responsible for a clinical

---

Dr. Pinzur or an immediate family member is a member of a speakers' bureau or has made paid presentations on behalf of Orthofix, Inc. and Stryker.

scenario of limb salvage versus amputation also need to be appreciated. When the decision is made to proceed with partial, or whole foot, amputation, both the functional effect and prosthetic implications associated with the projected level of amputation need to be considered, along with recent advances in endovascular and reconstructive plastic surgery. Whatever the etiology, the goals of modern amputation surgery are to remove all nonviable and infected tissue, followed by creation of a functional terminal organ of weight bearing. At least 80% of lower extremity amputations are secondary to antecedent diabetes and peripheral vascular disease. High-energy trauma, both civilian and military, is responsible for most of the foot and ankle amputations in younger individuals. Amputation secondary to infection, congenital deformity, and neoplastic disease are the most common etiologies. The most favorable clinical outcomes are achieved when a multidisciplinary team is involved in the preoperative assessment and perioperative and rehabilitative phases of care.

THE LOWER EXTREMITY AS AN ORGAN OF WEIGHT BEARING

The normal human foot is composed of 28 bones that allow the dual functions of a shock absorber at heel strike and a stable platform to allow propulsion at push-off. The ligaments that connect the bones of the foot are relaxed when the foot is loaded at heel strike. This unlocked position of the joints, combined with the unique durable cushioned plantar skin and subcutaneous fibrous connective tissue, allows the foot to dampen the impact of weight bearing. As the foot transitions from the unlocked load acceptance position of ankle dorsiflexion and foot supination at heel strike to the stability-producing locked

---

This chapter is adapted from McGann MR, Van Dyke B, Simpson GA, Philbin TM: Amputations of the foot and ankle, in Chou LB, ed: *Orthopaedic Knowledge Update®: Foot and Ankle 6*. American Academy of Orthopaedic Surgeons, 2020, pp 277-286.

© 2025 American Academy of Orthopaedic Surgeons

position of ankle plantar flexion and foot pronation at push-off, the foot functions both as an organ of dampening weight acceptance and a stable platform.[1]

Partial foot amputation decreases the efficiency of this process by decreasing the length of the lever arm at push-off. The key function of the flexor hallucis longus and brevis muscles is the provision of medial column stability at push-off. Amputation of the hallux at the proximal metaphysis of the proximal phalanx allows retention of the flexor hallucis brevis insertion, thus retaining reasonable stability of the medial column. Amputation of the first ray through the metatarsal-phalangeal or ray resection levels disengages the flexor hallux longus and brevis and leads to a relatively apropulsive gait. The shortened lever associated with midfoot amputation (transmetatarsal or tarsal-metatarsal) level decreases the efficiency of gait. Very few amputees are willing to use an adaptive ankle-foot orthosis to accommodate for the lever-arm deficiency.[2] The so-called hindfoot amputee (talonavicular, Chopart) not only has no lever arm for stability at push-off, but the development of a late equinus deformity is highly likely because of muscle imbalance. This lever arm is restored with Syme ankle disarticulation amputation because of the necessity of using a prosthetic for walking.[2]

WOUND HEALING PARAMETERS

Diabetes and peripheral vascular disease are responsible for most lower extremity amputations.[3-5] Primarily because of the multiple organ system comorbidities in both the populations who have peripheral vascular disease with diabetes and peripheral vascular disease without diabetes, the 2-year mortality approaches 40%.[3,6,7] The clinical parameters that have been used historically to predict wound healing include tissue turgor, bleeding, and muscle contraction with electrical stimulation. These clinical tools predict amputation wound healing with a 70% reliability. Including healing parameters such as vascular inflow, tissue nutrition, and immunocompetence will increase the odds ratio to a more than 90% probability of predicting successful wound healing. The ultrasound Doppler ankle-brachial index is the most commonly used tool to predict adequate vascular inflow. The accepted minimum threshold for adequate perfusion is an ankle-brachial index (ratio of ultrasound Doppler ankle pressure to brachial blood pressure) of 0.5. Calcification of the dorsalis pedis and posterior tibial arterials makes the ankle-brachial index unmeasurable in approximately 15% of patients with diabetes. The best alternative measure in such patients is the ultrasound Doppler toe pressure taken from the hallux, where the key threshold value is 30 mm Hg.[8-10]

Tissue nutrition is most easily assessed with a threshold serum albumin level of 3.0 g/dL. This level is often depressed in the presence of infection and will often rise once initial débridement and resolution of infection have been achieved. Low serum albumin levels in patients with renal failure often lead to wound failure in partial foot amputations. The initial acceptance of total lymphocyte count as a predictive metric of immunocompetence has not been validated over time.[9,10]

INITIAL WOUND MANAGEMENT

Traumatic amputation is generally associated with some elements of crush injury. Following the principles of damage control orthopaedics, the first step of treatment is excisional débridement of all nonviable tissue. The same decision-making process should be applied when the pathophysiology is infection, gangrene, or a combination of both. Tissue culture at the margins of diseased tissue can be used to direct adjunctive antibiotic therapy. Ensuring viable tissue margins is best achieved by open wound treatment with negative-pressure wound therapy.

Once a viable noninfected base is achieved, reconstruction to create a terminal organ of weight-bearing can be achieved using sound biomechanical principles as well as an understanding of available shoe/orthotic options. The best method of avoiding late equinus deformity following foot and ankle amputation is performing either percutaneous Achilles tendon or gastrocnemius muscle lengthening at the time of amputation. This should be combined with a short leg cast in dysvascular amputations, and either effective splinting or external fixation in traumatic amputations.

FUNCTIONAL AMPUTATION LEVELS

Hallux Amputation

Amputation of the distal phalanx leaves minimal residual disability. The so-called terminal Syme amputation creates a durable residual hallux by removing the nail and involved bone of the distal phalanx through a dorsal approach. Adequate functional stability of the medial column of the foot is achieved by retention of the proximal metaphysis of the proximal phalanx and the insertion of the flexor hallucis brevis. The optimal soft-tissue envelope in hallux amputation is accomplished with a plantar-based flap, although fish-mouth or sagittal flaps have been demonstrated to provide adequate soft-tissue coverage (**Figure 1**). Patients with perceived weakness or instability at the terminal stance phase of gait can use a carbon graphite Morton extension orthosis to substitute for absent flexor hallucis function.[11]

Chapter 22: Amputations of the Foot and Ankle

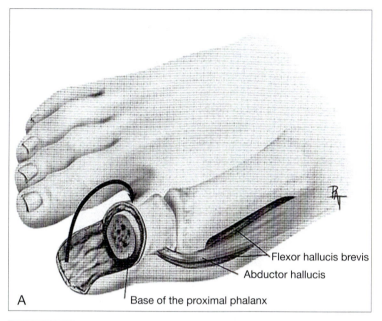
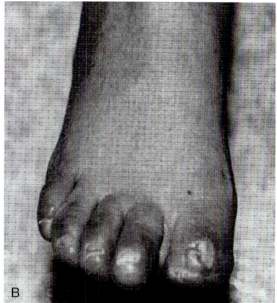

FIGURE 1 **A**, Illustration showing typical long posterior flap for hallux amputation. **B**, Clinical photograph at 1 year. (Reproduced with permission from Kelikian AS: *Operative Treatment of the Foot and Ankle*. Appelton and Lange Publishers, 1999, Figures 30-4, AB, p 613.)

Lesser Toe Amputation

There is little functional loss from lesser toe amputation. The one exception is second toe disarticulation, where the base of the proximal phalanx acts as a spacer, with disarticulation often being complicated by a late severe hallux valgus deformity with prominence of the medial border of the first metatarsal. This can be avoided by retaining the proximal metaphysis of the proximal phalanx (**Figure 2**). A better principle is to retain a parabola of the forefoot to avoid projections difficult to accommodate with footwear (**Figure 3**). Crumpled foot storage bags or neoprene toe fillers can be used to prevent the residual foot from sliding within the shoe.[11]

Ray Resection

Single outer (first or fifth) ray resection is generally used for osteomyelitis of an involved outer metatarsal. It is rarely indicated in dysvascular disease as it is unlikely to have adequate vascular inflow parallel to ischemic tissue. Oblique osteotomy of the first or fifth metatarsal

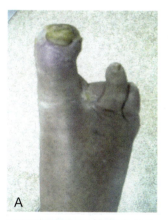
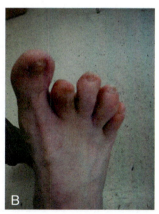
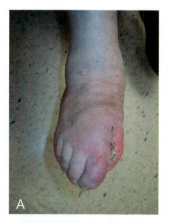
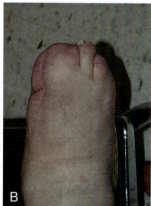

FIGURE 2 Clinical photographs from a patient who underwent second toe amputation for osteomyelitis. **A,** The patient is at increased risk for development of a severe hallux valgus leading to a pressure ulcer when the patient resumes wearing shoes. **B,** Late hallux valgus can be avoided by retaining even half of the proximal phalanx of the second toe.

FIGURE 3 **A**, Clinical photograph from a patient who recently underwent a first ray resection. The second toe became relatively long and a pressure-induced infection developed. **B**, Clinical photograph showing a more reasonable parabola allowing easy shoe fit accomplished following removal of the prominent second toe.

Section 6: Foot and Ankle Trauma

creates a smooth contour for shoe fitting. The potential consequences associated with lateral ray resection are due to the loss of motor influence of the disengaged muscle-tendon units. First ray resection disengages the flexor hallucis longus and brevis tendons, leading to medial column instability and an apropulsive gait pattern. Resection of the entire fifth metatarsal disengages the peroneus brevis and may lead to a late dynamic varus deformity.

The surgical procedure is performed with the so-called tennis racquet incision. Wound management can be accomplished with primary or delayed primary wound closure, open wound management, or loose approximation of wound edges to allow sufficient drainage during the perioperative period (**Figure 4**).

Central ray resections can be accomplished as a primary method of débridement of infection. When used as a definitive treatment, the resultant narrow or poorly contoured residual forefoot may create an unstable platform for terminal stance push-off and/or lead to difficult shoe fitting.[12]

Midfoot Amputation

Midfoot amputation can be performed at the transmetatarsal or tarsal-metatarsal levels. This amputation level creates an excellent contour for shoe fitting, at the cost of a shortened lever arm at push-off. The most durable soft-tissue envelope for midfoot amputation uses a plantar-based flap. This flap will generally require performing the bony transection at the level of the proximal metaphysis of each of the metatarsals. A longer lever arm can be accomplished by using fish-mouth dorsal-plantar flaps and performing the bony transection through the distal metatarsal shafts. The trade-off to achieve this improved lever arm for push-off is the need for less durable fish-mouth dorsal-plantar flaps and the risk of late plantar

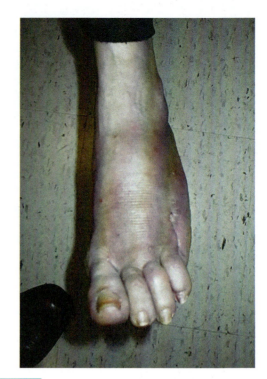

FIGURE 4 Photograph showing how a lateral ray resection leaves minimal deformity if the base of the metatarsal and the attachment of the peroneus brevis are retained.

pressure ulcers developing under the residual metatarsal shafts. Surgeons should almost always include either a percutaneous Achilles tendon lengthening or open gastrocnemius muscle lengthening to avoid the development of a late equinus deformity. Postoperative management should include a short leg cast to avoid heel ulcers secondary to overlengthening of the Achilles tendon with either Achilles tendon lengthening or gastrocnemius muscle lengthening[9,11,13] (**Figure 5**).

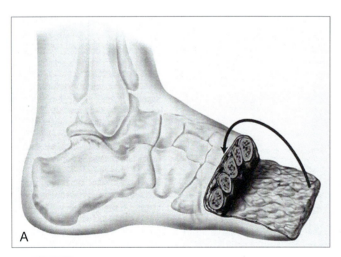
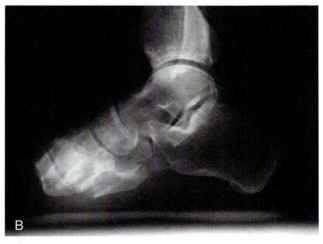

FIGURE 5 **A**, Illustration showing a long plantar flap used in transmetatarsal amputation. **B**, Radiograph showing a platform for weight bearing. (Panel A reproduced with permission from Kelikian AS: *Operative Treatment of the Foot and Ankle*. Appelton and Lange Publishers, 1999, Figure 30-7, p 616.)

A neoprene toe filler enhances comfort in standard oxford, or depth-inlay, shoes. Orthotists argue that a prosthetic combining a toe filler with an ankle-foot orthosis compensates for the shortened lever arm at push-off. Although this is functionally correct, most patients reject using the complex prosthosis.[11]

Hindfoot Amputation

Hindfoot amputation is generally performed as a method of accomplishing débridement of infected gangrene of the forefoot. As a definitive amputation level, amputation through the transverse tarsal joint, that is, Chopart joint, or the so-called Boyd and Pirogoff modifications should be avoided because of the high risk for the development of a late equinus deformity even when a section of the Achilles tendon is removed. Even when successful, the patient is left without a forefoot to act as a lever arm during terminal stance, leaving the patient with a propulsive gait pattern. These patients are functionally far better served with the Syme ankle disarticulation, which allows end bearing and space for a dynamic elastic response prosthetic foot (**Figure 6**).

Syme Ankle Disarticulation

The Syme ankle disarticulation is an end-bearing amputation that retains the weight-bearing surface of the distal tibia and the normal soft-tissue envelope of the retained heel pad.

The metabolic cost of walking is close to that for age-matched control patients, and far less than that for patients with a transtibial amputation. Patients require minimal gait training and rarely require hospitalization in a rehabilitation unit.[2,10,14,15]

The apices of the fish-mouth incision are placed at the anterior midpoints of the medial and lateral malleoli. The incision is taken down to the bone, followed by removal of the talus and calcaneus via sharp dissection. Care is taken to protect the posterior tibial artery, which is the primary blood supply of the flap. The malleoli are removed flush with the articular surface of the retained tibia, and the metaphysical flares of the distal tibia and fibula are removed with a small power saw. Migration of the heel pad is avoided by securing the heel pad to the retained tibia with a nonabsorbable suture placed through a drill hole in the anterior corner of the residual tibia (**Figure 7**).

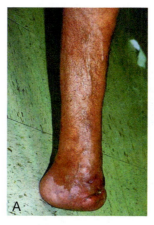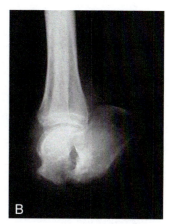

FIGURE 6 **A**, Photograph showing a successful hindfoot amputation. Even when a plantigrade residual foot can be achieved, the patient has an inadequate lever arm for propulsion. **B**, Lateral radiograph demonstrates late equinus that developed despite resection of 1 cm of Achilles tendon and cast immobilization for 1 month.

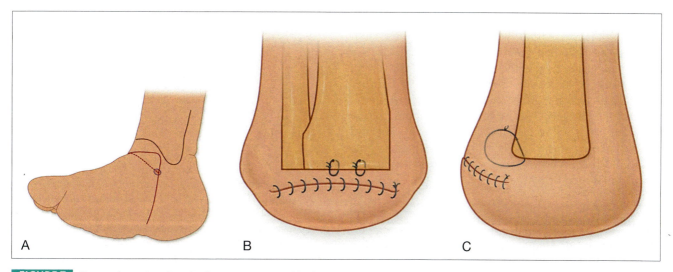

FIGURE 7 Illustrations showing single-stage Syme ankle disarticulation amputation. **A**, The incision is shown. **B** and **C**, The heel pad is secured to the distal tibia via drill holes and nonabsorbable suture. (Reproduced with permission from Pinzur MS, Stuck R, Sage R, Hunt N, Rabinovich Z: Syme's ankle disarticulation in patients with diabetes. *J Bone Joint Surg* 2003;85A[9]:1667-1672.)

Section 6: Foot and Ankle Trauma

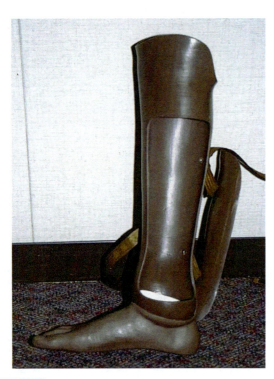

FIGURE 8 Photograph shows a Syme prosthesis.

Weight bearing with a walking cast with a rubber heel can be initiated as early as 2 weeks if the surgical wound appears secure. Early prosthetic fitting can be accomplished with a preparatory prosthesis as soon as 2 weeks following surgery (**Figure 8**).

Transtibial Amputation

Transtibial amputation is the most common amputation performed with the goal of restoring functional walking. The Burgess long posterior flap affords the most optimal soft-tissue envelope. The most functional residual tibial bone length is approximately 10 to 12 cm below the joint. The length of the flap should be equal to the diameter of the limb at the level of the tibial bone cut, plus 1 cm. The incision should be one-third to one-half the diameter of the leg, depending on the bulkiness/size of the limb.[16]

There has been increasing interest in support of the so-called Ertl bone-bridge fusion of the distal tibia and fibula. Although much has been written in support of the technique, there is little objective evidence to support an actual functional benefit.

POSTOPERATIVE CARE

Postoperative care should consider both wound healing and early functional ambulation. A protective cast is used in most partial foot amputations for both wound protection and early functional ambulation. Although there is little objective evidence, most experts advise the use of the rigid dressing following transtibial amputation. The timing of preparatory prosthetic limb fitting and weight bearing are generally dependent on the unique characteristics of the individual patient and the experience of the rehabilitation team. The most favorable clinical outcomes following amputation appear to be achieved when care is supervised by a multidisciplinary team.

SUMMARY

When performed properly, partial or whole-foot amputation allows retention of a reasonable platform for weight bearing and the normal soft-tissue envelope of the durable plantar skin. The energy cost of walking, that is, disability, can be minimized by good surgical technique.

Early weight bearing can be achieved with a well-contoured short leg walking cast. Custom insoles and mild shoe modification can preserve a high level of functional independence.

KEY STUDY POINTS

- Amputation should be considered as a reconstructive option following removal of nonviable or nonfunctional tissue.
- Amputation should be considered as the first step of reconstruction following removal of nonviable or nonfunctional tissue.
- The amputation residuum should be surgically constructed as a terminal organ of weight bearing.

ANNOTATED REFERENCES

1. Queen RM, Orendurff M: Amputee gait: Normal and abnormal, in Krajbich JI, Pinzur MS, Potter BK, Stevens PM, eds: *Atlas of Amputations and Limb Deficiencies*. American Academy of Orthopaedic Surgeons, 2016, pp 69-80.

2. Pinzur MS, Wolf B, Havey RM: Walking pattern of midfoot and ankle disarticulation amputees. *Foot Ankle Int* 1997;18(10):635-638.

3. Centers for Disease Control and Prevention. *National Diabetes Statistics Report*. Available at: https://www.cdc.gov/diabetes/data/statistics-report/index.html#:~:text=Diabetes%20Total%3A%2037.3%20million%20people%20have%20diabetes%20%2811.3%25,Diagnosed%3A%2028.7%20million%20people%2C%20including%2028.5%20million%20adults. Accessed March 2, 2022.

   This Centers for Disease Control and Prevention report on diabetes provides current data on prevalence, incidence, risk factors, and complications. Level of evidence: IV.

4. Ramasamy A, Hill AM, Masouros S, et al: Outcomes of IED foot and ankle blast injuries. *J Bone Joint Surg Am* 2013;95(5):e25.

5. Pinzur MS, Cavanah Dart H, Hershberger RC, Lomasney LM, O'Keefe P, Slade DH: Team approach: Treatment of diabetic foot ulcer. *JBJS Rev* 2016;4(7):e5.

6. Pinzur MS, Gottschalk F, Smith D, et al: Functional outcome of below-knee amputation in peripheral vascular insufficiency. *Clin Orthop Relat Res* 1993;286:247-249.

7. Shah SK, Bena JF, Allemang MT, et al: Lower extremity amputations: Factors associated with mortality or contralateral amputation. *Vasc Endovascular Surg* 2013;47(8):608-613.

8. Dickhaut SC, DeLee JC, Page CP: Nutritional status: Importance in predicting wound healing after amputation. *J Bone Joint Surg Am* 1984;66(1):71-75.

9. Pinzur MS, Kaminsky M, Sage R, Cronin R, Osterman H: Amputations at the middle level of the foot. *J Bone Joint Surg Am* 1986;68:1061-1064.

10. Pinzur MS, Stuck R, Sage R, Hunt N, Rabinovich Z: Syme's ankle disarticulation in patients with diabetes. *J Bone Joint Surg Am* 2003;85:1667-1672.

11. Pinzur MS, Dart HC: Pedorthic management of the diabetic foot. *Foot Ankle Clin* 2001;6(2):205-214.

12. Pinzur MS, Sage R, Schwaegler P: Ray resection in the dysvascular foot. A retrospective review. *Clin Orthop Relat Res* 1984;191:232-234.

13. Landry GJ, Silverman DA, Liem TK, Mitchell EL, Moneta GL: Predictors of healing and functional outcome following transmetatarsal amputations. *Arch Surg* 2011;146(9):1005-1009.

14. Pinzur MS, Gold J, Schwartz D, Gross N: Energy demands for walking in dysvascular amputees as related to the level of amputation. *Orthopedics* 1992;15(9):1033-1036.

15. Finkler ES, Marchwiany DA, Schiff AP, Pinzur MS: Long term outcomes following Syme's amputation. *Foot Ankle Int* 2017;38(7):732-735.

16. Burgess EM, Romano RL, Zettl JH: *The Management of Lower Extremity Amputations.* Bulletin TR 10-6, US Government Printing Office, 1969.

SECTION 7

Tendon Disorders and Sports-Related Foot and Ankle Injuries

Section Editors:
MaCalus Vinson Hogan, MD, MBA, FAAOS
Kenneth J. Hunt, MD, FAAOS

CHAPTER 23

Disorders of the Achilles Tendon

AJAY N. GURBANI, MD

ABSTRACT

The Achilles tendon is the strongest tendon in the body and plays a significant functional role. Anatomic characteristics of the Achilles tendon contribute to the development of varied pathology, including rupture and tendinopathy. The treatment of acute Achilles tendon ruptures remains controversial. It is important to review surgical and nonsurgical options for both Achilles tendon rupture and Achilles tendinopathy, along with rehabilitation protocols. Chronic Achilles tendon ruptures represent a challenging clinical entity, with most of the literature focused on varied surgical approaches.

Keywords: Achilles tendinopathy; Achilles tendon; Achilles tendon rupture

INTRODUCTION

The functional importance of the Achilles tendon is suggested by its status as the strongest and thickest tendon in the body. The Achilles tendon is formed by the two heads of the gastrocnemius and the soleus and inserts into the posterior aspect of the calcaneus. The slightly

Neither Dr. Gurbani nor any immediate family member has received anything of value from or has stock or stock options held in a commercial company or institution related directly or indirectly to the subject of this chapter.

medial to midline insertion allows the tendon to provide some inversion in addition to its primary role of plantar flexion of the ankle. The tendon does not have a true synovial sheath; instead, it is surrounded by a paratenon, a thin gliding membrane continuous proximally with the fascial envelope of the muscle. The paratenon is a highly vascular structure that, along with the surrounding muscle complex, provides blood flow to the tendon. An area that is relatively hypovascular within the tendon 2 to 6 cm from the calcaneal insertion may be predisposed to degenerative changes and rupture. The Achilles tendon is subjected to forces as high as 6 to 10 times the body weight during activities such as running. These factors, combined with the function of the gastrocnemius-soleus complex in crossing the knee, ankle, and subtalar joint, may help explain the high incidence of degenerative changes and injuries to the Achilles tendon.

ACUTE ACHILLES TENDON RUPTURES

Achilles tendon rupture is most common in men between the ages of 30 to 50 years. A retrospective review of 331 patients with Achilles tendon rupture found that 83% of injuries were sustained by men with an average age of 46.4 years. The same study noted that 68% of the sustained injuries were due to sports-related activities.[1] Most Achilles tendon ruptures occur 2 to 6 cm from the insertion of the tendon, with proximal ruptures accounting for only 10% to 15% of all Achilles tendon ruptures.[2] Ruptures at the insertion are rare and are associated with factors such as a Haglund deformity, a history of insertional Achilles tendinosis, or prior steroid therapy in the area. The common mechanism of rupture is a forced eccentric loading of the plantarflexed foot. The exact cause of Achilles tendon rupture remains unclear, but it

---

This chapter is adapted from Padanilam TG: Disorders of the anterior tibial, peroneal, and Achilles tendons, in Chou LB, ed: *Orthopaedic Knowledge Update®: Foot and Ankle 6*. American Academy of Orthopaedic Surgeons, 2020, pp 377-391.

© 2025 American Academy of Orthopaedic Surgeons

Orthopaedic Knowledge Update®: Foot and Ankle 7

has been associated with inflammatory or autoimmune disorders, systemic or injectable steroid use, collagen abnormality, exposure to fluoroquinolones, repetitive microtrauma, metabolic disorders, and overpronation of the foot.

An acute rupture usually can be diagnosed on the basis of the patient's history and physical examination. Most patients have a history of a traumatic event and describe a feeling of being kicked in the heel. Walking and climbing or descending stairs may be difficult. Examination reveals decreased plantar flexion strength, swelling around the tendon and loss of tendon contour, a palpable gap, lack of ankle movement when the calf is squeezed (the Thompson test), and an increased dorsiflexion position of the ankle when the patient is prone and the knee is bent to 90° (**Figure 1**). Imaging is rarely needed to confirm diagnosis of an acute Achilles tendon rupture. In fact, a retrospective study comparing patients with confirmed intraoperative Achilles tendon ruptures who had undergone preoperative MRI with those who did not undergo preoperative MRI found that a positive physical examination was more sensitive in diagnosing Achilles tendon rupture than radiologists' interpretation of MRI. The authors suggest that MRI evaluation be reserved for patients with equivocal examination findings, or in the setting of chronic injuries for preoperative planning.[3]

The treatment of an acute Achilles tendon rupture remains controversial. Nonsurgical treatment traditionally has consisted of prolonged immobilization in plantar flexion, with avoidance of weight bearing. Advocates of nonsurgical treatment emphasize the complications of surgical treatment, including wound healing–related issues. Surgical treatment traditionally has been recommended for active patients because of the belief that rerupture rates are higher after nonsurgical treatment. Many studies have attempted to answer the question of whether surgical or nonsurgical treatment is superior.

In a retrospective study of 945 patients with a nonsurgically treated Achilles tendon rupture, the decision for nonsurgical treatment was based on a palpation finding that the tendon ends were well approximated.[4] Patients were treated with an equinus cast for 4 weeks, a walker boot for the subsequent 4 weeks, and finally physical therapy. All patients were able to return to work and a preinjury level of sports activity. The rerupture rate was 2.8%. Almost all of the patients (99.4%) reported a good or excellent result. A historical control group of surgically treated patients was studied for comparison.

A retrospective study of 363 patients who underwent an identical functional rehabilitation program after surgical or nonsurgical treatment found a rerupture rate of 1.4% after surgical treatment and 8.6% after nonsurgical treatment.[2] The study was limited by the absence of standardized criteria for assignment to a treatment group. The patients who were surgically treated tended to be younger and have higher physical demands than those who were nonsurgically treated, or they had sought treatment more than 24 hours after injury. The study findings included no functional or outcome measures. Another study evaluated the functional outcomes of 80 patients who were randomly assigned to surgical or nonsurgical treatment.[5] No significant between-group difference was found in peak torque or total work at 1-year follow-up. Patients in both groups had decreased peak torque in the injured leg, however, in comparison with the uninjured leg. Cast immobilization was used for 6 weeks after surgery and for 10 weeks in nonsurgical treatment. The rerupture rates (5.4% in the patients who were surgically treated and 10.3% in those who were nonsurgically treated) were not considered to be statistically significantly different.

Early mobilization has been emphasized in the treatment of Achilles tendon ruptures. A randomized study of 97 patients evaluated functional outcomes when early mobilization was used after surgical or nonsurgical treatment.[6] All treatment was initiated within 72 hours of injury, and patients in both groups used a removable boot after 2 weeks of immobilization in a short leg equinus cast. The rerupture rate was 4% in patients who were surgically treated and 12% in those who were nonsurgically treated. Functional testing at 6-month follow-up revealed much better results in the patients who were surgically treated, but at 12-month follow-up

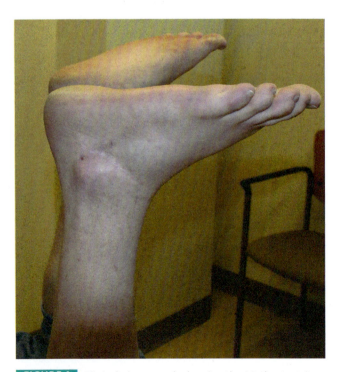

FIGURE 1 Clinical photograph showing the Matles test, in which the leg with an Achilles tendon rupture has greater dorsiflexion than the normal leg in the background.

the only significant between-group difference was that patients in the surgical group performed better in the heel-rise test. A study reported results on the first 45 of these 97 patients in whom an ultrasonography was performed before the initiation of treatment. Nonsurgical management of ruptures with more than 10 mm of diastasis between the tendon ends led to significantly higher rerupture rates than with surgical management.[7] Another randomized study of surgical and nonsurgical treatment in 144 patients evaluated functional outcomes after an accelerated functional rehabilitation program that began 2 weeks after injury.[8] No significant between-group difference was found in range of motion, strength, or rerupture rate. A meta-analysis of 10 randomized studies concluded that the risk of rerupture was equivalent after surgical or nonsurgical treatment of an Achilles tendon rupture if early motion was used during nonsurgical treatment.[9] If early motion was not used, the risk reduction with surgery was 8.8%. No significant difference was found in range of motion, strength, calf circumference, or functional outcome. A 2021 network meta-analysis of 19 randomized controlled trials compared outcomes of treatment with primary immobilization, function rehabilitation, minimally invasive repair, and open repair. No difference in rerupture risk was found between modern treatment techniques (functional rehabilitation, minimally invasive repair, and open repair), whereas traditional primary immobilization was associated with higher rerupture risk compared with open repair (odds ratio, 4.06). Minimally invasive surgery was associated with a lower risk of complication that resulted in additional procedures.[10]

This is a different result than was previously reported in a meta-analysis of level I and level II studies comparing surgical and nonsurgical treatment of acute Achilles tendon ruptures.[11] A 3.7% rerupture rate in the surgical group and 9.8% in the nonsurgical group were noted. No significant difference was found in return to sport, incidence of deep vein thrombosis, or physical activity scale. These results were similar to those found in a 2022 multicenter randomized controlled trial of 526 patients who were assigned to nonsurgical treatment, open repair, or minimally invasive repair. Although no difference in functional outcomes was reported between groups at 12 months, nonsurgical management was associated with a higher rate of rerupture (6.2% versus 0.6% in each of the surgical groups).[12]

With regard to trends in choice of treatment method, there may be geographic variability. A review of a large healthcare database suggested that surgical management is the preferred method of treatment for acute Achilles tendon ruptures in the United States.[13] A review of a Denmark national registry from 1994 to 2013 showed a statistically significant increase in incidence of Achilles tendon ruptures and a noticeable decline in surgical treatment from 2009 to 2013.[14]

Recent research on the surgical treatment of Achilles tendon ruptures has focused on the use of minimally invasive repair techniques and early mobilization (**Figure 2**). Historically, minimally invasive and percutaneous techniques have been criticized as leading to relatively high rates of rerupture and sural nerve injury.[15-17] A retrospective study evaluated the use of immediate weight bearing in 52 patients.[15] After surgery using a modified percutaneous approach, the limb was placed in a cast, and immediate weight bearing was allowed. A boot with a heel lift was substituted after 2 weeks, and exercises were started. At an average 28-month final follow-up, 47 patients (90%) were able to return to their desired level of activity, and the average American Orthopaedic Foot and Ankle Society score was 90. Four patients had sural neuritis, which resolved within 6 months. No reruptures were observed. A study of 15 elite athletes found that all were able to return to their sport after a minimally invasive repair.[17] Thirteen patients had no pain but did have a subjective perception of reduction in calf strength, two had wound-healing difficulty, and none had sural nerve injuries. The study concluded that percutaneous repair is safe and effective for treating Achilles tendon rupture in elite athletes. In a randomized prospective study comparing open repair with the use of a commercially available percutaneous repair device, all 40 patients regained Achilles tendon function.[16] No between-group difference was found in maximal calf circumference, ankle dorsiflexion, or the ability to perform heel rises. The complication rate was 5% in the patients treated with a percutaneous repair and 35% in those treated with an open repair. No reruptures or sural nerve injuries were found in either group of patients. There were fewer incidences of local tenderness, skin adhesion, and tendon

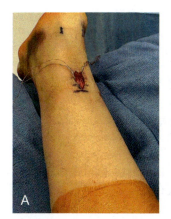 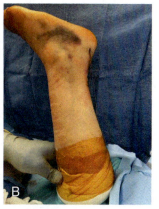

FIGURE 2 **A**, Intraoperative photograph showing a minimally invasive Achilles tendon repair. **B**, Photograph showing resting tension of the Achilles tendon restored after repair.

Section 7: Tendon Disorders and Sports-Related Foot and Ankle Injuries

thickening in the patients who received a percutaneous repair. A retrospective study of 270 patients compared open repair with percutaneous repair and found no statistically significant difference between the two approaches with regard to complications.[18]

Early motion was evaluated after open repair in a retrospective study of 107 patients, 96 of whom (90%) received no immobilization and started exercise 3 to 5 days after surgical repair.[19] Patients were able to resume heavy labor and sports activity 13 weeks after surgery on average. No rerupture, gap formation, or tendon elongation was noted. The study concluded that early motion may facilitate the proliferation, transportation, and alignment of tendon cells, thereby leading to an improvement in the overall reconstruction of the tendon. However, those results are somewhat contradictory to the results found in a separate 2022 prospective study of 60 patients who underwent percutaneous Achilles tendon repair that compared the outcomes of a traditional accelerated rehabilitation program to a slower rehabilitation protocol. In this study, both groups were allowed immediate weight bearing; however, the patients with the slower rehabilitation protocol were immobilized for a longer period and started eccentric exercises at a later time (approximately 12 weeks after surgery). The slower rehabilitation group was found to have improved patient-reported functional outcomes, calf circumference, isometric strength, and Achilles tendon tension as measured by resting angle at a 12-month follow-up. These results suggest that the added benefits of earlier mobilization may potentially be offset by an increased risk of tendon elongation during the healing process.[20]

In addition to tendon elongation, another marker that has been identified as a potential correlate to functional outcomes is the Achilles tendon cross-sectional area. A 2020 prospective study of 22 patients evaluated tendon structure using ultrasonography and patient functional outcomes at multiple time points up to 1 year after Achilles tendon rupture. In this study, which did not control for treatment provided, tendon cross-sectional area at 12 weeks was found to be the strongest predictor of improved performance on heel-rise testing at 1 year.[21] The effect of various rehabilitation protocols on Achilles tendon cross-sectional area after rupture continues to be explored.

CHRONIC ACHILLES TENDON RUPTURES

An estimated 10% to 25% of Achilles tendon ruptures are neglected or not immediately identified.[22] The patient risk factors for delayed diagnosis include age older than 55 years, a high body mass index, and injury unrelated to sports activity.[1] Although there is no clear demarcation between acute and chronic rupture, a rupture estimated to have been present for 4 to 6 weeks is likely to have

characteristics consistent with chronic rupture. Chronic rupture is more challenging to treat than acute rupture because of the presence of a gap between the tendon ends, retraction and scarring of the calf muscle, and loss of muscle contractility.

The patient may have vague symptoms that are not specific to the Achilles tendon region. There may be a sense of weakness or unsteadiness in gait, rather than pain. Difficulty in stair climbing and walking uphill is common. Loss of tendon contour is seen on examination. Some patients have sufficient reparative tissue to make palpation of a gap difficult. The Thompson test usually is positive but is less reliable than with acute rupture. The Matles test also usually is positive. Most patients are unable to perform a single-leg heel rise.

Retraction and scarring of the tendon ends means that nonsurgical restoration of the physiologic tension of the gastrocnemius-soleus complex is difficult. The use of an ankle-foot orthosis should be considered for a patient who is a poor surgical candidate because of significant comorbidities. A patient with minimal functional deficits also may benefit from nonsurgical treatment. The benefit of physical therapy is in recruiting other muscle groups to compensate for the loss of Achilles tendon function. There is limited evidence regarding the outcomes of nonsurgical management of chronic Achilles tendon ruptures in the literature.[23]

Surgical treatment of a chronic rupture involves the restoration of continuity to tendon ends that have retracted and created irreducible gaps. The available surgical techniques include tendon mobilization, turndown flaps, tendon advancement, tendon transfer, free tissue transfer, and synthetic graft.[22] A 2- to 3-cm gap can be effectively treated using tendon mobilization and stretching of the proximal musculature, followed by end-to-end repair. The use of turndown flaps involves freeing a strip of tendon from the proximal residual tendon and weaving it through the distal and proximal tendon ends. A study reported on the treatment of chronic ruptures with removal of a section of scar tissue and direct primary repair of the remaining scar tissue without the use of any graft in 30 patients.[24] At 33 months average follow-up, there were no reruptures and all patients were able to use stairs. Fourteen patients who were involved in sports were able to return to their sport. Histologic evaluation of the interposed scar tissue showed the biologic potential for healing. A V-Y tendon advancement can be used for gaps smaller than 5 cm and patients have reported satisfactory outcomes; however, the cosmetic results may be unsatisfactory and persistent plantar flexion weakness is seen.[25] Tendon transfers are an option for the treatment of chronic ruptures. Tendon transfer provides not only material to fill gaps between rupture ends but also additional strength with its associated musculotendinous unit. The most common donor sites are the flexor hallucis longus (FHL), peroneal tendons, and flexor digitorum longus. Peroneus brevis tendon transfers were performed through a limited approach in 32 patients and all were able to work and participate in leisure activities.[26] Six were rated as having an excellent outcome, and 24 had a good outcome. Loss of eversion strength was found objectively on examination but was not subjectively reported by patients. The FHL tendon transfer has several reported advantages including limited donor morbidity, greater strength than a peroneus brevis transfer, an axis of pull similar to that of the Achilles tendon, and improved vascularity of the reconstruction with presence of the low-lying muscle belly[27] (**Figure 3**). The use of a free tissue transfer such as a semitendinosus graft has had good results for the treatment of tendon gaps larger than 6 cm.[28] A study reported excellent results in 62 of 72 patients with a chronic rupture at the insertion of the Achilles tendon when the gastrocnemius aponeurosis was used to reconstruct the insertion.[29] Most studies of synthetic grafts have been small, and comparative evaluation therefore is difficult. Although surgical treatment of chronic ruptures has led to improved outcomes, patients continue to have strength deficits in comparison with the contralateral limb. A variety of techniques have been studied, but the small numbers of patients, combined with variations in patient selection, gap measurements, postoperative regimens, and outcome measurements, create difficulty in comparing data and making firm recommendations.

ACHILLES TENDINOPATHY

Achilles tendinopathy is described as insertional or noninsertional. Noninsertional tendinopathy is further classified as peritendinitis, peritendinitis with tendinosis, or tendinosis. Tendinosis is a chronic, noninflammatory, degenerative process of the tendon that is associated with decreased vascularity, repetitive microtrauma, and aging. The associated etiologic factors can include diabetes, hypertension, steroid use, obesity, and estrogen exposure. Patients range from relatively young and active patients with peritendinitis caused by overuse to patients older than 50 years with tendinosis combined with peritendinitis of varying severity. Patients with peritendinitis have diffuse swelling and tenderness along the course of the tendon. Patients with tendinosis typically have pain and swelling along a nodular area within the tendon. Tenderness to palpation often is present along the area of tendon thickening. The patient may have difficulty performing a single-leg heel rise. MRI and ultrasonography can be useful for defining the location and extent of disease.

Nonsurgical management is effective in 70% to 75% of patients.[30,31] Modalities including rest, NSAIDs,

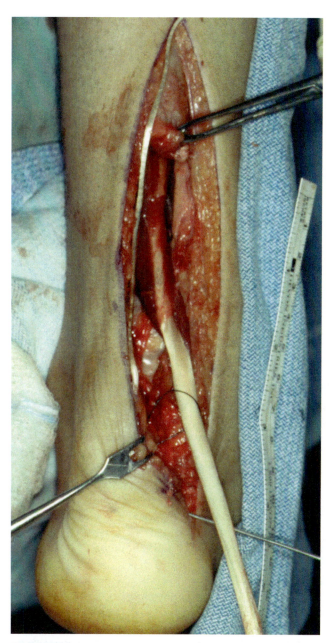

FIGURE 3 Intraoperative photograph showing the use of a harvested flexor hallucis longus tendon to treat a chronic Achilles tendon rupture.

activity modification, and eccentric strengthening frequently are used. Immobilization in a short leg cast or boot may be beneficial if the condition is recalcitrant. Injectable therapies are gaining popularity for treating Achilles tendinosis, using agents such as platelet-rich plasma, autologous blood, sclerosing agents, protease inhibitors, hemodialysate, corticosteroids, and prolotherapy. A systematic review of nine randomized controlled studies involving the use of injectable therapies found only one study meeting the quality criteria.[31] Most patients treated with an injectable therapy were found to have mild to moderate clinical benefit, but patients in placebo and control groups had similar improvements. In regard to platelet-rich plasma, a 2021 meta-analysis of four randomized controlled trials with 170 patients found no specific added benefit of platelet-rich plasma compared with saline injections when combined with an eccentric training program for the treatment of chronic midsubstance Achilles tendinopathy.[32]

The effectiveness of extracorporeal shock wave therapy was evaluated in a systematic meta-analysis of four randomized controlled studies and two pre-post studies.[33] The studies were inconsistent in participant characteristics as well as dosages and impulses per session. Four studies found statistically significant improvement in functional outcomes, and the meta-analysis concluded that the evidence was satisfactory to show the effectiveness of extracorporeal shock wave therapy for treating chronic Achilles tendinopathy.

Surgical treatment may be indicated for refractory Achilles tendinosis after 6 months of unsuccessful nonsurgical treatment. The traditional surgical treatment consists of removing diseased portions of the tendon. Augmentation with FHL tendon transfer may be needed if more than 50% of the tendon is removed. A prospective study of 56 patients who had FHL transfer for insertional or noninsertional Achilles tendinopathy found significant improvement in functional outcome scores at 24-month follow-up, and 32 patients (57%) had no hallux weakness.[34] Most of the patients in this study were described as sedentary. The study authors expressed concern that relatively young, active patients might notice functional deficits associated with great toe weakness.

Minimally invasive paratenon release also has been suggested for treating Achilles tendinopathy. In a retrospective case study of 26 patients, percutaneous release of adhesions between the paratenon and tendon was followed by instillation of methylprednisolone and bupivacaine into the paratenon.[35] At an average 13-month follow-up, 73% of tendons were pain free or had significant improvement in pain. The study authors suggested that the release of adhesions in this procedure disrupts the neovascularization process and allows tendon healing. A retrospective review of the outcomes of 39 runners found that 30 runners (77%) reported a good or excellent outcome an average 17 years after ultrasound-guided multiple percutaneous tenotomies for Achilles tendinosis.[36] Several studies of isolated gastrocnemius lengthening for Achilles tendinopathy found clinical improvement in all patients without loss of plantar flexion strength.[37-39] Comparison with other studies is difficult, however, because of the limited characterization of the extent of tendon involvement.

Insertional Achilles tendinopathy ranges from peritendinitis to tendinosis. Isolated peritendinitis tends to occur in relatively young and athletic individuals and can be caused by overuse, hill running, an interval training program, or a training error. Insertional tendinosis is more common in individuals older than 50 years with varying levels of activity. Patients often have concomitant symptoms from retrocalcaneal bursitis and Haglund deformity. Inflammatory arthropathies may contribute to the etiology and especially should be considered in a younger patient with bilateral symptoms. The initial symptoms usually are morning stiffness, posterior heel pain, and swelling with activity, progressing to constant pain. Often the patient has swelling along the posterior heel. Active and passive limitation of dorsiflexion may be present. The location of the tenderness can help distinguish among retrocalcaneal bursitis, Haglund deformity, and insertional tendinosis; all three sometimes are present. Radiographs may show calcification within the insertion of the tendon. Traditionally, a Haglund deformity was considered to be most common in patients with insertional tendinopathy, but a recent retrospective radiographic study challenged this belief.[40] No significant difference was found in the radiographic parameters of Haglund deformity between patients with or without insertional Achilles tendinosis. Calcification of the tendon insertion was present in 73% of patients.

The initial treatment, often including rest, NSAIDs, and activity modification, is effective in most patients.[30] Eccentric exercises are less effective for treating insertional tendinopathy than noninsertional tendinopathy.[33] A randomized controlled study found a 28% improvement in patients treated with eccentric exercise, compared with a 64% improvement in those treated with extracorporeal shock wave therapy.[41] A prospective study of 103 patients treated using an ankle-foot orthosis and a home stretching program found improvement in 91 patients (88%). The average duration of treatment was 163 days.[42]

Surgical treatment may be indicated if symptoms are not relieved after 6 to 12 months of nonsurgical management. Surgical treatment is directed toward the underlying pathologic changes. The techniques include débridement of the Achilles tendon insertion, débridement of the retrocalcaneal bursa, and posterosuperior calcaneal ostectomy (**Figure 4**). Several approaches have been described, including medial, lateral, combined medial and lateral, endoscopic, J-shaped, transverse, and central tendon splitting; there are insufficient data that suggest the superiority of one approach over another. A study reported on the results of dorsal closing wedge osteotomy in a group of recreational and professional athletes.[43] This was performed on 52 patients who showed signs of a Haglund deformity and less than 50% degenerative tendinopathy at the Achilles tendon insertion on magnetic resonance images. All professional athletes returned to the same

Chapter 23: Disorders of the Achilles Tendon

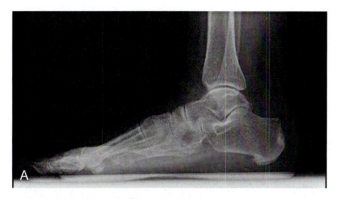

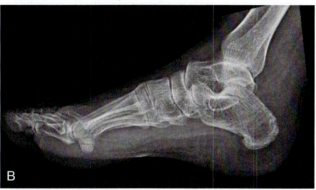

FIGURE 4 **A**, Preoperative lateral foot radiograph from a patient with chronic insertional Achilles tendinopathy with associated Haglund deformity. **B**, Postoperative lateral foot radiograph after posterosuperior calcaneal ostectomy, débridement of retrocalcaneal bursitis, Achilles tendon insertion débridement, and repair.

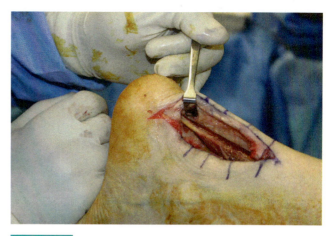

FIGURE 5 Intraoperative photograph showing the use of a harvested flexor hallucis longus tendon to augment the Achilles tendon after extensive débridement.

level of competition and 22 of the 29 recreational athletes returned to the same level of competition. Consistent with recent trends, newer minimally invasive approaches to surgical management of chronic insertional tendinopathy have been described. A 2021 retrospective case series of 27 patients reported the outcomes of percutaneous calcaneoplasty in patients who presented with evidence of distal Achilles tendon inflammation and retrocalcaneal bursitis, without associated advanced tendinopathy or intratendinous calcification. The study authors found improvement in patient-reported outcomes at an average of 26.5-month follow-up, with 22 patients (84.5%) reporting complete satisfaction and two additional patients (7.4%) reporting moderate satisfaction.[44]

In regard to débridement, it is thought that as much as 50% of the Achilles tendon insertion can be detached without significantly increasing the risk of rupture. With additional detachment and exposure, suture anchors may be needed to secure the tendon. Although clinical data are lacking to determine the ideal number and configuration of anchors, a study suggested better outcomes with the use of two-suture anchors or double row fixation when compared with a single anchor.[45] Patients with significant degenerative changes of the tendon may require extensive débridement and augmentation with FHL tendon transfer (**Figure 5**). A randomized prospective study compared patients with insertional Achilles tendinopathy treated with débridement alone with those who were augmented with an FHL transfer.[46] At 1-year follow-up, no significant difference in American Orthopaedic Foot and Ankle Society and visual analog scale scores was noted between the two groups. The FHL group was noted to have greater plantar flexion strength in the ankle. No assessment of the severity of tendinosis was provided for either group. The lack of a standardized method for assessing the severity of the condition makes it difficult to compare studies and provide firm recommendations.

SUMMARY

Acute and chronic injuries of the Achilles tendon can cause significant pain and disability. Physical examination usually allows an accurate diagnosis in cases of acute Achilles tendon rupture, but MRI may be helpful if the diagnosis is questionable or in the case of chronic pathology. Both surgical and nonsurgical management of acute Achilles tendon ruptures have been advocated, with recent evidence supporting early functional rehabilitation regardless of the approach taken. Most chronic Achilles tendon ruptures are managed surgically; however, nonsurgical management may be indicated in patients unfit for surgery or with low physical demands. A trial of nonsurgical management is indicated in the initial management of insertional and noninsertional Achilles tendinopathy. If surgical treatment is required, an open or minimally invasive procedure can be chosen, depending on the type and severity of the pathology. A return to occupational and recreational activities is possible for most patients; however, recovery may take 6 to 12 months.

KEY STUDY POINTS

- The Achilles tendon is the thickest and strongest tendon in the body and is subjected to high forces during activity. The central area of relative hypovascularity in the tendon is prone to the development of pathology.
- Controversy exists as to whether acute Achilles tendon ruptures are best managed surgically or nonsurgically. Functional rehabilitation is important in optimizing outcomes with both forms of treatment, with recent evidence indicating that early weight bearing may be more beneficial than early motion.
- Management of chronic Achilles tendon ruptures depends on the size of the gap between tendon ends. Tendon transfers provide both graft material to fill the gap and power from its associated muscle unit.
- Surgical management of Achilles tendinopathy may be warranted after failure of nonsurgical treatment. A variety of surgical techniques have been described with insufficient evidence to show clear superiority of one over the other.

ANNOTATED REFERENCES

1. Raikin SM, Garras DN, Krapchev PV: Achilles tendon injuries in a United States population. *Foot Ankle Int* 2013;34(4):475-480.

2. Gwynne-Jones DP, Sims M, Handcock D: Epidemiology and outcomes of acute Achilles tendon rupture with operative or nonoperative treatment using an identical functional bracing protocol. *Foot Ankle Int* 2011;32(4):337-343.

3. Garras DN, Raikin SM, Bhat SB, Taweel N, Karanjia H: MRI is unnecessary for diagnosing acute Achilles tendon ruptures: Clinical diagnostic criteria. *Clin Orthop Relat Res* 2012;470(8):2268-2273.

4. Wallace RGH, Heyes GJ, Michael ALR: The non-operative functional management of patients with a rupture of the tendo Achillis leads to low rates of re-rupture. *J Bone Joint Surg Br* 2011;93(10):1362-1366.

5. Keating JF, Will EM: Operative versus non-operative treatment of acute rupture of tendo Achillis: A prospective randomised evaluation of functional outcome. *J Bone Joint Surg Br* 2011;93(8):1071-1078.

6. Nilsson-Helander K, Silbernagel KG, Thomeé R, et al: Acute Achilles tendon rupture: A randomized, controlled study comparing surgical and nonsurgical treatments using validated outcome measures. *Am J Sports Med* 2010;38(11):2186-2193.

7. Westin O, Nilsson Helander K, Gravare Silbernagel K, Moller M, Kalebo P, Karlsson J: Acute ultrasonography investigation to predict reruptures and outcomes in patients with an Achilles tendon rupture. *Orthop J Sports Med* 2016;4(10):2325967116667920.

8. Willits K, Amendola A, Bryant D, et al: Operative versus nonoperative treatment of acute Achilles tendon ruptures: A multicenter randomized trial using accelerated functional rehabilitation. *J Bone Joint Surg Am* 2010;92(17):2767-2775.

9. Soroceanu A, Sidhwa F, Aarabi S, Kaufman A, Glazebrook M: Surgical versus nonsurgical treatment of acute Achilles tendon rupture: A meta-analysis of randomized trials. *J Bone Joint Surg Am* 2012;94(23):2136-2143.

10. Meulenkamp B, Woolnough T, Cheng W, et al: What is the best evidence to guide management of acute Achilles tendon ruptures? A systematic review and network meta-analysis of randomized controlled trials. *Clin Orthop Relat Res* 2021;479(10):2119-2131.

    A meta-analysis of 19 randomized controlled trials compared two or more of the following interventions for treatment of acute Achilles tendon rupture: primary immobilization, functional rehabilitation, open surgical repair, minimally invasive repair. The authors found an increased risk of rerupture with primary immobilization compared with open repair (odds ratio, 4.06); however, no difference in rerupture rates was found among the other treatments. Minimally invasive repair was associated with the lowest rate of complications that resulted in additional surgery in this analysis. Level of evidence: I.

11. Deng S, Sun Z, Zhang C, Chen G, Li J: Surgical treatment versus conservative management for acute Achilles tendon rupture: A systematic review and meta-analysis of randomized controlled trials. *J Foot Ankle Surg* 2017;56(6):1236-1243.

12. Myhrvold SB, Brouwer EF, Andresen TKM, et al: Nonoperative or surgical treatment of acute Achilles' tendon rupture. *N Engl J Med* 2022;386(15):1409-1420.

    This is a randomized controlled trial of 526 patients who underwent treatment for an acute Achilles tendon rupture with nonsurgical management, open repair, or minimally invasive surgery. No difference in patient-reported outcome (Achilles Tendon Total Rupture Score) was found between groups at 12 months. Nonsurgical treatment was associated with higher risk of rerupture (6.2%) than either surgical group (0.6% in each), and a lower risk of nerve injury. Level of evidence: I.

13. Wang D, Sandlin MI, Cohen JR, Lord EL, Petrigliano FA, SooHoo NF: Operative versus nonoperative treatment of acute Achilles tendon rupture: An analysis of 12,570 patients in a large healthcare database. *Foot Ankle Surg* 2015;21(4):250-253.

14. Ganestam A, Kallemose T, Troelsen A, Barfod KW: Increasing incidence of acute Achilles tendon rupture and a noticeable decline in surgical treatment from 1994 to 2013. A nationwide registry study of 33,160 patients. *Knee Surg Sports Traumatol Arthrosc* 2016;24(12):3730-3737.

15. Patel VC, Lozano-Calderon S, McWilliam J: Immediate weight bearing after modified percutaneous Achilles tendon repair. *Foot Ankle Int* 2012;33(12):1093-1097.

16. Aktas S, Kocaoglu B: Open versus minimal invasive repair with Achillon device. *Foot Ankle Int* 2009;30(5):391-397.

17. Maffulli N, Longo UG, Maffulli GD, Khanna A, Denaro V: Achilles tendon ruptures in elite athletes. *Foot Ankle Int* 2011;32(1):9-15.

18. Hsu AR, Jones CP, Cohen BE, Davis WH, Ellington JK, Anderson RB: Clinical outcomes and complications of percutaneous Achilles repair system versus open technique for acute Achilles tendon ruptures. *Foot Ankle Int* 2015;36(11):1279-1286.

19. Jielile J, Sabirhazi G, Chen J, et al: Novel surgical technique and early kinesiotherapy for acute Achilles tendon rupture. *Foot Ankle Int* 2012;33(12):1119-1127.

20. Maffulli N, Gougoulias N, Maffulli GD, Oliva F, Migliorini F: Slowed-down rehabilitation following percutaneous repair of Achilles tendon rupture. *Foot Ankle Int* 2022;43(2):244-252.

This is a prospective cohort study of 60 patients who underwent either traditional accelerated rehabilitation or a slowed-down rehabilitation (longer immobilization postoperatively with delay of eccentric exercises to 12 weeks postoperatively), both with immediate weight bearing. The slowed-down rehabilitation group was found to have improved outcomes as measured by Achilles tendon resting angle and Achilles Tendon Total Rupture Score at 12-month follow-up. The slowed-down rehabilitation group was also found to have improved isometric strength and calf circumference that were more similar to those of the contralateral leg. Level of evidence: II.

21. Zellers JA, Pohlig RT, Cortes DH, Grävare Silbernagel K: Achilles tendon cross-sectional area at 12 weeks post-rupture relates to 1-year heel-rise height. *Knee Surg Sports Traumatol Arthrosc* 2020;28(1):245-252.

This is a prospective cohort study of 22 patients with Achilles tendon ruptures, which examined tendon structure (length, cross-sectional area) using ultrasonography as well as functional outcomes at various time points up to 1 year postinjury. Treatment was not controlled in this study. Both tendon cross-sectional area and length were found to correlate with assessed function, with cross-sectional area at 12 weeks being the greatest predictor of heel rise at 1-year follow-up. Level of evidence: II.

22. Padanilam TG: Chronic Achilles tendon ruptures. *Foot Ankle Clin* 2009;14(4):711-728.

23. Arshad Z, Lau EJS, Leow SH, Bhatia M: Management of chronic Achilles ruptures: A scoping review. *Int Orthop* 2021;45(10):2543-2559.

This is a systematic review of the literature examining current described techniques and outcomes for treatment of chronic Achilles tendon ruptures. Only one article described nonsurgical management, whereas the remaining articles discussed various surgical approaches with improvement in patient outcomes reported with all techniques. A wide variety of outcomes were reported, however, making comparison between techniques difficult. Level of evidence: III.

24. Yasuda T, Shima H, Mori K, Kizawa M, Neo M: Direct repair of chronic Achilles tendon ruptures using scar tissue located between the tendon stumps. *J Bone Joint Surg Am* 2016;98(14):1168-1175.

25. Steginsky BD, Van Dyke B, Berlet GC: The missed Achilles tear. Now what? *Foot Ankle Clin* 2017;22(4):715-734.

26. Maffulli N, Spiezia F, Longo UG, Denaro V: Less-invasive reconstruction of chronic Achilles tendon ruptures using a peroneus brevis tendon transfer. *Am J Sports Med* 2010;38(11):2304-2312.

27. Jeng CL, Thawait GK, Kwon JY, et al: Relative strengths of the calf muscles based on MRI volume measurements. *Foot Ankle Int* 2012;33(5):394-399.

28. Sarzaeem MM, Lemraski MMB, Safdari F: Chronic Achilles tendon rupture reconstruction using a free semitendinosus tendon graft transfer. *Knee Surg Sports Traumatol Arthrosc* 2012;20(7):1386-1391.

29. Pavan Kumar A, Shashikiran R, Raghuram C: A novel modification of Bosworth's technique to repair zone I Achilles tendon ruptures. *J Orthop Traumatol* 2013;14(1):59-65.

30. Paavola M, Kannus P, Paakkala T, Pasanen M, Järvinen M: Long-term prognosis of patients with Achilles tendinopathy: An observational 8-year follow-up study. *Am J Sports Med* 2000;28(5):634-642.

31. Gross CE, Hsu AR, Chahal J, Holmes GB Jr: Injectable treatments for noninsertional Achilles tendinosis: A systematic review. *Foot Ankle Int* 2013;34(5):619-628.

32. Nauwelaers AK, Van Oost L, Peers K: Evidence for the use of PRP in chronic midsubstance Achilles tendinopathy: A systematic review with meta-analysis. *Foot Ankle Surg* 2021;27(5):486-495.

This is a systematic review of literature for platelet-rich plasma treatment of chronic midsubstance Achilles tendinopathy, with four randomized controlled trials meeting the criteria for inclusion in the meta-analysis. Pooled data from 170 patients demonstrated no difference in Victorian Institute of Sports Assessment–Achilles scores for patients undergoing platelet-rich plasma versus saline injection at 3, 6, and 12 months follow-up. No clear improvement in tendon structure among patients who underwent platelet-rich plasma was demonstrated. Level of evidence: I.

33. Al-Abbad H, Simon JV: The effectiveness of extracorporeal shock wave therapy on chronic Achilles tendinopathy: A systematic review. *Foot Ankle Int* 2013;34(1):33-41.

34. Schon LC, Shores JL, Faro FD, Vora AM, Camire LM, Guyton GP: Flexor hallucis longus tendon transfer in treatment of Achilles tendinosis. *J Bone Joint Surg Am* 2013;95(1):54-60.

35. Naidu V, Abbassian A, Nielsen D, Uppalapati R, Shetty A: Minimally invasive paratenon release for non-insertional Achilles tendinopathy. *Foot Ankle Int* 2009;30(7):680-685.

36. Maffulli N, Oliva F, Testa V, Capasso G, Del Buono A: Multiple percutaneous longitudinal tenotomies for chronic Achilles tendinopathy in runners: A long-term study. *Am J Sports Med* 2013;41(9):2151-2157.

37. Kiewiet NJ, Holthusen SM, Bohay DR, Anderson JG: Gastrocnemius recession for chronic noninsertional Achilles tendinopathy. *Foot Ankle Int* 2013;34(4):481-485.

38. Duthon VB, Lübbeke A, Duc SR, Stern R, Assal M: Non-insertional Achilles tendinopathy treated with gastrocnemius lengthening. *Foot Ankle Int* 2011;32(4):375-379.

39. Molund M, Lapinskas SR, Nilsen FA, Hvaal KH: Clinical and functional outcomes of gastrocnemius recession for chronic Achilles tendinopathy. *Foot Ankle Int* 2016;37(10):1091-1097.

40. Kang S, Thordarson DB, Charlton TP: Insertional Achilles tendinitis and Haglund's deformity. *Foot Ankle Int* 2012;33(6):487-491.

41. Rompe JD, Furia J, Maffulli N: Eccentric loading compared with shock wave treatment for chronic insertional Achilles tendinopathy: A randomized, controlled trial. *J Bone Joint Surg Am* 2008;90(1):52-61.

42. Johnson MD, Alvarez RG: Nonoperative management of retrocalcaneal pain with AFO and stretching regimen. *Foot Ankle Int* 2012;33(7):571-581.

43. Georgiannos D, Lampridis V, Vasiliadis A, Bisbinas I: Treatment of insertional Achilles pathology with dorsal wedge calcaneal osteotomy in athletes. *Foot Ankle Int* 2017;38(4):381-387.

44. Ferranti S, Migliorini F, Liuni FM, et al: Outcomes of percutaneous calcaneoplasty for insertional Achilles tendon problems. *Foot Ankle Int* 2021;42(10):1287-1293.

This is a retrospective case series of 27 patients who underwent percutaneous calcaneoplasty for insertional Achilles tendinopathy. The authors reported an improvement in visual analog scale and Victorian Institute of Sports Assessment–Achilles scores at an average of 26.5 months follow-up. Twenty-two patients (84.5%) reported complete satisfaction, whereas two patients (7.4%) reported moderate satisfaction and three patients (11.1%) reported being unsatisfied with results. Level of evidence: III.

45. Ettinger S, Razzaq R, Waizy H, et al: Operative treatment of the insertional Achilles tendinopathy through a Transtendinous approach. *Foot Ankle Int* 2016;37(3):288-293.

46. Hunt KJ, Cohen BE, Davis WH, Anderson RB, Jones CP: Surgical treatment of insertional Achilles tendinopathy with or without flexor hallucis longus tendon transfer: A prospective randomized study. *Foot Ankle Int* 2015;36(9):998-1005.

CHAPTER 24

Sports-Related Injuries of the Foot and Ankle

CHRISTOPHER E. GROSS, MD, FAAOS

ABSTRACT

The foot and ankle are often injured during athletic activities, and even when appropriately managed, such injuries can progress to become chronic conditions affecting both sports participation and routine activity. Although the most common athletic injury to the ankle is an acute sprain of the lateral ankle, several other pathologies regularly occur. Midfoot sprains are less common and require careful assessment to avoid a delay in diagnosis. Stable injuries are successfully treated nonsurgically, whereas unstable injuries require surgical intervention. Stress fractures of the foot and ankle are common in athletes and can be associated with vitamin D deficiency. Most stress fractures can be successfully treated nonsurgically. Anterior tibial tendon ruptures are relatively uncommon injuries, with spontaneous ruptures usually seen in men aged 50 to 70 years. Treatment includes surgical and nonsurgical options depending on the patient's activity level. Peroneal tendon pathology includes tenosynovitis, instability, and tears of the tendons; prompt recognition and treatment are important. Instability and tears often require surgical management in an active patient population.

Keywords: anterior tibial tendon; midfoot sprain; peroneal tendon; stress fracture

---

Dr. Gross or an immediate family member serves as a paid consultant to or is an employee of DJ Orthopaedics, Novastep, and Paragon 28; has received research or institutional support from Paragon 28 and Wright Medical Technology, Inc.; and serves as a board member, owner, officer, or committee member of American Academy of Orthopaedic Surgeons and American Orthopaedic Foot and Ankle Society.

INTRODUCTION

Acute traumatic injuries and cumulative stress injuries involving the foot and ankle can affect the sports participation and performance of both elite competitive athletes and people engaged in recreational or fitness activities. A thorough understanding of common injuries of the foot and ankle allows a logical and organized approach to managing these injuries and facilitates the patient's return to play.

This chapter is adapted from Palanca A, Gross CE: Forefoot, sesamoid, and turf toe injuries; Padanilam TG: Disorders of the anterior tibial, peroneal and Achilles tendons; and Lin J: Sports-related injuries of the foot and ankle, in Chou LB, ed: *Orthopaedic Knowledge Update®: Foot and Ankle 6*. American Academy of Orthopaedic Surgeons, 2020, pp 361-373, 377-391, 393-408.

ANKLE ANATOMY

The stability of the ankle is the result of a combination of osseous, ligamentous, and musculotendinous components. The ankle generally is described as a mortise in which the talus is housed in the dome-shaped tibial plafond and the medial, lateral, and posterior malleoli. The talus is wider anteriorly than posteriorly so that the ankle intrinsically is most stable in the dorsiflexed position when the wider portion of the talus is engaged in the mortise. Conversely, in the plantarflexed position, the narrower posterior talus is engaged in the mortise and the ankle therefore is more unstable. Therefore, in the plantarflexed position, the stability of the ankle is more dependent on the lateral ligament complex. Not surprisingly, most acute inversion sprains occur when the ankle is somewhat plantarflexed.

The peroneal musculotendinous unit is an important contributor to ankle stability. The peroneal tendons rapidly contract to resist and prevent excessive inversion. The peroneal complex is also part of an important proprioceptive feedback loop that enables an athlete to instinctively sense and control the position of the foot and ankle in space.

ANTERIOR TIBIAL TENDON DISORDERS

The anterior tibial tendon originates along the anterolateral tibia and inserts onto the medial aspect of the first metatarsal and medial cuneiform. It functions concentrically during the swing phase of gait to dorsiflex the ankle and allow clearance of the foot. At heel strike, the tendon works in an eccentric manner to control the progression to the foot's flat position. The anterior tibial tendon also assists with inversion of the foot.

Rupture of the anterior tibial tendon is relatively uncommon, and most studies involved only a small number of patients.[1,2] A normal anterior tibial tendon rarely ruptures except as a result of a laceration or sudden trauma. Spontaneous rupture occurs secondary to a degenerative process, usually in men aged 50 to 70 years.[1] The causes of degeneration include impingement, inflammatory arthritis, diabetes mellitus, infection, chronic microtrauma, ischemia, hyperparathyroidism, systemic lupus erythematosus, gout, obesity, and oral or local steroid therapy.[3] The usual site of an anterior tibial tendon rupture is 0.5 to 3 cm proximal to its insertion, where the tendon passes under the inferior extensor retinaculum. Formerly, this location was thought to be a vascular watershed area within the tendon, but microvascular studies have not found such an area.[4]

As described in a 2021 study, anterior tibial tendon rupture appears in two forms.[5] In relatively young patients, an acute onset of symptoms occurs after penetrating injury or severe trauma; in patients older than 50 years, a moderately forceful plantar flexion stress can bring on symptoms. The second form is seen in relatively sedentary patients older than 50 years with a several-month history of atraumatic footdrop. The rupture may have a prodrome of swelling and pain, or it may follow a minor misstep or a twisting injury of the ankle. The signs and symptoms of the second form of anterior tibial tendon injury can be perplexing.[1] The injury may be masked by a rapid resolution of any initial pain followed by compensation by the other extensor muscles. As a result, the diagnosis of rupture often is missed or delayed.[3] Pain may be minimal after the initial episode and is not a major factor for many patients who seek treatment. A patient is likely to report a foot slap or unsteady gait, limping, or increased fatigue with walking. Some patients may experience persistent anterior ankle pain as the extensor tendons compensate for decreased dorsiflexion strength.

Physical examination findings include gait abnormalities such as a foot slap or footdrop. It may be possible to palpate the proximal residuum of the anterior tibial tendon as a mass along the anteromedial aspect of the ankle. Dorsiflexion of the ankle reveals eversion of the foot and a loss of tendon contour compared with the contralateral limb. Most patients are able to use the functioning tendons that remain for dorsiflexion, but careful testing will reveal a strength deficit in comparison with the contralateral limb. Increased extension at the metatarsophalangeal (MTP) joint of the toes may be observed as the extensor tendons attempt to compensate for loss of dorsiflexion power.

Both surgical and nonsurgical treatment strategies have been recommended, but the optimal treatment remains controversial. One study found no difference in outcomes after surgical or nonsurgical treatment.[6] The patients treated nonsurgically had an average age of 74 years and had low physical demands; most of the patients treated surgically had an average age of 55 years and were more physically active. The available research is primarily composed of case reports and small studies, most of which recommended early direct repair to restore function.[6-8] This procedure may be particularly beneficial for a relatively young, active patient with a traumatic injury to the tendon. Direct tendon repair may be possible within the first few months after injury.[3] The retracted tendon end usually becomes entrapped at the distal extent of the superior extensor retinaculum.[2,7] Direct repair can be performed end to end with a grasping stitch using a Krackow, Kessler, or Bunnell technique. If the tendon is avulsed off the insertion site, suture anchors or soft-tissue interference screws can be used for reattachment.

Late treatment after an atraumatic rupture should be individualized based on the patient's activity level. A patient with low physical demands or a significant medical comorbidity may benefit from nonsurgical treatment, as discussed in a 2020 systematic review.[9] The use of an ankle-foot orthosis can facilitate foot clearance during the swing phase of gait and decrease fatigue during prolonged ambulation. Some patients find brace treatment overly restrictive and opt not to use it.[3] In a delayed surgical procedure, end-to-end repair may not be feasible because of adhesions and lack of excursion of the tendon ends, and an interpositional graft is likely necessary. A variety of methods have been described for managing chronic ruptures, including Achilles tendon grafting or transfer of the extensor hallucis longus, extensor digitorum longus, plantaris, or peroneus tertius tendon.[2,3,7,8]

A retrospective review evaluated the results of surgical treatment of 19 anterior tibial tendon ruptures in 18 patients.[7] Eight tendons underwent early repair, and 11 underwent delayed repair, 7 underwent direct repair, and 12 required the use of an interpositional graft. The plantaris tertius tendon was most commonly used for grafting, followed by the extensor digitorum longus tendon. Patients in both the early repair group and the late repair group had significant improvement in American Orthopaedic Foot and Ankle Society scores. Manual testing revealed normal dorsiflexion strength in 15 of the 19 ankles. Tendon repair was recommended for all patients with an unsteady gait, weakness, or fatigability because of lack of dorsiflexion strength. Another retrospective review of 15 surgically treated anterior tibial tendon ruptures in 14 patients found significant improvement in postoperative American Orthopaedic Foot and Ankle Society and Medical Outcomes Study 36-Item Short Form scores.[8] Five tendons were repaired primarily, and 10 had a tendon transfer; 9 of the transfers used the extensor hallucis longus tendon. There was no difference in the outcomes of patients with a primary repair and those who required a tendon transfer. Strength testing using a dynamometer and comparison with the uninjured contralateral limb found deficits in dorsiflexion strength in all patients. A retrospective study of 11 patients with chronic anterior tibial tendon ruptures evaluated the use of allograft in those with greater than a 4-cm gap between tendon ends.[10] Significant improvements in strength, visual analog scale pain score, and functional outcome scores were noted. The study authors thought allografts offered the advantages of shorter surgical times, absence of donor site complications, and greater options in regard to size and types of grafts.

PERONEAL TENDON DISORDERS

The peroneal tendons originate as muscle bellies in the lateral compartment of the leg and become tendinous as they pass through a fibro-osseous tunnel posterior to the lateral malleolus. The peroneal tendons share a sheath that bifurcates at the level of the peroneal tubercle of the lateral calcaneus. The peroneus longus runs posterolateral to the peroneus brevis and turns sharply at the tip of the fibula, passing under the trochlear process of the calcaneus and along a groove in the plantar surface of the cuboid to insert on the plantar base of the first metatarsal. The peroneus brevis muscle belly is lower and lies between the posterior fibula and the peroneus longus tendon in the fibro-osseous tunnel before sharply turning under the tip of the fibula to insert on the fifth metatarsal base. The peroneal tendons function as the major evertors and pronators of the ankle. In addition, the peroneus longus plantarflexes the first metatarsal.

A typical peroneal tendon disorder is classified as peroneal tendinitis without subluxation of the tendons, peroneal tendinitis with subluxation of the peroneal tendons at the level of the superior retinaculum, or stenosing tenosynovitis of the peroneus longus in the area of the peroneal tubercle, os peroneum, or cuboid tunnel. Peroneal tendon injuries can be missed because they often occur in conjunction with a lateral ankle sprain or chronic ankle instability, with only vague symptoms along the lateral ankle.[11] A patient with an acute injury may report having twisted the ankle. Symptoms of subluxation can often be concealed by the pain and swelling associated with a lateral ankle sprain. Swelling posterior to the lateral malleolus occurs with peroneal instability, tearing, and synovitis. Symptoms of tenosynovitis can be brought on by a change in activity level. A patient with a dislocation often reports pain and a popping sensation along the lateral retromalleolar area.

A careful physical examination often is the most important step in making the appropriate diagnosis. Acute subluxation may present with ecchymosis posterior to the lateral malleolus, and it may be associated with tenderness over the insertion of the superior retinaculum. Pain and a sensation of instability in the lateral retromalleolar area can be reproduced with active eversion, dorsiflexion, or circumduction of the ankle.[12] Palpable snapping or crepitus may be evident during these maneuvers. Synovitic thickening appears to be the most reliable sign of a peroneal tendon tear.[13] Pain with forced plantar flexion and inversion may be seen with synovitis. Pain is not always present with a peroneal tendon tear, but it may be possible to elicit pain with resisted eversion. A tear may cause tenderness along the course of the tendon. A longitudinal tear can cause early fatigability without apparent weakness.[14] A peroneus longus tear can cause pain with resisted plantar flexion of the first metatarsal. A patient with suspected peroneal tendon pathology should undergo an assessment for concomitant ankle instability and evaluation of the alignment of the hindfoot. Varus alignment may be seen with long-standing peroneal tendon pathology or may be a precursor to it. An excessively valgus hindfoot may cause subfibular impingement because the tendons are compressed between the tip of the fibula and the calcaneus.

A plain radiograph may reveal an avulsion fracture of the lateral aspect of the distal fibula, which suggests a peroneal tendon subluxation. Hypertrophy of the peroneal tubercle suggests peroneal tendon impingement. Fracture or migration of the os peroneum proximal to the calcaneocuboid joint may indicate a peroneus longus tear. The role of MRI in the evaluation of peroneal tendon pathology is unclear. A normal peroneus brevis tendon can appear to be partially torn because of an increase in signal intensity on T1-weighted images (called the magic angle effect). Tendon subluxation may be difficult to detect on MRI, especially if the subluxation is intermittent. A study of MRI performed in 133 patients found that radiologists detected only 56% of the peroneus brevis tears present at surgery.[15] In 82 patients who underwent surgery for lateral ankle instability, the positive predictive value of MRI for peroneal tendons was 66.7%.[16] Overreliance on MRI was found to lead to unnecessary surgical procedures. A retrospective review of 294 magnetic resonance images obtained in individuals without any lateral ankle symptoms found that 35% of the studies were interpreted as having some peroneal tendon pathology.[17] As described in a 2022 study, in-office needle tendoscopy is currently being investigated in diagnosing and treating several peroneal tendon pathologies.[18]

PERONEAL TENDON SUBLUXATION

Acute peroneal tendon dislocation usually is associated with a traumatic event during an athletic activity involving rapid changes in direction. The mechanism of injury is somewhat controversial; both inversion and extreme dorsiflexion have been suggested as the ankle position at the time of injury. An eccentric contraction of the peroneal tendons against resistance causes avulsion of the superior peroneal retinaculum off the fibula, often with periosteum or a cortical bone fragment off the lateral aspect of the fibula. The periosteum is elevated, creating a pouch in which the dislocated tendons sit.

The onset of chronic peroneal tendon subluxation usually is insidious and occurs after an untreated acute dislocation or a long-standing brevis or longus tear.[12] Recurrent subluxation from behind the lateral malleolus attenuates the superior retinaculum and often is associated with a split tear of the peroneus brevis tendon as it is caught between the fibrocartilaginous rim and the peroneus longus tendon. Often there is associated tenosynovitis.

Acute peroneal tendon dislocation that spontaneously reduces can be managed with immobilization. The reported success rate of nonsurgical treatment is approximately 50%.[19] Relatively young patients with high physical demands are treated surgically. Recurrent subluxation of the peroneal tendons can be associated with longitudinal tearing in the peroneus brevis, which should be repaired during the instability surgery. Surgical treatment options for peroneal tendon subluxation include reconstruction of the superior peroneal retinaculum, rerouting of the tendons under the calcaneofibular ligament, reconstruction of the retinaculum with a portion of the Achilles tendon, and a groove-deepening procedure. An isolated repair or reconstruction of the retinaculum is ideal for an acute dislocation in which the tissue is unlikely to be compromised.[19] In chronic dislocation, compromised retinacular tissue may require augmentation of the retinaculum with additional tissue or routing of the tendon under the calcaneofibular ligament.

The retromalleolar groove, in which the tendons rest, usually is concave, but it is flat or convex in 10% to 20% of patients.[20] The flat or convex shape contributes to peroneal tendon instability, and a groove-deepening procedure is considered if the patient has a flat or convex configuration of the posterior fibula. The extent of impaction or deepening is adjusted until it is sufficient to prevent dislocation of the tendons with ankle manipulation. A variety of techniques have been described. One technique uses tendoscopy to deepen the groove.[12] Seven patients with peroneal dislocation had the retromalleolar groove deepened with a burr and tendoscopy. Four patients had detachment of the superior retinaculum at the site of the fibular insertion, but surgical repair was not attempted. At an average 15.4-month follow-up, none of the patients had recurrent subluxation, and five reported an excellent outcome. Although the procedure was supposed to lead to less morbidity and more rapid recovery than an open procedure, the study included no control group for comparison.

Recent research has questioned the association between groove morphology and peroneal subluxation.[20-22] A retrospective MRI study of 39 ankles after surgical treatment of peroneal tendon dislocation classified the shape of the retromalleolar groove as concave, convex, or flat.[22] No significant difference was found on MRI between the treated ankles and 39 ankles without peroneal tendon dislocation. The superior peroneal retinaculum inserts into a fibrocartilaginous rim on the posterolateral fibula, which helps to deepen the retromalleolar groove, and the study authors suggested that this rim has a significant role in stabilizing the tendons. A cadaver study found that the peroneal tunnel has two components: an osseous component is formed by the retromalleolar groove, and

Chapter 24: Sports-Related Injuries of the Foot and Ankle

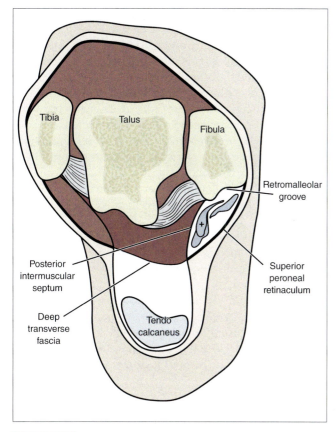

FIGURE 1 Illustration showing a horizontal section through the superior peroneal tunnel. The boundaries of the tunnel are the superior peroneal retinaculum, the retromalleolar groove, and the posterior intermuscular septum. (Redrawn with permission from Athavale SA, Vangara SV: Anatomy of the superior peroneal tunnel. *J Bone Joint Surg Am* 2011;93[6]:564-571.)

a medial soft-tissue component is formed by the posterior intermuscular septum of the leg[21] (**Figure 1**). The study concluded that the retromalleolar groove is shallow and unable to accommodate the peroneal tendons and suggested that splitting the soft-tissue component may be as effective as groove deepening. Another study prospectively compared peroneal tendon stabilization with and without fibular groove deepening. It was a consecutive series of 29 patients where 13 patients had groove deepening and 16 did not. The study authors found no significant difference in the outcome between the two groups and noted those without groove deepening had significantly decreased surgical time and the procedure was easier.[23] A healthcare database review concluded that soft-tissue procedures offer a satisfactory method of managing peroneal tendon dislocation without increased risk of revision surgery when compared with osteotomy techniques.[24] A 2023 systematic review that evaluated 25 studies showed that inferior results were demonstrated for bony procedures and rerouting procedures.[25]

PERONEAL TENOSYNOVITIS

Peroneal tenosynovitis, also called peritendinitis, usually results from repetitive or prolonged activity or from trauma to the peroneal tendons. Peroneal tenosynovitis may be the result of stenosis of the synovial sheath, which can occur in the presence of a hypertrophied peroneal tubercle or other anatomic factors as a cavovarus foot, osseous calcaneal tunnel, the presence of a peroneus quadratus muscle, or an incompetent superior peroneal retinaculum. Tenosynovitis usually occurs at a location where the tendon changes direction, such as behind the lateral malleolus, at the trochlear process, or under the cuboid. Tenosynovitis can be exacerbated by the presence of a space-occupying structure such as a low-lying peroneus brevis muscle belly or peroneus quartus tendon.

The initial treatment often is nonsurgical and may include activity modification, NSAIDs, physical therapy, a lateral wedge orthotic device, or an ankle brace. If the condition does not improve, short-term immobilization with a boot or a short leg cast can be considered. A 2019 study of 96 patients with peroneal tendinopathy, tears, or subluxation demonstrated that after an ultrasound-guided corticosteroid injection, only 25% of patients needed surgery.[26] Nonsurgical treatment is effective in most patients, but surgical treatment may be indicated if nonsurgical treatment is unsuccessful. Surgical treatment involves débridement of inflamed tenosynovium, release of any areas of stenosis or compression around the tendon, removal of any space-occupying structures such as a low-lying peroneus brevis muscle belly or peroneus quartus tendon, and repair or débridement of pathologic tendon. In addition, any associated ankle or tendon instability or hindfoot malalignment should be corrected.

PERONEAL TENDON TEARS

Peroneal tendon tears may be associated with chronic ankle instability, peroneal tendon subluxation or dislocation, cavovarus hindfoot, a prominent peroneal tubercle, or an accessory tendon. These tears are thought to be caused by acute or repetitive mechanical trauma. Peroneus brevis tears are reported to be more common than peroneus longus tears.[11] Peroneus brevis tears most often occur at the distal portion of the lateral malleolus, where the peroneus longus tendon compresses the peroneus brevis tendon against the lateral malleolus.[19]

In the absence of an acute rupture, usually the treatment is nonsurgical and of 2 to 6 months' duration.[14] In a cadaver study of partial acute peroneal tendon tears, 33% of peroneal tendons could resist supraphysiologic loads.[27] If surgical treatment is indicated, it is important to recognize that peroneal tendon injuries can be associated with other injuries, such as chronic ankle instability. All 30 patients who had arthroscopic evaluation of the ankle at the same time as peroneal tendon repair were found to have intra-articular pathology.[11] Extensive scar tissue was the most common diagnosis, followed by synovitis and soft-tissue impingement. The absence of a comparison group in this study makes it difficult to determine the true benefit of arthroscopy.

Peroneal tendon tears typically are longitudinal rather than transverse, although transverse tears can occur.[13] The low-lying muscle belly of the peroneus brevis has been implicated as a contributor to peroneal tendon tears. A study of 115 cadaver specimens found that peroneus brevis tears were more common if the peroneus musculotendinous junction was relatively proximal.[28] The traditional recommendation is for débridement and tubularization of tears involving less than 50% of the tendon diameter and for débridement and tenodesis of larger tears.[13] A retrospective study of 18 patients who underwent débridement and primary repair reported that 17 patients returned to full sports activity without limitations.[29] A retrospective study of 71 patients who underwent primary repair of the peroneus brevis tears showed that 83% were able to return to regular exercise and sports at final follow-up and 91% would undergo the same procedure again.[30] If one of the peroneal tendons has tears involving greater than 50% of the diameter and the other is relatively intact, then débridement of the unhealthy segment and tenodesis to the healthy tendon has been recommended.[13] A cadaver study has questioned this recommendation.[31] It evaluated allograft versus tenodesis for irreparable peroneus brevis tears and found allograft to be superior in regard to restoration of peroneus brevis tension. Currently, there are no clinical studies comparing allograft reconstruction with tenodesis.

An algorithm for the management of peroneal tendon tears has been suggested[32] (**Figure 2**). Rupture of both tendons is less common and may present additional challenges for reconstruction (**Figure 3**). Factors such as the presence of deformity (typically varus), quality of the tissue bed, and viability of the muscle unit must be taken into consideration and addressed. If the deformity is flexible, orthotic management may be adequate; otherwise, osteotomy may be needed. The presence of excursion of the residual proximal tendon has been used as an indicator that the muscle unit is still functional.[32]

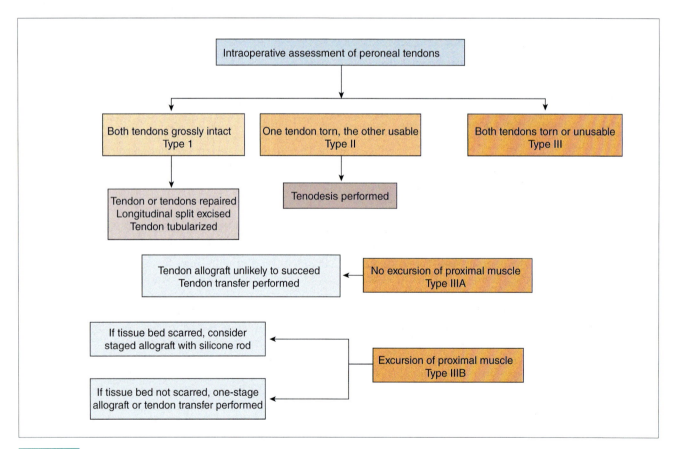

FIGURE 2 Algorithm for the surgical repair of peroneal tendon tears. (Redrawn with permission from Redfern D, Myerson M: The management of concomitant tears of the peroneus longus and brevis tendons. *Foot Ankle Int* 2004;25:697-707.)

Chapter 24: Sports-Related Injuries of the Foot and Ankle

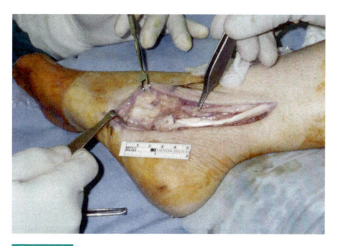

FIGURE 3 Intraoperative photograph showing ruptured peroneus longus and peroneus brevis tendons. The tendon ends are retracted, with gapping between the ends.

chronic concomitant peroneal ruptures with good results in six of seven patients.[38]

STRESS FRACTURES OF THE FOOT AND ANKLE

Athletes in training are susceptible to overuse injuries of the foot and ankle, including stress fracture. A stress fracture is distinguished from a traumatic fracture by its origin in repetitive, cumulative stress rather than in a single traumatic event. The most common sites of stress fracture in the foot and ankle are the distal tibia, malleoli, navicular, metatarsals, and sesamoids.[39]

Patient History and Physical Examination

The clinician should seek clues in the patient history that suggest a stress fracture. A change in the character, duration, or intensity of training is a major risk factor for stress fracture in athletes. Examples include the addition of hills or sprints for a jogger or a rapid increase in mileage for a distance runner. Similarly, an important change in shoewear, such as an abrupt switch to a minimalist-type running shoe, should raise the examiner's suspicion for a stress fracture.[40] A case-control study of 37 athletes (18 with zone 2 or zone 3 fifth metatarsal fractures and 19 control patients) clearly identified vitamin D deficiency as an independent risk factor for fifth metatarsal fracture.[41] The physician should ask whether the patient has a history of osteoporosis or osteopenia and obtain a baseline 25-hydroxy vitamin D level if stress fracture is strongly suspected.[42]

The character of the pain caused by a stress fracture experiences variable. Some patients experience pain primarily during training and are relatively pain free during activities of daily living. The symptoms may have been present for several weeks to months. This type of pain suggests a slowly evolving stress fracture. Early in the process, focal tenderness to palpation may be minimal, and the patient must run or jump to reproduce the symptoms.

Some patients describe mild prodromal symptoms that have become acutely worse during training. Often these patients have pain with activities of daily living or may be unable to tolerate any weight bearing. Palpation of the affected bone reliably reproduces the pain. This level of pain suggests a complete stress fracture.

In addition to the location of tenderness, the examiner should look for evidence of malalignment, which can predispose an individual to stress fracture. For example, fibular stress fracture may be associated with hindfoot valgus. More commonly, cavovarus malalignment is associated with medial malleolar or fifth metatarsal stress fracture. A plantarflexed first ray, as often is present in cavovarus malalignment, can have a role in

Some authors have found this determination difficult to make intraoperatively.[33] The proximal extension of MRI above the ankle to evaluate for fatty infiltration of the peroneal muscle may be a way to assess muscle function.[34] In the presence of a functioning muscle unit, graft reconstruction of the tendon can be performed. Good results have been reported with the use of allograft in a small series of 14 patients.[35]

In the absence of functioning muscle units, a tendon transfer may be indicated. One study in which eight patients with concomitant tears of both tendons were treated with a single-stage flexor digitorum longus (FDL) or flexor hallucis longus (FHL) transfer found significant postoperative improvement in functional outcome and pain scores; seven patients rated their outcome as excellent.[36] The study authors concluded that, although both transfers were successful, the FHL transfer provided greater strength and a better outcome. This finding is consistent with that of a study to compare the relative strength of the calf muscles; the FHL transfer was found to be stronger than the peroneus longus or peroneus brevis transfer and much stronger than the FDL transfer.[37] Another study reported outcomes in nine patients who underwent either FHL or FDL tendon transfer for concomitant tears of both tendons.[33] All patients were satisfied with the procedure and demonstrated at least 4/5 eversion strength and returned to the desired activity. Testing did reveal that eversion peak force and power were reduced by greater than 55% compared with the normal extremity. The study authors also recommended the use of FHL tendon to avoid injuries to the tibial neurovascular bundle seen with FDL transfer. In cases where the tissue bed is significantly scarred, a staged procedure in which a Hunter rod placement is followed by FHL tendon transfer 3 months later has been used for sesamoid stress fracture. Identifying these predisposing factors early in the treatment increases the likelihood of a successful outcome.

Radiographic Evaluation

It is critical to understand that radiographs may be negative during the early stages of a stress fracture. Follow-up radiographs 2 to 4 weeks after treatment is initiated generally are more revealing. If a stress fracture is present, the follow-up radiographs will show early callus formation and periosteal reaction consistent with initial bone healing (**Figure 4**). However, if the follow-up radiographs remain negative for fracture, another diagnosis should be considered, or more sophisticated imaging studies should be performed. MRI is particularly useful because it can show intraosseous edema consistent with stress reaction in a bone before progression to a radiographically detectable stress fracture.

Treatment

Most stress fractures about the foot and ankle can be successfully managed with a combination of relative rest, activity modification, immobilization, and restricted weight bearing. Immobilization in a prefabricated fracture boot and the use of crutches usually are successful for treating the initial pain while maintaining an acceptable level of function and fitness. If the patient's vitamin D level is found to be low, supplementation with 50,000 IU weekly is initiated.[42] In general, symptoms substantially improve 3 to 4 weeks after initiation of treatment. The use of the fracture boot can be gradually discontinued at this time, and a low-impact aerobic program can be initiated. For most fractures, clinical healing is achieved at 6 to 8 weeks, when a cautious return to a sports rehabilitation program can be started. As activity is resumed, it is critical to correct any training errors that may have precipitated the stress fracture. If malalignment is thought to have played a role in the development of the stress injury, appropriate shoe inserts should be prescribed. A patient with a sesamoid stress fracture benefits from wearing a shoe insert that incorporates relief beneath the first metatarsal head. A full return to sports generally requires 3 to 6 months of recovery, depending on the severity of the fracture and the specific physical demands of the sport.

Although nonsurgical management is indicated for most stress fractures of the foot and ankle, surgical intervention should be considered in specific situations. The most difficult-to-treat stress fractures in the foot and ankle are those of the medial malleolus, navicular, fifth metatarsal, and sesamoid bones.[39] These fractures have a relatively high risk of delayed healing or nonunion. In addition, the prolonged period of immobilization and restricted weight bearing necessary for successful nonsurgical treatment of these injuries often is poorly tolerated by athletic patients.

Stress fracture of the medial malleolus or navicular involves the ankle or talonavicular joint, respectively, and warrants consideration of early surgical treatment. CT is used to accurately assess fracture completeness and displacement. A complete and/or displaced fracture should be managed surgically. Because most medial malleolar stress fractures are vertically oriented, they are best treated with compression screws and buttress plating. Débridement of the fracture and/or bone grafting may be necessary for a chronic injury, particularly if sclerosis or cystic change is noted on preoperative CT.

Navicular stress fractures are stabilized with compression lag screws. Because the fracture line typically is lateral, screws must be placed from lateral to medial to achieve adequate purchase and stability (**Figure 5**). An investigation into the intraosseous blood supply of the navicular challenged the traditional belief that the fracture line corresponds to a relatively avascular portion of the navicular.[43] If preoperative CT reveals substantial diastasis, displacement, cystic change, or sclerosis, open reduction and internal fixation through a dorsal approach is required, with liberal use of bone graft. A systematic literature review questioned the need for aggressive surgical treatment of navicular stress fractures.[44] No evidence was found to indicate that surgical treatment was superior over nonsurgical treatment without weight bearing; both treatment options were more successful than nonsurgical treatment with permitted weight bearing.

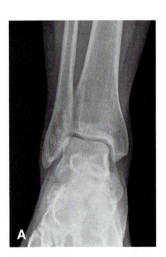 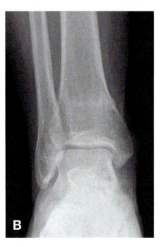

FIGURE 4 Radiographs from a patient with acute distal leg pain after running. **A**, Initial AP ankle radiograph showing no abnormality. The patient was found to have vitamin D deficiency and was treated with restricted weight bearing and vitamin D supplementation. **B**, Follow-up AP ankle radiograph after 3 weeks of restricted weight bearing showing evidence of bone reaction consistent with a healing metaphyseal stress fracture.

Chapter 24: Sports-Related Injuries of the Foot and Ankle

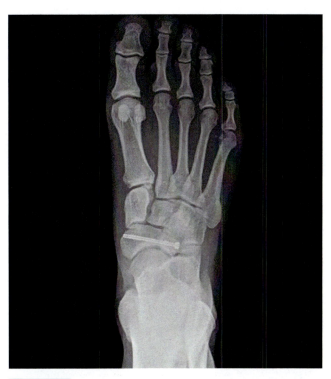

FIGURE 5 Postoperative AP radiograph of the foot showing a navicular stress fracture managed using lateral-to-medial lag screw.

Indications for surgical management of a fifth metatarsal stress fracture include nonunion or delayed union as well as a desire to facilitate healing while minimizing the need for casting. A fifth metatarsal stress fracture is managed using the same intramedullary screw technique as for an acute Jones fracture. Intramedullary or extramedullary bone grafting can be considered for a chronic fracture with substantial sclerosis. However, bone grafting was found to be unnecessary in most fractures, even with a nonunion.[45] A sesamoid stress fracture can be managed with open reduction and internal fixation, partial excision, or complete excision, depending on the size of the fragments, the chronicity of the fracture, and the presence of avascular changes.

MIDFOOT SPRAINS

Injuries of the tarsometatarsal joint complex range in severity from a mild sprain to a severe crush injury. Although a midfoot sprain lies on the less severe end of the spectrum, this injury has the potential to render the midfoot unstable and cause lingering morbidity in an athlete.

Soccer and football players are particularly susceptible to a midfoot sprain because of the high-intensity sprinting, jumping, and cutting maneuvers involved in these sports. The mechanism of injury usually involves a dorsally directed abduction force applied to the plantarflexed foot, resulting in an awkward twisting motion. Particularly in football, another player may fall onto the back of the foot and ankle, again causing a dorsiflexion-abduction force to be applied to the foot. In either scenario, the indirect force exerted on the foot produces injury of variable severity to the osseoligamentous structure of the midfoot. The ligamentous stability of the tarsometatarsal joint complex primarily is provided by the stout plantar ligaments, including the interosseous Lisfranc ligament that connects the medial cuneiform to the base of the second metatarsal. In a mild midfoot sprain, the relatively weak dorsal ligaments may be injured, producing pain but no subluxation or loss of stability. In a more severe sprain, injury to both the dorsal and plantar ligaments leads to tarsometatarsal joint subluxation and instability.

Patient History and Physical Examination

An athlete with a midfoot sprain has pain primarily on the dorsum of the midfoot. If the patient also reports significant pain in the lateral midfoot, the possibility of an associated cuboid fracture should be considered. Swelling, tenderness, and ecchymosis tend to occur dorsally over the midfoot. The presence of plantar midfoot ecchymosis particularly suggests a significant ligament injury to the tarsometatarsal joint complex. Dorsoplantar stressing of the metatarsals also may reproduce pain. Weight bearing may be difficult or impossible.

Radiographic Evaluation

No radiographic abnormalities are seen with a ligamentously stable midfoot sprain. On an AP radiograph of the foot, there is no widening between the medial cuneiform and the base of the second metatarsal, and the medial cortex of the second metatarsal base is collinear with the medial cortex of the middle cuneiform. On an oblique radiograph, the medial cortex of the fourth metatarsal is aligned with the medial border of the cuboid. The lateral radiograph also should show the dorsal cortices of the first and second metatarsals aligned with their respective cuneiforms. Widening of the Lisfranc joint, a fleck sign adjacent to the second metatarsal base, and/or lateral or dorsal subluxation of the tarsometatarsal joints are each diagnostic of an unstable midfoot sprain.

Good-quality weight-bearing radiographs are essential. Obtaining weight-bearing radiographs can be particularly challenging after an acute injury, when weight bearing may be extremely painful, but non–weight-bearing radiographs are insufficiently sensitive for showing the subtle subluxations that can occur after a midfoot sprain.

A combined cadaver and clinical study demonstrated that the Lisfranc ligament is well imaged along its entire course in a single slice on magnetic resonance images.[46] If plain radiographs are inconclusive, MRI should be considered. MRI can demonstrate the integrity or failure of the ligaments and, in cases of chronic injury, can demonstrate healing of torn ligaments. Moreover, a high correlation was found between MRI and surgical findings after a suspected midfoot injury.[47] Weight-bearing CT provides even greater osseous detail than MRI. Small avulsion fracture and subtle subluxation about the midfoot can be readily seen on CT. If static imaging studies are equivocal, stress fluoroscopy under local or general anesthesia can be used to assess the stability of the tarsometatarsal joint complex.

Treatment

The management of a midfoot sprain is dictated by the severity of the ligamentous injury. A dorsal sprain without instability or subluxation is treated nonsurgically with 4 to 6 weeks of immobilization in a cast or prefabricated boot and restricted weight bearing. As symptoms improve, weight bearing is begun with the use of a fracture boot for protection and support. For an athlete, a semirigid custom orthotic device subsequently can be used to facilitate the transition to regular shoes and resumption of activity. Return to sports typically is achieved 3 to 6 months after injury.

Unstable midfoot sprains, defined by the presence of any detectable subluxation, are treated surgically. The options for surgical treatment include open reduction and internal fixation as well as primary tarsometatarsal joint fusion. Prospective randomized studies found superior outcomes after primary fusion for primarily ligamentous midfoot injuries.[48,49] The benefits of primary fusion include reliable bony healing, decreased need for hardware removal, and decreased incidence of posttraumatic arthritis.

Open reduction and internal fixation remains a viable alternative for athletes who want to return to competitive sports. Although flexibility of the tarsometatarsal joints is widely thought to be expendable, the putative benefits of open reduction and internal fixation include preservation of joint motion with improved balance, proprioception, and athletic performance. The traditional implants are transarticular metal screws. To avoid iatrogenic joint damage associated with transarticular screws, some surgeons have also begun to use joint-spanning plates and staples to stabilize the tarsometatarsal joint complex (**Figure 6**). These devices are also useful if the bone is osteoporotic or associated fractures compromise traditional screw fixation. After anatomic reduction and screw fixation, immobilization without weight bearing is required for 6 to 8 weeks, with gradual resumption of protected weight bearing in a prefabricated boot. Hardware generally is removed 3 to 6 months after surgery and before initiation of a rehabilitation program. Return to sports after surgical treatment of an unstable midfoot sprain generally is achieved within 6 to 12 months.

Nonabsorbable suture button devices have been used for fixation of unstable Lisfranc joint injuries.[50] The proposed benefits of suture stabilization include flexible fixation, which may allow an earlier return to weight bearing with a decreased risk of implant failure, as well as avoidance of routine hardware removal. Additional clinical studies are needed to evaluate the success of these implants in managing unstable midfoot injuries.

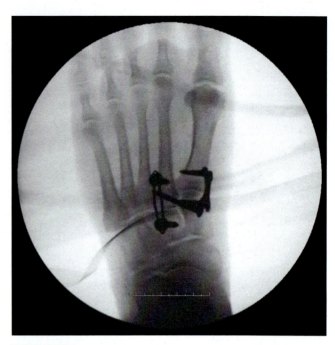

FIGURE 6 Intraoperative fluoroscopic image showing a midfoot sprain managed with a plate spanning the first tarsometatarsal joint and a staple spanning the second tarsometatarsal joint. The Lisfranc joint was stabilized with a lag screw.

SUMMARY

The foot and ankle are often injured during athletic activities, and acute or chronic ankle ligament injury can severely affect athletic performance and participation. Patients with these injuries can be challenging to treat, especially high-level athletes for whom a rapid return to peak performance is of paramount importance. The initial treatment of an acute injury generally is nonsurgical. Midfoot sprains, which can cause significant disability in athletes, range from a mild sprain to a severe crush injury. Treatment of a midfoot sprain depends on its severity; a stable sprain is treated with immobilization and avoidance of weight bearing, and an unstable strain is treated surgically. Stress fractures are most common in the distal tibia, malleoli, navicular, and metatarsals. Most stress fractures of the foot and ankle can be successfully treated using a combination of relative rest, activity modification, immobilization, and restricted weight bearing. A stress fracture of the medial malleolus and navicular has a relatively high risk of nonunion and requires lengthy immobilization for healing. Surgical treatment may be preferred in a high-performance athlete.

KEY STUDY POINTS

- Management of midfoot sprains depends on severity: a stable sprain is managed with immobilization and avoidance of weight bearing, and an unstable strain is managed surgically.
- Stress fractures of the foot and ankle are often associated with vitamin D deficiency. Most of these injuries can be successfully managed using a combination of activity modification, immobilization, and restricted weight bearing.
- Traumatic anterior tibial tendon ruptures in young patients should be repaired. Atraumatic ruptures in sedentary patients can be treated nonsurgically and those in active patients may require the use of a graft.
- Techniques for peroneal tendon repair depend on the degree of tendon involvement, the presence of associated deformity, quality of the tissue bed, and viability of the muscle unit.

ANNOTATED REFERENCES

1. Khoury NJ, el-Khoury GY, Saltzman CL, Brandser EA: Rupture of the anterior tibial tendon: Diagnosis by MR imaging. *AJR Am J Roentgenol* 1996;167(2):351-354.

2. Tucker S, Sammarco GJ, Sammarco VJ: Surgical repair of tibialis anterior tendon rupture. *Tech Foot Ankle Surg* 2012;11:39-44.

3. Ouzounian TJ, Anderson R: Anterior tibial tendon rupture. *Foot Ankle Int* 1995;16(7):406-410.

4. Geppert MJ, Sobel M, Hannafin JA: Microvasculature of the tibialis anterior tendon. *Foot Ankle* 1993;14(5):261-264.

5. Levitsky MM, Freibott CE, Greisberg JK, Vosseller JT: Risk factors for anterior tibial tendon pathology. *Foot Ankle Int* 2021;42(3):329-332.

   Traumatic ruptures tend to occur in younger patients, whereas older patients are more likely to suffer atraumatic ruptures. Level of evidence: II.

6. Markarian GG, Kelikian AS, Brage M, Trainor T, Dias L: Anterior tibialis tendon ruptures: An outcome analysis of operative versus nonoperative treatment. *Foot Ankle Int* 1998;19(12):792-802.

7. Sammarco VJ, Sammarco GJ, Henning C, Chaim S: Surgical repair of acute and chronic tibialis anterior tendon ruptures. *J Bone Joint Surg Am* 2009;91(2):325-332.

8. Ellington JK, McCormick J, Marion C, et al: Surgical outcome following tibialis anterior tendon repair. *Foot Ankle Int* 2010;31(5):412-417.

9. McHale S, Williams M, Ball T: Retrospective cohort study of operatively treated ankle fractures involving the posterior malleolus. *Foot Ankle Surg* 2020;26(2):138-145.

   Patients with fragments >10% have an intra-articular injury. They recommend direct anatomic reduction and rigid internal fixation. Level of evidence: III.

10. Huh J, Boyette D, Parekh S, Nunley J: Allograft reconstruction of chronic tibialis anterior tendon ruptures. *Foot Ankle Int* 2015;36(10):1180-1189.

11. Bare A, Ferkel RD: Peroneal tendon tears: Associated arthroscopic findings and results after repair. *Arthroscopy* 2009;25(11):1288-1297.

12. Vega J, Batista JP, Golanó P, Dalmau A, Viladot R: Tendoscopic groove deepening for chronic subluxation of the peroneal tendons. *Foot Ankle Int* 2013;34(6):832-840.

13. Krause JO, Brodsky JW: Peroneus brevis tendon tears: Pathophysiology, surgical reconstruction, and clinical results. *Foot Ankle Int* 1998;19(5):271-279.

14. Crates J, Barber FA: Treatment of longitudinal mid-substance tears of peroneal tendons. *Curr Orthop Pract* 2012;23(2):86-90.

15. O'Neill PJ, Van Aman SE, Guyton GP: Is MRI adequate to detect lesions in patients with ankle instability? *Clin Orthop Relat Res* 2010;468(4):1115-1119.

16. Park HJ, Cha SD, Kim HS, et al: Reliability of MRI findings of peroneal tendinopathy in patients with lateral chronic ankle instability. *Clin Orthop Surg* 2010;2(4):237-243.

17. O'Neil J, Pedowitz D, Kerbel Y, Codding JL, Zoga AC, Raikin SM: Peroneal tendon abnormalities on routine magnetic resonance imaging of the foot and ankle. *Foot Ankle Int* 2016;37(7):743-747.

18. Kanakamedala A, Chen JS, Kaplan DJ, et al: In-office needle tendoscopy of the peroneal tendons. *Arthrosc Tech* 2022;11(3):e365-e371.

In-office needle tendoscopy can be used for the diagnosis and treatment of several peroneal tendon pathologies including peroneal tendon tendinopathy, tears, and instability. Level of evidence: V.

19. Philbin TM, Landis GS, Smith B: Peroneal tendon injuries. *J Am Acad Orthop Surg* 2009;17(5):306-317.

20. Grear B, Richardson D: Morphology of the malleolar fibular groove: Implications in peroneal tendon pathology. *Curr Orthop Pract* 2012;23(2):91-93.

21. Athavale SA, Swathi, Vangara SV: Anatomy of the superior peroneal tunnel. *J Bone Joint Surg Am* 2011;93(6):564-571.

22. Adachi N, Fukuhara K, Kobayashi T, Nakasa T, Ochi M: Morphologic variations of the fibular malleolar groove with recurrent dislocation of the peroneal tendons. *Foot Ankle Int* 2009;30(6):540-544.

23. Cho J, Kim J, Song D, Lee W: Comparison of outcome after retinaculum repair with and without fibular groove deepening for recurrent dislocation of the peroneal tendons. *Foot Ankle Int* 2014;35(7):683-689.

24. Yasui Y, Vig K, Tonogai I, et al: Incidence of reoperation and wound dehiscence in patients treated for peroneal tendon dislocations: Comparison between osteotomy versus soft tissue procedures. *Knee Surg Sports Traumatol Arthrosc* 2018;26(3):897-902.

25. Lootsma J, Wuite S, Hoekstra H, Matricali GA: Surgical treatment options for chronic instability of the peroneal tendons: A systematic review and proportional meta-analysis. *Arch Orthop Trauma Surg* 2023;143(4):1903-1913.

    Surgical treatment results in excellent clinical and functional outcomes in patients with chronic peroneal instability. More inferior results were demonstrated for rerouting and bony procedures. Level of evidence: III.

26. Fram BR, Rogero R, Fuchs D, Shakked RJ, Raikin SM, Pedowitz DI: Clinical outcomes and complications of peroneal tendon sheath ultrasound-guided corticosteroid injection. *Foot Ankle Int* 2019;40(8):888-894.

    US-guided PTS corticosteroid injection was safe and relatively effective in patients with symptomatic peroneal tendon tears or tendinopathy, including those who had undergone prior surgery. Level of evidence: IV.

27. Wagner E, Wagner P, Ortiz C, Radkievich R, Palma F, Guzmán-Venegas R: Biomechanical cadaveric evaluation of partial acute peroneal tendon tears. *Foot Ankle Int* 2018;39(6):741-745.

28. Unlu MC, Bilgili M, Akgun I, Kaynak G, Ogut T, Uzun I: Abnormal proximal musculotendinous junction of the peroneus brevis muscle as a cause of peroneus brevis tendon tears: A cadaveric study. *J Foot Ankle Surg* 2010;49(6):537-540.

29. Demetracopoulos C, Vineyard J, Kiesau C, Nunley J: Long term results of debridement and primary repair of peroneal tendon tears. *Foot Ankle Int* 2014;35(3):252-257.

30. Steginsky B, Riley A, Lucas D, Philbin T, Berlet G: Patient reported outcomes and return to activity after peroneus brevis repair. *Foot Ankle Int* 2016;37(2):178-185.

31. Pellegrini M, Glisson R, Matsumoto T, et al: Effectiveness of allograft reconstruction vs tenodesis for irreparable peroneus brevis tears: A cadaveric model. *Foot Ankle Int* 2016;37(8):803-808.

32. Redfern D, Myerson M: The management of concomitant tears of the peroneus longus and brevis tendons. *Foot Ankle Int* 2004;25(10):695-707.

33. Seybold J, Campbell J, Jeng C, Short K, Myerson M: Outcome of lateral transfer of the FHL or FDL for concomitant peroneal tendon tears. *Foot Ankle Int* 2016;37(6):576-581.

34. Hamid K, Amendola A: Chronic rupture of the peroneal tendons. *Foot Ankle Clin* 2017;22(4):843-850.

35. Mook W, Parekh S, Nunley J: Allograft reconstruction of peroneal tendons: Operative technique and clinical outcomes. *Foot Ankle Int* 2013;34(9):1212-1220.

36. Jockel JR, Brodsky JW: Single-stage flexor tendon transfer for the treatment of severe concomitant peroneus longus and brevis tendon tears. *Foot Ankle Int* 2013;34(5):666-672.

37. Jeng CL, Thawait GK, Kwon JY, et al: Relative strengths of the calf muscles based on MRI volume measurements. *Foot Ankle Int* 2012;33(5):394-399.

38. Wapner KL, Taras JS, Lin SS, Chao W: Staged reconstruction for chronic rupture of both peroneal tendons using Hunter rod and flexor hallucis longus tendon transfer: A long-term followup study. *Foot Ankle Int* 2006;27(8):591-597.

39. Shindle MK, Endo Y, Warren RF, et al: Stress fractures about the tibia, foot, and ankle. *J Am Acad Orthop Surg* 2012;20(3):167-176.

40. Salzler MJ, Bluman EM, Noonan S, Chiodo CP, de Asla RJ: Injuries observed in minimalist runners. *Foot Ankle Int* 2012;33(4):262-266.

41. Shimasaki Y, Nagao M, Miyamori T, et al: Evaluating the risk of a fifth metatarsal stress fracture by measuring the serum 25-hydroxy vitamin D levels. *Foot Ankle Int* 2016;37(3):307-311.

42. McCabe MP, Smyth MP, Richardson DR: Current concept review: Vitamin D and stress fractures. *Foot Ankle Int* 2012;33(6):526-533.

43. McKeon KE, McCormick JJ, Johnson JE, Klein SE: Intraosseous and extraosseous arterial anatomy of the adult navicular. *Foot Ankle Int* 2012;33(10):857-861.

44. Torg JS, Moyer J, Gaughan JP, Boden BP: Management of tarsal navicular stress fractures: Conservative versus surgical treatment. A meta-analysis. *Am J Sports Med* 2010;38(5):1048-1053.

45. Habbu RA, Marsh RS, Anderson JG, Bohay DR: Closed intramedullary screw fixation for nonunion of fifth metatarsal Jones fracture. *Foot Ankle Int* 2011;32(6):603-608.

46. Kitsukawa K, Hirano T, Niki H, Tachizawa N, Nakajima Y, Hirata K: MR imaging evaluation of the Lisfranc ligament in cadaveric feet and patients with acute to chronic Lisfranc injury. *Foot Ankle Int* 2015;36(12):1483-1492.

47. Raikin SM, Elias I, Dheer S, Besser MP, Morrison WB, Zoga AC: Prediction of midfoot instability in the subtle Lisfranc injury: Comparison of magnetic resonance imaging with intraoperative findings. *J Bone Joint Surg Am* 2009;91(4):892-899.

48. Ly TV, Coetzee JC: Treatment of primarily ligamentous Lisfranc joint injuries: Primary arthrodesis compared with open reduction and internal fixation. A prospective, randomized study. *J Bone Joint Surg Am* 2006;88(3):514-520.

49. Henning JA, Jones CB, Sietsema DL, Bohay DR, Anderson JG: Open reduction internal fixation versus primary arthrodesis for Lisfranc injuries: A prospective randomized study. *Foot Ankle Int* 2009;30(10):913-922.

50. Panchbhavi VK, Vallurupalli S, Yang J, Andersen CR: Screw fixation compared with suture-button fixation of isolated Lisfranc ligament injuries. *J Bone Joint Surg Am* 2009;91(5):1143-1148.

CHAPTER 25

Ankle Ligament Injuries

CHIRAG S. PATEL, MD, FAAOS

ABSTRACT

The foot and ankle are often injured during athletic activities. Even when appropriately managed, such injuries can progress to become chronic conditions affecting both sports participation and routine activity. The most common athletic injury to the ankle is an acute sprain of the lateral ankle ligament complex. The initial treatment of an acute lateral ankle sprain is a combination of walking boot immobilization, functional brace treatment, and neuromuscular rehabilitation. Chronic ankle instability can also be debilitating to the athlete and is initially managed nonsurgically, but often ultimately requires surgical intervention. Assessing and correcting deformity of the hindfoot, in addition to ligament reconstruction, is necessary to optimize results. Acute syndesmotic ankle sprains are typically more severe than lateral ankle sprains and require longer treatment before return to sport. High-grade injuries require immediate surgical reduction and stabilization. Deltoid ligament injuries usually occur with fracture and/or with osteochondral injury about the ankle. However, isolated injuries are becoming more prevalent in athletes. Without appropriate nonsurgical treatment, surgical intervention may be necessary to stabilize the ankle.

Keywords: acute ankle sprain; chronic ankle instability; deltoid ligament sprain; high ankle sprain; medial ankle sprain

---

Dr. Patel or an immediate family member serves as an unpaid consultant to Dunamis.

INTRODUCTION

Acute traumatic injuries and cumulative stress injuries involving the foot and ankle can affect the sports participation and performance of both elite competitive athletes and people engaged in recreational or fitness activities. A thorough understanding of common injuries of the foot and ankle allows a logical and organized approach to treating these injuries and facilitates the patient's return to play.

The stability of the ankle is the result of a combination of osseous, ligamentous, and musculotendinous components. The ankle generally is described as a mortise in which the talus is housed in the dome-shaped tibial plafond and the medial, lateral, and posterior malleoli. The talus is wider anteriorly than posteriorly so that the ankle intrinsically is most stable in the dorsiflexed position when the wider portion of the talus is engaged in the mortise. Conversely, in the plantarflexed position, the narrower posterior talus is engaged in the mortise and the ankle therefore is more unstable. Therefore, in the plantarflexed position, the stability of the ankle is more dependent on the lateral ligament complex. Not surprisingly, most acute inversion sprains occur when the ankle is somewhat plantarflexed.

The lateral ankle ligament complex primarily is composed of the anterior talofibular ligament (ATFL), the calcaneofibular ligament (CFL), and the posterior talofibular ligament. The ATFL prevents anterior translation of the plantarflexed ankle. The CFL is a collateral ligament that stabilizes both the ankle and the subtalar joint, preventing varus of the ankle and subtalar joint. In more severe inversion sprains, the CFL is injured along with the ATFL.

The peroneal musculotendinous unit is an important contributor to ankle stability. The peroneal tendons

---

This chapter is adapted from Lin J: Sports-related injuries of the foot and ankle, in Chou LB, ed: *Orthopaedic Knowledge Update®: Foot and Ankle 6*. American Academy of Orthopaedic Surgeons, 2020, pp 393-408.

LATERAL ANKLE INJURIES

Acute Lateral Ankle Ligament Injuries

Acute lateral ankle sprain is one of the most common injuries sustained during sports activity. An epidemiologic study of ankle sprains reported that more than three million sprains occurred during the 4-year study period and that more than half of these injuries occurred during athletic activity.[1] Acute ankle sprain was most common in individuals aged 10 to 19 years. Boys and men aged 15 to 24 years sustained more ankle sprains than girls and women in the same age range, but women older than 30 years sustained more sprains than their male counterparts.

An acute ankle sprain causes a variable amount of mechanical injury to the lateral ligament complex of the ankle. Such an injury can lead to lingering symptoms such as instability and pain, which can impede or preclude return to play. Proper initial management and detection of concomitant injuries (ie, talar chondral injuries, peroneal tendon pathology, fractures) minimizes the risk of long-term morbidity and speeds the resumption of athletic participation.

Patient History and Physical Examination

Successful treatment of an acute ankle sprain begins with a careful history and meticulous physical examination. Important components of the history include the time since injury, the ability to tolerate weight bearing, whether the injury is improving, or if there have been previous sprains of the same ankle. The physical examination should document the location and severity of swelling and ecchymosis. Probably the most important component of the physical examination is assessing the location of tenderness to palpation. After an acute lateral ankle ligament injury, swelling, ecchymosis, and tenderness usually are noted over the ATFL and CFL in the region just anterior and distal to the tip of the fibula. However, tenderness should be checked over several different structures to look for signs that could implicate an alternative or concomitant diagnosis. Laterally, the distal syndesmosis, lateral malleolus, peroneal tendons, fifth metatarsal, anterior process of the calcaneus, and lateral process of the talus should be palpated in addition to the lateral ligament complex. Medially, the medial malleolus, deltoid ligament, sustentaculum tali, and navicular should be examined and assessed for tenderness. Routine palpation of the Achilles tendon, tibialis anterior tendon, and midfoot articulations should also be included; injury to these structures sometimes is neglected when a diagnosis of ankle sprain is presumed. Manual muscle testing is also performed despite the effects of acute swelling and pain to verify continuity of these structures and to aid in the detection of acute peroneal dislocation. Resistance to inversion with the ankle in a dorsiflexed everted position and circumduction of the ankle are used to improve the sensitivity of detecting peroneal dislocation. Despite the use of a careful physical examination, many findings can still be obscured by diffuse swelling and poorly localized tenderness during the first 10 to 14 days after an acute ankle inversion injury. As a result, it is important to repeat the examination 10 to 14 days later, when the findings will be more specific and revealing.

Instability tests such as the anterior drawer and talar tilt tests have a role in the evaluation of an acute ankle sprain if performed acutely. Once the ankle is too swollen and uncomfortable to allow an unguarded and accurate assessment of stability, it can be more difficult to use these tests to confirm instability. The results of these tests generally do not affect the initial treatment of an acute sprain, and they should be reserved for evaluating chronic ankle instability.

Radiographic Evaluation

Appropriate radiographic studies are helpful for avoiding a misdiagnosis and facilitating a prompt diagnosis of associated injuries. In the emergency department, the Ottawa ankle rules provide guidance as to whether radiographs are necessary or can be deferred. Ankle radiographs are indicated if the presence of a fracture is suggested by tenderness along the distal 6 cm of the posterior edge of the fibula or the tip of the lateral malleolus, tenderness along the distal 6 cm of the posterior edge of the tibia or the tip of the medial malleolus, or inability to tolerate weight bearing for at least four steps. In the absence of these findings, the diagnosis usually is an acute sprain, and radiographs are unnecessary. Adherence to these guidelines reduces the patient's cost, time in the emergency department, and exposure to radiation.

The Ottawa ankle rules were designed for implementation and use in the emergency department. However, many patients who sustain an acute lateral ankle ligament injury are evaluated by an orthopaedic surgeon in an outpatient clinical office several days to a few weeks after injury. In this more specialized environment, the threshold for radiographic evaluation is lower because the definitive diagnosis and treatment plan are based on the evaluation. An orthopaedic surgeon should attempt to obtain a series of weight-bearing ankle radiographs for most patients with an acute lateral ankle sprain. Additional weight-bearing radiographs of the foot can be added when there is suspicion for a concomitant foot injury based on either the history or physical examination. Weight-bearing views provide substantially better imaging of relevant osseous structures than non–weight-bearing views and thereby minimize the possibility of missing an injury. Simulated weight-bearing views can be obtained at the initial evaluation if full weight bearing is too painful. Obtaining full weight-bearing views is deferred until symptoms improve.

The AP and mortise radiographs of the ankle should be evaluated for medial clear space and syndesmotic widening, malleolar fracture, lateral process of talus fracture, and talar osteochondral fracture (**Figure 1**). The lateral views of the ankle and foot can reveal dorsal talar avulsion fractures, anterior process of the calcaneus fractures, or the presence of an os trigonum injury. The AP and oblique foot views can reveal navicular fractures, midfoot injuries, cuboid fractures, or fifth metatarsal fractures. Radiographic and physical examination findings always must be correlated to provide an accurate and complete diagnosis.

CT and MRI have limited indications in the evaluation of an acute ankle sprain. CT is used to detect an associated fracture suspected on the basis of plain radiographs; these include fracture of the lateral process of the talus and the anterior process of calcaneus, posterior talar fracture, and osteochondral fracture. CT provides an accurate assessment of fracture size, displacement, and comminution that ultimately can guide treatment. CT, preferably weight-bearing, can also detect malalignment or displacement of the syndesmosis through visualizing the clear space in the axial plane. MRI rarely is indicated to evaluate an acute ankle sprain and should be obtained only if suspicion is high for an osteochondral lesion of the talus or an associated soft-tissue injury such as an Achilles tendon rupture or peroneal tendon tear or dislocation. MRI is useful for distinguishing a preexisting chronic osteochondral lesion from an acute osteochondral fracture. MRI has also been found to be superior to physical examination for the detection of syndesmotic injuries in the setting of ambiguous plain radiographs.[2]

Classification and Treatment

Acute lateral ankle sprains are graded based on the involved ligaments and the severity of the structural injury to the lateral ligament complex. A grade I acute sprain is a minor injury to the ATFL characterized by microscopic tears in the ligament fibers without gross structural damage. In a grade II sprain, partial macroscopic structural damage has occurred without complete loss of integrity; a grade II sprain primarily affects the ATFL, but the CFL may be involved to a lesser extent. A grade III sprain involves complete rupture of the lateral ligament complex, with loss of integrity of both the ATFL and the CFL.

The severity of a lateral ankle sprain affects both its treatment and prognosis. Patients with a grade I or II sprain typically do not require crutches and are able to perform activities of daily living with minimal discomfort. A grade I or II sprain appears to recover best when an early rehabilitation regimen is implemented. In fact, a randomized controlled study demonstrated that grade I and II sprains achieve earlier recovery when an immediate functional range-of-motion protocol is initiated compared with early immobilization.[3] The timing of the patient's return to sports activity primarily is based on the level of discomfort and ability to perform necessary sport-specific activities. Generally, the patient can return to sports 2 to 6 weeks after a grade I or II ankle sprain, with the use of a protective brace and initiation of peroneal strengthening and proprioceptive exercises aimed at preventing reinjury.

Patients with a grade III injury often initially experience discomfort during ambulation and while performing activities of daily living. A period of immobilization and protected weight bearing often is beneficial. However, the optimal length of time and the exact method of immobilization are not well established, as there have been conflicting results in various studies. A prospective randomized study compared the efficacy of four different modes of immobilization (tubular compression sleeve, walking boot, stirrup brace, and cast) for the initial treatment of an acute grade III ankle sprain.[4] Somewhat surprisingly, the results favored initial cast immobilization for a severe ankle sprain. Patients who had initial casting experienced the most rapid overall

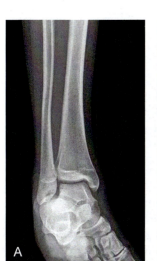
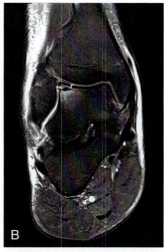

FIGURE 1 **A**, Mortise ankle radiograph from a patient with an acute ankle sprain. Lucency in the lateral talar dome suggests a fracture. **B**, MRI confirms that the patient has an acute unstable lateral talar osteochondral fracture.

recovery, with less pain and an earlier return to activity. The use of a walking boot was found to confer no significant benefit over that of a tubular compression sleeve. In another randomized trial of acute management of lateral ankle sprains, the use of a walking boot for 3 weeks followed by progression to a functional brace was compared with immediate initiation of functional bracing treatment without any period of immobilization.[5] There was no observed difference between groups in pain or instability; however, the immediate functional bracing treatment group had better functional scores and a more rapid recovery period. In a related randomized study comparing functional bracing treatment, neuromuscular training, and a combination of these interventions for lateral ankle sprains, authors found that bracing treatment was the most cost-effective of these interventions.[6]

After the initial pain, swelling, and discomfort have resolved over 2 to 4 weeks, a patient with a grade III sprain receives a functional brace, and formal physical therapy is initiated to decrease swelling, improve range of motion, and restore strength to the ankle. With symptom improvement, the therapeutic exercises gradually advance to proprioceptive exercises and sport-specific functional drills. Plyometric drills should be incorporated into the rehabilitation program because they are superior to standard peroneal strengthening exercises for restoration of subjective ankle stability and resumption of athletic participation.[7] The return to sport after a grade III sprain typically requires 6 to 12 weeks of rehabilitation. Although nonsurgical functional rehabilitation for a grade III ankle sprain remains the standard of care in North America, a body of evidence from Europe suggests that superior results are possible when an acute grade III sprain is surgically treated.[8,9] A meta-analysis of 27 studies revealed less giving way and overall better functional results when the initial treatment of grade III sprains was surgical rather than nonsurgical.[8] A subsequent prospective, randomized comparison of surgical treatment and functional rehabilitation in grade III ankle sprains found comparable functional results and fewer recurrent sprains in the patients treated surgically.[9] Additional high-quality studies are necessary before surgical treatment can supplant functional rehabilitation as the treatment of choice for grade III ankle sprains.

CHRONIC LATERAL ANKLE LIGAMENT INSTABILITY

With proper treatment, most patients who sustain an acute lateral ankle sprain successfully recover and return to their desired sports and preinjury level of activity. However, the outcome of a lateral ankle sprain, particularly a grade III injury, is not always favorable. A multiple database study of acute ankle sprains found that as many as 33% of patients still had pain 1 year after injury, and as many as 34% of patients sustained a recurrent sprain within a 3-year period after the initial injury.[10] The evaluation of a patient with chronic symptoms after ankle ligament injury must help identify the source of the lingering symptoms and initiate appropriate nonsurgical treatment. When necessary, surgical intervention is required to facilitate a return to sports.

Patient History

The history should elicit details of the initial injury, subsequent reinjury, and current symptoms. It is important to assess whether the patient's symptoms primarily involve instability, pain, or both. A detailed characterization of the instability and pain components of the patient's symptoms should be sought. The duration, frequency, and severity of instability episodes should be recorded and should include the number of sprains per month or year. The examiner should assess whether the recurrent sprains occur only during sports activities or also during activities of daily living. Patients with severe chronic instability may report frequent sprains with seemingly innocuous mechanisms such as stepping on a pebble, a curb, or a crack in a sidewalk. The examiner should document the extent of earlier treatment, including physical therapy, and to what extent bracing treatment controls the instability. Previous or recurrent sprains are strongest predictors of future ankle injuries as noted in a 2021 level II study.[11]

The timing, severity, and location of the pain component should also be assessed. The patient should be asked whether pain is present constantly or only after a sprain. Patients sometimes report surprisingly little pain after recurrent ankle sprains because of the overall laxity of the ligaments. Other patients report pain as the primary symptom and describe pain that precipitates the giving way episode. This type of pain should alert the examiner to the possibility that functional instability symptoms may be the result of concomitant mechanical pathology. It is particularly important for the patient to identify the location of the pain as specifically as possible. Determining whether the pain primarily is medial, anterolateral, or retrofibular will suggest the most likely causes and guide the choice of imaging.

Physical Examination

The goals of the physical examination of a patient with symptoms of chronic instability are to characterize the severity of ligament laxity, identify sources of pain, and assess for anatomic factors that predispose the patient to instability or affect the response to treatment. Ankle ligament laxity is assessed using the anterior drawer and talar tilt maneuvers. The anterior drawer test is used to assess the integrity of the ATFL and is performed with the ankle in a resting equinus position. This position of relative plantar flexion orients the fibers of the ATFL in line with the examiner's pull. The examiner stabilizes the tibia above the ankle with one hand, wraps the other hand around the heel, and translates the foot and ankle anteriorly on the stationary tibia. The examiner can feel the extent of anterior translation and can see a dimpling of the skin over the ATFL if significant laxity is present. The talar tilt maneuver assesses the laxity of the CFL. It is important to perform this maneuver with the ankle in a relatively neutral position to orient the CFL vertically and allow it to be tested as a true collateral ligament of the ankle. Failure to adequately dorsiflex the ankle during the talar tilt test can make it difficult to distinguish normal subtalar motion from true talar tilt. Again, the examiner secures the tibia with one hand, positions the ankle in neutral with the other hand, and exerts an inversion stress on the ankle and hindfoot. Placing a thumb beneath the fibula allows the examiner to feel the talus tilt within the ankle mortise. With both of these tests, it is crucial to examine the contralateral side as well as the general laxity of other joints. Although anterior drawer is the gold standard examination for ATFL insufficiency, electromagnetic sensors have been shown to quantitate the insufficiency with high intraexaminer and interexaminer reliability.[12] Hyperextension of knees, elbows, and fingers can point to the presence of general ligamentous laxity, which can predispose a patient to recurrent instability. The Beighton criteria for joint hypermobility are used in identifying patients with signs of generalized laxity, which can significantly affect the outcome of specific treatments.[13] A 2018 study noted Beighton criteria to be a predictor of arthralgia, dislocation, and subluxation.[14]

The foot and ankle should be examined for strength, range of motion, tenderness, swelling, and gait, in addition to ligament laxity. The presence of claw toes or weak ankle dorsiflexion and eversion may suggest the presence of a neurologic condition such as Charcot-Marie-Tooth disease. Isolated peroneal weakness with painful resisted eversion often accompanies a peroneal tendon tear. Tenderness, swelling, popping, subluxation, or frank dislocation of the peroneal tendons provides further evidence of peroneal tendon pathology. Decreased passive ankle dorsiflexion may result from the presence of distal tibial osteophytes or a gastrocnemius-soleus complex contracture. Limited passive subtalar inversion can be a clue to the presence of a tarsal coalition.

It is critical to assess for cavovarus deformity while the patient is standing and walking. The importance of early diagnosis of cavovarus deformity cannot be overstated because these patients are at substantially increased risk for ankle inversion injury, are more likely than other patients to experience chronic symptoms, and are less likely to have a successful outcome after standard nonsurgical or surgical treatment. When a patient with cavovarus alignment is examined standing and facing the clinician, a so-called peek-a-boo heel sign can be seen, in which the medial portion of the heel pad is visible (**Figure 2**). When examined from the back, the heel rests in varus relative to the axis of the tibia, with weight bearing concentrated on the lateral border of the foot. A Coleman block test is then performed to determine the flexibility of the hindfoot. The patient is observed from behind while standing on a 1-inch block under the lateral heel and foot with the first ray allowed to hang off the edge of the block. Improvement in hindfoot varus during this test suggests that first ray plantar flexion is driving the hindfoot deformity and that correcting the first ray will produce adequate correction of the hindfoot. If the hindfoot varus is not corrected or only partially corrected during Coleman block testing, the varus deformity is coming primarily from the hindfoot, possibly necessitating an additional hindfoot procedure to obtain full correction of the deformity.

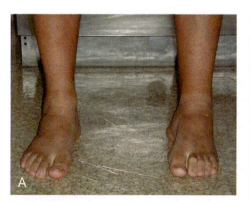 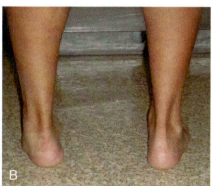 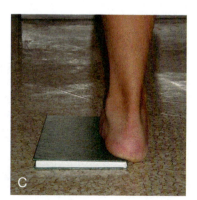

FIGURE 2 Clinical photographs from a patient with chronic left ankle instability and cavovarus. **A**, The so-called peek-a-boo heel sign. **B**, Hindfoot varus as seen from behind, with weight bearing on the outer border of the heel. **C**, Correction of hindfoot varus with the Coleman block test.

Radiographic Evaluation

Standard weight-bearing radiographs of the ankle and foot are used to evaluate a patient for chronic lateral ligament injury. AP and mortise views of the ankle should be scrutinized for lucent lesions in the talar dome that may signify osteochondral injury. The physician also should look for a large avulsion fracture off the distal tip of the fibula, which may accompany chronic ATFL injury. The lateral radiograph allows detection of anterior distal tibial osteophytes that can cause anterior ankle impingement. Radiographs can provide confirmation of subtle cavovarus malalignment. On a lateral radiograph of the foot, a cavus arch is suggested by a positive Meary angle formed by the axis of the talus and the axis of the first metatarsal. In cavovarus, a lateral radiograph fails to capture the talus in true profile, the fibula appears posterior, and the posterior facet is extremely well visualized, as in a Broden view. An AP foot radiograph may reveal so-called stacking of the metatarsals or metatarsus adductus. A hindfoot alignment view can determine the presence and severity of hindfoot varus or valgus. Each of these radiographic signs should raise the examiner's suspicion for concomitant malalignment.

Stress evaluation of the ankle involves the anterior drawer and talar tilt maneuvers done with fluoroscopy or plain radiography. Stress images are useful if it is desirable to quantify the severity of the instability, as for a research study. Stress fluoroscopy also is helpful for distinguishing true talar tilt from subtalar motion (**Figure 3**).

MRI has a more common role in chronic lateral ankle ligament injuries than in acute injuries. MRI is recommended if the patient's history, physical examination, or plain radiographs suggest the possibility of osteochondral lesions of the talus or peroneal tendon injury. MRI also is indicated if the patient has poorly defined ankle pain because it can reveal conditions such as anterolateral soft-tissue impingement lesions, loose bodies, or subtle fractures.[13] If possible, 1.5- or 3.0-T MRI should be obtained; the image resolution of open MRI is inadequate to provide meaningful information.

A retrospective cohort study compared MRI with stress radiographs among 187 patients.[15] Although MRI was highly sensitive compared with stress radiographs (83% versus 66%), the specificity of MRI was lower (53% versus 97%). The overall accuracy of stress radiographs was 74%, whereas the overall accuracy of MRI was 71%. The authors concluded that although MRI is a useful screening tool for concomitant ankle pathology associated with lateral ankle instability, it should not be used on its own for the diagnosis of chronic ankle instability.

Ultrasonography can be a useful tool. There are advantages and disadvantages to this mode of evaluation. Ultrasonography can be portable and does not

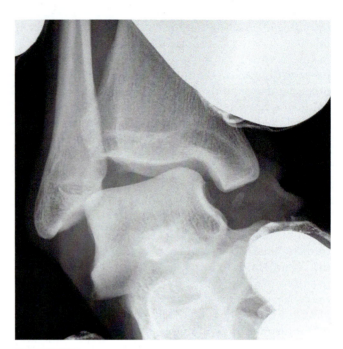

FIGURE 3 Stress fluoroscopic view showing laxity of the calcaneofibular ligament with a resulting increase in talar tilt.

expose anyone to radiation. The soft-tissue structures can be visualized in adequate detail in various parts of the extremity. The images can be repeated to allow prospective follow-up because of lower cost than MRI and portability. Where radiographs and MRI are static studies, ultrasonography can provide dynamic imaging. The scope of the ultrasonography may be limited because of its inability to visualize deeper structures in adequate detail. There is also operator variability as its biggest disadvantage. A 2022 study noted that the anterior drawer test was 81% sensitive and 80% specific for ATFL injury. Ultrasonography was 89% to 100% sensitive and 90% to 100% specific. Calcaneofibular injury was detected with 93% sensitivity and deltoid ligament injury was 90% sensitive with ultrasonography. Ultrasonography may be a useful tool to augment clinical examination.[16,17]

Treatment

The treatment of a patient with chronic lateral ankle ligament injury begins with nonsurgical interventions designed to improve ankle stability and decrease pain. Brace treatment should be implemented for a high-risk sports activity, such as basketball, volleyball, or tennis, or for any activity performed on uneven ground, such as hiking or lawn mowing. A course of neuromuscular physical therapy designed to optimize peroneal tendon strength, balance, and proprioception should be used unless previously completed.[18] Range of motion has been a key indicator in return to play as noted by a 2021 study. It was also noted that during immobilization, isometric exercise combined with electrical muscle stimulation increased range of motion and decreased return to play.[19] A 2021 randomized blind study showed Mulligan mobilization-with-movement was an effective therapy in more than 80% of the treatment group with subacute grade 1 to 2 sprains compared with sham treatment.[20] Early dynamic training after acute sprain decreased time to return to sport, increased functional performance, and decreased self-reported reinjury per a 2022 study.[21] Activation of tibialis anterior and peroneus longus muscles and coactivation of the quadriceps and hamstring muscles can enhance ankle and knee stability as shown by remodeled bicycle pedal training.[22] Unfortunately, nonsurgical treatments often do not adequately control symptoms, particularly in patients who desire to return to an active athletic lifestyle. A 2021 study correlated worse clinical outcomes in combined ligamentous injury (ATFL and CFL) versus isolated ATFL injury. There was decreased return to full sports activities with combined injury in this analysis.[23]

Surgical intervention may be indicated if nonsurgical treatment (which is the primary choice) does not provide sufficient stability and pain relief. The four types of lateral ligament reconstruction techniques are anatomic, anatomic-augmented, nonanatomic tenodesis, and anatomic free tendon graft. The goals of all surgical strategies and techniques are to improve mechanical ankle stability, decrease pain, and facilitate return to sports. A 2022 study indicated that lymphocyte-to-monocyte ratio greater than 3.824 may predict better American Orthopaedic Foot and Ankle Society score of open or arthroscopic repair for ATFL injury.[24,25]

The preferred technique for lateral ankle ligament reconstruction remains the anatomic Broström repair technique. This is the most commonly used technique, and it is successful in treating chronic instability in most patients.[26,27] This technique involves incising and reefing the ATFL alone or both the ATFL and CFL to eliminate the laxity and elongation produced by chronic inversion injuries[28] (**Figure 4**). The ligament can be reefed midsubstance in a vest-over-pants fashion or reefed directly to the fibula using drill holes or suture anchors.[29] The inferior extensor retinaculum can be advanced to the fibula (the Gould modification) to further stabilize the ligament repair[30] (**Figure 5**). A 2022 study noted that distal tears about the talar or calcaneal attachment have delayed return to sport and inferior performance in resuming preinjury sports level.[31] Although this modification has been often-advocated, a study compared patients undergoing isolated and modified Broström procedures and found no difference in clinical or radiographic outcomes.[32] The authors concluded that an isolated ligament reconstruction (ie, without the Gould modification) may be sufficient to restore stability. In a related study, authors

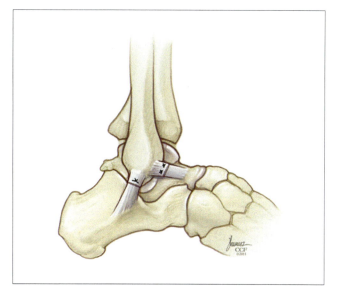

FIGURE 4 Illustration showing reefing of the anterior talofibular and calcaneofibular ligaments during a Broström reconstruction. (Reprinted with permission, Cleveland Clinic © 2011-2014. All Rights Reserved.)

compared attachment of the ligaments to the fibula using suture anchors versus suture bridges, finding that both options showed similar functional outcomes with the suture bridge being more expensive.[33]

Because the Broström procedure relies on maturation of the native tissue, immobilization of the ankle for as long as 6 weeks and a delay in return to sport for as long as 4 to 6 months may be required. A more recent variation of the Broström procedure is augmentation with anchor-to-anchor suture tape.[34] In a study of 81 patients with lateral ankle instability undergoing this procedure, mean return to sport was 84.1 days, potentially representing an advantage over nonreinforced anatomic repair.[34] Functional outcomes were excellent and similar to those reported for other anatomic repair techniques. These data suggest that athletes who are motivated to rapidly return to play may benefit from Broström augmentation with anchor-to-anchor suture tape.

All-inside arthroscopic techniques have also been developed. In a randomized study comparing all-inside to open procedures, one set of authors found no difference in clinical or radiographic outcomes at 12 months minimum follow-up.[35] Given these similar outcomes and the corresponding increases in the use of arthroscopy to treat conditions in the knee and shoulder, it is likely that arthroscopic treatment of chronic ankle instability may become increasingly common.[36] A 2020 study concluded arthroscopic anatomic repair of ATFL for chronic lateral ankle instability had good clinical outcomes at 24 to 45 months postoperatively.[37] A 2021 retrospective study also demonstrated improved American Orthopaedic Foot and

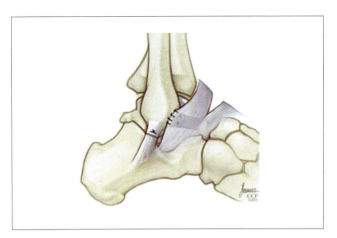

FIGURE 5 Illustration showing the Gould modification of the Broström reconstruction, in which the extensor retinaculum is incorporated into the ligament repair. (Reprinted with permission, Cleveland Clinic © 2011-2014. All Rights Reserved.)

Ankle Society scores with arthroscopic double band anatomic reconstruction of the ATFL.[38] A 2022 study noted shorter time and higher rate of return to sport activities and better clinical scores, posture control, and muscle strength in arthroscopic modified Broström group versus open modified Broström group 6 months postoperatively and no difference at 1 or 2 years postoperatively.[39]

The modified Broström-Evans anatomic-augmented procedure also has achieved excellent clinical results, particularly in high-level athletes.[40] Stability is added to a standard modified Broström procedure by transferring half of the peroneus brevis tendon to the fibula. The orientation of this tendon transfer is approximately midway between the axes of the ATFL and the CFL. The tendon is placed through a bone tunnel in the fibula and is stabilized with an interference screw to serve as a checkrein against excessive ankle and hindfoot inversion (**Figure 6**). This procedure is particularly useful in a patient who is a high-demand athlete, is undergoing revision surgery, or has tenuous ligamentous tissue.

The modified Broström-Evans technique has been much more successful than older, nonanatomic tenodesis procedures such as the traditional Evans tenodesis, in which the entire peroneus brevis tendon is transferred to the fibula at a right angle to the axis of the subtalar joint (**Figure 7**). This type of nonanatomic tenodesis procedure has largely been abandoned because it produces excessive peroneal weakness and stiffness of the subtalar joint. The current use of a nonanatomic tenodesis procedure is limited to patients with a neurologic condition and low functional demands.

Anatomic free tendon graft procedures generally use autograft or allograft hamstring tendon placed through bone tunnels in the talus, fibula, and calcaneus.[41-43] A 2021 study has described a quadruped plantaris tendon

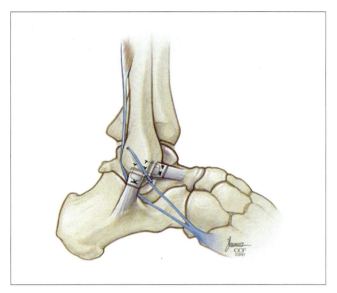

FIGURE 6 Illustration showing the modified Broström-Evans procedure, in which the anterior half of the peroneus brevis serves as a checkrein against excessive inversion. (Reprinted with permission, Cleveland Clinic © 2011-2014. All Rights Reserved.)

graft technique to match the ATFL tensile strength.[44] The tendon is routed in such a way as to re-create the anatomic orientation of the ATFL and CFL (**Figure 8**). This preservation of anatomic ligament orientation provides maximal ankle stability while avoiding excessive subtalar stiffness. As in the modified Broström-Evans procedure, the tendon generally is secured in the bone tunnels using interference screws. A free tendon augmentation procedure is indicated for a patient who is a high-level athlete, is

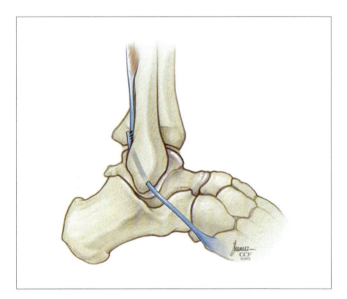

FIGURE 7 Illustration showing the traditional Evans procedure, in which the entire peroneus brevis is transferred. The result can be excessive stiffness. (Reprinted with permission, Cleveland Clinic © 2011-2014. All Rights Reserved.)

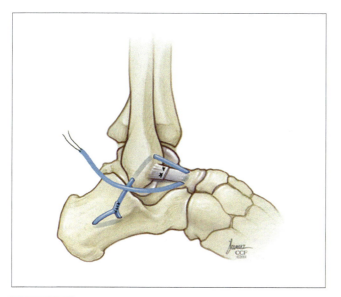

FIGURE 8 Illustration showing a free tendon graft reconstruction using hamstring autograft or allograft fixed in bone tunnels to re-create the orientation of the native anterior talofibular and calcaneofibular ligaments. (Reprinted with permission, Cleveland Clinic © 2011-2014. All Rights Reserved.)

undergoing revision surgery, or has generalized ligamentous laxity or severely attenuated ligamentous tissues. A 2022 retrospective analysis also showed significantly early rehabilitation and return to preinjury activity level compared with isolated modified Broström-Gould repair.[45]

If substantial cavovarus malalignment is identified before surgery, consideration should be given to including a realignment along with the lateral ligament reconstruction procedure. The threshold for a cavovarus realignment is poorly defined and ultimately is based on clinical judgment, but patients with uncorrected cavovarus are at significant risk of gradually stretching out even the stoutest lateral ligament reconstruction.[46] Thus, cavovarus malalignment should be included in the surgical plan if it is thought to be a significant contributor to the patient's instability or pain. Other commonly used procedures to correct cavovarus are plantar fascia release, dorsiflexion first metatarsal base closing wedge osteotomy, lateralizing calcaneal tuberosity osteotomy, and peroneus longus to peroneus brevis transfer.

Chronic lateral ankle ligament injuries rarely occur in isolation, and a high incidence of concomitant intra-articular and extra-articular pathology has been observed.[47-50] These concomitant abnormalities often explain the pain that accompanies chronic ankle instability and must be considered during surgical reconstruction. Intra-articular pathology such as soft-tissue impingement lesions, distal tibial osteophytes, loose bodies, synovitis, and osteochondral lesions of the talus are best treated arthroscopically. Thus, many surgeons routinely perform ankle arthroscopy in conjunction with lateral ankle ligament reconstruction.[47,48]

Peroneal tendon abnormalities are common in patients with chronic ankle instability.[49] In 28% of patients undergoing lateral ligament reconstruction, abnormalities such as a peroneal tendon tear, tenosynovitis, or peroneal tendon subluxation or dislocation were found as well as symptomatic anatomic variants such as a low-lying peroneus brevis muscle belly or a peroneus quartus.[49] Untreated peroneal tendon abnormalities also were found to be associated with unsuccessful surgical treatment. Therefore, a low threshold is recommended for exploring the peroneal tendons during ligament reconstruction.

SYNDESMOSIS INJURIES

Most ankle sprains are caused by inversion injury that primarily involves the lateral ankle ligaments. A mechanism of injury primarily involving eversion and external rotation changes the anatomy, character, and severity of the injury. Visual video analysis of acute ankle syndesmosis injury in rugby players confirmed rotational mechanism with a fixed externally rotated foot with posterior collapse of the body's center of mass.[51] Therefore, a high ankle sprain must be distinguished from a lateral ankle sprain and treated in a different manner. Up to 10% of ankle sprains are high ankle sprains with syndesmotic injury.[52]

Patient History and Physical Examination

Obtaining an accurate history is critical to diagnosis of a high ankle sprain. The patient should be prompted to describe the mechanism of injury if possible, and it may be helpful to ask the patient to demonstrate the perceived mechanism of injury on the contralateral side. The clinician should suspect a high ankle sprain if the patient describes the ankle having turned or rotated outward rather than inward. The location of maximal discomfort must be identified. Pain usually is localized to the lateral ankle after an inversion injury, but with a high ankle sprain the patient may describe more pain in the medial ankle as well as more proximally along the anterolateral leg.

During the physical examination, the clinician should attempt to elicit pain by palpating along the deltoid ligament and the distal tibiofibular syndesmosis as well as more proximally along the interosseous membrane and the proximal fibula. A syndesmotic sprain can be revealed by a positive squeeze test, in which the examiner compresses the tibiofibular joint in a mediolateral direction approximately 5 to 6 cm proximal to the ankle joint. Pain at the syndesmosis with this maneuver strongly suggests a syndesmotic injury. Similarly, external rotation stress applied to the ankle can be used to evaluate for injury to the deltoid ligament and syndesmosis, with reproduction of pain suggesting a high ankle sprain.

These maneuvers have high specificity for syndesmotic injury when positive but have overall low sensitivity.[2] A 2021 meta-analysis noted high sensitivity with palpation and dorsiflexion lunge. The authors concluded that other studies are required to demonstrate stable versus unstable injury and therefore confirm the optimal management (nonsurgical versus surgical).[53] Thus, the examiner cannot rule out syndesmotic injury based on physical examination alone as sagittal, coronal, and rotational stability have confirmed.[52]

Radiographic Evaluation

The radiographic evaluation of a suspected high ankle sprain includes the standard three ankle views, preferably while the patient is bearing weight. Simulated weight bearing can be used if the pain is severe. The lateral radiograph should be closely scrutinized for evidence of a posterior malleolar avulsion fracture, which can accompany a high ankle sprain. Similarly, AP and mortise radiographic views must be assessed for signs of syndesmotic widening. Stress imaging can be performed under fluoroscopy to determine whether there is dynamic widening of the ankle mortise during lateral translation stress. This test is most accurate immediately following injury.

On the AP radiograph, the tibiofibular overlap should be at least 5 mm. On the mortise view, the tibiofibular clear space should be less than 5 mm. Abnormalities in these measurements suggest syndesmotic instability. A full-length tibiofibular radiograph should be included to evaluate for a proximal fibular fracture, as in a Maisonneuve-type injury. Because of variability in the shape of the incisura between individuals, contralateral comparison of the uninjured ankle is reasonable internal control.[52]

Additional imaging is indicated if suspicion is high for syndesmotic instability despite inconclusive radiographs.

Axial weight-bearing CT of both ankles side by side can reveal even small amounts of widening or incongruity of the tibiofibular articulation. Dynamic change in area between weight bearing and non–weight bearing with the contralateral uninjured ankle can provide two key data points for surgeons to predict if an injury is stable or not.[54] Alternatively, axial MRI can reveal structural injury to the anterior tibiofibular ligament as well as to the posterior syndesmotic ligaments and posterior malleolus.[2] Fluid-sensitive axial sequences reveal substantial edema within the interosseous membrane in the setting of a high ankle sprain. High-resolution studies such as CT and MRI may identify other concomitant injury, which may require surgical treatment.[52] Although the objective of surgical treatment is to restore anatomy, a 2021 study concluded that in vivo analysis of syndesmosis repair failed to restore static and dynamic distal tibiofibular anatomy, even in patients who reported good to excellent clinical outcomes.[55]

CT and MRI provide more information than plain radiographs, but they are static studies that may miss dynamic instability of the syndesmosis. External rotation stress radiography or stress fluoroscopy is recommended if suspicion of instability remains high. To ensure an accurate test, a stress examination requires adequate relaxation and pain control, which can be challenging to achieve in the clinic. Thus, examination after administration of a local anesthetic or in the operating room under anesthesia should be considered if suspicion is high for an unstable syndesmosis (**Figure 9**).

Classification

High ankle sprains are classified based on the severity of injury to the deltoid ligament and the syndesmotic complex. A grade I sprain involves only microscopic structural damage. A grade II sprain involves macrostructural

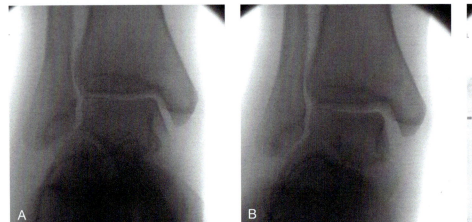
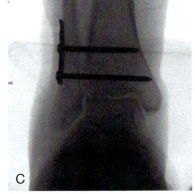

FIGURE 9 Fluoroscopic images from a patient with a syndesmotic sprain. **A**, Static image reveals no displacement. **B**, External rotation stress image, taken with the patient under anesthesia, reveals mortise and syndesmotic instability. **C**, Image after stabilization with syndesmotic screws.

damage without loss of stability or subluxation. In a grade III sprain, complete ligamentous injury, including injury to the deltoid ligament, is accompanied by demonstrable widening of the syndesmosis and typically medial joint space widening. A 2020 prospective analysis of military recruits at West Point noted quick return to play following surgical stabilization of unstable syndesmosis injury. Moreover, concomitant cartilage injury and older age were associated with longer return to play.[56]

Treatment

The treatment of a grade I or II syndesmotic sprain resembles that of an acute lateral ankle sprain, with several important differences. Because pain and swelling are often more severe and weight bearing takes longer to reestablish after a high ankle sprain than after an acute lateral sprain, a period of immobilization as long as 4 to 6 weeks should be considered. Initial cast immobilization may provide greater initial pain relief than the use of a prefabricated removable boot and can facilitate early recovery.[4] When the initial pain and swelling have subsided and weight bearing has resumed, standard functional rehabilitation protocols are initiated to restore range of motion, strength, balance, gait, and proprioception. Return to sports usually takes twice as long as after a lateral ankle sprain, and early in the treatment the patient should be counseled about the long recovery period. A 2020 retrospective study investigated the effect of acute versus delayed treatment (longer than 6 months) of unstable syndesmotic injuries. The authors concluded that delayed treatment resulted in significantly lower Foot and Ankle Outcome Score and quality of life.[57]

A grade III syndesmotic injury is unstable and requires surgical stabilization. Stabilization procedures traditionally used solid metal tibiofibular transfixion screws to immobilize the syndesmosis and mortise in an anatomic position so as to facilitate subsequent healing of the deltoid and syndesmotic ligaments. Recent evidence confirms that ankle dorsiflexion leads to increased external rotation and translation of the fibula on MRI; hence, the ankle should be placed in neutral dorsiflexion during syndesmotic fixation.[58] Despite extensive research, there is no consensus as to the size and number of screws to be used, the number of cortices to engage, and whether or when to remove the screws.[59]

A nonabsorbable suture button device is commonly used to stabilize the tibiofibular joint.[60] Suture stabilization theoretically avoids several difficulties associated with screw fixation. Proponents argue that suture devices provide more flexible fixation, thus facilitating restoration of normal tibiofibular biomechanics without implant removal or the potential for implant breakage.[61] A 2019 study concluded that anatomic reduction of the syndesmosis results in better outcomes in terms of arthritis changes.[62] A study also found that syndesmotic malreduction was less common when a suture button device was used, compared with traditional metal screws.[63] A meta-analysis of randomized controlled trials comparing screws to suture button showed improved functional outcomes and less malreduction with suture buttons, providing a grade A recommendation for suture buttons.[64] A 2022 international survey of foot and ankle and sports orthopaedic surgeons indicated that most respondents prefer suture buttons or hybrid constructs over screws alone for ligamentous syndesmosis disruption.[65,66] However, it is important to note that complications have been reported with the use of suture button devices, including stitch abscesses, loss of reduction, and osteolysis around the suture.[67] The repair construct used is at the surgeon's discretion based on a number of factors.

A 6- to 12-week period of protected avoidance of weight bearing is required to facilitate ligament healing after surgical stabilization of a grade III high ankle sprain.[56] Results from a 2020 study suggest that 10 days of partial weight bearing with pneumatic boot and unrestricted running and strengthening at 3 weeks is sufficient to return to sports.[56] Syndesmotic screws generally are left in place a minimum of 3 to 4 months. At that time, the surgeon must decide whether to remove or retain the screws. Removal requires a second surgical procedure and risks loss of reduction if ligament healing is incomplete. Retention may lead to restriction of ankle motion, screw breakage, or osteolysis around the screws. One study found no negative effect with retention of syndesmotic screws, even if a screw later broke.[64] Although tibiofibular screws may be retained without consequence in nonathletes, consideration should be given to planned removal approximately 4 months after surgery in a patient who is an athlete.[64] This timing avoids the risk of broken hardware or ankle motion restriction while allowing adequate time for ligament healing. A 2019 meta-analysis noted equal outcomes between static (screw) and dynamic (suture button) fixation. However, the authors noted less need for second surgeries with dynamic fixation.[65] Functional rehabilitation is subsequently initiated, with a return to sports typically expected between 8 weeks and 6 months after surgical treatment.[65]

DELTOID LIGAMENT INJURIES

In contrast to lateral ankle injury, medial ankle injury is less common. Isolated deltoid ligament without lateral ligamentous or fibular injury is rare.[68] The medial structures are at most risk with the foot supinated and the talus externally rotated. If untreated, medial ankle injury can cause instability and arthrosis. Up to 15% of ankle sprains involve the deltoid ligament.[69] Deltoid ligament injury is being increasingly identified especially in athletes and individuals involved in sports.[70] An observational study at West Point noted football, basketball, and soccer were

Section 7: Tendon Disorders and Sports-Related Foot and Ankle Injuries

the sports most commonly related to injury, with 4% incidence of medial ankle sprain. Tibial and saphenous nerve traction injury may be present in these injuries as well.[68]

Anatomy

The deltoid comprises superficial and deep fibers. The superficial fibers are on tension with eversion or supination. These fibers originate at the anterior malleolus without any distinct bands and a broad insertion footprint. The tibionavicular portion (strongest) of the superficial deltoid attaches to the navicular and acts as a strut for the spring or plantar calcaneonavicular ligament. The tibiocalcaneal portion of the superficial deltoid attaches to the sustentaculum tali. The posterior tibiotalar portion is the final part of the superficial deltoid ligament.[68] The deep fibers are tight with external rotation. The deltoid ligament has a robust blood supply with two intraosseous sources from the medial malleolus and medial talus and three extraosseous sources—medial tarsal artery, posterior tibialis artery, and anterior tibialis artery.[69] Ligament repair should address the specific injury, such as ligament avulsion, bone avulsion, or midsubstance tear.[70]

Deltoid Ligament Injuries

Typically, deltoid ligament injury is concomitant with ankle fractures and syndesmosis injury. Medial instability is not expected after these injuries. With adequate restoration of fibular alignment, stability, and immobilization, the deltoid injury heals without much sequelae in these settings. Acute-on-chronic injury of the deltoid is likely a result of repetitive microtrauma and discrete trauma. Although eversion is the likely mechanism for acute injuries, inversion injuries can also be implicated in the pathomechanics.[70] Deltoid rupture can occur with pronation-eversion, internal rotation, forced plantar flexion, or forced dorsiflexion.[68] The deep deltoid can be impinged between the medial malleolus and the talus. This can lead to hypertrophy and degeneration. This has been known to occur in an isolated (inversion injury) manner without injury to the lateral ligament or articular surface. An inversion injury can lead to occult deltoid ligament injury resulting in partial tearing and degeneration. Associated posterior tibialis tendon dysfunction can lead to ligament degeneration and rupture leading to progressive flatfoot and ankle instability.[70]

Radiographic Evaluation

Radiography can identify associated injuries. A valgus stress radiograph can show talar tilt. Sometimes radiographs can be normal with incomplete ligament injury. MRI is the preferred study to evaluate acute deltoid ligament tear. The tibionavicular and anterior tibiotalar components are best seen in the coronal plane with the foot in 40° to 50° plantar flexion. The tibiocalcaneal

and posterior tibiotalar components are best seen in the coronal plate with the foot in 10° to 20° of dorsiflexion.[68]

Classification and Treatment

The American Medical Association classification of ligament injury consists of grades 1 to 3 (3 being most severe). Grade 1 is described as a ligament stretch. Grade 2 is described as a partial tear. Grade 3 is a complete tear of the ligament. Medial ankle instability is described based on the location of the injury: type 1 lesion is a proximal tear or avulsion, type 2 lesion is an intrasubstance injury, and type 3 is located distally (being the most common).[68,71]

Nonsurgical treatment has a role in most medial ankle injuries. In conjunction with treatment-associated injuries, the prolonged immobilization period (8 to 10 weeks) should be sufficient. Immobilization in a walking cast or boot is necessary to prevent external rotation of the foot and allow healing. Nonsurgical treatment for chronic insufficiency includes taping, bracing, casting, physical therapy, and orthoses.[68]

The procedure for deltoid ligament repair consists of inspecting and treating the posterior tibialis tendon. The location, orientation, and extent of tear dictate the treatment procedure of the deltoid ligament. In patients with avulsion injury, a proximally based periosteal flap is elevated from the tip of the medial malleolus. A rongeur or burr is used to create a trough with bleeding bone. Drill holes are made with Kirschner wires and sutures (nonabsorbable braided sutures are recommended) are passed through. Alternatively, an anchor is used to secure the sutures in medial malleolus. The ligament is reduced into the trough and the sutures are tied similar to a horizontal mattress stitch. The periosteal flap is brought down over the ligament in a pants-over-vest fashion. Midsubstance tears can be repaired end to end with fresh edges on both sides. Any concurrent deformity should be corrected in the same setting. Chronic degenerative tears are especially beholden to this concept.

Many deltoid injuries go undiagnosed in patients with asymptomatic flatfoot. A medial displacing calcaneus osteotomy should be performed as part of a flatfoot reconstruction to alleviate tension on the deltoid ligament repair.[70] If the tissues are not adequate, flexor digitorum longus graft, hamstring tendon graft, a split posterior tibial tendon graft, or an allograft tendon can be used to reconstruct the injured portion of the ligament.[68] Arthroscopic evaluation may assist in confirming deltoid injury in subtle cases. A 2022 cadaver study concluded that arthroscopic medial clear space widening of more than 2.5 mm had greater accuracy for deltoid ligament injury than external rotation stress and gravity stress radiograph.[72] A 2020 study described arthroscopic technique to repair both lateral and medial collateral ligament injury to restore rotational ankle instability.[73] For subtle or persistent recalcitrant injury, arthroscopy may be a useful tool to evaluate the injury and treat it in the same setting. Although a 2022 meta-analysis noted a lack of high-quality studies guiding treatment of deltoid ligament injury, radiographic evidence supports deltoid ligament reconstruction.[74] Another 2021 meta-analysis showed benefit of deltoid ligament repair with concomitant fracture fixation compared with fracture fixation alone.[75]

SUMMARY

Ankle injuries may be more than meets the eye. Identification of the injury is key to adequate treatment. Despite appropriate treatment, chronic injury may result. Therefore, adequate and periodic assessment is warranted. This can allow for appropriate timing of surgical intervention and return to activity/sports. Lateral sprains may require soft-tissue and bony procedures, so alignment and preexisting or generalized conditions should be assessed. Deltoid injuries can be conspicuous and may require arthroscopy for evaluation. Syndesmosis injuries are common in athletes, and dynamic fixation with suture button seems to be advantageous compared with syndesmosis screws; this can allow for quicker return to sports.

KEY STUDY POINTS

- The initial treatment of acute lateral ankle sprains is immobilization, functional bracing, and neuromuscular rehabilitation, depending on severity and patient-specific factors.
- Chronic ankle instability can be initially managed with therapy and bracing but often requires surgical intervention. Stabilization can be in the form of anatomic reconstruction, anatomic-augmented reconstruction, nonanatomic tenodesis, or anatomic free tendon graft. Most patients should be treated with anatomic reconstruction.
- Acute syndesmotic ankle sprain is a more severe injury than acute lateral ankle ligament sprain. Unstable injuries require syndesmotic fixation. Flexible fixation with nonabsorbable suture buttons show better outcomes likely because of restoration of biomechanics.
- Deltoid ligament injuries are rare and can be concomitant with ankle fracture and syndesmosis injury. Posterior tibialis tendon dysfunction and progressive flatfoot can also lead to medial ankle instability. Anatomic reconstruction can be performed when alignment is normal. In the face of a flatfoot deformity a medial displacing calcaneal osteotomy should be performed to relieve tension on the repair.

ANNOTATED REFERENCES

1. Waterman BR, Owens BD, Davey S, Zacchilli MA, Belmont PJ Jr: The epidemiology of ankle sprains in the United States. *J Bone Joint Surg Am* 2010;92(13):2279-2284.

2. de Cesar PC, Avila EM, de Abreu MR: Comparison of magnetic resonance imaging to physical examination for syndesmotic injury after lateral ankle sprain. *Foot Ankle Int* 2011;32(12):1110-1114.

3. Bleakley CM, O'Connor SR, Tully MA, et al: Effect of accelerated rehabilitation on function after ankle sprain: Randomised controlled trial. *BMJ* 2010;340:1964.

4. Lamb SE, Marsh JL, Hutton JL, Nakash R, Cooke MW, Collaborative Ankle Support Trial (CAST Group): Mechanical supports for acute, severe ankle sprain: A pragmatic, multicentre, randomised controlled trial. *Lancet* 2009;373(9663):575-581.

5. Prado MP, Mendes AAM, Amodio DT, Camanho GL, Smyth NA, Fernandes TD: A comparative, prospective, and randomized study of two conservative treatment protocols for first-episode lateral ankle ligament injuries. *Foot Ankle Int* 2014;35:201-206.

6. Janssen KW, Hendriks MRC, van Mechelen W, Verhagen E: The cost-effectiveness of measures to prevent recurrent ankle sprains: Results of a 3-arm randomized controlled trial. *Am J Sports Med* 2014;42(7):1534-1541.

7. Ismail MM, Ibrahim MM, Youssef EF, El Shorbagy KM: Plyometric training versus resistive exercises after acute lateral ankle sprain. *Foot Ankle Int* 2010;31(6):523-530.

8. Pijnenburg AC, Van Dijk CN, Bossuyt PM, Marti RK: Treatment of ruptures of the lateral ankle ligaments: A meta-analysis. *J Bone Joint Surg Am* 2000;82(6):761-773.

9. Pihlajamaki H, Hietaniemi K, Paavola M, Visuri T, Mattila VM: Surgical versus functional treatment for acute ruptures of the lateral ligament complex of the ankle in young men: A randomized controlled trial. *J Bone Joint Surg Am* 2010;92(14):2367-2374.

10. van Rijn RM, van Os AG, Bernsen RMD, Luijsterburg PA, Koes BW, Bierma-Zeinstra SMA: What is the clinical course of acute ankle sprains? A systematic literature review. *Am J Med* 2008;121(4):324-331.e6.

11. Pourgharib Shahi MH, Selk Ghaffari M, Mansournia MA, Halabchi F: Risk factors influencing the incidence of ankle sprain among elite football and basketball players: A prospective study. *Foot Ankle Spec* 2021;14(6):482-488.

    History of recurrent and acute ankle sprain was the strongest predictor for ankle injuries. Level of evidence: II.

12. Kataoka K, Hoshino Y, Nagamune K, et al: The quantitative evaluation of anterior drawer test using an electromagnetic measurement system. *Sports Biomech* 2022;21(4):550-561.

    The intraexaminer and interexaminer reliability was 0.99 and 0.89. The electromagnetic sensor could quantify the anterior translation during the anterior drawer test, which corresponds to fluoroscopic evaluation.

13. Ferkel RD, Tyorkin M, Applegate GR, Heinen GT: MRI evaluation of anterolateral soft tissue impingement of the ankle. *Foot Ankle Int* 2010;31(8):655-661.

14. Armstrong R, Greig DM: The Beighton score as a predictor of Brighton criteria in sport and dance. *Phys Ther Sport* 2018;32:145-154.

15. Johan S, Robbins J, Lewis L, Wilkes M, Ryan P: Comparison of magnetic resonance imaging and stress radiographs in the evaluation of chronic lateral ankle instability. *Foot Ankle Int* 2017;38(4):397-404.

16. Hosseinian SHS, Aminzadeh B, Rezaeian A, Jarahi L, Naeini AK, Jangjui P: Diagnostic value of ultrasound in ankle sprain. *J Foot Ankle Surg* 2022;61(2):305-309.

    Ultrasonography is an effective complementary tool for primary evaluation of ankle injuries, which leads to early diagnosis and efficient quality of care. Clinical tests are not reliable to rule out the ankle ligaments injury and the results should be interpreted with caution. Level of evidence: III.

17. Cao M, Liu S, Zhang X, et al: Imaging diagnosis for anterior talofibular ligament injury: A systemic review with meta-analysis. *Acta Radiol* 2023;64(2):612-624.

    The pooled sensitivity rates of chronic ATFL injuries were 86.3% (82.5% to 89.5%) by MRI, 98.7% (95.3% to 99.8%) by ultrasonography, 74.4% (63.6% to 83.4%) by stress radiography, and 100% (87.7% to 100.0%) for magnetic resonance arthrography. In conclusion, ultrasonography may be a valuable imaging technique with high sensitivity for diagnosing chronic lateral ankle ligament injuries.

18. de Vries JS, Krips R, Sierevelt IN, Blankevoort L, van Dijk CN: Interventions for treating chronic ankle instability. *Cochrane Database Syst Rev* 2011;(8):CD004124.

19. Toyoshima Y, Akagi R, Nabeshima K: Isometric exercise during immobilization reduces the time to return to play after lateral ankle sprain. *Phys Ther Sport* 2021;52:168-172.

    Increased deficiency in ankle range of motion led to a longer time to return to play, and isometric exercise combined with electrical muscle stimulation during immobilization increased the total ankle range of motion and shortened the time to return to play.

20. Nguyen AP, Pitance L, Mahaudens P, et al: Effects of Mulligan mobilization with movement in subacute lateral ankle sprains: A pragmatic randomized trial. *J Man Manip Ther* 2021;29(6):341-352.

    More than 80% of participants with subacute lateral ankle sprains responded well to the Mulligan mobilization-with-movement approach. Three sessions of pragmatically determined Mulligan mobilization-with-movement provided a significant and clinically meaningful benefit in dorsiflexion range of motion and Y-balance test performance compared with a sham treatment.

21. Tee E, Melbourne J, Sattler L, Hing W: Evidence for rehabilitation interventions after acute lateral ankle sprains in athletes: A scoping review. *J Sport Rehabil* 2022;31(4):457-464.

Early dynamic training after an acute lateral ankle sprain in athletes results in a shorter time to return to sport, increased functional performance, and decreased self-reported reinjury. The results of this scoping review support an early functional and dynamic rehabilitation approach when compared with passive interventions for athletes returning to sport after a lateral ankle sprain.

22. Wu HW, Chang YS, Arefin MS, You YL, Su FC, Lin CF: Six-week remodeled bike pedal training improves dynamic control of lateral shuffling in athletes with functional ankle instability. *Sports Health* 2022;14(3):348-357.

    Remodeled bicycle pedal training facilitates the tibialis anterior and peroneus longus activation and the coactivation of the quadriceps and hamstring muscles during lateral shuffling and resulted in enhanced ankle and knee joint stability. In addition, a better ankle movement strategy during a dynamic task can be achieved via a 6-week remodeled pedal training program. Level of evidence: II.

23. Pacheco J, Guerra-Pinto F, Araújo L, et al: Chronic ankle instability has no correlation with the number of ruptured ligaments in severe anterolateral sprain: A systematic review and meta-analysis. *Knee Surg Sports Traumatol Arthrosc* 2021;1129:3512-3524.

    A significant statistical correlation between a combined ATFL-CFL rupture and chronic ankle instability, compared with an isolated ATFL rupture, was not found. There is, however, fair evidence showing a worse clinical outcome score in the combined ruptures, as well as a decreased return to full sports activities. The use of reliable and accessible diagnostic methods to determine the number of ruptured ligaments might have a role in managing severe ankle sprains. Level of evidence: III.

24. Yuan C, Wang Z, Zhu G, Wang C, Ma X, Wang X: Preoperative lymphocyte-to-monocyte ratio can indicate the outcomes in repair of I-III degree injury of lateral ankle ligament. *Biomed Res Int* 2022;2022:6234561.

    The clinical outcomes of open or arthroscopic repair for ATFL injury are satisfactory. As a marker of systemic inflammation, preoperative lymphocyte-to-monocyte ratio can be used as a prognostic indicator for ankle lateral ligament repair. Level of evidence: IV.

25. Altomare D, Fusco G, Bertolino E, et al: Evidence-based treatment choices for acute lateral ankle sprain: A comprehensive systematic review. *Eur Rev Med Pharmacol Sci* 2022;26(6):1876-1884.

    Nonsurgical treatment should be the first choice for severe acute lateral ankle sprains, because it provides satisfactory functional outcomes without the risks and costs of surgery. It was not possible to identify the best external support, but a preference toward flexible braces emerged because they allow an earlier return to daily activities. The paucity of studies comparing different rehabilitation protocols precluded the possibility of defining the ideal one.

26. Tourné Y, Mabit C, Moroney PJ, Chaussard C, Saragaglia D: Long-term follow-up of lateral reconstruction with extensor

retinaculum flap for chronic ankle instability. *Foot Ankle Int* 2012;33(12):1079-1086.

27. Bell SJ, Mologne TS, Sitler DF, Cox JS: Twenty-six-year results after Broström procedure for chronic lateral ankle instability. *Am J Sports Med* 2006;34(6):975-978.

28. Lee KT, Park YU, Kim JS, Kim JB, Kim KC, Kang SK: Long-term results after modified Brostrom procedure without calcaneofibular ligament reconstruction. *Foot Ankle Int* 2011;32(2):153-157.

29. Cho BK, Kim YM, Kim DS, Choi ES, Shon HC, Park KJ: Comparison between suture anchor and transosseous suture for the modified-Broström procedure. *Foot Ankle Int* 2012;33(6):462-468.

30. Behrens SB, Drakos M, Lee BJ, et al: Biomechanical analysis of Brostrom versus Brostrom-Gould lateral ankle instability repairs. *Foot Ankle Int* 2013;34(4):587-592.

31. Du M, Li J, Jiao C, Guo Q, Hu Y, Jiang D: Distal insertion rupture of lateral ankle ligament as a predictor of weakened and delayed sports recovery after acute ligament repair: Mid-term outcomes of 117 cases. *BMC Musculoskelet Disord* 2022;23(1):294.

    Ankle arthroscopy followed by open anatomic ligament repair is a reliable procedure for patients requiring return to high-demand sports after severe acute ankle sprains. Distal rupture near the talar or calcaneal end was associated with delayed return to sport and inferior performance in resuming preinjury sports level.

32. Jeong BO, Kim MS, Song WJ, SooHoo NF: Feasibility and outcome of inferior extensor retinaculum reinforcement in modified Broström procedures. *Foot Ankle Int* 2014;35(11):1137-1142.

33. Cho BK, Kim YM, Park KJ, Park JK, Kim DK: A prospective outcome and cost-effectiveness comparison between two ligament reattachment techniques using suture anchors for chronic ankle instability. *Foot Ankle Int* 2015;36(2):172-179.

34. Coetzee JC, Ellington JK, Ronan JA, Stone RM: Functional results of open Broström ankle ligament repair augmented with a suture tape. *Foot Ankle Int* 2018;39(3):304-310.

35. Yeo ED, Lee KT, Sung IH, Lee SG, Lee YK: Comparison of all-inside arthroscopic and open techniques for the modified Broström procedure for ankle instability. *Foot Ankle Int* 2016;37(10):1037-1045.

36. Atilano Carvalho P, Fradet J, Oliveira F, Charpail C, Guillo S: Searching for an endoscopic all-inside classic Broström-Gould technique. *Arthrosc Tech* 2022;11(4):e697-e703.

    In the Broström-Gould technique, lateral ankle endoscopy provides a clear view and access to these structures, allowing for an all-inside Broström-Gould procedure using three portals. The procedure is safe and reproducible, resulting in a repair that mostly resembles the classical open technique.

37. Feng SM, Sun QQ, Wang AG, Chang BQ, Cheng J: Arthroscopic anatomical repair of anterior talofibular ligament for chronic lateral instability of the ankle: Medium- and long-term functional follow-up. *Orthop Surg* 2020;12(2):505-514.

Arthroscopic anatomic repair of ATFL for chronic lateral ankle instability is precise, with less surgical trauma and reliable medium-term and long-term effect.

38. Chen H, Zhang T, Qu J, et al: Treatment of chronic lateral ankle instability by double-band anatomical reconstruction of the anterior talofibular ligament's fibular enthesis. *J Cent South Univ Med Sci* 2021;46(12):1354-1362.

    Arthroscopic débridement and double-band anatomic reconstruction of the ATFL's fibular enthesis for the treatment of chronic lateral ankle instability gains beneficial short-term effects for its minimal invasion and quick recovery.

39. Hou ZC, Su T, Ao YF, et al: Arthroscopic modified Broström procedure achieves faster return to sports than open procedure for chronic ankle instability. *Knee Surg Sports Traumatol Arthrosc* 2022;30(10):3570-3578.

    Shorter period and higher rates of return to sport activities and better clinical scores, posture control, and muscle strength were achieved in the arthroscopic group at 6 months postoperatively, and no clinical differences were found between arthroscopic and open modified Broström procedure 1 year or 2 years postoperatively. Arthroscopic modified Broström procedure is a reliable procedure for chronic lateral ankle instability injuries with the demand for fast exercise recovery. Level of evidence: II.

40. Girard P, Anderson RB, Davis WH, Isear JA, Kiebzak GM: Clinical evaluation of the modified Brostrom-Evans procedure to restore ankle stability. *Foot Ankle Int* 1999;20(4):246-252.

41. Wang B, Xu XY: Minimally invasive reconstruction of lateral ligaments of the ankle using semitendinosus autograft. *Foot Ankle Int* 2013;34(5):711-715.

42. Coughlin MJ, Schenck RC Jr, Grebing BR, Treme G: Comprehensive reconstruction of the lateral ankle for chronic instability using a free gracilis graft. *Foot Ankle Int* 2004;25(4):231-241.

43. Jeys LM, Harris NJ: Ankle stabilization with hamstring autograft: A new technique using interference screws. *Foot Ankle Int* 2003;24(9):677-679.

44. Lopes R, Andrieu M, Molinier F, Colin F, Morin V: PT4: New arthroscopic technique for isolated reconstruction of the anterior talofibular ligament using a quadrupled plantaris tendon. *Orthop Traumatol Surg Res* 2021;107(6):102995.

    Typical gracilis tendon graft is not always appropriate. Interest in using the plantaris tendon as a graft has increased because a biomechanics study found the tensile strength of a quadrupled plantaris tendon is comparable to that of the ATFL. The authors described an original arthroscopic technique for isolated ATFL reconstruction using a quadrupled plantaris tendon graft.

45. Jain NP, Ayyaswamy B, Griffiths A, Alderton E, Kostusiak M, Limaye RV: Is internal brace augmentation a gold standard treatment compared to isolated modified Brostrom Gould repair for chronic lateral ligament ankle instability? Effect on functional outcome and return to preinjury activity: A retrospective analysis. *Foot (Edinb)* 2022;50:101865.

The use of internal brace augmentation with modified Broström-Gould repair showed significantly better outcomes in terms of early rehabilitation and return to preinjury activity level compared with isolated modified Broström-Gould repair. The functional outcome and visual analog scale score were better in internal brace group compared with modified Broström-Gould group with no significant difference. Level of evidence: IV.

46. Fortin PT, Guettler J, Manoli A II: Idiopathic cavovarus and lateral ankle instability: Recognition and treatment implications relating to ankle arthritis. *Foot Ankle Int* 2002;23(11):1031-1037.

47. Sugimoto K, Takakura Y, Okahashi K, Samoto N, Kawate K, Iwai M: Chondral injuries of the ankle with recurrent lateral instability: An arthroscopic study. *J Bone Joint Surg Am* 2009;91(1):99-106.

48. Ferkel RD, Chams RN: Chronic lateral instability: Arthroscopic findings and long-term results. *Foot Ankle Int* 2007;28(1):24-31.

49. Strauss JE, Forsberg JA, Lippert FG III: Chronic lateral ankle instability and associated conditions: A rationale for treatment. *Foot Ankle Int* 2007;28(10):1041-1044.

50. Crim JR, Beals TC, Nickisch F, Schannen A, Saltzman CL: Deltoid ligament abnormalities in chronic lateral ankle instability. *Foot Ankle Int* 2011;32(9):873-878.

51. Delahunt E, Farrell G, Boylan A, et al: Mechanisms of acute ankle syndesmosis ligament injuries in professional male rugby union players: A systematic visual video analysis. *Br J Sports Med* 2021;55(12):691-696.

    Injuries incurred while tackling were exclusively the result of suboptimal tackle mechanics. A majority of injuries incurred while being tackled involved a posterior tackle, which often resulted in a posterior collapse of the injured player's centre of mass over a fixed externally rotated foot.

52. Bejarano-Pineda L, DiGiovanni CW, Waryasz GR, Guss D: Diagnosis and treatment of syndesmotic unstable injuries: Where we are now and where we are headed. *J Am Acad Orthop Surg* 2021;29(23):985-997.

    Several fixation methods have been described, but the foremost aspect is to achieve an anatomic reduction. Identifying any associated injuries and characteristics of the syndesmotic instability will lead to the appropriate treatment that restores the anatomy and stability of the distal tibiofibular joint.

53. Netterström-Wedin F, Bleakley C: Diagnostic accuracy of clinical tests assessing ligamentous injury of the ankle syndesmosis: A systematic review with meta-analysis. *Phys Ther Sport* 2021;49:214-226.

    The ATFL is best assessed using a cluster of palpation (rule out) and anterior drawer testing (rule in). The talar tilt test can rule in injury to the CFL, but a sensitive clinical test for the ligament is lacking. It is unclear if ligamentous injury grading can be done beyond the binary (injured vs uninjured), and clinical tests of the subtalar joint ligaments are not well researched. Level of evidence: IIIA.

54. Del Rio A, Bewsher SM, Roshan-Zamir S, et al: Weightbearing cone-beam computed tomography of acute ankle syndesmosis injuries. *J Foot Ankle Surg* 2020;59(2):258-263.

    Syndesmosis area measurement was reliable and reproducible. Dynamic change in area and weight-bearing comparison with the contralateral uninjured ankle are two parameters that may prove useful in the future for predicting syndesmotic instability. Level of evidence: III.

55. Canton SP, Gale T, Onyeukwu C, Hogan MV, Anderst W: Syndesmosis repair affects in vivo distal interosseous tibiofibular ligament elongation under static loads and during dynamic activities. *J Bone Joint Surg Am* 2021;103(20):1927-1936.

    This study provides the first in vivo evidence of postfixation changes in biomechanics after syndesmosis repair. Syndesmosis repair fails to restore healthy static and dynamic distal tibiofibular anatomy, even in patients who report good to excellent clinical outcomes. Level of evidence: IV.

56. D'Hooghe P, Grassi A, Alkhelaifi K, et al: Return to play after surgery for isolated unstable syndesmotic ankle injuries (West Point grade IIB and III) in 110 male professional football players: A retrospective cohort study. *Br J Sports Med* 2020;54(19):1168-1173.

    In this cohort of professional football players, surgical stabilization of isolated unstable syndesmosis injuries (West Point grade ≥IIB) allowed for relatively quick return to play. High-grade injury (West Point grade III), concomitant cartilage injury, and greater age were associated with longer return-to-play times. Level of evidence: II.

57. Kent S, Yeo G, Marsland D, et al: Delayed stabilisation of dynamically unstable syndesmotic injuries results in worse functional outcomes. *Knee Surg Sports Traumatol Arthrosc* 2020;28(10):3347-3353.

    The results of this study suggest that delayed surgical stabilization (>6 months) is associated with significantly worse clinical function, and thus timely identification and early referral of those patients with potentially unstable syndesmotic injuries is recommended. Level of evidence: III.

58. Nault ML, Marien M, Hebert-Davies J, et al: MRI quantification of the impact of ankle position on syndesmosis anatomy. *Foot Ankle Int* 2017;38(2):215-219.

59. White TO, Bugler KE: Ankle fractures, in Court-Brown CM, Heckman JD, McQueen MM, Ricci WM, Tornetta P III, McKee MD, eds: *Rockwood and Green's Fractures in Adults*, ed 8. Lippincott, Williams & Wilkins, 2015.

60. DeGroot H, Al-Omari AA, El Ghazaly SA: Outcomes of suture button repair of the distal tibiofibular syndesmosis. *Foot Ankle Int* 2011;32(3):250-256.

61. Klitzman R, Zhao H, Zhang LQ, Strohmeyer G, Vora A: Suture-button versus screw fixation of the syndesmosis: A biomechanical analysis. *Foot Ankle Int* 2010;31(1):69-75.

62. Akoh CC, Phisitkul P: Anatomic ligament repairs of syndesmotic injuries. *Orthop Clin North Am* 2019;50(3):401-414.

Indications for surgical intervention for isolated syndesmotic injuries include frank syndesmosis diastasis, medial clear space widening on plain radiographs, significant radiographic syndesmosis diastasis during stress examination, or subtle syndesmotic diastasis detected by arthroscopic evaluation. Complications after syndesmosis repair include symptomatic hardware, malreduction, and arthritis. Anatomic reduction of the syndesmosis leads to better outcomes following surgery.

63. Naqvi GA, Cunningham P, Lynch B, Galvin R, Awan N: Fixation of ankle syndesmotic injuries: Comparison of tightrope fixation and syndesmotic screw fixation for accuracy of syndesmotic reduction. *Am J Sports Med* 2012;40(12):2828-2835.

64. Moore JA Jr, Shank JR, Morgan SJ, Smith WR: Syndesmosis fixation: A comparison of three and four cortices of screw fixation without hardware removal. *Foot Ankle Int* 2006;27(8):567-572.

65. Gan K, Zhou K, Hu K, Lu L, Gu S, Shen Y: Dynamic fixation versus static fixation for distal tibiofibular syndesmosis injuries: A meta-analysis. *Med Sci Monit* 2019;25:1314-1322.

    The dynamic fixation and static fixation methods are equal in clinical outcomes, with dynamic fixation needing fewer second interventions for distal tibiofibular syndesmosis injuries. Level of evidence: IA.

66. Hunt KJ, Bartolomei J, Challa SC, et al: Significant variations in surgical construct and return to sport protocols with syndesmotic injuries: An ISAKOS global perspective. *J ISAKOS* 2022;7(1):13-18.

    A Research Electronic Data Capture survey of 742 surgeons (457 American and 285 international) was conducted to gather demographics, indications for treatment of syndesmotic injuries, preferred treatment and technique, and postoperative management. The most common elements used as surgical indications were syndesmosis widening greater than 2 mm on radiographs, an anterior inferior talofibular ligament injury in combination with a posterior inferior talofibular ligament or deltoid ligament involvement on MRI, and widening of the distal tibiofibular joint during arthroscopic evaluation. Overall, flexible fixation (eg, suture button) was the preferred device choice for the repair of an injured syndesmosis. Most respondents did not alter their rehabilitation protocol or anticipated return-to-play timeline based on the injury severity. However, there was considerable variability between respondents on the time to weight bearing, running, and full participation. Further pragmatic outcomes data are necessary to guide safe return to play protocols for syndesmotic injuries. Level of evidence: IV.

67. Storey P, Gadd RJ, Blundell C, Davies MB: Complications of suture button ankle syndesmosis stabilization with modifications of surgical technique. *Foot Ankle Int* 2012;33(9):717-721.

68. Clanton TO, McGarvey W: Athletic injuries to the soft tissues of the foot and ankle, in Coughlin MJ, Mann RA, Saltzman CL, eds: *Surgery of the Foot and Ankle*. Mosby Elsevier, 2007, pp 1485-1489.

69. Haynes JA, Gosselin M, Cusworth B, McCormick J, Johnson J, Klein S: The arterial anatomy of the deltoid ligament: A cadaveric study. *Foot Ankle Int* 2017;38(7):785-790.

70. Myerson MS: Ankle instability and impingement syndrome, in *Reconstructive Foot and Ankle Surgery: Management of Complications*. Elsevier Saunders, 2010, pp 385-388.

71. Hintermann B: Medial ankle instability. *Foot Ankle Clin* 2003;8:723-738.

72. Chiang CC, Lin CFJ, Tzeng YH, Teng MH, Yang TC: Arthroscopic quantitative measurement of medial clear space for deltoid injury of the ankle: A cadaveric comparative study with stress radiography. *Am J Sports Med* 2022;50(3):778-787.

    Arthroscopic medial clear space measurement can differentiate intact deltoid ligament, partial deltoid ligament injury, and complete deltoid ligament injury. Compared with external rotation stress and gravity stress radiography, arthroscopic medial clear space measurement has greater accuracy with excellent interrater reliability.

73. Vega J, Allmendinger J, Malagelada F, Guelfi M, Dalmau-Pastor M: Combined arthroscopic all-inside repair of lateral and medial ankle ligaments is an effective treatment for rotational ankle instability. *Knee Surg Sports Traumatol Arthrosc* 2020;28(1):132-140.

    Rotational ankle instability can be successfully treated by an arthroscopic all-inside repair of the lateral and medial ligaments of the ankle. Level of evidence: IV.

74. James M, Dodd A: Management of deltoid ligament injuries in acute ankle fracture: A systematic review. *Can J Surg* 2022;65(1):E9-E15.

    High-quality evidence guiding treatment of deltoid ligament injury in acute ankle fractures is lacking; currently available evidence appears to support deltoid ligament repair. Given recent increased interest in deltoid ligament repair and syndesmotic fixation, a comprehensive multicenter randomized controlled trial is warranted. Although radiographic evidence indicates the potential benefit of deltoid ligament repair, further research is required to establish the superiority of deltoid ligament repair versus clinical equipoise. Level of evidence: I.

75. Guo W, Lin W, Chen W, Pan Y, Zhuang R: Comparison of deltoid ligament repair and non-repair in acute ankle fracture: A meta-analysis of comparative studies. *PLoS One* 2021;16(11):e0258785.

    In this meta-analysis of comparative studies, deltoid ligament repair offered great advantages in terms of the postoperative medial clear space, final medial clear space, American Orthopaedic Foot and Ankle Society score, and rate of complications compared with nonrepair. The repair of the deltoid ligament in patients with acute ankle fractures might be beneficial to ankle joint stability and assist in improving the quality of ankle reduction. More high-quality and prospective studies with long follow-up durations are needed to further demonstrate the superiority of deltoid ligament repair over nonrepair. Level of evidence: I.

CHAPTER 26

Arthroscopy of the Foot and Ankle and Osteochondral Lesions of the Talus

ERIC I. FERKEL, MD, FAAOS • CHRISTOPHER L. RULAND, MD, MS

ABSTRACT

Arthroscopy offers the orthopaedic surgeon a unique surgical technique for diagnosis and treatment of conditions of the foot and ankle. By providing the ability to perform procedures in a manner that minimizes soft-tissue disruption, arthroscopy has changed the practice of orthopaedics. As familiarity with local anatomy and proficiency with arthroscopy continue to increase, the indications and techniques are also expanding in the foot and ankle. Arthroscopic treatment of ankle impingement, osteochondral lesions, arthritis, ligamentous instability, tendinopathies, and fractures continues to develop. Osteochondral lesions of the talus are common and difficult problems to treat and typically are associated with a history of trauma; however, nontraumatic etiologies have been described. There are many options for surgical intervention, typically categorized as primary repair, reparative techniques, replacement techniques, and restorative techniques. The size, type, location, stability, and displacement of the lesion should be taken into consideration when deciding on the appropriate surgical intervention.

Dr. Ferkel or an immediate family member is a member of a speakers' bureau or has made paid presentations on behalf of Arthrex, Inc. and Ferring Pharmaceuticals; serves as a paid consultant to or is an employee of Arthrex, Inc., Ferring Pharmaceuticals, Medartis, Mitek, Ossio, and Smith & Nephew; has received research or institutional support from DJ Orthopaedics, Mitek, Össur, and Smith & Nephew; and serves as a board member, owner, officer, or committee member of American Academy of Orthopaedic Surgeons, American Orthopaedic Foot and Ankle Society, American Orthopaedic Society for Sports Medicine, and Arthroscopy Association of North America. Neither Dr. Ruland nor any immediate family member has received anything of value from or has stock or stock options held in a commercial company or institution related directly or indirectly to the subject of this chapter.

Keywords: ankle arthroscopy; ankle impingement; osteochondral allograft transplantation; osteochondral lesions of the talus; tendoscopy

INTRODUCTION

Ankle arthroscopy, along with subtalar arthroscopy, tendoscopy, hindfoot endoscopy and forefoot arthroscopy, has given orthopaedic surgeons minimally invasive access to diagnose and treat a multitude of pathologies. There have been substantial developments over the past 100 years in arthroscopy that now allow the surgeon to directly inspect and treat joint, tendon, ligament, and cartilage injuries that may decrease morbidities for the patient, leading to a decrease in

This chapter is adapted from Miniaci-Coxhead SL: Osteochondral lesions of the talus; and Jockel JR: Arthroscopy of the foot and ankle, in Chou LB, ed: *Orthopaedic Knowledge Update®: Foot and Ankle 6*. American Academy of Orthopaedic Surgeons, 2020, pp 409-430.

postoperative pain and ideally faster rehabilitation and return to sports and daily activities. It is important to discuss the basics of ankle and foot arthroscopy, tendoscopy and endoscopy, including the indications, techniques and approach to a variety of pathologies.

Osteochondral lesions in the ankle and foot, specifically the talus, are a relatively uncommon injury; however, they can often be seen in patients with ankle sprains and associated trauma. These lesions are challenging to treat, which highlights the importance of clinical diagnosis by the physician. Improved imaging studies and greater technologic advancements in treating this pathology make earlier diagnosis and management of osteochondral lesions critical. The physician needs the most up-to-date information to better understand the best evidence-based diagnosis and treatment methods for osteochondral lesions.

ARTHROSCOPY OF THE FOOT AND ANKLE

Arthroscopy is an essential aspect of orthopaedic foot and ankle practice, originating primarily as a diagnostic tool and evolving from simple evaluations. Arthroscopy has advanced from a tool of débridement and documentation to more advanced diagnostic and reconstruction procedures. Although anterior ankle arthroscopy continues to be the most common type of procedure, posterior ankle arthroscopy is gaining popularity. Furthermore, the roles of tendoscopy and small joint arthroscopy in the foot continue to expand. Moreover, the indications for arthroscopy continue to expand from diagnostic to treatment and management of trauma, instability, reconstruction, and cartilage restoration. The skill of arthroscopy allows for minimally invasive access, potentially leading to faster rehabilitation and less morbidity.

Anterior Ankle Arthroscopy

Anterior ankle arthroscopy is essential to a foot and ankle arthroscopist's practice. Low complication rates can be expected when modern methods of anterior ankle arthroscopy are used. In general, complication rates are higher than average for patients with a workers' compensation claim, and patients who do not have a specific preoperative diagnosis are likely to have a relatively poor outcome.[1,2] There are numerous indications that will be described in the next several paragraphs. Damage to the superficial peroneal nerve is the most common complication following anterior ankle arthroscopy. The use of noninvasive distraction, preoperative identification of the superficial peroneal nerve, and careful portal placement all will help reduce the rate of complications following ankle arthroscopy.[1] Proper education about portal-related complications has been shown in a 2020 study to decrease the rate of injury to the superficial peroneal nerve.[3]

Indications

Conditions commonly managed with anterior ankle arthroscopy include anterolateral or anteromedial impingement, osteochondral lesions of the talus (OLTs) and tibial plafond, synovitis, and symptomatic loose bodies (**Figure 1**). Anterior ankle arthroscopy also is used for arthroscopically assisted arthrodesis, medial and lateral ankle ligament stabilization, and fracture reduction. Arthroscopy is a great option in evacuation, irrigation, and débridement of a septic ankle joint. Arthroscopic treatment of impingement lesions and arthrofibrosis after total ankle arthroplasty is likely to become more common with the increasing popularity of total ankle arthroplasty procedures.[4]

Technique

Most ankle arthroscopic procedures can be performed as outpatient ambulatory surgery. The modern setup for ankle arthroscopy includes a small joint 2.7- or 1.9-mm arthroscope; a 4.0-mm arthroscope is rarely used, and routine use is not recommended because its larger size prevents safe maneuverability within the joint. Gravity or an arthroscopic pump at a low pressure (40 mm Hg) and flow can be used to control the fluid inflow and help obtain hemostasis and improve visualization.

A general and regional block anesthetic agent is routinely used for ankle arthroscopy. A prospective randomized study evaluated the influence of a preoperative intra-articular injection of a local anesthetic agent on postoperative pain following ankle arthroscopy. In addition to a general or spinal anesthetic agent, patients receiving a preoperative intra-articular anesthetic injection reported significantly lower pain levels during the first 24 hours following surgery. Lower amounts of

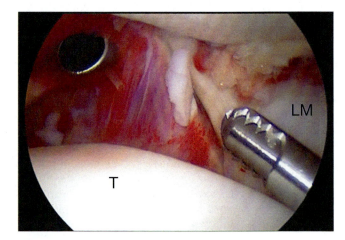

FIGURE 1 Anterior ankle arthroscopic image, with visualization from the anteromedial portal, demonstrating a loose body in the lateral joint space. LM = lateral malleolus, T = talus

supplemental analgesic agents also were required when a preemptive anesthetic injection was administered. No significant differences in pain were seen on postoperative days 2 or 3.[5]

Traditionally, a thigh tourniquet has been used during arthroscopy to minimize bleeding, improve surgeon visibility, and decrease surgical time. A prospective randomized controlled trial evaluated anterior ankle arthroscopy with and without the use of a tourniquet. Although the quality of visualization was statistically different between the two groups, there was no difference in surgical time or blood loss. Because the tourniquet did not need to be inflated for procedure completion in any of the patients not using a tourniquet, it was concluded that ankle arthroscopy could be performed adequately without the use of a tourniquet.[6]

Noninvasive ankle distraction can be used to improve visualization of the joint space, and a padded thigh holder is useful for providing countertraction. Distraction improves visualization of the central and posterior compartments, as well as the medial gutter and deltoid ligament (**Figure 2**). A cadaver study demonstrated that posterior structures such as the deep fascicle of the posterior tibiofibular ligament and the intermalleolar ligament could be observed better with distraction-assisted anterior arthroscopy.[2] Because most complications are neurologic in nature, prolonged use of traction should be avoided to prevent neurapraxia.

Dorsiflexion of the ankle without traction also can be performed. By increasing the volume of the anterior joint pouch, this technique is advantageous for evaluating the anterior compartment and lateral gutter, including inspection of the lateral ankle and syndesmotic ligaments.[2] A 2020 cadaver study also demonstrated that ankle dorsiflexion and nondistraction arthroscopic technique allows full visualization of the medial and lateral ankle collateral ligaments: the superior fascicle of the anterior talofibular ligament, the distal fascicle of the anterior tibiofibular ligament, and the anterior tibiotalar ligament.[7]

Typically, a two-portal or three-portal technique is used along with an anteromedial, anterolateral, and/or posterolateral portal (**Figure 3**). An anteromedial portal is created at the joint level just medial to the tibialis anterior tendon. A No. 11 blade scalpel is used to nick the skin, and a small hemostat is used to vertically spread the underlying soft tissue for entering the joint capsule. The saphenous nerve and vein can be at risk of injury with establishment of the anteromedial portal. The anterolateral portal is created just lateral to the peroneus tertius at the joint line with care to avoid injury to the superficial peroneal nerve, which frequently can be seen through the skin, and is at risk of injury during establishment of the anterolateral portal. The superficial peroneal nerve moves 4 mm laterally when the ankle is brought from plantar flexion to neutral, and the anterolateral incision should be made medial to the visualized nerve to avoid iatrogenic damage.[8] Although skin closure can be performed according to surgeon preference as discussed in a 2019 study, an improperly placed suture can irritate the intermediate branch of the superficial peroneal nerve.[9] The posterolateral portal, which is placed at the soft spot just lateral to the Achilles tendon, 1.2 cm above a parallel line drawn from the fibular tip, can be used for inflow and as a safe additional working portal.

Ankle Impingement

Ankle impingement can be described as soft tissue or bony. Anterolateral soft-tissue impingement by the anterior inferior tibiofibular ligament is common.[10] These lesions are

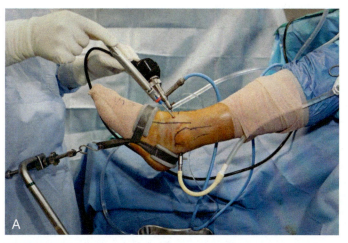
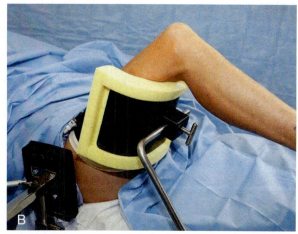

FIGURE 2 Anterior ankle arthroscopy. Clinical photographs show all three portals used for visualization (**A**) and the working portal and inflow with thigh holder distraction (**B**).

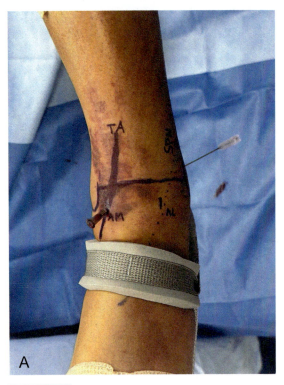
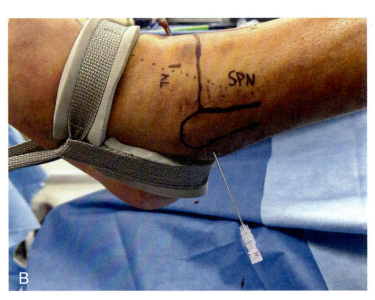

FIGURE 3 Supine ankle arthroscopy. Clinical photographs show anterolateral (AL) and anteromedial (AM) (**A**) and posterolateral (**B**) portals. SPN = superficial peroneal nerve, TA = tibialis anterior

thought to be caused by multiple inversion injuries that lead to the formation of hypertrophy at either the superior portion of the anterior inferior tibiofibular ligament, inferior portion of the anterior inferior tibiofibular ligament or at separate fascicle, or Bassett ligament after resorption of hematoma after an ankle sprain. The patient commonly reports a history of ankle sprains and swelling, with pain during palpation at the anterolateral ankle that is worse with dorsiflexion. Pain with single-leg squatting and ankle eversion or dorsiflexion is shown to best correlate with positive findings on ankle arthroscopy. MRI can be useful for ruling out other entities, but often the MRI findings do not contribute to making a correct diagnosis of anterolateral soft-tissue impingement. A diagnostic intra-articular injection may be useful in this regard.

Anteromedial impingement lesions can occur after repeated capsular traction injuries or deltoid injuries that lead to scarring and hypertrophy of the synovium. The typical patient is a soccer player or a martial artist. Anteromedial osseous abnormality, if present, often can be seen on oblique radiographs of the foot. Arthroscopic resection of anteromedial impingement lesions was found to have a satisfactory outcome in 93% of patients.[11]

Arthroscopic Ankle Arthrodesis

Arthroscopic ankle arthrodesis is a minimally invasive way to treat patients with end-stage ankle arthritis. Purported advantages of the arthroscopic approach include less disruption of the soft-tissue envelope, shorter time to bone union, preservation of bony anatomy allowing potential conversion to future ankle arthroplasty, and the ability to perform surgery on high-risk patients as well as those with compromised soft tissues (**Figure 4**).

A multicenter study evaluated open and arthroscopic arthrodesis using a validated Ankle Osteoarthritis Scale score measuring disability and pain. Although both groups had significant improvements after surgery, the arthroscopic group had significantly better scores than the open arthrodesis group at both 1- and 2-year follow-up, as well as a more rapid rate of postoperative improvement. No difference in tourniquet times between open and arthroscopic techniques was reported, and equivalent deformity correction and nonunion rates were achieved.[12] A 2020 systematic review demonstrated a significantly higher fusion rate, less blood loss, shorter tourniquet time, and shorter length of hospitalization following arthroscopic arthrodesis compared with open surgery.[13]

Ankle Ligament Repair

Lateral ankle sprains are one of the most common injuries seen by the orthopaedic surgeon (approximately 300,000 ankle sprains annually).[14] Because of the high rate of associated intra-articular pathology, arthroscopy often is performed in the same surgical setting as treatment

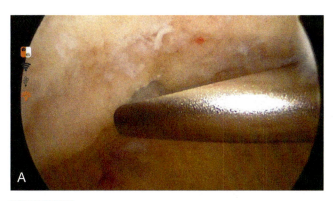 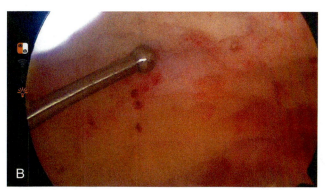

FIGURE 4 Final preparation of bone surfaces with a burr during arthroscopic ankle arthrodesis. Arthroscopic images showing punctate bleeding of the tibia (**A**) and talus (**B**).

of chronic lateral ankle instability,[15] and arthroscopically assisted ankle stabilization procedures are being reported with increasing frequency. These techniques primarily focus on the repair and reconstruction of the anterior talofibular ligament and less commonly include the calcaneofibular ligament.

The open modified Broström technique incorporates the extensor retinaculum into the ankle ligament repair. A randomized controlled trial found no significant clinical differences between arthroscopic all-inside repair and open modified Broström technique procedures at 1-year follow-up. Furthermore, there were no radiographic differences in talar tilt and anterior drawer test results between the two techniques 1 year postoperatively.[16]

A long-term study reported a 95% rate of good to excellent outcomes with a three-portal technique for reconstruction of the anterior talofibular ligament with extensor retinaculum reinforcement at an average follow-up of 9.8 years; the calcaneofibular ligament was not surgically treated. Eighty-seven percent of active patients were able to return to sports activities at their preoperative level, whereas 13% changed to a lower level or gave up sports participation.[17]

As a developing technique, the reported complication rate of arthroscopic ankle stabilization in some studies has approached 30%.[16] To avoid soft-tissue and nerve entrapment during arthroscopic ligament repair, a safe zone has been described. This quadrant includes the 51-mm intertendinous safe zone from peroneus tertius to peroneus brevis, 43-mm internervous zone between the sural and superficial peroneal nerves, and 15 mm from the tip of the fibula to the inferior extensor retinaculum.[18] A 2020 meta-analysis comparing arthroscopic versus open repair of lateral ankle ligament demonstrated significant difference in favor of arthroscopic repair with regard to American Orthopaedic Foot and Ankle Society (AOFAS) functional outcome score, but no significant difference with regard to Karlsson score. There was also no difference in total, nerve, or wound complications with at least 12 months of follow-up in each group. It was concluded that current evidence is still limited with regard to open versus arthroscopic management of lateral ankle instability, and further prospective trials with longer follow-up are needed.[19] Similarly, a 2020 systematic review and meta-analysis comparing open versus arthroscopic management of lateral ankle instability demonstrated improvement in AOFAS scores in the arthroscopic group compared with the open treatment group, with no differences in stress radiograph outcomes or total and nerve complication rates.[20]

Arthroscopy-Assisted Fracture Management

Intra-articular injuries are common with acute ankle fractures, and these injuries may be underdiagnosed or misdiagnosed with traditional radiographic evaluation alone. Arthroscopy in the setting of an ankle fracture allows for evaluation of the ligamentous injury, degree of instability, chondral surface of the talus and tibial plafond for osteochondral lesions, and assessment of the reduction of the articular surfaces of the tibia and talus and also allows for removal of loose bodies. Caution should be exercised with arthroscopy in the setting of an acute ankle fracture to avoid excessive fluid extravasation and swelling to minimize the risk of potential compartment syndrome and is contraindicated in the setting of an open fracture or severe swelling. Arthroscopy also can be used for assistance with reduction, and evaluation of restoration of articular alignment and syndesmotic congruity (**Figure 5**).

There are relatively few studies directly comparing ankle fracture open reduction and internal fixation (ORIF) with and without arthroscopy. One study compared functional outcomes following ankle fracture ORIF with and without simultaneous arthroscopy at an average follow-up of 67 months. Using a validated Patient-Reported Outcomes Measurement Information System score, the study authors found no significant

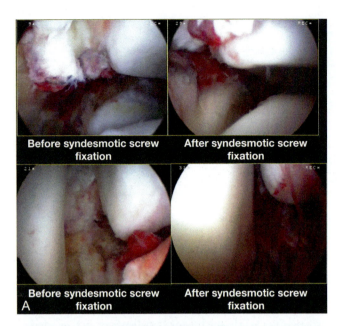
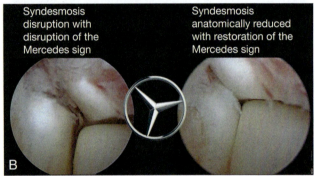

FIGURE 5 Arthroscopic evaluation of an ankle fracture with syndesmosis disruption with evidence of reduction of the syndesmosis as confirmed arthroscopically postreduction (**A** and **B**).

differences between the two groups despite 21% of the patients who underwent ankle ORIF with ankle arthroscopy having removal of loose bodies and 62% having associated cartilage lesions of the tibia or talus. Notably, the surgical time was significantly longer in patients who underwent ankle ORIF with ankle arthroscopy. The results of this study did not support the routine use of arthroscopy to improve functional outcomes of ankle ORIF.[21]

A 2019 study looked at the use of arthroscopic reduction and minimally invasive surgery (ARMIS) plating compared with standard ORIF. ARMIS was followed by arthroscopy for detection of syndesmotic injuries and arthroscopic reduction of medial malleolar fracture or mini-open repair of the deltoid ligament. More syndesmotic injuries were detected in the ARMIS group, and visual analog scale pain score was lower in the ARMIS group in comparison with the ORIF group. The postoperative hospital stay was shorter in the ARMIS group. However, in a 2019 study, longer surgical time and higher irradiation doses were found in the ARMIS group in comparison with the ORIF group.[22]

A 2020 retrospective cohort study compared results of ORIF without arthroscopy and ORIF with ankle arthroscopy. In this study, ankle arthroscopy at the time of ORIF led to significant improvements in patient-reported outcomes for Weber B fibula fractures and ankle dislocations. There was no difference in complication rates and the arthroscopy took 10 minutes longer to perform on average.[23]

Posterior Ankle Arthroscopy and Hindfoot Endoscopy

Posterior ankle arthroscopy is not performed as often as anterior ankle arthroscopy, and many orthopaedic surgeons are less experienced with this procedure.[24] The increasing number of reports on posterior ankle arthroscopy reflects an evolving interest among foot and ankle orthopaedic surgeons. Hindfoot arthroscopy and endoscopy have been popularized as a safe way to evaluate and treat patients with a multitude of posterior ankle pathology.

Anatomy

Knowledge of hindfoot anatomy is crucial to avoid injury to the surrounding neurovascular structures. The relevant posterior anatomy of the talus includes the posterior bony tubercles, flexor hallucis longus (FHL) tendon, multiple ligamentous attachments, and the ankle and subtalar joints. The posterior process of the talus includes the medial tubercle, or Cedell process, which is the attachment for the posterior tibiotalar/deltoid ligament. The lateral tubercle, or Stieda process, is the attachment for the posterior talofibular ligament. An os trigonum results from the unossified posterior lateral tubercle forming a synchondrosis, as opposed to complete bone fusion with the talus, at its secondary ossification center (**Figure 6, A**).

The FHL tendon courses between the medial and lateral tubercles of the posterior process of the talus at the ankle joint level and serves as a major landmark during ankle arthroscopic procedures. The neurovascular structures should be safe from injury if arthroscopic surgery is lateral to the FHL. However, the occasional presence of an accessory muscle called the peroneocalcaneus internus muscle, or false FHL, can disorient an inexperienced arthroscopic surgeon and jeopardize the neurovascular structures.

Indications

Several indications for posterior ankle arthroscopy have been described: débridement of posterior soft-tissue impingement of the ankle, microfracture of osteochondral

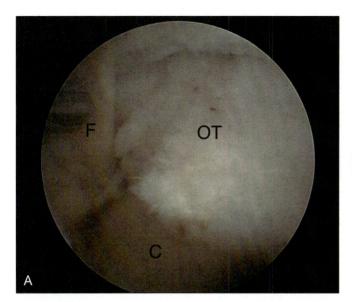 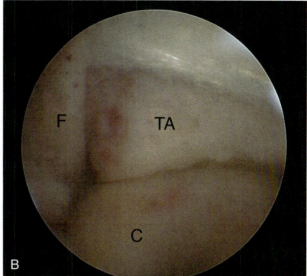

FIGURE 6 **A,** Arthroscopic image demonstrating the management of posterior ankle impingement caused by symptomatic os trigonum (OT). Flexor hallucis longus (F) is the critical safety landmark medially. **B,** Arthroscopic image demonstrating endoscopic excision of os trigonum using a burr for débridement. C = calcaneus, TA = talus

lesions, excision of a symptomatic os trigonum—Stieda process, removal of loose bodies, visualization of structures not well seen in anterior ankle arthroscopy, and visualization during fracture reduction or arthrodesis.[2] Hindfoot endoscopy is indicated for retrocalcaneal bursitis, Haglund deformity, and FHL tenosynovitis.

Contraindications include an inadequate period of appropriate nonsurgical treatment, infection, and an earlier open procedure that may have caused scarring around the vital structures. Relative contraindications include the presence of vascular disease and severe edema.

Technique

Isolated posterior ankle arthroscopy usually is performed with the patient lying in a prone position. After induction of general or spinal anesthesia and proper padding to prevent iatrogenic injury, the patient is positioned with the ankle distal to the edge of the operating table. A bump-type positioning device can be used under the distal tibia. A thigh tourniquet is applied and inflated. A 4.0-mm arthroscope and shaver can be used outside the joint capsule to clear the soft-tissue envelope and create working space. A small joint arthroscope then can be used if needed. An arthroscopic pump, if used, should be set at 30 to 40 mm Hg. Although a minimally invasive distraction technique has been described, most routine setups do not include distraction.[25,26]

The posterolateral portal is created at the level of the tip of the fibula, along the lateral border of the Achilles tendon. The medial portal is created at the same level at the medial border of the Achilles tendon. The initial skin incision should be superficial and should be followed by vertical spreading of the underlying soft tissues to prevent iatrogenic injury to nearby structures. Fluoroscopy should be available to assist in portal placement, if needed. The arthroscope initially is introduced through the lateral portal. A blunt probe is introduced through the medial portal and directed toward the arthroscope until the instruments are in contact. The probe then follows the arthroscope to the posterior ankle joint.[26] An alternative technique has been described for introducing the instruments toward the fibula to avoid inadvertently damaging the medial neurovascular structures.[27] An anatomic study suggested keeping the ankle in neutral position and making the portals at the level of the tip of the fibula to avoid iatrogenic neurovascular injury.

Combined anterior and posterior ankle arthroscopy may be indicated for some patients. As complete repositioning disrupts the procedure and requires an intraoperative delay, an experienced arthroscopic surgeon can consider other positioning options including the lateral decubitus, supine, and prone positions. In the lateral decubitus position, the leg is externally rotated over a leg holder for anterior ankle arthroscopy; the leg holder then is removed and the hip is internally rotated to facilitate posterior ankle arthroscopy.[28] After anterior ankle arthroscopy is performed with the patient supine, the leg holder is removed and the leg is then externally rotated at the hip to allow access to the medial ankle. Two medial portals are created to accomplish posterior ankle arthroscopy.[29] When the prone position is used, the ankle is suspended on a shoulder-holding traction frame to allow combined anterior and posterior arthroscopy without repositioning the patient.[30]

Posterior Ankle Impingement

Posterior ankle impingement can be either bony or soft tissue in nature and is a common cause of posterior ankle pain in athletes. Posterior talar compression can occur in extreme plantar flexion when the posterior lip of the tibia closes against the superior border of the calcaneus. This condition most commonly occurs as a result of repetitive injury to these structures in dancers and soccer players. The patient often reports having posterior ankle pain while running downhill, wearing high heels, or dancing in the en pointe or demi pointe ballet position. In dancers, posterior impingement also can be caused by pseudomeniscal transformation of the posterior transverse ligament.[31]

Posterior ankle soft-tissue impingement is seen most commonly in the posterolateral corner at the posterior talofibular ligament and transverse ligament. Posteromedial impingement can develop after ankle sprains with injury to the deep deltoid ligament, leading to entrapment of fibrotic scar tissue in the posteromedial gutter of the ankle. In some cases, inadequate healing of posteromedial soft tissue leads to the formation of thickened and disorganized fibrous tissue within the posteromedial ankle joint, which impinges between the posterior aspect of the medial malleolus and the medial talus.

Hypertrophy of the posterior tibiotalar/deltoid ligament after an injury that caused intra-articular impingement can be managed with posterior ankle arthroscopy. Other causes of posteromedial ankle pain include FHL tendon pathology and missed fracture of the Cedell process.[32] Because of the proximity of neurovascular structures, open management of these extra-articular conditions is recommended. No conclusive data exist to support all-arthroscopic management of these conditions, and it should be avoided until the safety profile of the arthroscopic approach to medial pathology is firmly established.

The goal of surgery for posterior ankle impingement is to remove the offending soft tissue or osseous structures. Isolated treatment of patients with extra-articular pathology is with hindfoot endoscopy by definition; however, the ankle and subtalar joints can be routinely assessed in the same surgical setting. An os trigonum causing posterior impingement can be débrided with a large burr or excised in its entirety (**Figure 6, B**).

Endoscopic management of posterior ankle impingement may lead to an earlier return to activities than an open procedure. A randomized controlled trial compared open and endoscopic excision of os trigonum for the management of posterior ankle impingement in athletes. All patients were able to achieve their previous level of sports participation at 5-year final follow-up and had good outcomes in regard to pain and function. The group undergoing endoscopic excision, however, had a significantly shorter return to training by 5 weeks and return to prior sports participation level by 4 weeks, compared with patients undergoing an open procedure. The number of complications with the endoscopic approach for os trigonum excision also was significantly lower.[33] Other studies also have shown early return to athletics with this approach for posterior impingement.[34]

Subtalar Arthroscopy

Indications

Subtalar arthroscopy is used to assist with diagnosis and treatment of the various pathologies of the subtalar joint, some of which may be difficult to fully diagnose without arthroscopic evaluation. The conditions that may warrant subtalar arthroscopy include osteochondral lesions, excision of painful os trigonum from a supine approach, excision of synovitis, sinus tarsi syndrome, loose bodies, and arthrofibrosis. If pain, swelling, catching, and locking continue despite a course of nonsurgical treatment, subtalar arthroscopy can be considered.[35] Confirmation of the diagnosis with an injection of either a corticosteroid or a local anesthetic to the subtalar joint may be considered as part of the preoperative workup. Subtalar arthroscopy also has been described for excision of tarsal coalitions, subtalar arthrodesis, and assistance with fracture reduction[35]

Technique

The procedure can be performed with the patient in either the lateral or prone position. Small joint equipment and setup for subtalar arthroscopy are similar to those for anterior tibiotalar joint arthroscopy, using 1.9-mm, 30° and 2.7- to 3.0-mm, 70° short arthroscopes. A 70° arthroscope should be available to improve visualization in the confined space.

Three portals are typically used primarily (anterolateral, central, posterolateral). The anterolateral subtalar arthroscopy portal is created 2.5 to 3 cm anterior to the fibular tip, the central portal is created just inferior to the fibular tip and approximately a thumb's breadth anterior to the fibular tip, and the posterolateral portal is created 2 cm posterior and 1 cm proximal to the fibular tip in the soft spot lateral to the Achilles tendon. An accessory portal may be necessary. Alternatively, two-portal subtalar arthroscopy can be performed using a posterior portal technique with the patient lying in the prone position, as in a posterior ankle arthroscopy setup.

Subtalar Arthrodesis

Subtalar arthrodesis can be used to treat patients with subtalar arthritis. Traditional open arthrodesis has a fusion rate of 84% to 95%, and a similar success rate can be expected after arthroscopic subtalar arthrodesis by an experienced arthroscopic surgeon. The arthroscopic approach may offer advantages important for surgical success, especially in patients at high risk, including preservation of the talar blood supply and protection of the soft tissues from intraoperative damage. Although the limits of deformity correction have not yet been defined, patients with a severe deformity should not be treated with the arthroscopic approach.

A retrospective review compared outcomes in 121 patients (129 feet) following open or arthroscopic subtalar arthrodesis. With an almost 2-year mean follow-up, there were no significant differences in 36-Item Short Form (SF-36) scores, Foot Function Index, visual analog scale pain scores, or union rates between the groups. The time to union, however, was significantly shorter in the arthroscopic group by approximately 4 weeks. Furthermore, the time to return to activities of daily living, sports, and work was also significantly less following arthroscopic fusion. Because there were no differences in overall complications or surgical time between the groups, it was suggested that arthroscopic and open arthrodesis are of comparable technical difficulty following learning curve progression and advanced experience.[36] A 2021 systematic review demonstrated similar results, and it was concluded that arthroscopic subtalar fusion was a safe and effective alternative to open subtalar arthrodesis with high patient satisfaction scores, high union rates, and low complication rates.[37]

Arthrofibrosis

Arthroscopic débridement of the joint can be considered as an alternative to subtalar arthrodesis for the management of arthrofibrosis after calcaneal fracture. In a retrospective study, 17 patients with painful stiffness after a Sanders type II or III calcaneal fracture underwent arthroscopic débridement of the subtalar joint. The mean AOFAS score had increased from 50 to 80 points at 17-month follow-up. Although no immediate complications were noted, two patients subsequently underwent arthrodesis.[38]

First Metatarsophalangeal Joint Arthroscopy

Arthroscopy of the great toe metatarsophalangeal (MTP) joint is an excellent minimally invasive treatment approach. The theoretical advantages of the procedure include less bleeding, lower infection rate, less scarring, better cosmesis, and more rapid recovery than with an open procedure. No studies have directly compared open and arthroscopic treatment of pathology of the first MTP joint.[39]

Indications and Contraindications

The reported indications for first MTP joint arthroscopy include unsuccessful nonsurgical management of hallux rigidus, focal chondral lesions, loose bodies, arthrofibrosis, synovitis, and arthritis. The contraindications include local infection, severe joint disease, severe edema, and severe joint space narrowing. The indications and contraindications continue to evolve.[35]

Technique

Traction can be provided using a sterile finger trap device or suspension holder commonly used in wrist arthroscopic procedures. Because of the small joint size, a short 1.9- to 2.7-mm arthroscope is used. Relatively small-diameter shavers (2.0 to 2.3 mm) are recommended. Dorsomedial and dorsolateral portals are created at the joint, avoiding the extensor hallucis longus tendon and the dorsomedial cutaneous branch of the superficial peroneal nerve. A straight medial portal can also be used midway between the dorsal and plantar aspect and created under direct visualization. As in arthroscopy of other joints, a nick-and-spread technique is used to enter the MTP joint capsule from portals at the joint. A straight medial portal can be used to improve the ability to see the sesamoid–metatarsal head articulation (**Figure 7**).

Hallux Rigidus

Arthroscopic cheilectomy of the first MTP joint can be considered for removal of small osteophytes. The

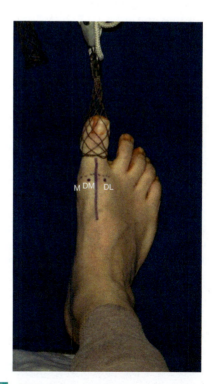

FIGURE 7 Clinical photograph showing first metatarsophalangeal joint arthroscopy with distraction. The dorsal medial (DM), dorsolateral (DL), and medial (M) portals are marked and identified.

arthroscopic shaver can be used from the dorsomedial portal to improve visualization. The arthroscopic burr is used to remove the dorsal spur.[35] There are several reports reviewing the results of the great toe arthroscopy. Published reports on small cohorts reflect overall good to excellent results in up to 74% of patients.[40]

First MTP Joint Arthrodesis

To preserve the soft-tissue envelope in patients who have a high risk of poor wound healing, arthroscopic fusion of the first MTP joint can be considered. Only anecdotal reports and small studies have been published. A cadaver study found that the use of a third accessory medial portal led to more complete cartilage débridement than the two-portal technique.[41] Intraoperative fluoroscopy and a high-angled small joint arthroscope should be readily available. Percutaneous screws can be placed for stabilization in this procedure.

Tendoscopy

Tendsocopic management of foot and ankle tendon pathology can lead to faster recovery times and quicker mobilization. Although the intra-articular portion of the FHL is routinely seen during ankle arthroscopic procedures, true diagnostic and interventional tendoscopy of the ankle and hindfoot is uncommon.

A systematic review attempted to determine on which tendons of the foot and ankle tendoscopy is supported by the current literature. The outcomes and complications for generally accepted indications of tendoscopy were evaluated and an evidence-based recommendation was assigned. Poor-quality (grade C_f) evidence was assigned in support of tendoscopy of peroneal, FHL, and Achilles tendons. There was insufficient (grade I) evidence to recommend for or against tendoscopy of tibialis anterior, tibialis posterior, flexor digitorum longus, extensor hallucis longus, and extensor digitorum longus tendons. Despite the paucity of studies, it was concluded that foot and ankle tendoscopy can be performed as an effective and safe procedure.[42]

Although most of the existing studies are from a limited number of institutions, tendoscopy may become more common as further scientific studies and techniques are reported.

Posterior Tibial Tendon

Patients with medial hindfoot pain who have tenderness directly over the tendon sheath may have pathology involving the posterior tibial tendon. Clinical suspicion is further elevated if the patient has difficulty or pain with single-toe heel raises. After an unsuccessful course of nonsurgical treatment, described indications for posterior tibial tendoscopy include tenosynovitis, tendinopathy, dislocation, and posttraumatic adhesions.[42]

Posterior tibial tendoscopy portals can be created approximately 2 cm proximal and 2 cm distal to the tip of the medial malleolus, directly superficial to the posterior tibial tendon. With the use of a small joint arthroscope and shaver, tenosynovitis, vincula thickening, and partial tears can be débrided.

Peroneal Tendons

The peroneal tendons are the primary dynamic lateral stabilizers of the ankle. Patients with reported ankle instability symptoms and pain located directly over the tendons are suspected to have pathology of the peroneal tendons. Pain, snapping, and swelling over the tendons may be noted on clinical examination; however, true weakness of the peroneal tendons is atypical unless there is a complete tear. Cavus alignment, peroneal tendon subluxation, and ankle instability should be assessed clinically. Intra-articular ankle pathology may exist concurrently and needs to be managed.[43]

The indications for tendoscopy may include peroneal tenosynovitis, postoperative adhesions and scarring, small partial tears, snapping, and tendon instability.[42] The setup for peroneal tendoscopy is such that the patient lies in a supine or lateral position, and an ankle distractor is not recommended. The distal portal is created 2 cm distal to the tip of the fibula, and the proximal portal is created 3 cm proximal to the tip of the fibula. Small shavers and low inflow are used.

Intrasheath subluxation of the peroneal tendon can be difficult to diagnose clinically, and MRI findings often are negative. Dynamic ultrasonography can be important for making the correct diagnosis. The common causes of intrasheath subluxation include the presence of a peroneus quartus or another accessory muscle, a low-lying muscle belly of the peroneus brevis, and a nonconcave configuration of the posterior fibular surface. Endoscopic evaluation and groove deepening have been recommended, and a favorable outcome was reported in a study of six patients.[44]

Achilles Tendon

The primary indications for tendoscopy of the Achilles tendon include the management of noninsertional tendinopathy and peritendinopathy, as well as assistance with repair of tendon ruptures.[42]

A retrospective case series reported high patient satisfaction following management of noninsertional tendinopathy by endoscopic release of the paratenon of the Achilles tendon and plantaris transection, at a median follow-up of almost 5 years. With prone positioning, the distal portal was initially created 2 to 3 cm below the pathologic region on the lateral edge of the Achilles tendon. The proximal portal was created 2 to 4 cm above the tendinopathy along the medial tendon border. A shaver was then used to resect the anterior Achilles tendon paratenon at the level of tendon nodularity to remove areas of neovascularization.[45]

Distal procedures in proximity to the Achilles tendon also continue to be developed. Endoscopic retrocalcaneal bursectomy and calcaneoplasty can also be performed with the patient lying in a prone position. With a 4.0-mm arthroscope to provide inflow for visualization, intraoperative mini-fluoroscopy is used to confirm the adequacy of bone removal, if needed.[46] The endoscopic technique may be preferred for treating some patients at high risk for wound dehiscence with an open technique.

OSTEOCHONDRAL LESIONS OF THE TALUS

Osteochondritis dissecans was originally described as a process of loose body formation associated with articular cartilage and subchondral bone fracture in the hip and knee. Historically, a variety of terms including osteochondritis dissecans, transchondral talar fracture, and osteochondral talar fracture have been used to describe what are now universally referred to as OLTs, a term that was introduced in 1994.[47]

Incidence

OLTs represent approximately 4% of all osteochondral lesions. An epidemiologic study of active-duty US military personnel found the overall occurrence of OLTs to be 27 per 100,000 patient-years over a 10-year period.[48] This finding suggests that OLTs may be more common than previously considered. Several authors have reported that the incidence of bilateral lesions is approximately 10%.[49] In a 2022 study, in patients presenting with symptomatic OLT, the prevalence of bilateral OLT was 15%, with 33% of these patients having bilateral symptomatic OLT. Patients with bilateral symptomatic OLTs were younger and more likely to present with nontraumatic etiology in comparison with patients with unilateral symptoms.[50]

Medial osteochondral lesions are more common than lateral osteochondral lesions. Medial lesions have been described as deeper with extension into subchondral bone, and they often develop into cystic lesions. Lateral lesions, which are more commonly associated with a traumatic injury, are described as shallow and have the tendency to become displaced.[51]

A grid system was used to identify the precise location of talar dome lesions in an MRI study of 428 ankles with OLTs. In contrast to the historically described anterolateral and posteromedial locations, the midtalar dome was involved in 80% of lesions. It was determined that the midmedial zone was the most common location (53%). The lesions in this location were the largest and deepest. The midlateral zone was the second most common zone (26%).[52]

Clinical Presentation

An OLT diagnosis is rarely made immediately after an acute ankle injury, although radiographs at initial presentation can show an osteochondral fracture of the talus. In most cases, the condition is associated with chronic ankle pain, especially after inversion injury to the lateral ligamentous complex. Patients presenting with an OLT often describe prolonged pain, recurrent ankle swelling, weakness, and continued subjective instability. Patients also may report mechanical symptoms including catching, clicking, and locking. The physical examination may reveal tenderness at the level of the ankle mortise anteriorly or posteriorly. The differential diagnosis is wide, but a high index of suspicion must be maintained for an OLT when evaluating patients with chronic ankle pain.[53]

Etiology/Pathoanatomy/Natural History

The etiology of an OLT may be nontraumatic or traumatic. Most authors think that trauma has an integral role in the pathogenesis of most OLTs and that OLTs most likely represent the chronic phase of a compressed talar dome fracture. A single event of macrotrauma or repetitive microtrauma may elicit initiation of the lesion in a person who is already predisposed to talar dome ischemia.

Subchondral cysts with overlying chondromalacia, osteochondral fragments, and loose bodies all represent various stages in the progression of OLTs. The development of a symptomatic OLT depends on various factors. The primary mechanism is damage and insufficient repair of the subchondral bone plate. One study theorized that water from compressed cartilage is forced into the microfractured subchondral bone during loading, which subsequently leads to localized increased fluid pressure within the subchondral bone. Local osteolysis can then predispose to the development of a subchondral cyst. The pain is thought to be a result of stimulation of the highly innervated subchondral bone under the cartilage defect.[53]

The precise natural history of OLTs is unclear. In a review of serial MRI studies from 29 patients with OLTs treated nonsurgically, 45% showed progression, 24% improved, and 31% remained unchanged. Bone marrow edema and subchondral cysts were found not to be reliable indicators of lesion progression.[54]

Imaging and Classification

The first staging system based on radiographic findings was described in 1959.[51] This classification system was later modified with the addition of stage V to describe lesions with a cystic component[55] (**Figure 8**).

Advanced imaging modalities have significantly increased the ability to accurately diagnose OLTs. CT is used predominantly as an adjunct for a more comprehensive evaluation of and preoperative planning for known

Section 7: Tendon Disorders and Sports-Related Foot and Ankle Injuries

Section 7: Tendon Disorders and Sports-Related Foot and Ankle Injuries

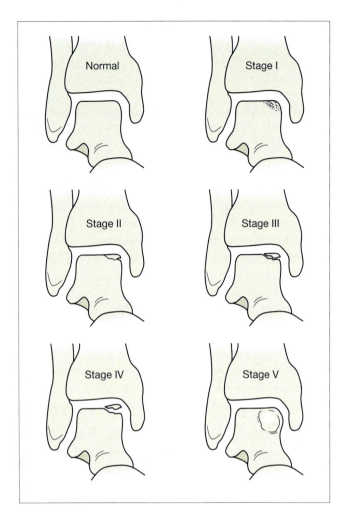

FIGURE 8 Illustrations showing Loomer and associates' modification of the Berndt and Harty radiographic classification of osteochondral lesions of the talus. Stage I: Compression of subchondral bone. Stage II: Partially detached osteochondral fragment. Stage III: Completely detached osteochondral fragment remaining in fragment bed. Stage IV: Displaced osteochondral fragment. Stage V: Presence of a cystic component. (Redrawn with permission from Loomer R, Fischer C, Lloyd-Schmidt R, et al: Osteochondral lesions of the talus. *Am J Sports Med* 1993;21:13-19.)

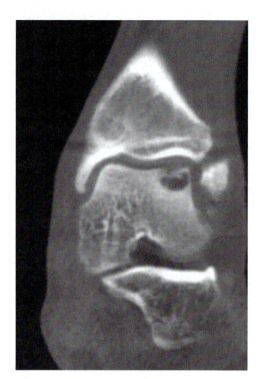

FIGURE 9 Coronal CT image of the ankle demonstrating an osteochondral defect of the lateral talar dome with cystic involvement.

lesions[56] (**Figure 9**). A four-stage system of classifying the lesions based on CT findings has been described[57] (**Figure 10**). This system not only corresponds to stages described in the original classification but also considers subchondral cyst formation, fragmentation, and the overall extent of osteonecrosis.

MRI is the preferred imaging study for detection of suspected OLTs that are not seen on initial plain radiographs[58] (**Figure 11**), although it may find lesions that are incidental. MRI also is useful for further evaluation of known OLTs and provides improved three-dimensional localization and sizing of a lesion. It also aids in the assessment of stability and identification of a cystic component. MRI also is used to stage OLTs. An MRI classification system based on the original classification system was described and later revised, primarily by subdividing stage 2 based on the presence or absence of surrounding edema.[59] Lesions with subchondral cysts were reclassified as stage 5. An MRI grading system based on an earlier arthroscopic grading system, the Mintz classification, was described[60] (**Table 1**). CT (thin slice and weight bearing preferably) should also be performed to better evaluate cystic changes in the setting of an osteochondral defect or osteochondral fracture of the talus.

Nonsurgical Treatment

A trial of nonsurgical management may be appropriate for OLTs, with the literature recommending a trial period of minimum 3 months.[61] Nonsurgical treatment consists of 4 to 6 weeks of immobilization with touch-down weight bearing, especially in patients with asymptomatic lesions, incidental findings, nondisplaced acute cartilage/bone injury, and those patients of older age with lower functional status, those who have advanced arthritic joint changes, or those who are skeletally immature.[62] Nonsurgical treatment ranges from no weight bearing in a cast to protected weight bearing in a boot.[62] An updated systematic review demonstrated that the use of immobilization over a period ranging from 3 weeks

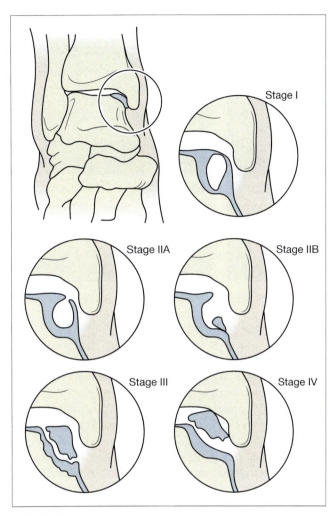

FIGURE 10 Illustrations showing the Ferkel and Sgaglione CT classification of osteochondral lesions of the talus. Stage I: Cystic lesion within the dome of the talus, intact roof on all views. Stage IIA: Cystic lesion with communication to the talar dome surface. Stage IIB: Open articular surface lesion with overlying nondisplaced fragment. Stage III: Nondisplaced lesion with lucency. Stage IV: Displaced fragment. (Redrawn from Feinblatt J, Graves SC: Osteochondral lesions of the talus: Acute and chronic, in Pinzur MS, ed: *Orthopaedic Knowledge Update®: Foot and Ankle 4*. American Academy of Orthopaedic Surgeons, 2008, pp 147-158.)

to 4 months demonstrated a 53% success rate. In addition, rest or activity modification alone was reported in three studies, with a 45% success rate.[63] A study of 142 patients who were treated nonsurgically found that at a mean follow-up of 6 years, CT findings were decreased or unchanged in 89%, the mean visual analog scale pain score was decreased, and the mean AOFAS ankle-hindfoot score and SF-36 both were increased, and no patients had osteoarthritis progression.[64]

Surgical Treatment

Surgical intervention is indicated for acute displaced OLTs and for those refractory to nonsurgical care. The approach and objectives of surgery are variable and are determined by the type of lesion. Goals may range from removal of a loose fragment to securing a larger fragment anatomically. Alternatively, the primary objective may be to create an environment amenable to fibrocartilaginous proliferation or resurfacing with hyaline cartilage.

The primary approach to evaluation and management of osteochondral defects includes ankle arthroscopy, although open ankle arthrotomy remains a treatment modality in the setting of autograft and allograft transplantation.

Ankle arthroscopy has been established as a useful tool in OLT diagnosis and treatment (**Figures 12** and **13**). When compared with an extensive open approach, arthroscopy provides superior visualization of the talar dome and improved access to the lesion. As a result of recent advances, including small joint arthroscopes and instrumentation, arthroscopic management of OLTs is now the preferred technique.[65] With the advent of small joint arthroscopes and instrumentation as well as careful placement of both anterior and posterior portals, all lesions can be accessed and addressed arthroscopically.[66]

Numerous open exposure methods have been described, including several variations of medial malleolar osteotomies and distal tibial osteotomies along with combined anterior and posterior arthrotomies.[51] Open approaches produce significant tissue trauma and, as a result, may be associated with postoperative stiffness, prolonged rehabilitation time, and poor cosmetic appearance. In addition, nonunion or malunion of the malleoli is a risk with approaches involving a malleolar osteotomy. Inadequate visualization of talar dome lesions, particularly posterior lesions, remains a primary limitation of any open approach.[51]

A wide variety of procedures that vary in complexity have been described for the management of OLTs. Treatment strategies generally are categorized as primary repair, reparative techniques, restorative techniques, or replacement techniques. Marrow-inducing reparative treatment strategies include abrasion arthroplasty, microfracture, and drilling techniques. Restorative techniques primarily include autologous chondrocyte implantation (ACI), osteochondral autologous transfer system and mosaicplasty, and osteochondral allograft. Future directions in restorative techniques for OLTs include matrix/membrane ACI (MACI), collagen-covered ACI, arthroscopic allograft/autograft with platelet-rich plasma (PRP) implantation, hyaluronic acid, stem cell–mediated cartilage implants, and scaffolds.[61]

A systematic review of 52 published reports describing the results of 65 treatment groups indicated that most recent publications on management of OLTs involve arthroscopic excision or curettage, and bone marrow

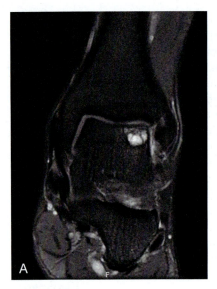 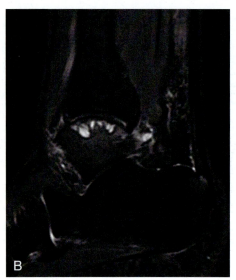 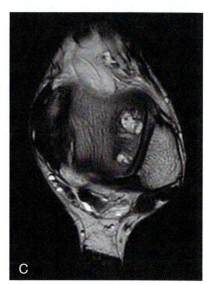

FIGURE 11 Sagittal (**A**), axial (**B**), and coronal (**C**) magnetic resonance images of the ankle demonstrating an osteochondral defect of the lateral talar dome with cystic involvement.

stimulation (BMS), ACI, or osteochondral autologous transfer system with success rates of 85%, 76%, and 87%, respectively.[63] As a result, arthroscopic excision, curettage, and BMS were recommended as initial treatment because they are relatively inexpensive and associated with low morbidity and a high success rate. However, because of diversity in the literature and highly variable treatment results, definitive conclusions could not be drawn.[63]

When selecting the appropriate treatment option, several important variables should be considered. It is imperative to delineate, primarily from advanced imaging, the type, stability, and displacement of the lesion. Chronicity, size, location, and containment are other important factors to consider.

The prime variable to consider when choosing between a reparative and a restorative technique is the size of the lesion. The prognostic significance of defect size on MRI was examined in a large series of patients treated using arthroscopic marrow stimulation techniques. A cutoff point of 150 mm^2 for a defect size was identified, at which risk factors for poor outcomes became evident.[67] A systematic review attempted to review all available literature on lesion size and outcomes after BMS. Literature quality was quite poor: 88% were level of evidence III or IV, and 96% did not have good-quality evidence. However, it was concluded that BMS should be reserved for lesions smaller than 107.4 mm^2 or 10.2 mm in diameter because lesions larger than this have significantly poorer outcomes.[68] It was later demonstrated that patients with an uncontained shoulder-type osteochondral lesion, whether medial or lateral, have worse clinical outcomes with arthroscopic marrow stimulation techniques than those who have a contained nonshoulder-type lesion.[69] This was true even when the increased size of the shoulder-type lesion was taken into account.

Surgical Procedures

Primary Repair

Primary repair of the OLT with internal fixation is indicated after acute osteochondral fracture of the talus and for larger lesions with intact articular cartilage. A systematic review of treatment strategies for patients with an osteochondral defect revealed a 73% success rate with this method.[61] In a 2022 study, clinical outcomes and

Table 1

Mintz and Associates' MRI Classification Compared With Cheng's Arthroscopic Staging System for Osteochondral Lesions of the Talus

MRI	Arthroscopic
Grade 0: Normal	Stage A: Smooth, intact but soft
Grade I: Hyperintense but intact cartilage surface	Stage B: Rough surface
Grade II: Fibrillation of fissures not extending to bone	Stage C: Fibrillation or fissuring
Grade III: Flap present or exposed bone	Stage D: Flap present or exposed bone
Grade IV: Loose, nondisplaced fragment	Stage E: Loose, nondisplaced fragment
Grade V: Displaced fragment	Stage F: Displaced fragment

Chapter 26: Arthroscopy of the Foot and Ankle and Osteochondral Lesions of the Talus

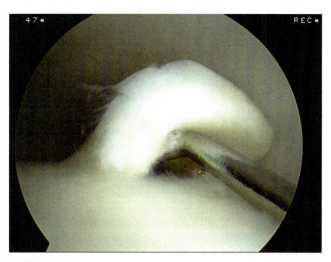

FIGURE 12 Arthroscopic image demonstrating an osteochondral flap identified via arthroscopy.

AOFAS scores of patients who underwent osteochondral defect fixation were found to be superior to BMS alone, even for lesions smaller than 100 mm². In a 2022 study, fixation was recommended for small lesions when possible, especially with bony involvement, and more centralized lesions in the medial and lateral sides of the talus.[70] Multiple different approaches are available to address the fracture depending on the location (**Figure 14**).

Arthroscopic Débridement With or Without BMS

For symptomatic OLTs that are smaller than 150 mm², the current recommendation is arthroscopic BMS with débridement, drilling, and microfracture or curettage of the lesion. The purpose of this procedure is to excise the loose or delaminated articular cartilage and to

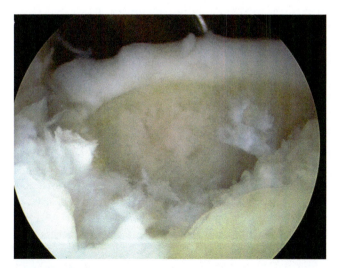

FIGURE 13 Arthroscopic image of osteochondral lesion of the talus with cystic involvement defined on CT and MRI and intraoperatively noted with the cystic membrane lining the defect.

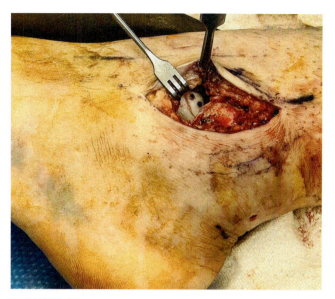

FIGURE 14 Intraoperative photograph showing fixation of an osteochondral fracture of the talus with biointegrative nails.

promote fibrocartilage formation over the defect. The fibrocartilaginous material is composed of mostly type I collagen rather than hyaline cartilage. The literature was reviewed to determine the prognostic factors affecting the clinical outcome after arthroscopic BMS, and it was concluded that inferior clinical outcome is associated with lesions larger than 150 mm² and uncontained lesions.[71] In addition, advancing age and cystic formation may not influence the outcome after surgery. A study of 50 patients who underwent arthroscopic BMS for OLTs smaller than 150 mm² was conducted.[72] It was concluded that medial lesions, especially uncovered medial lesions, were associated with worse outcomes than lateral lesions. Patients who were older than 40 years had inferior outcomes. No correlation was found between lesion size or body mass index and clinical outcome. Another study examined the various techniques of arthroscopic BMS for the management of OLTs ranging in size from 0.9 to 4.5 cm² in 198 patients.[73] All procedures involved excising the unstable cartilage and performing microfracture to depths of 2 to 4 mm and 3 to 4 mm apart. Excellent or good results were obtained in 81% of patients. Another study investigated the results of arthroscopic microfracture of OLTs in 22 patients, 18 of whom had no or mild occasional pain 2 years after surgery. MRI showed that most defects were completely or partially filled.[49,53,74] The effect of early weight-bearing protocols after arthroscopic BMS for OLTs has been compared with non–weight-bearing protocols. The authors of a 2021 study demonstrated that there was no difference in pain, complications, or functional scores between the two protocols.[75] Medial uncontained lesions have a worse prognosis than lateral lesions after arthroscopic BMS. Postoperative MRI can show evidence of filling of the defect. Another 2021 study examined long-term outcome after arthroscopic débridement and BMS, noting a 93.3% survival rate and 85.7% return to sports participation.[76]

Although arthroscopic débridement with BMS remains the first-line surgical treatment strategy for OLT, a 2021 systematic review suggests there is no superiority between arthroscopic débridement alone or arthroscopic débridement with BMS. Arthroscopic débridement alone has several advantages, including preservation of the subchondral plate, and therefore not compromising the outcome of secondary procedures, shorter rehabilitation time, and no donor site morbidity. Despite the success of BMS, midterm radiology joint changes, poor outcomes after revision procedures in patients who undergo primary BMS, and inconsistent return to sports remain concerns. Arthroscopic débridement alone showed satisfactory short-term and midterm outcomes for the primary management of OLTs regardless of size or depth.[77]

Osteochondral Autograft Transplantation

Osteochondral autograft usually is obtained from the superior medial edge of the medial femoral condyle, and bone plugs are transplanted into the prepared OLT defect. For lesions that are too large (>1.5 cm^2), especially with a large cystic component involving the shoulder of the talus, osteochondral allograft can be used. When more than one plug is used, the technique is known as mosaicplasty. A new method with which to harvest periosteum-covered plugs from the iliac crest for transplantation into OLTs has been described.[78] Thirteen patients experienced improvement of AOFAS scores from a mean score of 47 preoperatively to 81 postoperatively. At the time of follow-up, plug consolidation was present in 9 of 11 ankles based on plain radiographic evaluation; however, arthroscopic evaluation revealed fibrocartilage formation in only four ankles and periosteal hypertrophy in five ankles. One study reported 95% good to excellent results in 52 patients with osteochondral autograft transplants.[79] The osteochondral plugs were harvested from the lateral edge of the lateral trochlea of the femoral condyle. At the second-look arthroscopy a mean of 13 months after surgery, the incongruency at the medial malleolar osteotomy, presence of soft-tissue impingement, and uncovered areas around the graft were associated with poor results. No donor site morbidity at the ipsilateral knee was reported. In an evaluation of long-term follow-up (mean follow-up of 62.8 months), 11 studies involving 500 ankles were reviewed. Good or excellent

results were reported in 87.4%. There was a 10.6% complication rate, with donor site morbidity reported as the most common complication. Revision surgery was performed in 6.2% of patients, but only 1% were considered failures.[80] In a study on clinical results after osteochondral autograft transplantation procedures in primary and secondary settings, there was no difference between patients who previously underwent a BMS procedure compared with those who did not. There was a significantly increased failure rate in those patients with lesion size larger than 225 mm^2.[81] Contained osteochondral lesions had better clinical outcomes than noncontained lesions.[82] In 2022, 11 studies with 207 ankles were reviewed and a high rate of return to play (86.3%) was demonstrated in an athletic population treated with osteochondral autograft, citing increasing age as a negative prognostic factor for return to play. It was also noted that there was no correlation with OLT size and return to play.[83]

Recent literature has demonstrated that augmenting osteochondral autograft transplantation with cartilage extracellular matrix and bone marrow aspirate concentrate improves clinical and radiologic outcomes.[84] Furthermore, in 2022, a case series documented promising results when using vascularized free flaps from femoral trochlea as an interesting alterative to the usual nonvascularized plugs; therefore, they could potentially be used when previous osteochondral autograft has failed.[85]

Autologous Chondrocyte Implantation

ACI for the management of OLTs involves implantation of viable chondrocytes into the defect. ACI for the management of osteochondral knee lesions is a two-stage procedure in which chondrocytes are harvested from the donor site and cells are implanted into the osteochondral defect. The 10-year follow-up results of ACI using MRI T2 mapping in 10 patients were reviewed, and it was determined that the regenerated cartilage had T2 mapping values similar to those of healthy hyaline cartilage.[86]

Matrix/Membrane Autologous Chondrocyte Implantation

The second generation of ACI, MACI, involves imbedding harvested and expanded autologous chondrocytes into a type I/III collagen bilayer or hyaluronic acid scaffold before implantation. As with ACI, MACI has been shown to result in formation of hyalinelike cartilage;[87] however, unlike ACI, MACI does not require a periosteal patch and the associated morbidity of periosteal harvest and possible hypertrophy. Moreover, there is no risk of chondrocyte cell leakage or uneven cell distribution within the talar defect because the chondrocytes are evenly embedded within the stable matrix and affixed to the defect with fibrin glue.[88] As a salvage procedure for ankles not affected by arthritis, kissing lesions, instability, or axial defects that occur after failed débridement and curettage or microfracture, results to date are promising. One study reported that 10 patients with full-thickness talar dome osteochondral lesions who underwent MACI had improvement in physical function and pain as measured by the SF-36 and improved AOFAS hindfoot scores at 1 and 2 years in all patients. It was noted that, unlike ACI, the MACI technique offers the advantage of no required malleolar osteotomy.[88] In another study, 46 patients were treated arthroscopically; 80% experienced good or excellent results that were maintained over time and the return to sport rate was 86%.[89] An investigation of the rate of return to sport in 26 patients after an arthroscopic MACI procedure found that 80.8% of patients returned to the same preinjury sport at a mean follow-up of 42.6 months, with significant improvements in their AOFAS, SF-12, Halasi, and University of California, Los Angeles Activity Scale scores.[90] One study reported on the use of fibrin matrix–mixed gel-type ACI in the management of 38 OLTs, 34 of which had excellent, good, or fair subjective results. Analysis of chondrocyte regeneration by second-look arthroscopy at 12 months and MRI at 24 months after surgery revealed that 75% of OLTs were graded as normal or nearly normal.[91]

Osteochondral Allograft Transplantation

Allograft transplantation, like ACI, can be used for treatment of larger lesions in patients who are too young or active for arthroplasty or arthrodesis; unlike ACI, however, this intervention obviates the need for a two-stage procedure and potential for donor site morbidity and it can be used to treat patients with lesions involving large volumes of subchondral bone.[92] The use of both frozen and fresh talar allograft has been described.[93] One long-term study with an average follow-up of 11 years reported that 6 of 9 patients who underwent allograft transplantation retained functional grafts, with the remaining 3 requiring conversion to arthrodesis.[94] A subsequent study reported 4-year midterm results in 13 patients with an average age of 30 years who underwent fresh allograft transplantation. Although five of these patients required additional surgeries because of prominent implants and soft-tissue impingement, all eventually had good results with 100% graft incorporation, improved pain and function, return to at least low-demand activities of daily living, and, in 11 patients, return to high-impact activities by 1 year.[95] Although showing promising results, these two studies may be limited by their small sample size. In contrast,

one study reported an average follow-up of just over 3 years in 38 of 42 patients who underwent fresh allograft transplantation. Although four grafts failed, the average pain and functional scores improved significantly, and 74% of the patients reported satisfaction with the procedure as good to excellent.[96] Tempering these positive clinical results, posttransplant MRI performed on a subset of 15 of these patients revealed that, although there was little graft subsidence, instability, or loss of articular congruence, 80% of the grafts appeared to be unincorporated into surrounding native bone.[96] Other disadvantages of allograft transplantation include the cost and inconvenience of obtaining grafts from a tissue bank and the potential for transmission of disease and immunologic rejection, although preparation of grafts with pulsatile lavage to remove donor immunogenic cells may decrease this risk.[95]

Particulated Juvenile Cartilage

For OLTs larger than 100 mm², ACI/MACI and allograft transplant are particularly useful because they involve restoration of a hyaline or hyalinelike articular surface; however, these techniques are technically challenging and, for ACI, necessitate a two-stage procedure. An alternative is particulated juvenile cartilage implantation, in which prepackaged cartilage allograft from juvenile donors is placed directly into the talar lesion in a single-stage procedure. One study reported the use of this technique for 24 OLTs judged unlikely to respond well to BMS alone.[97] The average lesion size and depth were 125 mm² and 7 mm, respectively, and 16 of the 24 lesions were uncontained. Lesions were approached according to surgeon preference, either arthroscopically or by limited arthrotomy. The technique involved applying a thin layer of fibrin glue to the prepared lesion surface, followed by the particulated juvenile cartilage, and finally covering the cartilage with a second thin layer of fibrin glue after which the ankle was ranged to mold the construct. Although the retrospective nature of the study precluded comparison with preoperative functional outcome scores, postoperative results at an average of 16.2 months are encouraging, with 92% good or excellent results in lesions 10 to 15 mm in the largest dimension. In contrast, these investigators found only 56% good or excellent results in lesions at least 15 mm in size in the largest dimension, suggesting that particulated juvenile cartilage may offer a good gap strategy for lesions larger than 100 mm² but smaller than 150 mm². A smaller retrospective series reported 15 patients with a mean 34.6-month follow-up after particulated juvenile cartilage allograft transplantation. A 40% failure rate, defined as no change or worsening of symptoms and/or the need for a subsequent procedure, was reported. Patients with lesions larger than 125 mm² had a significantly increased risk for failure. Patients with successful surgeries had a significant improvement in their functional outcome scores.[98] A 2020 retrospective series demonstrated clinically significant improvements in pain and function and cited behavioral health diagnoses as a negative prognostic factor.[99]

A 2021 systematic review of 10 studies and 132 total patients demonstrated promising functional outcomes with particulated juvenile cartilage. However, postoperative MRI demonstrated a heterogeneous picture of regenerate cartilaginous tissue and lack of repair in subchondral bone and subchondral lamina.[100]

Disadvantages of particulated juvenile cartilage include limited supply of allograft, theoretical risk of disease transmission, and lack of long-term data.

Micronized Cartilage Extracellular Matrix

Micronized allogeneic cartilage extracellular matrix is derived from allograft cartilage and is composed of multiple extracellular constituents such as proteoglycans, cartilage growth factors, and type II cartilage that serve as a scaffold to help promote autologous cellular interactions and repair. This can be enhanced further when mixed with bone marrow aspirate concentrate to deliver growth factors and increase the infill of the lesion (**Figure 15**).

A 2021 study examining the radiographic and functional improvement when using bone marrow aspirate concentrate with extracellular matrix showed superior MRI results as evidenced by Magnetic Resonance Observation of Cartilage Repair Tissue scores and lower rate of revisions surgery when compared with microfracture.[101]

Stem Cell Therapy

Stem cell therapy holds great promise for management of OLT but currently has limited applicability; it may be used as an adjunct to marrow stimulation treatment, however. Microfracture relies on penetration through the subchondral plate to underlying bone marrow with subsequent release of mesenchymal stem cells (MSCs) into the cartilage defect where they may differentiate into chondrocytes. Because density of MSCs within a patient's marrow appears to decline with age, the addition of MSCs previously harvested from other sites into the microfractured lesion may benefit older patients. One study compared the outcomes of OLTs in older patients treated with either microfracture alone or with microfracture plus the addition of MSCs harvested from the gluteal fat pad. Patients older than 50 years experienced better improvement in pain, level of activity, and satisfaction when MSCs were used as an adjunct to microfracture compared with microfracture alone.[102]

Autologous Matrix-Induced Chondrogenesis

One of the major drawbacks of ACI and MACI is that they are two-stage procedures. Autologous matrix-induced chondrogenesis (AMIC) attempts to achieve the same goal of ACI/MACI but with a one-step procedure. AMIC combines microfracture with autologous iliac crest bone marrow aspirate concentrate or PRP delivered on a collagen matrix scaffold in an attempt to allow hyaline cartilage in the defect rather than fibrocartilage that results from microfracture alone.

A prospective study of 48 patients who underwent AMIC with lesions larger than 150 mm² and less than 5 mm deep resulted in improved AOFAS scores within a range comparable with that achieved with other widely used treatment techniques.[103] Moreover, second-look arthroscopy in three asymptomatic patients demonstrated complete integration of the graft and macroscopic appearance of new cartilage that was similar to surrounding native cartilage. Two more patients had arthroscopic chondroplasty to treat MRI-demonstrated cartilage hypertrophy; histologic analysis of these two patients showed varying degrees of tissue remodeling toward a hyaline cartilage lineage. MRI T2 mapping corroborates the success of this technique in regenerating articular cartilage; as much as 78% of regenerated tissue demonstrated relaxation times comparable with that achieved with hyaline as opposed to fibrocartilage.[104] A retrospective study compared clinical outcomes and MRI results in patients with BMS plus concentrated bone marrow aspirate (BMS/CBMA) with

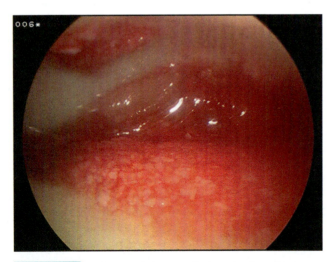

FIGURE 15 Arthroscopic image of micronized cartilage extracellular matrix mixed with bone marrow aspirate concentrate laid over the osteochondral defect of the talus with fibrin glue.

those in patients with BMS alone. Both groups demonstrated significant improvement in their Foot and Ankle Outcome Score and SF-12 physical component scores, but the Magnetic Resonance Observation of Cartilage Repair Tissue scores were significantly higher in the BMS/CBMA group. The MRI results demonstrated improved border repair tissue integration and less fissuring/fibrillation in the BMS/CBMA group.[105] In a systematic review of the AMIC procedure, the authors stated that the current literature supports the use of AMIC as an effective treatment for OLT. It was noted that the literature showed great heterogeneity and no comparative studies were found.[106]

Platelet-Rich Plasma

In vitro studies demonstrate that PRP may increase chondrocyte proliferation and production of collagen and stimulate MSC migration, proliferation, and chondrogenic differentiation.[107] In addition, PRP has been shown to suppress many of the catabolic mediators present in inflammatory intra-articular environments that would otherwise add to further cartilage injury and inhibit cartilage regeneration. In a 2020 systematic review of clinical trials, PRP was demonstrated to improve function and reduce pain when compared with microfracture surgery alone.[108]

Hyaluronic Acid

Hyaluronic acid has been used as an adjunct to microfracture in the management of OLTs. A systematic review of randomized controlled trials conducted in 2022 demonstrated improvements in function and pain at-short term follow-up compared with microfracture alone. Future studies are needed to investigate this possible adjunct therapy.[109]

SUMMARY

The indications and applications of foot and ankle arthroscopy, tendoscopy, and endoscopy continue to expand. Foot and ankle orthopaedic surgeons can anticipate further refinement of arthroscopic procedures and their use in managing conditions of the bone, ligaments, tendons, and relatively small joints. Nonsurgical and surgical management strategies of OLT continue to pose challenges. The success rate of surgical treatment is dependent on many variables such as lesion size, location, and containment and patient age. Continued research on articular cartilage restoration will lead to improved future management strategies.

KEY STUDY POINTS

- Arthroscopic ankle arthrodesis may result in improved patient outcomes compared with traditional open arthrodesis.
- Although arthroscopically assisted ORIF can be safely performed for ankle fractures, the current literature has not demonstrated improved patient outcomes.
- Endoscopic management of posterior ankle impingement caused by symptomatic os trigonum may result in an earlier return to activities compared with open treatment.
- OLTs are likely more common than initially thought and typically occur with a history of ankle fracture or sprain, although nontraumatic etiologies also occur. Lesions typically are located in the midmedial or midlateral zones.
- Osteochondral lesions should be in the differential diagnosis of a patient who presents with chronic ankle pain, swelling, and perhaps mechanical symptoms. Advanced imaging in the form of MRI typically is required.
- In patients with OLT in whom nonsurgical treatment fails, the first-line surgical option typically is ankle arthroscopy, osteochondral excision, curettage, and BMS (microfracture).

ANNOTATED REFERENCES

1. Young BH, Flanigan RM, DiGiovanni BF: Complications of ankle arthroscopy utilizing a contemporary non-invasive distraction technique. *J Bone Joint Surg Am* 2011;93(10):963-968.

2. van Dijk CN, van Bergen CJ: Advancements in ankle arthroscopy. *J Am Acad Orthop Surg* 2008;16(11):635-646.

3. Malagelada F, Vega J, Guelfi M, Kerkhoffs G, Karlsson J, Dalmau-Pastor M: Anatomic lectures on structures at risk prior to cadaveric courses reduce injury to the superficial peroneal nerve, the commonest complication in ankle arthroscopy. *Knee Surg Sports Traumatol Arthrosc* 2020;28(1):79-85.

   The effectiveness of cadaver ankle arthroplasty courses in reducing iatrogenic injuries was studied, with hindfoot endoscopy found to be safer than anterior ankle arthroscopy in terms of injury to anatomic structures. Level of evidence: V.

4. Shirzad K, Viens NA, DeOrio JK: Arthroscopic treatment of impingement after total ankle arthroplasty: Technique tip. *Foot Ankle Int* 2011;32(7):727-729.

5. Liszka H, Gądek A: Preemptive local anesthesia in ankle arthroscopy. *Foot Ankle Int* 2016;37(12):1326-1332.

6. Dimnjaković D, Hrabač P, Bojanić I: Value of tourniquet use in anterior ankle arthroscopy: A randomized controlled trial. *Foot Ankle Int* 2017;38(7):716-722.

7. Dalmau-Pastor M, Malagelada F, Kerkhoffs GM, Karlsson J, Guelfi M, Vega J: Redefining anterior ankle arthroscopic anatomy: Medial and lateral ankle collateral ligaments are visible through dorsiflexion and non-distraction anterior ankle arthroscopy. *Knee Surg Sports Traumatol Arthrosc* 2020;28(1):18-23.

   Ankle dorsiflexion and nondistraction anterior arthroplasty techniques allow clear visualization of medial and lateral collateral ankle ligaments to assess pathology. Level of evidence: V.

8. de Leeuw PA, Golanó P, Sierevelt IN, van Dijk CN: The course of the superficial peroneal nerve in relation to the ankle position: Anatomical study with ankle arthroscopic implications. *Knee Surg Sports Traumatol Arthrosc* 2010;18(5):612-617.

9. Zekry M, Shahban SA, El Gamal T, Platt S: A literature review of the complications following anterior and posterior ankle arthroscopy. *Foot Ankle Surg* 2019;25(5):553-558.

   Complication rates associated with anterior and posterior ankle arthroscopy are outlined. According to the literature, superficial peroneal nerve injury and temporary Achilles tendon tightness are the most common complications associated with anterior and posterior ankle arthroscopy, respectively. Level of evidence: V.

10. Bassett FH 3rd, Gates HS 3rd, Billys JB, Morris HB, Nikolaou PK: Talar impingement by the anteroinferior tibiofibular ligament: A cause of chronic pain in the ankle after inversion sprain. *J Bone Joint Surg Am* 1990;72(1):55-59.

11. Murawski CD, Kennedy JG: Anteromedial impingement in the ankle joint: Outcomes following arthroscopy. *Am J Sports Med* 2010;38(10):2017-2024.

12. Townshend D, Di Silvestro M, Krause F, et al: Arthroscopic versus open ankle arthrodesis: A multicenter comparative case series. *J Bone Joint Surg Am* 2013;95(2):98-102.

13. Mok TN, He Q, Panneerselavam S, et al: Open versus arthroscopic ankle arthrodesis: A systematic review and meta-analysis. *J Orthop Surg Res* 2020;15(1):187.

    In comparison with open surgery, arthroscopic arthrodesis was associated with a higher fusion rate, less estimated blood loss, shorter tourniquet time, and shorter length of hospitalization. Level of evidence: V.

14. Ferran NA, Oliva F, Maffulli N: Ankle instability. *Sports Med Arthrosc Rev* 2009;17(2):139-145.

15. Komenda GA, Ferkel RD: Arthroscopic findings associated with the unstable ankle. *Foot Ankle Int* 1999;20(11):708-713.

16. Yeo ED, Lee KT, Sung IH, Lee SG, Lee YK: Comparison of all-inside arthroscopic and open techniques for the modified Broström procedure for ankle instability. *Foot Ankle Int* 2016;37(10):1037-1045.

17. Nery C, Raduan F, Del Buono A, Asaumi ID, Cohen M, Maffulli N: Arthroscopic-assisted Broström-Gould for chronic ankle instability: A long-term follow-up. *Am J Sports Med* 2011;39(11):2381-2388.

18. Acevedo JI, Ortiz C, Golano P, Nery C: ArthroBroström lateral ankle stabilization technique: An anatomic study. *Am J Sports Med* 2015;43(10):2564-2571.

19. Brown AJ, Shimozono Y, Hurley ET, Kennedy JG: Arthroscopic versus open repair of lateral ankle ligament for chronic lateral ankle instability: A meta-analysis. *Knee Surg Sports Traumatol Arthrosc* 2020;28(5):1611-1618.

    In an analysis of comparative studies of arthroscopic and open techniques for management of chronic lateral ankle instability, AOFAS functional scores were substantially improved with arthroscopic lateral repair in comparison with open repair. Level of evidence: III.

20. Zhi X, Lv Z, Zhang C, Kong C, Wei S, Xu F: Does arthroscopic repair show superiority over open repair of lateral ankle ligament for chronic lateral ankle instability: A systematic review and meta-analysis. *J Orthop Surg Res* 2020;15(1):355.

    In comparison with open repair, arthroscopic repair for lateral ankle instability exhibits excellent clinical results. Level of evidence: III.

21. Fuchs DJ, Ho BS, LaBelle MW, Kelikian AS: Effect of arthroscopic evaluation of acute ankle fractures on PROMIS intermediate-term functional outcomes. *Foot Ankle Int* 2016;37(1):51-57.

22. Chiang CC, Tzeng YH, Jeff Lin CF, Wang CS, Lin CC, Chang MC: Arthroscopic reduction and minimally invasive surgery in supination-external rotation ankle fractures: A comparative study with open reduction. *Arthroscopy* 2019;35(9):2671-2683.

    Using an algorithm for ARMIS, surgical outcomes with standard ORIF for supination–external rotation ankle fractures were compared. These techniques were found to be reliable and effective. Level of evidence: III.

23. Smith KS, Drexelius K, Challa S, Moon DK, Metzl JA, Hunt KJ: Outcomes following ankle fracture fixation with or without ankle arthroscopy. *Foot Ankle Orthop* 2020;5(1):2473011420904046.

    The authors assessed the clinical effect of performing an ankle arthroscopy during ankle fracture ORIF and found that patient-reported outcomes were significantly improved. Level of evidence: III.

24. Ferkel RD: In which position do we perform arthroscopy of the hindfoot – Supine or prone? Commentary on an article by Florian Nickisch, MD, et al.: "Postoperative complications of posterior ankle and hindfoot arthroscopy". *J Bone Joint Surg Am* 2012;94(5):e33.

25. Beals TC, Junko JT, Amendola A, Nickisch F, Saltzman CL: Minimally invasive distraction technique for prone posterior ankle and subtalar arthroscopy. *Foot Ankle Int* 2010;31(4):316-319.

26. van Dijk CN, de Leeuw PA, Scholten PE: Hindfoot endoscopy for posterior ankle impingement: Surgical technique. *J Bone Joint Surg Am* 2009;91(suppl 2):287-298.

27. Yoshimura I, Naito M, Kanazawa K, Ida T, Muraoka K, Hagio T: Assessing the safe direction of instruments during posterior ankle arthroscopy using an MRI model. *Foot Ankle Int* 2013;34(3):434-438.

28. Hampton CB, Shawen SB, Keeling JJ: Positioning technique for combined anterior, lateral, and posterior ankle and hindfoot procedures: Technique tip. *Foot Ankle Int* 2010;31(4):348-350.

29. Allegra F, Maffulli N: Double posteromedial portals for posterior ankle arthroscopy in supine position. *Clin Orthop Relat Res* 2010;468(4):996-1001.

30. Kim HN, Park YJ, Lee SY, Park YW: Three-portal ankle arthroscopy in prone position with ankle suspended: Technique tip. *Foot Ankle Int* 2012;33(11):1027-1030.

31. Hamilton WG: Posterior ankle pain in dancers. *Clin Sports Med* 2008;27(2):263-277.

32. Kim DH, Berkowitz MJ, Pressman DN: Avulsion fractures of the medial tubercle of the posterior process of the talus. *Foot Ankle Int* 2003;24(2):172-175.

33. Georgiannos D, Bisbinas I: Endoscopic versus open excision of os trigonum for the treatment of posterior ankle impingement syndrome in an athletic population: A randomized controlled study with 5-year followup. *Am J Sports Med* 2017;45(6):1388-1394.

34. Noguchi H, Ishii Y, Takeda M, Hasegawa A, Monden S, Takagishi K: Arthroscopic excision of posterior ankle bony impingement for early return to the field: Short-term results. *Foot Ankle Int* 2010;31(5):398-403.

35. Ferkel RD, Hammen JP: Arthroscopy of the ankle and foot, in Coughlin MJ, Mann RA, Saltzman CL, eds: *Surgery of the Foot and Ankle*, ed 8. Mosby Elsevier, 2007, pp 1641-1726.

36. Rungprai C, Phisitkul P, Femino JE, Martin KD, Saltzman CL, Amendola A: Outcomes and complications after open versus posterior arthroscopic subtalar arthrodesis in 121 patients. *J Bone Joint Surg Am* 2016;98(8):636-646.

37. Loewen A, Ge SM, Marwan Y, Berry GK: Isolated arthroscopic-assisted subtalar fusion: A systematic review. *JBJS Rev* 2021;9(8).

    The safety and efficacy of isolated arthroscopic subtalar fusion was assessed. Level of evidence: IV.

38. Lee KB, Chung JY, Song EK, Seon JK, Bai LB: Arthroscopic release for painful subtalar stiffness after intra-articular fractures of the calcaneum. *J Bone Joint Surg Br* 2008;90(11):1457-1461.

39. Carreira DS: Arthroscopy of the hallux. *Foot Ankle Clin* 2009;14(1):105-114.

40. van Dijk CN, Veenstra KM, Nuesch BC: Arthroscopic surgery of the metatarsophalangeal first joint. *Arthroscopy* 1998;14(8):851-855.

41. Vaseenon T, Phisitkul P: Arthroscopic debridement for first metatarsophalangeal joint arthrodesis with a 2- versus 3-portal technique: A cadaveric study. *Arthroscopy* 2010;26(10):1363-1367.

42. Cychosz CC, Phisitkul P, Barg A, Nickisch F, van Dijk CN, Glazebrook MA: Foot and ankle tendoscopy: Evidence-based recommendations. *Arthroscopy* 2014;30(6):755-765.

43. Bare A, Ferkel RD: Peroneal tendon tears: Associated arthroscopic findings and results after repair. *Arthroscopy* 2009;25(11):1288-1297.

44. Vega J, Golanó P, Dalmau A, Viladot R: Tendoscopic treatment of intrasheath subluxation of the peroneal tendons. *Foot Ankle Int* 2011;32(12):1147-1151.

45. Opdam KTM, Baltes TPA, Zwiers R, Wiegerinck JI, van Dijk CN: Endoscopic treatment of mid-portion Achilles tendinopathy: A retrospective case series of patient satisfaction and functional outcome at a 2- to 8-year follow-up. *Arthroscopy* 2018;34(1):264-269.

46. van Dijk CN: Hindfoot endoscopy for posterior ankle pain. *Instr Course Lect* 2006;55:545-554.

47. Ferkel RD, Fasulo GJ: Arthroscopic treatment of ankle injuries. *Orthop Clin North Am* 1994;25(1):17-32.

48. Orr JD, Dawson LK, Garcia EJ, Kirk KL: Incidence of osteochondral lesions of the talus in the United States military. *Foot Ankle Int* 2011;32(10):948-954.

49. Hermanson E, Ferkel RD: Bilateral osteochondral lesions of the talus. *Foot Ankle Int* 2009;30(8):723-727.

50. Rikken QGH, Wolsink LME, Dahmen J, Stufkens SAS, Kerkhoffs GMMJ: 15% of talar osteochondral lesions are present bilaterally while only 1 in 3 bilateral lesions are bilaterally symptomatic. *J Bone Joint Surg Am* 2022;104(18):1605-1613.

    The authors determined the prevalence of osteochondral lesions of the contralateral talus in patients with osteochondral lesions confirmed using CT and whether the contralateral lesions were symptomatic. Level of evidence: III.

51. Berndt AL, Harty M: Transchondral fractures (osteochondritis dissecans) of the talus. *J Bone Joint Surg Am* 1959;41-A:988-1020.

52. Elias I, Zoga AC, Morrison WB, Besser MP, Schweitzer ME, Raikin SM: Osteochondral lesions of the talus: Localization and morphologic data from 424 patients using a novel anatomical grid scheme. *Foot Ankle Int* 2007;28(2):154-161.

53. van Dijk CN, Reilingh ML, Zengerink M, van Bergen CJ: Osteochondral defects in the ankle: Why painful? *Knee Surg Sports Traumatol Arthrosc* 2010;18(5):570-580.

54. Elias I, Jung JW, Raikin SM, Schweitzer MW, Carrino JA, Morrison WB: Osteochondral lesions of the talus: Change in MRI findings over time in talar lesions without operative intervention and implications for staging systems. *Foot Ankle Int* 2006;27(3):157-166.

55. Loomer R, Fisher C, Lloyd-Smith R, Sisler J, Cooney T: Osteochondral lesions of the talus. *Am J Sports Med* 1993;21(1):13-19.

56. Zinman C, Wolfson N, Reis ND: Osteochondritis dissecans of the dome of the talus. Computed tomography scanning in diagnosis and follow-up. *J Bone Joint Surg Am* 1988;70(7):1017-1019.

57. Ferkel RD, Sgaglione NA, Del Pizzo W, et al: Arthroscopic treatment of osteochondral lesions of the talus: Long-term results. *Orthop Trans* 1990;14:172-173.

58. Loredo R, Sanders TG: Imaging of osteochondral injuries. *Clin Sports Med* 2001;20(2):249-278.

59. Hepple S, Winson IG, Glew D: Osteochondral lesions of the talus: A revised classification. *Foot Ankle Int* 1999;20(12):789-793.

60. Mintz DN, Tashjian GS, Connell DA, Deland JT, O'Malley M, Potter HG: Osteochondral lesions of the talus: A new magnetic resonance grading system with arthroscopic correlation. *Arthroscopy* 2003;19(4):353-359.

61. Verhagen RA, Struijs PA, Bossuyt PM, van Dijk CN: Systematic review of treatment strategies for osteochondral defects of the talar dome. *Foot Ankle Clin* 2003;8(2):233-242, viii-ix.

62. Dombrowski M, Yasui Y, Murawski C, et al: Conservative management and biological treatment strategies: Proceedings of the international consensus meeting on cartilage repair of the ankle. *Foot Ankle Int* 2018;39(1 suppl):9S-15S.

63. Zengerink M, Struijs PA, Tol JL, van Dijk CN: Treatment of osteochondral lesions of the talus: A systematic review. *Knee Surg Sports Traumatol Arthrosc* 2010;18(2):238-246.

64. Seo SG, Kim JS, Seo DK, Kim YK, Lee SH, Lee HS: Osteochondral lesions of the talus: Few patients require surgery. *Acta Orthop* 2018;89(4):462-467.

65. Kim HN, Kim GL, Park JY, Woo KJ, Park YW: Fixation of a posteromedial osteochondral lesion of the talus using a three-portal posterior arthroscopic technique. *J Foot Ankle Surg* 2013;52(3):402-405.

66. Wodicka R, Ferkel E, Ferkel R: Osteochondral lesions of the ankle. *Foot Ankle Int* 2016;37(9):1023-1034.

67. Choi WJ, Park KK, Kim BS, Lee JW: Osteochondral lesion of the talus: Is there a critical defect size for poor outcome? *Am J Sports Med* 2009;37(10):1974-1980.

68. Ramponi L, Yasui Y, Murawski CD, et al: Lesion size is a predictor of clinical outcomes after bone marrow stimulation for osteochondral lesions of the talus: A systematic review. *Am J Sports Med* 2017;45(7):1698-1705.

69. Choi WJ, Choi GW, Kim JS, Lee JW: Prognostic significance of the containment and location of osteochondral lesions of the talus: Independent adverse outcomes associated with uncontained lesions of the talar shoulder. *Am J Sports Med* 2013;41(1):126-133.

70. Nakasa T, Ikuta Y, Sumii J, Nekomoto A, Kawabata S, Adachi N: Clinical outcomes of osteochondral fragment fixation versus microfracture even for small osteochondral lesions of the talus. *Am J Sports Med* 2022;50(11):3019-3027.

Clinical outcomes of osteochondral fragment fixation are superior to those of the BMS technique in managing OLTs. Fixation is recommended even for small lesions. Level of evidence: III.

71. Choi WJ, Jo J, Lee JW: Osteochondral lesion of the talus: Prognostic factors affecting the clinical outcome after arthroscopic marrow stimulation technique. *Foot Ankle Clin* 2013;18(1):67-78.

72. Yoshimura I, Kanazawa K, Takeyama A, et al: Arthroscopic bone marrow stimulation techniques for osteochondral lesions of the talus: Prognostic factors for small lesions. *Am J Sports Med* 2013;41(3):528-534.

73. Kok AC, Dunnen Sd, Tuijthof GJ, van Dijk CN, Kerkhoffs GM: Is technique performance a prognostic factor in bone marrow stimulation of the talus? *J Foot Ankle Surg* 2012;51(6):777-782.

74. Kuni B, Schmitt H, Chloridis D, Ludwig K: Clinical and MRI results after microfracture of osteochondral lesions of the talus. *Arch Orthop Trauma Surg* 2012;132(12):1765-1771.

75. Danilkowicz RM, Grimm NL, Zhang GX, et al: Impact of early weightbearing after ankle arthroscopy and bone marrow stimulation for osteochondral lesions of the talus. *Orthop J Sports Med* 2021;9(9):23259671211029883.

In patients undergoing ankle arthroscopy with concomitant BMS, there was no difference in pain level, range of motion, or complications when immediate and full weight bearing as tolerated was allowed. Level of evidence: III.

76. Corr D, Raikin J, O'Neil JO, Raikin S: Long-term outcomes of microfracture for treatment of osteochondral lesions of the talus. *Foot Ankle Int* 2021;42(7):833-840.

In patients undergoing isolated arthroscopic microfracture for talar osteochondral defects followed up for a minimum of 10 years, there was a 93.3% survival rate and 85.7% return to sports participation. Level of evidence: IV.

77. Marín Fermín T, Hovsepian JM, D'Hooghe P, Papakostas ET: Arthroscopic debridement of osteochondral lesions of the talus: A systematic review. *Foot (Edinb)* 2021;49:101852.

The authors evaluated current evidence on clinical outcomes of arthroscopic débridement for managing OLT. Level of evidence: V.

78. Leumann A, Valderrabano V, Wiewiorski M, Barg A, Hintermann B, Pagenstert G: Bony periosteum-covered iliac crest plug transplantation for severe osteochondral lesions of the talus: A modified mosaicplasty procedure. *Knee Surg Sports Traumatol Arthrosc* 2014;22(6):1304-1310.

79. Kim YS, Park EH, Kim YC, Koh YG, Lee JW: Factors associated with the clinical outcomes of the osteochondral autograft transfer system in osteochondral lesions of the talus: Second-look arthroscopic evaluation. *Am J Sports Med* 2012;40(12):2709-2719.

80. Shimozono Y, Hurley ET, Myerson CL, Kennedy JG: Good clinical and functional outcomes at mid-term following

autologous osteochondral transplantation for osteochondral lesions of the talus. *Knee Surg Sports Traumatol Arthrosc* 2018;26(10):3055-3062.

81. Park KH, Hwang Y, Han SH, et al: Primary versus secondary osteochondral autograft transplantation for the treatment of large osteochondral lesions of the talus. *Am J Sports Med* 2018;46(6):1389-1396.

82. Shimozono Y, Donders JCE, Yasui Y, et al: Effect of the containment type on clinical outcomes in osteochondral lesions of the talus treated with autologous osteochondral transplantation. *Am J Sports Med* 2018;46(9):2096-2102.

83. Seow D, Shimozono Y, Gianakos AL, et al: Autologous osteochondral transplantation for osteochondral lesions of the talus: High rate of return to play in the athletic population. *Knee Surg Sports Traumatol Arthrosc* 2021;29(5):1554-1561.

   In a systematic review of data, there was a high rate of return to play following autologous osteochondral transplantation in the athletic population. Level of evidence: IV.

84. Drakos MC, Hansen OB, Eble SK, et al: Augmenting osteochondral autograft transplantation and bone marrow aspirate concentrate with particulate cartilage extracellular matrix is associated with improved outcomes. *Foot Ankle Int* 2022;43(9):1131-1142.

   The addition of adjuncts such as cartilage extracellular matrix with bone marrow aspirate concentrate to osteochondral autograft transplantation helped improve radiographic and patient-reported outcomes. Level of evidence: IV.

85. Windhofer CM, Orthner E, Bürger HK: Vascularized osteochondral free flaps from the femoral trochlea as versatile procedure for reconstruction of osteochondral lesions of the talus. *Foot Ankle Surg* 2022;28(7):935-943.

   In a study of 19 patients with symptomatic OLT, vascularized transfer of osteochondral flaps from the femoral trochlea is a reliable treatment option. Level of evidence: IV.

86. Giannini S, Battaglia M, Buda R, Cavallo M, Ruffilli A, Vannini F: Surgical treatment of osteochondral lesions of the talus by open-field autologous chondrocyte implantation: A 10-year follow-up clinical and magnetic resonance imaging T2-mapping evaluation. *Am J Sports Med* 2009;37(suppl 1):112S-118S.

87. Ronga M, Grassi FA, Montoli C, et al: Treatment of deep cartilage defects of the ankle with matrix-induced autologous chondrocyte implantation (MACI). *Foot Ankle Surg* 2005;11:29-33.

88. Giza E, Sullivan M, Ocel D, et al: Matrix-induced autologous chondrocyte implantation of talus articular defects. *Foot Ankle Int* 2010;31(9):747-753.

89. Giannini S, Buda R, Vannini F, Di Caprio F, Grigolo B: Arthroscopic autologous chondrocyte implantation in osteochondral lesions of the talus: Surgical technique and results. *Am J Sports Med* 2008;36(5):873-880.

90. D'Ambrosi R, Villafañe JH, Indino C, Liuni FM, Berjano P, Usuelli FG: Return to sport after arthroscopic autologous matrix-induced chondrogenesis for patients with osteochondral lesion of the talus. *Clin J Sport Med* 2019;29(6):470-475.

   Nearly 81% of the patient group who underwent arthroscopic autologous matrix-induced chondrogenesis (AT-AMIC) returned to the same preinjury sport with a mean follow-up was 42.6 months. Level of evidence: IV.

91. Lee KT, Kim JS, Young KW, et al: The use of fibrin matrix-mixed gel-type autologous chondrocyte implantation in the treatment for osteochondral lesions of the talus. *Knee Surg Sports Traumatol Arthrosc* 2013;21(6):1251-1260.

92. Winters BS, Raikin SM: The use of allograft in joint-preserving surgery for ankle osteochondral lesions and osteoarthritis. *Foot Ankle Clin* 2013;18(3):529-542.

93. Raikin SM: Stage VI: Massive osteochondral defects of the talus. *Foot Ankle Clin* 2004;9(4):737-744, vi.

94. Gross AE, Agnidis Z, Hutchison CR: Osteochondral defects of the talus treated with fresh osteochondral allograft transplantation. *Foot Ankle Int* 2001;22(5):385-391.

95. Hahn DB, Aanstoos ME, Wilkins RM: Osteochondral lesions of the talus treated with fresh talar allografts. *Foot Ankle Int* 2010;31(4):277-282.

96. El-Rashidy H, Villacis D, Omar I, Kelikian AS: Fresh osteochondral allograft for the treatment of cartilage defects of the talus: A retrospective review. *J Bone Joint Surg Am* 2011;93(17):1634-1640.

97. Coetzee JC, Giza E, Schon LC, et al: Treatment of osteochondral lesions of the talus with particulated juvenile cartilage. *Foot Ankle Int* 2013;34(9):1205-1211.

98. Dekker TJ, Steele JR, Federer AE, Easley ME, Hamid KS, Adams SB: Efficacy of particulated juvenile cartilage allograft transplantation for osteochondral lesions of the talus. *Foot Ank Int* 2018;39(3):278-283.

99. Heida KA, Tihista MC, Kusnezov NA, Dunn JC, Orr JD: Outcomes and predictors of postoperative pain improvement following particulated juvenile cartilage allograft transplant for osteochondral lesions of the talus. *Foot Ankle Int* 2020;41(5):572-581.

   In a study reporting outcomes and predictors of success with particulated juvenile cartilage allograft transplantation in the management of OLT, 40% to 50% improvement in ankle pain and disability within 3.5 years was reported. Level of evidence: IV.

100. Aldawsari K, Alrabai HM, Sayed A, Alrashidi Y: Role of particulated juvenile cartilage allograft transplantation in osteochondral lesions of the talus: A systematic review. *Foot Ankle Surg* 2021;27(1):10-14.

   In a systematic literature review, particulated juvenile cartilage allograft transplantation was found to have promising clinical and radiologic outcomes in the management of OLT. Level of evidence: III.

101. Drakos MC, Eble SK, Cabe TN, et al: Comparison of functional and radiographic outcomes of talar osteochondral lesions repaired with micronized allogenic cartilage

extracellular matrix and bone marrow aspirate concentrate vs microfracture. *Foot Ankle Int* 2021;42(7):841-850.

Superior MRI results were observed in patients with OLT treated with extracellular matrix marrow aspirate concentrate than with traditional microfracture. Level of evidence: III.

102. Kim YS, Park EH, Kim YC, Koh YG: Clinical outcomes of mesenchymal stem cell injection with arthroscopic treatment in older patients with osteochondral lesions of the talus. *Am J Sports Med* 2013;41(5):1090-1099.

103. Giannini S, Buda R, Vannini F, Cavallo M, Grigolo B: One-step bone marrow-derived cell transplantation in talar osteochondral lesions. *Clin Orthop Relat Res* 2009;467(12):3307-3320.

104. Battaglia M, Rimondi E, Monti C, et al: Validity of T2 mapping in characterization of the regeneration tissue by bone marrow derived cell transplantation in osteochondral lesions of the ankle. *Eur J Radiol* 2011;80(2): e132-e139.

105. Hannon CP, Ross KA, Murawski CD, et al: Arthroscopic bone marrow stimulation and concentrated bone marrow aspirate for osteochondral lesions of the talus: A case-control study of functional and magnetic resonance observation of cartilage repair tissue outcomes. *Arthroscopy* 2016;32(2):339-347.

106. Jantzen C, Ebskov LB, Johansen JK: AMIC procedure for treatment of osteochondral lesions of talus –

A systematic review of the current literature. *J Foot Ankle Surg* 2022;61(4):888-895.

According to a literature review, AMIC was found to be effective for the treatment of patients with OLT. Level of evidence: V.

107. Smyth NA, Murawski CD, Haleem AM, Hannon CP, Savage-Elliott I, Kennedy JG: Establishing proof of concept: Platelet-rich plasma and bone marrow aspirate concentrate may improve cartilage repair following surgical treatment for osteochondral lesions of the talus. *World J Orthop* 2012;3(7):101-108.

108. Yausep OE, Madhi I, Trigkilidas D: Platelet rich plasma for treatment of osteochondral lesions of the talus: A systematic review of clinical trials. *J Orthop* 2020;18:218-225.

In a systematic review of clinical trials, the authors found that PRP improves joint function and reduces pain in patients with OLT regardless of the method of implementation. Level of evidence: II.

109. Dilley JE, Everhart JS, Klitzman RG: Hyaluronic acid as an adjunct to microfracture in the treatment of osteochondral lesions of the talus: A systematic review of randomized controlled trials. *BMC Musculoskelet Disord* 2022;23(1):313.

In comparison with arthroscopic microfracture alone, hyaluronic acid injection as an adjunct in the treatment of patients with OLT provides clinically important improvements in function and pain at short-term follow-up. Level of evidence: II.

SECTION 8

Contemporary Surgical Techniques

Section Editor:
Ariel A. Palanca, MD, FAAOS

CHAPTER 27

Surgical Management of Charcot Neuroarthropathy

IAN M. FORAN, MD • DAVID J. DALSTROM, MD, FAAOS

ABSTRACT

The surgical management of Charcot neuroarthropathy presents multiple challenges to the foot and ankle surgeon. These include social factors and medical comorbidities, poor soft tissues and bone quality, rigid deformity, and ulcers/infection. The timing and techniques of surgical management are controversial and vary by surgeon preference and experience. However, the common end goal of a stable, infection-free, plantigrade foot remains the same. Research is limited to case series and reports, and ongoing efforts are being made to clarify the best treatment.

Keywords: Charcot; deformity; diabetes; neuroarthropathy; superconstruct

INTRODUCTION

Charcot neuroarthropathy of the foot and ankle is a challenging and often disabling disease. The number of affected patients is rising. Early stages of disease generally present with pain, swelling, and instability, whereas later stages involve rigid deformity, ulcer formation, and progressive infection. These problems often result in substantial disability, are an indication for amputation, and contribute to increases in

---

Dr. Foran or an immediate family member has stock or stock options held in Aesclepius LLC and serves as a board member, owner, officer, or committee member of American Orthopaedic Foot and Ankle Society. Dr. Dalstrom or an immediate family member serves as a paid consultant to or is an employee of Stryker.

mortality. Traditional treatment has largely focused on early nonsurgical management with immobilization and weight-bearing restrictions followed by late ostectomy for patients with residual deformity, risk for skin breakdown, or infected ulcers. Historically, efforts at deformity correction with internal fixation were met with a high rate of failure. More recently, stronger internal fixation constructs, minimally invasive soft-tissue sparing techniques, and advances in external fixation have generated renewed interest by demonstrating more promising results. In all cases, successful treatment depends on patient compliance and a coordinated multidisciplinary team approach, in which the orthopaedic surgeon plays a critical role. However, complication rates still remain high.

NATURAL HISTORY, PATHOLOGY, AND EPIDEMIOLOGY

Charcot neuroarthropathy involves progressive destruction of bone and joints, most commonly in the feet and ankles. Although this was first described in patients with syphilis and dorsalis tabes, the most common contemporary patient population is those with diabetes with associated lower extremity neuropathy. The reported incidence of this complication is less than 1% in the general population of patients with diabetes and as high as 13% in high-risk patients with diabetes. As the number of patients in whom diabetes is diagnosed continues to steadily rise, consequently so does the number of patients with Charcot neuroarthropathy. Men and women are at equal risk. Thirty percent of patients with this complication have bilateral involvement.[1]

Two theories are proposed to explain the development of Charcot neuroarthropathy. The theory of neurotraumatic destruction states that joint destruction is the result of cumulative trauma unrecognized by an insensate foot. In contrast, the theory of neurovascular destruction states that bone resorption and ligament laxity are secondary to a neurally controlled vascular reflex. Most experts think that a combination of these pathways is responsible for the destruction seen in the affected diabetic foot or ankle.[2] Increased expression of nuclear transcription factor kappa B results in increased osteoclastogenesis, thus confirming the role of inflammatory cytokines.[3]

The severity of diabetes is not linearly correlated with the risk of Charcot neuroarthropathy.[4] Charcot neuroarthropathy can develop in patients with mild diabetes who are being treated with oral hypoglycemic medications and/or diet control. It is not understood why this develops in some patients and not in others. Peripheral neuropathy is necessary but not alone sufficient to cause Charcot neuroarthropathy.

The primary orthopaedic morbidity of Charcot neuroarthropathy is the lower extremity deformity and instability that results after severe destruction of the normal joint anatomy. Deformities of the foot alter normal plantar weight-bearing pressure, which leads to overload of the plantar soft tissues and ulceration. Ulceration may subsequently result in a portal for bacterial colonization leading to soft-tissue infection, and ultimately deep bony infection. Osteomyelitis often results in surgical treatment by amputation for cure. When Charcot neuroarthropathy involves the hindfoot or ankle, it results in severe instability with progressive malalignment and inability to bear weight (**Figure 1**).

The result of these problems on function and quality of life is profound. Patients with diabetes and Charcot neuroarthropathy have a 7% risk of amputation over their lifetime, and a 28% risk of amputation if they present with an ulcer.[1] Patients with diabetes and Charcot neuroarthropathy have physical functioning scores a full SD lower than patients with diabetes and without Charcot neuroarthropathy. Patients with Charcot neuroarthropathy have also been shown to have worse physical functioning scores than patients with cardiovascular disease, Parkinson disease, or end-stage renal disease.[5] Patients with Charcot neuroarthropathy have a worse self-reported quality of life than those with diabetes alone.[6,7]

Charcot neuroarthropathy can be classified either by temporal disease staging or by anatomic location. Temporal staging of Charcot neuroarthropathy was first described in three classic stages[8] in 1966, based on the natural history of the condition (**Table 1**). Stage I (fragmentation) is clinically characterized by hyperemia, edema, increased warmth, and erythema around the affected joint. Stage I is radiographically characterized by fragmentation of bone associated with fracture and joint subluxation. In stage II (coalescence), the acute inflammatory findings decrease. Radiographs demonstrate evidence of bone debris and new bone formation.

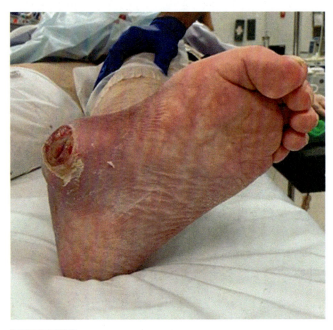

FIGURE 1 Photograph showing severe progressive Charcot neuroarthropathy of the hindfoot. Lateral subtalar and talonavicular dislocation resulting in collapse, deformity, and consequent soft-tissue ulceration/infection over the talar head.

Table 1

Eichenholtz Classification of Charcot Neuroarthropathy

Eichenholtz Classification	Clinical Presentation	Radiographic Findings
Stage 0 Prodromal	Swelling, warmth, pain, erythema	Normal
Stage I Fragmentation	Hyperemia, warmth, pain, edema	Fracture and joint subluxation/dislocation
Stage II Coalescence	Decreased inflammation, less swelling	Bony debris, new bone formation
Stage III Consolidation	Resolution of warmth and swelling	Bony healing, residual deformity, bone loss

Stages I-III described by Eichenholtz, Stage 0 added by Shibata et al in Shibata T, Tada K, Hashizume C: The results of arthrodesis of the ankle for leprotic neuroarthropathy. *J Bone Joint Surg Am* 1990;72:749-756.

Stage III (consolidation) is characterized by resolution of swelling and warmth surrounding the affected joints. At this stage, the joints will be more stable and the fragmentation will have consolidated; however, residual joint deformity and bone loss are evident. In 1990, Stage 0 (prodromal) was added to the classification because clinical signs often precede any radiographic changes.[9,10]

Several anatomic classifications have also been described for Charcot neuroarthropathy. In one classification system, Charcot involvement of the foot and ankle is described in terms of the four commonly affected anatomic areas[1] (**Figure 2**). Type I, which occurs in 60% of patients, affects the midfoot, tarsometatarsal, and naviculocuneiform joints. The subsequent collapse most commonly results in a residual deformity involving a plantarmedial bony exostosis that places the foot at risk of pressure ulceration. Type II, which affects 30% to 35% of patients, involves the hindfoot, with subsequent instability resulting in foot subluxation and ulcer formation. Type IIIA, which affects 5% of patients, involves the ankle joint and is the most unstable pattern. Type IIIB involves fracture of the calcaneal tuberosity and results in weak push-off, pes planus, and risk of ulceration associated with the avulsed bony prominence. In general, the more proximal the Charcot joint involvement, the higher the risk of subsequent joint instability.

In a second classification, type I is described as destruction of the tarsometatarsal joints, with medial plantar prominence and abduction deformity.[11] Type II involves the naviculocuneiform joint, with residual plantarlateral prominence under the fourth and fifth tarsometatarsal joints. Type III affects the navicular and the medial column, with collapse resulting in an adducted-supinated deformity and a plantarlateral prominence under the

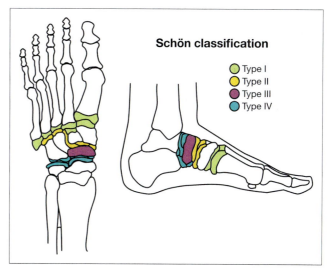

FIGURE 3 Illustration showing the Schön classification of midfoot Charcot Neuroarthropathy. (Courtesy of Shane Bass.)

cuboid. Type IV involves the transverse tarsal joints with associated prominence under the calcaneocuboid and talonavicular joints. Substage A, B, or C is assigned based on the progression of the rocker-bottom sole, with the most severe stage defined as progression of medial column collapse to below the plantar surface of the foot (**Figure 3**).

There are no imaging or laboratory markers in isolation that can diagnose Charcot neuroarthropathy. The early temporal stages (Eichenholtz stage 0 or I) can be confusing and misdiagnosis is common.[1] The swelling, warmth, and lack of clear antecedent trauma can lead clinicians to make an errant diagnosis of osteomyelitis, even when there is no ulceration present. In cases where ulcers are present, it is difficult to distinguish between the fragmentation stage of Charcot neuroarthropathy and osteomyelitis, and in some cases both may be present. A careful history and physical examination are essential. MRI and technetium bone scans can have a similar appearance in cases of infection or Eichenholtz stage I Charcot neuroarthropathy, although MRI can show an adjacent abscess. Use of tagged white blood cell scans is controversial but may help differentiate Charcot neuroarthropathy from osteomyelitis. A bone biopsy can be useful if imaging is not definitive.

Treatment Background

The treatment of Charcot neuroarthropathy is an active area of research and remains controversial. The goal of both nonsurgical and surgical options is to "achieve a stable, plantigrade functional foot that is resistant to ulceration, to prevent amputation, to improve performance in activities of daily living, and to allow the use of nonprescription footwear."[1]

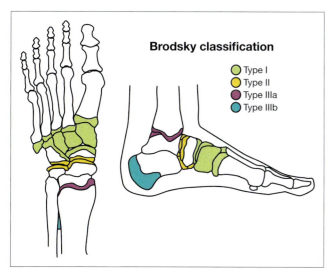

FIGURE 2 Illustration showing the Brodsky classification of Charcot neuroarthropathy. (Courtesy of Shane Bass.)

In cases of midfoot and hindfoot (Brodsky type I-II) Charcot neuroarthropathy, most clinicians favor an initial nonsurgical approach with total-contact casting or CROW (Charcot Restraint Orthotic Walker) use and weight-bearing limitations.[12] The goal is to maintain the shape of the foot until Eichenholtz stage III is reached, such that the foot remodels without severe rocker-bottom deformity. There is some controversy regarding whether weight-bearing restrictions are necessary, with some studies demonstrating comparable outcomes using weight-bearing total-contact casts.[13] Immobilization often requires several months until the foot both clinically and radiographically appears to exit the fragmentation phase. Hindfoot (Brodsky type II) disease generally takes longer to reach coalescence and remodeling than midfoot (Brodsky type I) Charcot neuroarthropathy.

Nonsurgical treatment is not completely benign. Prolonged immobilization and non–weight bearing results in deconditioning, osteopenia, and functional limitations. Casting or boot use can also result in ulceration, especially in patients with more severe neuropathy and/or poor-quality soft-tissue envelopes. Bony deformity develops in a substantial number of patients, requiring subsequent surgical intervention despite nonsurgical management. This has led some investigators to advocate for earlier surgical treatment of Charcot neuroarthropathy.[14] Studies of early treatment of midfoot Charcot neuroarthropathy are confined to small case studies but do show promising results, with earlier return of patients to function than would be expected with nonsurgical treatment and comparable rates of complication.

Notwithstanding those advocating early surgical intervention, most investigators suggest that indications for surgical treatment include ulceration with underlying bony prominence, infection, and deformity or instability that cannot be managed with bracing or commercial shoe wear. Ankle and some cases of hindfoot Charcot neuroarthropathy are often highly unstable and progressive despite nonsurgical treatment. In these cases, surgical management is often indicated for reconstruction and stabilization of the limb.

Multiple host factors must be taken into consideration when considering surgical management of Charcot neuroarthropathy. These include patient comorbidities and nutrition, quality of the soft-tissue envelope, bone quality, and the presence of infection. Vascular surgery consultation for consideration of revascularization should be obtained before orthopaedic surgery in cases where patients have absent or monophasic pulses. In patients with overwhelming infection, or where there is severe bone loss precluding ability to obtain stable internal fixation, amputation is the most reliable option to cure the patient and for a speedy recovery.

Surgical Techniques and Considerations

Once surgical management has been indicated, it must be emphasized that each case of Charcot neuroarthropathy is unique and presents different challenges.

Regardless of the surgical treatment chosen, soft-tissue management and placement of incisions is crucial to achieve a good result. The soft tissues in patients with Charcot neuroarthropathy are often traumatized, receive poor blood supply, and have decreased capacity for healing. In addition, when major deformities are corrected during reconstruction, regions of soft tissue that were initially contracted may suddenly be placed under significant tension. Incisions should be placed away from areas of anticipated postoperative high tension whenever possible, as wounds under tension are more likely to dehisce or necrose. Incisions on the plantar surface of the foot should be avoided when possible to avoid the possibility of painful plantar scarring or wound complication. Investigators advocate that exostectomy and deformity corrections should be performed through incisions separate from any ulcer or ulcers to avoid working through traumatized tissue that has bacterial colonization or infection.

SPECIFIC SURGICAL TECHNIQUES

Exostectomy

Exostectomy is a popular technique for management of midfoot Charcot neuroarthropathy in which plantar bony prominence has developed and is at risk for, or has already caused, ulceration. Candidates for exostectomy should have a stable foot in the late coalescence or the remodeling phase.[15] Plantar exostectomy typically involves making an incision on the lateral or medial border of the midfoot, elevating the soft tissues from the region of bony prominence with a periosteal elevator, and excising the region of plantar prominence with an osteotome or saw. More recently, minimally invasive techniques using low-speed, high-torque burrs have been described, which significantly reduce incision size.[16] Advantages to exostectomy include minimal soft-tissue violation, allowance of early weight bearing, and no need for internal or external fixation and the attendant-associated risks. A study on 27 exostectomy procedures performed for patients who have diabetes and Charcot neuroarthropathy with midfoot prominence and recurrent or chronic ulceration demonstrated satisfactory results, with 72% of patients achieving ulcer healing.[15] Patients with lateral plantar ulcers were less likely to achieve healing.

Reconstruction

Early attempts at reconstruction and fixation of Charcot neuroarthropathy were often met with failure. These early failures have led to the development of techniques that sometimes require the orthopaedic surgeon to suspend traditional orthopaedic principles that are applied in normal cases. Most commonly, some degree of bone removal and consequent shortening is necessary to adequately correct deformity and avoid undue tension on the soft tissue.

Superconstructs

One form of reconstruction that can be considered for patients with Charcot neuroarthropathy is the superconstruct. Superconstruct formation is a technique and not a specific implant type. Superconstructs have been described as having four features: (1) extending fusions past the area of injury to obtain stronger fixation, (2) performing liberal bony resection to decrease tension on the soft-tissue envelope, (3) using the strongest implant that will be tolerated by the soft tissues, and (4) placing implants in a way that maximizes their mechanical function.[17]

One major advantage of superconstructs is that they extend fixation to areas of bone that are not affected by the Charcot neuroarthropathy disease process. Bone in the affected region of Charcot neuroarthropathy is osteopenic and there is often bone loss due to bony resorption. Because superconstructs are more robust, they can also resist weight-bearing forces better than traditional constructs. Patients with Charcot neuroarthropathy often have medical comorbidities and full non–weight bearing can be very challenging (**Figure 4**).

Superconstructs can be created with standard plates, locking plates, beams, external fixation, or a combination

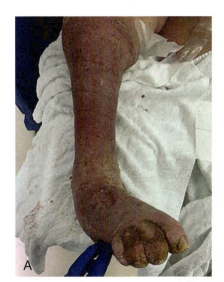
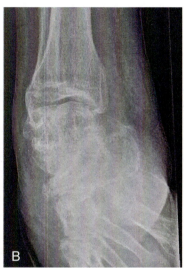
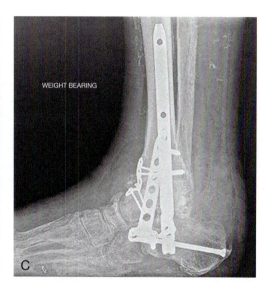
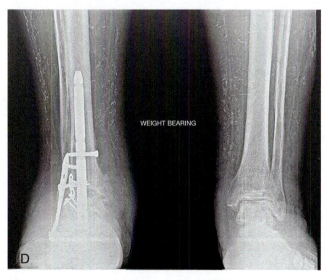

FIGURE 4 Superconstruct fixation used for the stabilization of a rigid neuropathic equinovarus deformity in a patient with morbid obesity and with severe lymphedema and osteopenia. **A**, Clinical photograph of the patient's deformity. **B**, AP radiograph demonstrating severe varus deformity. Standing lateral (**C**) and AP (**D**) radiographs demonstrating the superconstruct.

of these techniques. Locking plates carry the advantage of relying less on friction with osteopenic bony surfaces. Plantar plating has been suggested to be biomechanically superior to dorsal plating. One study of 34 patients treated with plantar plating for midfoot Charcot neuroarthropathy demonstrated a 90% satisfaction rate, with only one patient unable to wear commercial shoe wear.[18] Obtaining exposure for plantar plating however can be challenging.[18]

Although intramedullary fixation with axial screw placement has existed for many years, it has more recently gained increased traction as a technique option.[17-21] One advantage to this technique is that fixation can often be performed through small incisions without the need for extensive periosteal stripping or dissection for implant placement. However, studies have found several complications with these implants. One study of 22 patients who underwent intramedullary fixation for severe midfoot Charcot neuroarthropathy achieved limb salvage in all patients with maintenance of radiographic findings at final average follow-up of 52 months.[18] However, there were five nonunions, three patients with recurrent ulcers requiring surgical management, and eight cases of hardware failure. Another study of 25 patients with severe midfoot Charcot neuroarthropathy treated with midfoot osteotomy and intramedullary beams achieved an 84% ulcer-free rate at 1 year postoperatively. However, only 46% of osteotomies were united on radiograph; deep infection developed in 25% of patients, requiring surgical management; and four patients (16%) progressed to amputation because of infection.[19] In this study, presence of preoperative ulcer predicted the formation of a deep infection.

Ring external fixation is another method of fixation that has multiple advantages in the population with Charcot neuroarthropathy. External fixation allows rigid bony stability with minimal soft-tissue insult. It allows access to the soft-tissue envelope through which ulcers may be treated or monitored. External fixation can allow incremental correction of deformity, which in the case of large deformities can decrease the risk of neurovascular compromise or injury to the soft-tissue envelope. External fixation can be particularly useful in cases of infection because it avoids placement of deep implants where infection and biofilm can develop. Finally, external fixation has the advantage of allowing early weight bearing and can be used in combination with other constructs.[22] Some disadvantages to external fixation include the need for multiple patient office visits to monitor pin sites and potentially adjust the frame, pin site infections, and nonunion.

More recently, techniques have been described using minimally invasive high-torque, low-speed burr technology to perform percutaneous osteotomies, which are then fixated with percutaneous and/or intramedullary fixation.[16,23] Typically, a Shannon burr is first used to perform the osteotomy, followed by a wedge burr that morcellizes the bone, allowing it to be squeezed out

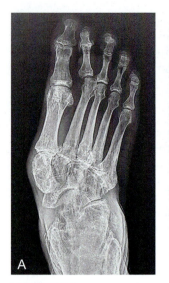 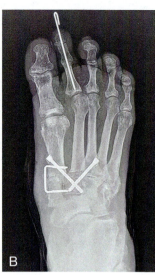

FIGURE 5 **A**, AP radiograph of a right foot with severe rigid planovalgus midfoot deformity. A 2.5-cm medial incision was used to perform the medial closing wedge plantar flexion osteotomy. A specialized water-cooled low-speed, high-torque burr is used to remove bone through the minimal surgical exposure. Supplemental percutaneous fixation was then placed for additional stability. **B**, At 6 weeks postoperatively, early bony healing is noted.

through small incisions. Deformity is then corrected and percutaneous fixation can be applied with axial screws, beams, or bolts. These techniques hold the promise of performing large deformity corrections through much smaller incisions, avoiding the increased risks of larger open incisions traditionally used for deformity correction. However, there are few reports detailing the results with these procedures (**Figure 5**).

One important consideration is that it may not always be necessary to achieve complete bony union in cases of arthrodesis. A stable incomplete union coupled with neuropathy is often asymptomatic and does not mandate further intervention.[24] The end goal of a painless stable plantigrade foot remains unchanged.

ANKLE AND HINDFOOT

Involvement of the ankle and/or subtalar joint in Charcot neuroarthropathy can be especially debilitating and challenging to treat. Ankle Charcot neuroarthropathy can develop after rotational ankle fractures, pilon fractures, or seemingly minimal trauma or avulsion fractures. It is now well established that patients with diabetes and rotational ankle fractures have a high risk of failure of traditional fixation methods and should be treated with robust internal fixation (eg, fibular locking plates with multiple syndesmosis screws) to prevent formation of Charcot neuroarthropathy.

Ankle and hindfoot Charcot neuroarthropathy often does not improve with nonsurgical management such as total-contact casting.[25] Instead, deformity and instability tends to worsen over time. Worsening deformity leads to high tension on the soft-tissue envelope and well as major bony prominences that can result in skin breakdown. In addition, the frank instability can make weight bearing impossible. Therefore, early surgical intervention is often indicated in these patients.

Several different patterns of ankle/hindfoot Charcot neuroarthropathy have been described. In general, the goal of deformity correction should be to obtain neutral axial hindfoot alignment. Typically, the ankle and subtalar joint are both fused. In cases of isolated ankle involvement, it is controversial whether the subtalar joint needs to be formally prepared or whether it can simply be spanned with the fixation construct.[26] Residual malalignment (eg, varus or valgus) can result in abnormal load bearing at the foot, resulting in ulceration. Specifics of surgical intervention depend on the anatomy of the deformity. If possible, corrective osteotomies should be made at the apex of the deformity as these will have the greatest power to correct the deformity. Soft-tissue releases including Achilles tendon lengthening or release of other joint capsules/tendons may be required on the tension side of the deformity to allow correction. As previously noted, an attempt should be made to keep incisions away from areas that are anticipated to have increased tension postoperatively. The surgeon should not hesitate to perform partial bony resection if it is required to obtain axial alignment and less tension on the soft tissues, even if this results in some shortening the limb (**Figure 6**).

Retrograde intramedullary nailing, external fixation, or a hybrid construct using both these fixation devices are the currently favored constructs for treatment. Intramedullary nails are a robust construct that can be placed through relatively small incisions. They can also provide some degree of compression across the fusion mass. External fixators have the advantage of avoiding placement of deep implant and are favored in cases of infection. Hybrid constructs can allow earlier weight bearing and additionally allow continuous compression as the external fixator can be adjusted at office visits to apply increasing compression.

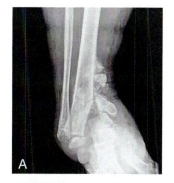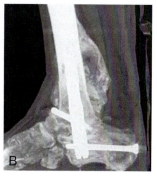

FIGURE 6 **A**, AP radiograph of showing severe chronic neuropathic ankle fracture-dislocation treated by lateral surgical approach, fibular osteotomy, partial distal tibial excision, and retrograde tibiotalocalcaneal fusion nail. In a chronic rigid deformity, it is advisable to avoid undue soft-tissue tension and incisions on the shortened side of the deformity. **B**, Lateral radiograph showing that salvage success depends on soft-tissue healing and achieving reduction of the calcaneus under the mechanical axis of the limb.

Outcomes after treatment with these constructs in the literature are mixed and likely reflect the heterogeneous patient population. A 2019 study of 56 patients with a mean follow-up of 7.5 years used intramedullary nails for noninfected patients (17 patients) and external fixation for those with infection (39 patients). The authors found that 28 patients (50%) achieved a favorable clinical outcome, and eight patients underwent amputation.[25] A 2020 study comparing intramedullary nailing with external fixation for 27 patients with ankle Charcot neuroarthropathy found similar rates of limb salvage between the two groups, with nine of 11 external fixation patients and 15 of 16 of intramedullary nail patients achieving limb salvage.[26] However, there were higher rates of complication in the intramedullary nailing group, with seven patients requiring revision surgical management for screw cutout or infection versus only one patient in the external fixation group. A study of 24 patients with ankle Charcot neuroarthropathy with a mean follow-up of 36 months found a 92% fusion rate with a hybrid construct and a 100% limb salvage rate.[27]

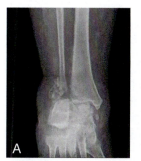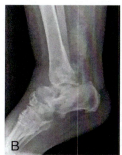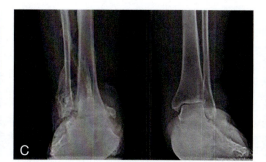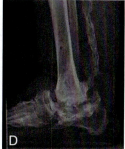

FIGURE 7 **A** and **B**, AP and lateral radiographs showing unstable neuropathic ankle and hindfoot fracture-dislocation. **C** and **D**, Stable plantigrade pain-free extremity after realignment, and ring external fixation for tibiotalocalcaneal fusion. Despite concern for incomplete union, the patient has remained well aligned, ambulatory, pain free, and ulcer free for over 2 years.

However, there were two plantar heel ulcerations from a backed-out nail and eight pin tract infections.

As noted for midfoot reconstruction, complete bony union is not always necessary to achieve lasting, stable improvement in alignment. Incomplete union in isolation is not a mandatory indication for return to the operating room. If the goals of surgery (a stable, plantigrade foot that can fit into commercial shoe wear) have been achieved, continued observation and regular follow-up is indicated (**Figure 7**).

SUMMARY

Charcot neuroarthropathy is one of the most challenging conditions that the foot and ankle surgeon can treat. Patients generally have multiple comorbidities, poor soft tissues, poor bone quality, and overall poor healing potential. When nonsurgical treatment is unsuccessful or not feasible, surgical intervention can be attempted. Surgical management often requires the suspension of normal orthopaedic surgical principles in favor of stronger superconstructs with stronger fixation that spans multiple joints. Limbs can often be salvaged, but complication rates can be high. Many patients, especially those with active infection or ulceration, will progress to amputation. More research is required to determine the optimal approach to this disabling disease process.

Acknowledgment

The authors wish to thank Shane Bass for his medical illustrations.

KEY STUDY POINTS

- Charcot disease of the foot is one of the most challenging entities to treat.
- The goal of nonsurgical and surgical treatment of Charcot neuroarthropathy is to obtain a stable, plantigrade foot that is free from ulcerations.
- The primary indications for surgery (change to surgical treatment) in Charcot neuroarthropathy of the foot and ankle are recurrent ulceration, significant deformity, deep infection, and pain.
- Surgical intervention should be approached methodically taking into account host factors, soft tissue, and bony considerations.
- In general, more robust constructs (superconstructs) should be used to decrease the probability of mechanical failure and loss of fixation. Incisions should be placed to avoid areas of expected postoperative tension. Union of fusions is not always needed to achieve a good result.

ANNOTATED REFERENCES

1. Brodsky JW: The diabetic foot, in Coughlin MJ, Mann RA, Saltzman CL, eds: *Surgery of the Foot and Ankle*, ed 8. Mosby, 2007, pp 1281-1368.

2. Schon LC, Easley ME, Weinfeld SB: Charcot neuroarthropathy of the foot and ankle. *Clin Orthop Relat Res* 1998;349:116-131.

3. Jeffcoate WJ, Game F, Cavanagh PR: The role of proinflammatory cytokines in the cause of neuropathic osteoarthropathy (acute Charcot foot) in diabetes. *Lancet* 2005;366(9502):2058-2061.

4. Sämann A, Pofahl S, Lehmann T, et al: Diabetic nephropathy but not HbA1c is predictive for frequent complications of Charcot feet - long-term follow-up of 164 consecutive patients with 195 acute Charcot feet. *Exp Clin Endocrinol Diabetes* 2012;120(6):335-339.

5. Dhawan V, Spratt KF, Pinzur MS, Baumhauer J, Rudicel S, Saltzman CL: Reliability of AOFAS diabetic foot questionnaire in charcot arthropathy: Stability, internal consistency, and measurable difference. *Foot Ankle Int* 2005;26(9):717-731.

6. Kroin E, Schiff A, Pinzur MS, Davis ES, Chaharbakhshi E, DiSilvio FA: Functional impairment of patients undergoing surgical correction for charcot foot arthropathy. *Foot Ankle Int* 2017;38(7):705-709.

7. Raspovic KM, Wukich DK: Self-reported quality of life in patients with diabetes: A comparison of patients with and without Charcot neuroarthropathy. *Foot Ankle Int* 2014;35(3):195-200.

8. Eichenholtz SN: *Charcot Joints*. Charles C. Thomas, 1966.

9. Rosenbaum AJ, Dipreta JA: Classifications in brief: Eichenholtz classification of Charcot arthropathy. *Clin Orthop Relat Res* 2015;473(3):1168-1171.

10. Shibata T, Tada K, Hashizume C: The results of arthrodesis of the ankle for leprotic neuroarthropathy. *J Bone Joint Surg Am* 1990;72(5):749-756.

11. Schon LC, Marks RM: The management of neuroarthropathic fracture-dislocations in the diabetic patient. *Orthop Clin North Am* 1995;26(2):375-392.

12. Pinzur M: Surgical versus accommodative treatment for Charcot arthropathy of the midfoot. *Foot Ankle Int* 2004;25(8):545-549.

13. Pinzur MS, Lio T, Posner M: Treatment of Eichenholtz stage 1 Charcot foot with a weight-bearing total contact cast. *Foot Ankle Int* 2006;27(5):324-329.

14. Mittlmeier T, Klaue K, Haar P, Beck M: Should one consider primary surgical reconstruction in Charcot arthropathy of the feet? *Clin Orthop Relat Res* 2010;468(4):1002-1011.

15. Catanzariti AR, Mendicino R, Haverstock B: Ostectomy for diabetic neuroarthropathy involving the midfoot. *J Foot Ankle Surg* 2000;39(5):291-300.

16. Botezatu I, Laptoiu D: Minimally invasive surgery of diabetic foot: Review of current techniques. *J Med Life* 2016;9(3):249-254.

17. Sammarco VJ: Superconstructs in the treatment of charcot foot deformity: Plantar plating, locked plating, and axial screw fixation. *Foot Ankle Clin* 2009;14(3):393-407.

18. Sammarco VJ, Sammarco GJ, Walker EW Jr, Guiao RP: Midtarsal arthrodesis in the treatment of Charcot midfoot arthropathy. *J Bone Joint Surg Am* 2009;91(1):80-91.

19. Doorgakant A, Davies MB: An approach to managing midfoot Charcot deformities. *Foot Ankle Clin* 2020;25(2):319-335.

    Expert review of approaches to Charcot foot deformity. Level of evidence: V.

20. Ford SE, Cohen BE, Davis WH, Jones CP: Clinical outcomes and complications of midfoot Charcot reconstruction with intramedullary beaming. *Foot Ankle Int* 2019;40(1):18-23.

    This is a retrospective review of 25 patients who underwent intramedullary beaming for Charcot with minimum 1-year follow-up. Level of evidence: IV.

21. Richman J, Cota A, Weinfeld S: Intramedullary nailing and external ring fixation for tibiotalocalcaneal arthrodesis in charcot arthropathy. *Foot Ankle Int* 2017;38(2):149-152.

22. Conway JD: Charcot salvage of the foot and ankle using external fixation. *Foot Ankle Clin* 2008;13(1):157-173, vii.

23. Miller RJ: Neuropathic minimally invasive surgeries (NEMESIS): Percutaneous diabetic foot surgery and reconstruction. *Foot Ankle Clin* 2016;21(3):595-627.

24. Lowery NJ, Woods JB, Armstrong DG, Wukich DK: Surgical management of Charcot neuroarthropathy of the foot and ankle: A systematic review. *Foot Ankle Int* 2012;33(2):113-121.

25. Harkin EA, Schneider AM, Murphy M, Schiff AP, Pinzur MS: Deformity and clinical outcomes following operative correction of Charcot ankle. *Foot Ankle Int* 2019;40(2):145-151.

    This is a retrospective review of 56 consecutive patients who underwent surgical treatment of Charcot deformities of the foot and ankle by a single surgeon. Level of evidence: IV.

26. Pinzur MS: Treatment of ankle and hindfoot Charcot arthropathy. *Foot Ankle Clin* 2020;25(2):293-303.

    This is an expert review of Charcot arthropathy comparing results of midfoot, hindfoot, and ankle disease. Level of evidence: V.

27. El-Mowafi H, Abulsaad M, Kandil Y, El-Hawary A, Ali S: Hybrid fixation for ankle fusion in diabetic Charcot arthropathy. *Foot Ankle Int* 2018;39(1):93-98.

CHAPTER 28

Minimally Invasive Surgery of the Foot and Ankle

ARIEL A. PALANCA, MD, FAAOS • MEGAN C. PAULUS, MD, FAAOS

ABSTRACT

Minimally invasive foot and ankle surgery has evolved over the past several decades and gained popularity worldwide, secondary to industry advancements of instrumentation and improvement of surgical technique. From exostectomies to osteotomies, a less invasive approach, when done in the proper setting, can achieve deformity correction and improvement in pain and function with faster recovery for the patient. It is important to be knowledgeable about current minimally invasive procedures that are commonly performed.

Keywords: calcaneal osteotomy; forefoot surgery; hallux valgus; minimally invasive surgery; MIS

INTRODUCTION

Foot and ankle surgery has gained importance as a subspecialty of orthopaedics over the past few decades. As with other fields in orthopaedic surgery, there have been efforts made to achieve the same goals of surgery with more minimally invasive techniques, from arthroscopy to tendoscopy to deformity correction through osteotomies and fusions. The theoretical advantages behind minimally invasive surgery (MIS) include decreased soft-tissue dissection through smaller incisions, potentially leading to faster recovery and less pain. More recent advances in techniques, instrumentation, and fixation methods have shown promise when incorporated intelligently with a

---

Dr. Palanca or an immediate family member serves as a paid consultant to or is an employee of DJ Orthopaedics and Stryker. Dr. Paulus or an immediate family member serves as a paid consultant to or is an employee of Arthrex, Inc.

thorough understanding of the anatomy and basic principles of surgical treatment of the pathology of the foot and ankle.

HISTORY

Diagnostic arthroscopy was first described in 1912, and the first arthroscopic partial meniscectomy was performed in Japan in 1962. Arthroscopy has revolutionized the approach to intra-articular pathologies; the procedure was first performed in North America around 1965. Continued improvements in the instruments and techniques have made arthroscopy the standard for many procedures.[1] In a similar way, arthroscopy of the ankle has led to interest in minimally invasive approaches to other foot and ankle pathology.

In the 1940s, the use of small instruments placed percutaneously for excision of exostoses was developed and later expanded on in the 1960s. This led to the use of electric motors to power instruments. By 1974, the first course in surgical techniques in MIS was held at the Pennsylvania College of Podiatric Medicine.[2]

In the 1980s, the so-called first generation of MIS surgeries of the forefoot for hallux valgus were described along with the advent of some of the procedures to correct bunions.[3] There was minimal internal fixation used and there were concerns for recurrent deformity and loss of range of motion, particularly with an intra-articular osteotomy.[4] In the 1990s, these techniques were Bosch modified and elaborated on in Europe as the second generation. Use of temporary fixation was performed in an extra-articular osteotomy with increased success, although not perfected. Significant rates of malalignment were noted, upward of 60% in some studies.[5,6] As discussed in a 2020 study, newer techniques with permanent internal fixation methods began to show improved outcomes with low recurrence and complication rates.[7]

Section 8: Contemporary Surgical Techniques

© 2025 American Academy of Orthopaedic Surgeons

Orthopaedic Knowledge Update®: Foot and Ankle 7

439

Section 8: Contemporary Surgical Techniques

In Spain in 2003, these techniques were expanded on and outlined in the text *Cirugía Percutánea del Pie*, which was later published in English in 2009 and titled *Minimally Invasive Foot Surgery*.[8] Poor results from the early procedures created an aversion to MIS in the foot and ankle. The combination of newer technology and instrumentation with stronger fixation methods using AO techniques has created promising results, redefining the third generation of minimally invasive foot and ankle surgery. Percutaneous osteotomies are performed with a 2-mm burr and the metatarsal head is shifted medially and held into place with headless screws to allow for faster rehabilitation. Promising results have been published, and these techniques are gaining popularity worldwide.[9]

INSTRUMENTATION

Instrumentation for MIS of the foot and ankle continues to evolve at a rapid pace. The creation of low-speed, high-torque burrs has minimized the risk of soft-tissue damage while being able to achieve deformity correction through minimal incisions (**Figure 1**). Most burrs are designed to operate at 6,000 rpm to minimize soft-tissue damage. Along with these burrs, some systems have built-in irrigation to mitigate the risk of necrosis from heat produced. Some surgeons advocate for refrigeration of irrigation fluids as a means to reduce risk of thermal injury.

Beaver blades, periosteal elevators, and rasps have been designed to work through the small incisions made for minimally invasive procedures. The burrs created for MIS can be categorized into two types: cutting burrs versus shaving burrs. Straight burrs of various diameters and lengths were developed to optimize use in specific osteotomies. Smaller burrs are used for lesser toe osteotomies; burr size can be increased to accommodate for larger bones, such as the calcaneus. There are wedge, side-cutting burrs, which are typically used for excision of exostoses and shaving down any remaining prominences following deformity correction. Headless screw systems, particularly beveled headless screws, are used to decrease the potential for painful prominent hardware, specifically for those screws that are put in at extremely oblique angles.

SURGICAL TECHNIQUE

MIS can be used for many different procedures, from bunion repair to exostectomies for decompression of diabetic pressure ulcers. Technique varies by procedure but many similar principles apply.

For all MIS procedures, patient positioning is key. Practice of surgical technique on cadavers multiple times is recommended until a high comfort level is achieved, and undergoing at least two formal trainings. Furthermore, it is helpful to have highly experienced surgical staff in the operating room for the first cases. As a standard, when using a mini C-arm, the C-arm should come in from the left side if the surgeon is right handed, or from the right if the surgeon is left handed, regardless of the side of the surgical foot. Also, the foot should be hanging off the end of the bed (**Figure 2**). The ideal first case would be a right hallux cheilectomy for a right-handed surgeon. Fluoroscopy should be checked before starting the case to ensure that the positioning is appropriate for imaging. Also, mini-open incisions can be used in the beginning as the surgeon becomes comfortable with the technique. Patients should be informed of the possible need for more extensile incisions.

Selection of burrs is based on procedure. For example, 2-mm straight burrs are typically used for hallux valgus osteotomies, whereas a wedge burr is used for cheilectomies and Haglund excisions because it is a side-cutting burr. The burr is held the way a pencil is held in the surgeon's dominant hand to enhance precision (**Figure 3**).

FOREFOOT

Hallux Cheilectomy

A minimally invasive cheilectomy for hallux rigidus is a great surgical procedure to begin with to get acquainted with MIS. As discussed in a 2019 study, cheilectomy is not technically challenging and results in excellent patient-reported outcomes of pain relief and early return to function.[10] Very few if any significant complications are reported in the literature. It should be noted that a 2020 study did show an increased reoperation rate in MIS cheilectomies compared with open approaches. As with all MIS procedures, there is a learning curve.[11]

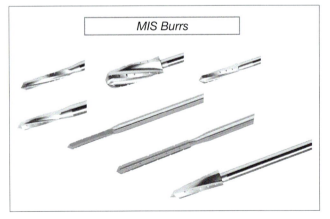

FIGURE 1 Photograph showing examples of new-generation minimally invasive surgery (MIS) burrs. (Courtesy of Arthex, Inc.)

Chapter 28: Minimally Invasive Surgery of the Foot and Ankle

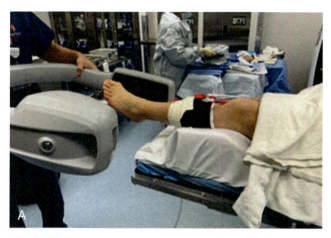
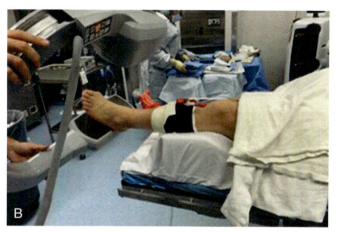

FIGURE 2 Photographs show the fluoroscopy setup for a minimally invasive forefoot procedure for (**A**) lateral and (**B**) AP images. This would be for a right-handed surgeon, because the C-arm is entering from the left side of the patient.

One (dorsomedial to the joint) to two incisions (a second may be needed for outflow) are used. The patient is positioned with the foot off the surgical table, first ensuring a lateral fluoroscopic view. It is important to fully elevate the capsule off the dorsal metatarsal. A wedge burr is advanced and sequentially shaves down the spur.

The bone shavings are milked out of the incision. The toe is flexed to prevent irritation of the proximal phalanx cartilage, and it is important not to notch or overresect. The bone shavings can be successfully irrigated with a 16-gauge angiocatheter and saline.[12,13] As discussed in a 2021 study, an arthroscopy can be performed at the end of the case to ensure complete removal of all bony debris[14] (**Figure 4**).

Postoperatively, a compression dressing is applied to help control edema. Immediate weight bearing is possible in a postoperative shoe.

Bunion and Bunionette Repair

There are more than 150 known open surgical procedures for hallux valgus; however, there is no obvious evidence that one technique surpasses the others, and each has its downfalls. MIS hallux valgus repair is becoming more and more common in the United States. Industry advanced with better instrumentation such as beveled screws, long headless screws, and low-torque burrs, and surgeon interest grew as well. High patient satisfaction and good clinical outcomes further encouraged the trend. Less prominent scars, faster wound healing, and less stiffness have been observed. However, as described in a 2019 study, moderate stiffness can still be expected after MIS correction.[15]

As discussed in a 2021 study, mild to severe hallux valgus can be accomplished by a distal metatarsal osteotomy often in conjunction with an Akin osteotomy.[16] The distal osteotomy can either be a transverse or a chevron fashion. The benefit of a chevron osteotomy is stability and the ability to translate the osteotomy in a lengthening fashion. The benefit of the transverse osteotomy is ease of the technique and ability to derotate the metatarsal head and reduce the sesamoid articulation, although fixation can be more challenging given the lack of stability.

FIGURE 3 Photograph showing a right-handed surgeon performing a bunion repair. Note the pencil grip of the burr.

Section 8: Contemporary Surgical Techniques

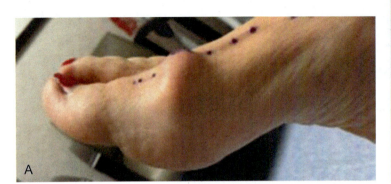
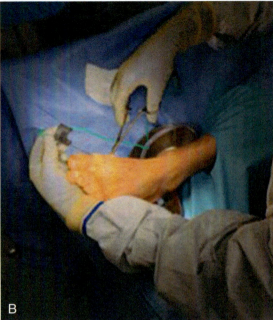
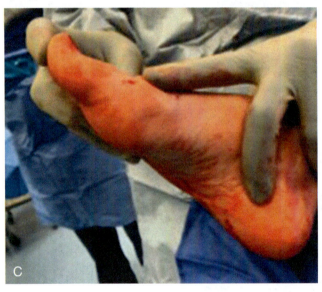

FIGURE 4 Preoperative (**A**), intraoperative (**B**), and postoperative (**C**) photographs of a hallux cheilectomy. Note that the surgeon intraoperatively made an accessory portal to help assist with the irrigation of the bone slurry.

Once the distal osteotomy is complete, the metatarsal head is translated laterally. The surgeon must take care not to dorsally or plantarly translate the metatarsal head (plantar is more common). Screw fixation is accomplished with cannulated headless screws, which lie flush to the cortex. Some find it easier to place the Kirschner wire before the osteotomy just shy of the lateral cortex of the metatarsal. A quadcortical Kirschner wire is then placed into the metatarsal head and the first screw is placed. Four-cortex fixation is very important for stabilization of the construct. A second smaller screw is then placed more distally. Often, the prominent medial wall (or "spike") of the metatarsal needs to be removed with a burr, rasp, or rongeur while taking care not to compromise the screw fixation. Patient satisfaction results of up to 95% have been reported[17] (**Figure 5**).

For severe hallux valgus and a very large intermetatarsal angle, a basal wedge osteotomy has also been described.[18] This removes a lateral wedge of proximal bone that allows for reduction of the intermetatarsal angle and fixation is also with two screws.

Chapter 28: Minimally Invasive Surgery of the Foot and Ankle

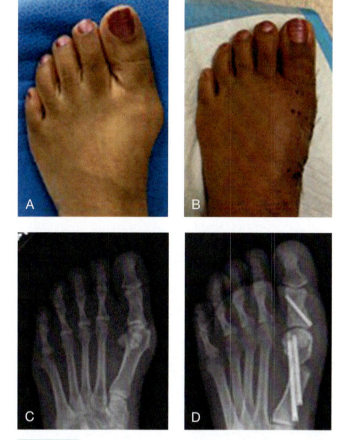

FIGURE 5 **A** and **B**, Preoperative clinical pictures, and **C** and **D**, radiographs 1 week after minimally invasive surgery for bunion repair.

A percutaneous adductor release is performed when necessary. Using a 15 blade scalpel, an incision is made in the first web space at the level of the first metatarsal joint.

As described in a 2020 study, the blade is progressed from a 45° to 60° angle until the blade enters the joint. External rotation and varus is applied to the toe until the tendon is released.[19]

Some authors cite immediate postoperative weight bearing in a postoperative shoe, whereas others advocate 2 weeks heel weight bearing. Postoperative stiffness can still occur with MIS surgery.

There are three types of bunionette deformity according to the bony aspect: type 1 presents as a prominent lateral condyle of the fifth metatarsal; type 2 is a lateral bowing of the fifth metatarsal shaft diaphysis; and type 3 is a divergence of the fourth and fifth metatarsals. Type 3 occurs most frequently.[20]

MIS correction of bunionettes can be achieved with all three types. For a true type 1 deformity, a wedge burr can be used to shave down the bony lateral prominence. For types 2 and 3, an oblique burr cut with a 2-mm burr can be used in a distal to proximal fashion and the metatarsal head is allowed to drift proximal and medial. Most techniques do not describe fixation; however, the most encountered complication after a percutaneous bunionette correction is delayed union[21,22] (**Figure 6**). Therefore, if there is concern, pinning or a percutaneous screw can be used. Protected and restricted weight bearing until radiographic evidence of callus is recommended. Also, toe strapping with tape can aid in healing. Other complications include hypertrophic callus formation that can cause symptoms until resorbed. To avoid nerve complications, a dorsomedial approach can be used as described in a 2019 study, because the nerve lies in the dorsolateral portion of the metatarsal neck.[23] Also, more distal approaches can preserve the blood supply as the nutrient artery enters around the junction of the middle and proximal thirds of the medial aspect of the fifth metatarsal. No nerve and/or vascular complications are known to have been reported in clinical studies.

MIS Arthrodesis

Small low-powered studies show high union rates for MIS and arthroscopic double and triple arthrodesis; most challenging is the talonavicular joint, which saw a union rate of 78%. Time to union has been reported to be between 8 and 26 weeks. Care must be taken in establishing working portals, and the rotary deformity must be addressed.[24] A two-portal sinus tarsi approach is sufficient for a triple arthrodesis, although accessory dorsal portals, particularly for the talonavicular joint, may need to be used.[25,26] Nerve injury is rare and can be avoided with a careful nick-and-spread technique.[27] Compression can be achieved via a percutaneous pin distractor on compression before screw insertion.

MIS first metatarsophalangeal arthrodesis is also becoming more popular. Recent cadaver studies show that joint preparation is comparable to arthroscopic joint preparation and patient outcomes are at least equivalent to open procedures.[28,29] Fixation is typically achieved with headless crossing screws through small incisions.

Metatarsalgia/Lesser Toe Deformities

Standard open distal metatarsal osteotomies have a high incidence of postoperative stiffness and floating, making improvement of technique an interest to surgeons.[30] Furthermore, these techniques can be used to offload diabetic forefoot ulcers.[31]

When performing distal metatarsal osteotomies using MIS, it is necessary to include the second, third, and fourth metatarsals to avoid a transfer lesion developing under the third or fourth metatarsal heads. The most common complication is a delayed union (no radiographic healing after 6 months), reported up to 5%, and usually involves the second metatarsal.[32] The procedure is performed with a 2-mm burr directed at a 45° angle perpendicular to the metatarsal in the coronal plane. Postoperatively, forefoot spica dressings are used to enhance stability.[33]

Section 8: Contemporary Surgical Techniques

Hammer, mallet, crossover, or claw toes can also be addressed using MIS. Each are accomplished via directed osteotomies, interphalangeal fusions, and soft-tissue balancing based on the deformity. Pinning may or may not be necessary and is typically decided intraoperatively based on the stability of the osteotomies, or whether an arthrodesis is required (**Figure 7**).

CALCANEAL OSTEOTOMY

Either a lateral or medial shift osteotomy can be accomplished via MIS technology. A key benefit of the minimally invasive technique is the ability to place other incisions nearby, including those required for access to the peroneal tendons or for lateral ankle ligament repair.[34] Typically a 3-mm burr is used, which resects a safe amount of bone and then also allows for impressive translation.

The authors of one study described a safe zone for a calcaneal osteotomy to avoid damage to the sural nerve. Using a lateral calcaneal fluoroscopic image, a line is

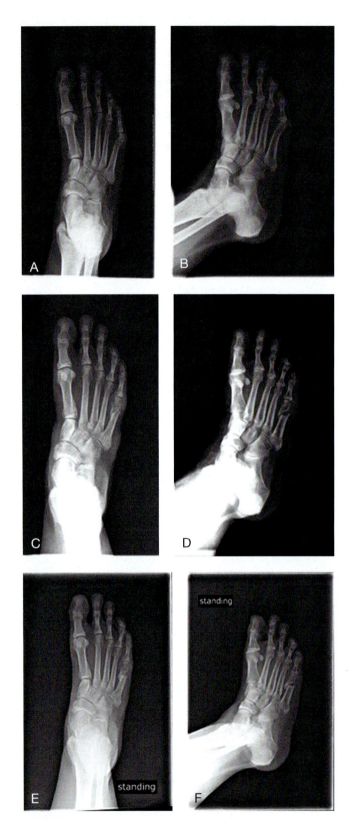

FIGURE 6 Anteroposterior and oblique radiographs at preoperative visit (**A** and **B**), 6 weeks postoperative visit (**C** and **D**), and 3 months postoperative visit (**E** and **F**). This case demonstrates a delayed callous formation, which is the most common complication with these procedures.

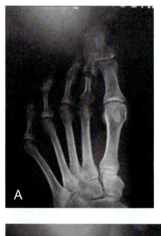
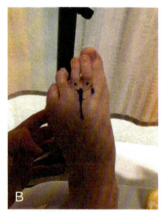
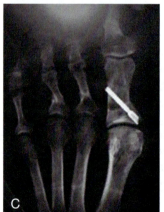
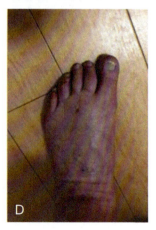

FIGURE 7 Preoperative (**A** and **B**) and postoperative (**C** and **D**) radiographs and clinical pictures showing minimally invasive surgery for lesser toe correction via closing-wedge proximal phalanx osteotomies. (Courtesy of Tyler Gonzales, MD, MBA, Assistant Professor of Orthopaedic Surgery at University of South Carolina.)

drawn from the plantar fascia origin to the posterosuperior apex of the calcaneus, which marks the center of the safe zone[35] (**Figure 8**).

Patient position can either be lateral or supine with a large hip bump if other incisions are planned. Radiographs should be obtained preoperatively to ensure that the contralateral leg will not impede imaging. If supine, the mini or large C-arm can be positioned from the foot of the bed with the surgeon standing in the middle. There should be a bump under the leg with the heel free. If lateral, the foot is positioned directly on the C-arm image intensifier. Some companies have implant systems with targeting devices, which can be assembled after the pilot hole is made, but many surgeons accomplish the osteotomy freehand. A small incision is made in the skin. Surgeons prefer to mark out the plane of the osteotomy on fluoroscopy first as a guide. Under fluoroscopic guidance, the burr should be placed center in the safe zone. The burr should barely penetrate the medial cortex to protect the medial structures. Typically, the osteotomy is then made in a quadrant approach with a fanlike cut, starting superior lateral, superior medial, inferior lateral, and then inferior medial. A laminar spreader can be used to open the osteotomy and remove any remaining bone and irrigate. Marrow and fat extruding from the incision site often is a marker that the osteotomy is complete. The osteotomy can be translated manually or with elevators and then secured with a screw in the typical fashion (**Figure 9**). Weight bearing can start between the fourth and sixth weeks after surgery depending on whether other procedures were also accomplished.[36-38]

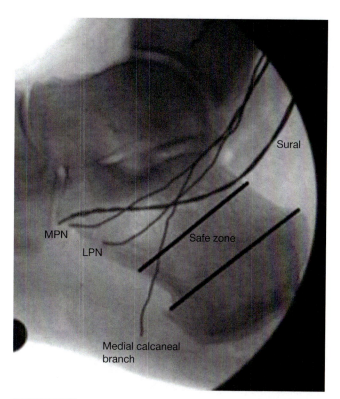

FIGURE 8 Lateral ankle radiograph demonstrating the safe zone for minimally invasive calcaneal osteotomy. LPN = lateral plantar nerve, MPN = medial plantar nerve. (Reproduced with permission from Talusan PG, Cata E, Tan EW, Parks BG, Guyton GP: Safe zone for neural structures in medial displacement calcaneal osteotomy: A cadaveric and radiographic investigation. *Foot Ankle Int* 2015;36[12]:1493-1498.)

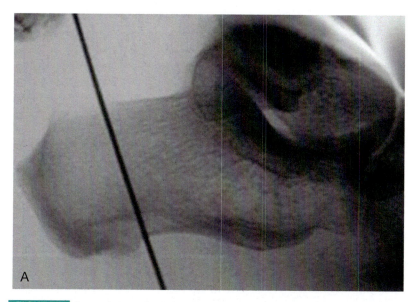
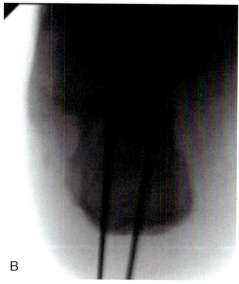

FIGURE 9 Lateral (**A**) and axial (**B**) intraoperative radiographs for a minimally invasive calcaneal osteotomy. First, the safe zone is marked and then an axial view is used to confirm adequate shift.

SUMMARY

For the correct patient and indication, common foot and ankle surgeries can be accomplished via minimally invasive techniques, affording faster recovery and fewer soft-tissue complications. MIS techniques have a steep learning curve, and proper training, setup, and understanding of common pitfalls are critical. Industry innovations continue to advance surgical indications while minimizing previously reported complications.

KEY STUDY POINTS

- Early results with minimally invasive foot and ankle surgery showed a high rate of complications, particularly with failure of fixation of osteotomies.
- Since the early 2000s, advancements in industry, including low-speed high-torque burrs and stronger internal fixation, have repopularized minimally invasive surgical techniques.
- Proper training and preoperative setup is imperative for successful execution of MIS techniques.

ANNOTATED REFERENCES

1. DeMaio M: Giants of orthopaedic surgery: Masaki Watanabe MD. *Clin Orthop Relat Res* 2013;471(8):2443-2448.

2. De Prado M, Ripoll P-L, Golan P: Minimally invasive foot surgery: A paradign shift, in de Prado M, ed: *Minimally Invasive Surgery of the Foot and Ankle*. Springer, 2011, pp 3-5.

3. Isham SA: The Reverdin-Isham procedure for the correction of hallux abducto valgus. A distal metatarsal osteotomy procedure. *Clin Podiatr Med Surg* 1991;8:81-94.

4. Bauer T, de Lavigne C, Biau D, De Prado M, Isham S, Laffenetre O: Percutaneous hallux valgus surgery: A prospective multicenter study of 189 cases. *Orthop Clin North Am* 2009;40(4):505-514, ix.

5. Magnan B, Pezze L, Rossi N, Bartolozzi P: Percutaneous distal metatarsal osteotomy for correction of hallux valgus. *J Bone Joint Surg Am* 2005;87:1191-1199.

6. Enan A, Abo-Hegy M, Seif H: Early results of distal metatarsal osteotomy through minimally invasive approach for mild-to-moderate hallux valgus. *Acta Orthop Belg* 2010;76:526-535.

7. Biz C, Crimì A, Fantoni I, Tagliapietra J, Ruggieri P: Functional and radiographic outcomes of minimally invasive intramedullary nail device (MIND) for moderate to severe hallux valgus. *Foot Ankle Int* 2020;42(4):409-424.

    This is a case series of 100 patients who underwent correction of their hallux valgus deformity with use of a minimally invasive intramedullary nail device. The study demonstrated significant correction radiographically with a low rate of complications and recurrence. Level of evidence: IV.

8. De Prado M, Ripoll PL, Golanó P: *Cirugía Percutánea del Pie*. Elsevier-Masson, 2003.

9. De Prado M, Ripoll PL, Golanó P: *Minimally Invasive Foot Surgery*. AYH Publishers, 2009.

10. Teoh KH, Tan WT, Atiyah Z, Ahmad A, Tanaka H, Hariharan K: Clinical outcomes following minimally invasive dorsal cheilectomy for hallux rigidus. *Foot Ankle Int* 2019;40(2):195-201.

    This was a retrospective study of patients treated with an MIS cheilectomy for hallux rigidus. The results showed improvement in patient-reported outcome measures and a safety profile similar to that of open cheilectomy, though there was evidence of a learning curve. Level of evidence: IV.

11. Stevens R, Bursnall M, Chadwick C, et al: Comparison of complication and reoperation rates for minimally invasive versus open cheilectomy of the first metatarsophalangeal joint. *Foot Ankle Int* 2020;41(1):31-36.

    This study is a retrospective analysis comparing open versus minimally invasive cheilectomies over a 5-year period. The authors found increased risks and need for reoperation in the MIS cohort, mainly conversion to a metatarsophalangeal joint fusion. Level of evidence: III.

12. De Prado M, Ripoll P-L, Golan P: Minimally invasive management of hallux rigidus, in Maffuli N, Easley M, eds: *Minimally Invasive Surgery of the Foot and Ankle*. Springer, 2011, pp 75-88.

13. Morgan S, Jones C, Palmer S: Minimally invasive cheilectomy (MIS): Functional outcome and comparison with open cheilectomy. *J Bone Joint Surg Br* 2012;94-B:93.

14. Glenn RL, Gonzalez TA, Peterson AB, Kaplan J: Minimally invasive dorsal cheilectomy and hallux metatarsal phalangeal joint arthroscopy for the treatment of hallux rigidus. *Foot Ankle Orthop* 2021;6(1):2473011421993103.

    This study looked at 20 patients who underwent MIS hallux cheilectomy and metatarsophalangeal arthroscopy. The procedure showed improved pain relief with minimal complications, as well as a high rate of intra-articular debris along with intra-articular pathology post cheilectomy. Level of evidence: IV.

15. Frigg A, Zaugg S, Maquieira G, Pellegrino A: Stiffness and range of motion after minimally invasive chevron-Akin and open scarf-Akin procedures. *Foot Ankle Int* 2019;40(5):515-525.

    This is a retrospective study comparing scarf with MIS bunion repairs. Outcomes were very similar, except for a higher need for reoperation in the MIS cohort and increased stiffness and higher wound complications in the scarf cohort. Level of evidence: II.

16. Schilde S, Delank KS, Arbab D, Gutteck N: Minimally invasive vs open akin osteotomy. *Foot Ankle Int* 2021;42(3):278-286.

    This is a retrospective study comparing open versus MIS Akin osteotomies. Deformity correction was equivalent in both groups as well as rates of infection and complication. Level of evidence: III.

17. Lam P, Lee M, Xing J, Di Nallo M: Percutaneous surgery for mild to moderate hallux valgus. *Foot Ankle Clin* 2016;21(3):459-477.

18. Vernois J, Redfern DJ: Percutaneous surgery for severe hallux valgus. *Foot Ankle Clin* 2016;21(3):479-493.

19. Del Vecchio JJ, Dalmau-Pastor M: Percutaneous lateral release in hallux valgus: Anatomic basis and indications. *Foot Ankle Clin* 2020;25(3):373-383.

    This is a technique article on how to perform a percutaneous lateral release for correction of hallux valgus. Level of evidence: IV.

20. Du Vries HL: *Surgery of the Foot*, ed 2. CV Mosby, 1965, pp 456-462.

21. Michels F, Van Der Bauwhede J, Guillo S, Oosterlinck D, de Lavigne C: Percutaneous bunionette correction. *Foot Ankle Surg* 2013;19:9-14.

22. Laffenêtre O, Millet-Barbé B, Darcel V, Lucas Y Hernandez J, Chauveaux D: Percutaneous bunionette correction: Results of a 49-case retrospective study at a mean 34 months' follow-up. *Orthop Traumatol Surg Res* 2015;101(2):179-184.

23. Tonogai I, Hayashi F, Tsuruo Y, Sairyo K: Direction and location of the nutrient artery to the fifth metatarsal at risk in osteotomy for bunionette. *Foot Ankle Surg* 2019;25(2):193-197.

    This report describes the direction and location of the nutrient artery entering the fifth metatarsal studied in 10 cadaver lower limbs. The nutrient artery enters the medial aspect of the fifth metatarsal around the junction of the middle and proximal thirds obliquely from a distal direction and medial-plantar in the axial plane. Level of evidence: V.

24. Jagodzinski NA, Parsons AM, Parsons SW: Arthroscopic triple and modified double hindfoot arthrodesis. *Foot Ankle Surg* 2015;21(2):97-102.

25. Lintz F, Guillard C, Colin F, Marchand JB, Brilhault J: Safety and efficiency of a 2-portal lateral approach to arthroscopic subtalar arthrodesis: A cadaveric study. *Arthroscopy* 2013;29(7):1217-1223.

26. Mouilhade F, Oger P, Roussignol X, Boisrenoult P, Sfez J, Duparc F: Risks relating to posterior 2-portal arthroscopic subtalar arthrodesis and articular surfaces abrasion quality achievable with these approaches: A cadaver study. *Orthop Traumatol Surg Res* 2011;97(4):396-400.

27. Walter R, Parsons S, Winson I: Arthroscopic subtalar, double, and triple fusion. *Foot Ankle Clin* 2016;21(3):681-693.

28. Angthong C, Rajbhandari P, Handoyo HR: Minimally invasive surgery versus an arthroscopic procedure for the first metatarsophalangeal arthrodesis: A comparative study of the effectiveness and safety profile. *Eur J Orthop Surg Traumatol* 2021;31(3):497-501.

This cadaver study reviewed arthroscopy versus MIS first metatarsophalangeal arthrodesis fusion techniques. There were no significant differences in the effectiveness of articular surface preparation between the MIS and arthroscopic groups. Level of evidence: V.

29. Hodel S, Viehöfer A, Wirth S: Minimally invasive arthrodesis of the first metatarsophalangeal joint: A systematic literature review. *Foot Ankle Surg* 2020;26(6):601-606.

    This is a systematic literature review of six studies (one level V, five level IV) reporting on minimally invasive arthrodesis of the first metatarsophalangeal joint. Results showed comparable clinical radiologic outcome and complication rates to open surgery. Level of evidence: IV.

30. Khurana A, Kadamabande S, James S, Tanaka H, Hariharan K: Weil osteotomy: Assessment of medium term results and predictive factors in recurrent metatarsalgia. *Foot Ankle Surg* 2011;17(3):150-157.

31. Biz C, Gastaldo S, Dalmau-Pastor M, Corradin M, Volpin A, Ruggieri P: Minimally invasive distal metatarsal diaphyseal osteotomy (DMDO) for chronic plantar diabetic foot ulcers. *Foot Ankle Int* 2018;39(1):83-92.

32. Haque S, Kakwani R, Chadwick C, Davies MB, Blundell CM: Outcome of minimally invasive distal metatarsal metaphyseal osteotomy (DMMO) for lesser toe metatarsalgia. *Foot Ankle Int* 2016;37(1):58-63.

33. Redfern DJ, Vernois J: Percutaneous surgery for metatarsalgia and the lesser toes. *Foot Ankle Clin* 2016;21(3):527-550.

34. Guyton GP: Minimally invasive osteotomies of the calcaneus. *Foot Ankle Clin* 2016;21(3):551-566.

35. Talusan PG, Cata E, Tan EW, Parks BG, Guyton GP: Safe zone for neural structures in medial displacement calcaneal osteotomy: A cadaveric and radiographic investigation. *Foot Ankle Int* 2015;36(12):1493-1498.

36. Di Domenico LA Jr. Joseph M, La Civita MD: Percutaneous calcaneal displacement osteotomy, in Maffuli N, Easley M, eds: *Minimally Invasive Surgery of the Foot and Ankle*. Springer, 2011, pp 231-244.

37. Kheir E, Borse V, Sharpe J, Lavalette D, Farndon M: Medial displacement calcaneal osteotomy using minimally invasive technique. *Foot Ankle Int* 2015;36:248-252.

38. Bruce BG, Bariteau JT, Evangelista PE, Arcuri D, Sandusky M, DiGiovanni CW: The effect of medial and lateral calcaneal osteotomies on the tarsal tunnel. *Foot Ankle Int* 2014;35:383-388.

CHAPTER 29

Revision Total Ankle Arthroplasty

GREGORY C. BERLET, MD, FRCS(C), FAAOS, FAOA • ROBERT D. SANTROCK, MD, FAAOS

ABSTRACT

The use of total ankle arthroplasty has been increasing at a rate similar to that of total knee arthroplasty. The availability of viable revision options is likely one factor that has led to this increase. However, it is still important to explore the causes of premature total ankle implant failure as well as long-term implant wear to minimize the need for revision surgery.

Keywords: malalignment; osteolysis; revision ankle arthroplasty; total ankle arthroplasty

---

Dr. Berlet or an immediate family member has received royalties from Artelon, In2Bone, Ossio, Stryker, and ZimmerBiomet; is a member of a speakers' bureau or has made paid presentations on behalf of Artelon, DJ Orthopaedics, Ossio, and Stryker; serves as a paid consultant to or is an employee of Artelon, CrossRoads, DJ Orthopaedics, Medline, Restor3d, and Stryker; has stock or stock options held in Curvebeam, Grammercy, Ossio, and Tissue Tech; and has received research or institutional support from Artelon and Zimmer. Dr. Santrock or an immediate family member has received royalties from Treace Medical Concepts; is a member of a speakers' bureau or has made paid presentations on behalf of Exactech, Inc. and Treace Medical Concepts; serves as a paid consultant to or is an employee of Exactech, Inc., Treace Medical Concepts, and Vilex; serves as an unpaid consultant to Epic Extremity and OREdMatters.com; has stock or stock options held in Epic Extremity, OREdMatters.com, and Treace Medical Concepts, Inc.; and has received research or institutional support from Treace Medical Concepts, Inc.

INTRODUCTION

Ankle arthritis is a unique yet disabling disease pattern resulting in poor quality of life and function. Compared with other arthritic conditions such as knee arthritis, ankle arthritis is complicated by an earlier onset and a traumatic etiology. Ankle arthrodesis delivers pain relief at the expense of motion and frequent patient dissatisfaction because of stiffness as well as adjacent joint arthritis. For this reason, ankle arthroplasty and the goal of motion preservation remain attractive to both surgeons and patients.

First-generation implants had inconsistent outcomes with instability, subsidence, and cyst formation, which limited their longevity.[1] Modern manufacturing techniques and better understanding of the biomechanics principles of ankle kinematics have allowed for the evolution to third-generation and fourth-generation implants.

The goal of treatment for ankle arthritis is pain relief with functional improvement in gait and quality of life. Gait analysis in patients undergoing total ankle arthroplasty rather than ankle fusion has shown ground reaction forces closer to those of normal control patients.[2]

Survivorship, as a measure of success, has continued to improve, with one study reporting 93.3% survivorship at 5 years and 80.3% at 10 years.[3] Looking at a younger patient cohort (younger than 55 years at implantation), a 2022 study reported implant survival of 94% for a total of 51 patients. However, follow-up was abbreviated with a mean follow-up of 31.2 months (SD = 16.2).[4]

As the popularity of total ankle arthroplasty increases so does the likelihood for revision total ankle arthroplasty.

There are several risk factors associated with total ankle arthroplasty failure, and it is important to know how to mitigate these risks. Also, a surgeon must be aware of options for preserving a functional ankle joint arthroplasty with revision components when possible, to avoid salvage arthrodesis or amputation.

MANAGEMENT OF MALALIGNMENT

Proximal (Tibial) Issues

Deformity or malalignment that is not accurately addressed at the time of the primary total ankle arthroplasty can lead to excessive implant damage or loosening, which may require a revision surgery. Many of the principles discussed in this section can serve to guide the surgeon dealing with deformity before implantation.

The overall guiding principles in dealing with proximal malalignment are to understand the mechanical axis of the lower leg and the center of rotation and angulation of the deformity. These two factors are influenced by structures above (hip and knee) as well as structures below (foot) the ankle. It is most sound practice to address these areas first, before revision if at all possible. Addressing deformities in the area of the ankle and distal third of the tibia can often be done simultaneously with the ankle arthroplasty revision. In general, altered joint mechanics occurs with alignment that is greater than 5° or greater than 2 cm displaced.[5]

For implants that have been in place for a substantial amount of time, correction of deformity above the ankle arthroplasty likely does not negate the need for revision of the implant, because the forces now may not be balanced as during primary surgery. Alternatively, the wear in the previous deformed state has now caused articular instability or poor function as a result of damage to the polyethylene insert.

Tibial deformity closer to the ankle joint (lower third) usually has a greater effect than more proximal deformity.[6] In other words, there is more forgiveness in the ankle/ankle arthroplasty to tolerate deformities above the lower third of the tibia. This is fortunate for the ankle arthroplasty surgeon who is familiar with this region and anatomy so that often corrections can proceed simultaneously at the time of the ankle replacement. However, patient-specific factors as well as surgeon experience may favor a staged approach.

Varus Malpositioning

Varus malpositioning of total ankle arthroplasty is a common technical mistake that can occur during implantation and can be intra-articular or extra-articular. In either situation, total ankle arthroplasty can fail because of increased forces on the implant. Intra-articular varus essentially leads to joint surface incongruency. The literature has reported that increased forces on the implant occur at 10° to 15° of varus malpositioning.[7,8] This deformity can be managed with a distal supramalleolar osteotomy. In a series of 22 patients, there was an average of 6° of improvement in the coronal plane alignment of postoperative radiographs, as well as improvements in the visual analog scale pain scores and American

---

Table 1

Steps for Intra-articular Correction of Varus Malpositioning

Removal of bony osteophytes
Thorough gutter débridement
Deltoid ligament complete peel or release
Talonavicular capsulotomy
Posterior tibial tendon sheath release
Posterior tibial tendon lengthening
Sliding medial malleolus osteotomy

Orthopaedic Foot and Ankle Society functional scores. However, there was a nonunion rate of 14%.[7] In cases where the varus is 10° or less, intra-articular adjustments (simple component repositioning) can suffice.

Intra-articular correction of varus malpositioning involves a well-described sequence of maneuvers, some of which are necessary for proper implant repositioning. These maneuvers are listed in **Table 1**.

There are three caveats to this process: (1) the risk of excessive deltoid and other medial releases can be mitigated with the placement of a lamina spreader or polyethylene trial in the joint set at the proper ligament tension or balance;[9] (2) the sliding tibial osteotomy medially is uncommonly used, and should be deployed with caution because of the thin medial malleolus bony architecture after total ankle arthroplasty;[10] and (3) after correction of varus malpositioning, a repair or reconstruction of the lateral ankle ligaments is usually necessary.[11]

Cavus Foot Issues (Varus)

Cavovarus foot deformity left untreated or undertreated is a common condition associated with poor outcome of primary total ankle arthroplasty. When performing revision total ankle arthroplasty in a patient with the foot in varus, the first decision to be made is whether to perform the revision and the foot correction simultaneously or to stage the surgical procedures. The literature over the past decade shows success in simultaneous varus foot correction and total ankle arthroplasty.[12,13] However, a staged approach is also reasonable and allows for the extensive reconstruction to be less taxing on both the surgeon and patient. When a staged approach for revision total ankle with cavovarus foot as a mechanism for failure is deployed, the first surgery is an explantation of the ankle implants and a proper corrective procedure on the foot. The ankle space is preserved with a cement spacer in the neutral (corrected) position for the necessary time until the foot reconstruction is healed, usually 12 to 16 weeks. The second stage is the removal of the spacer and revision total ankle implantation.

The second decision is determining the proper foot reconstruction necessary by assessing the amount of foot rigidity present. It is important that all of the involved regions of the foot be included in the reconstruction: hindfoot, midfoot, and forefoot. In rigid deformities, it will be necessary to perform bone reconstruction that includes some type of arthrodesis. The most severe cases will necessitate the triple arthrodesis and the Lapidus first tarsometatarsal arthrodesis. Less severe deformities may be accommodated by a subtalar arthrodesis. In flexible foot deformities, the reconstruction may be appropriate for joint-sparing procedures such as the valgus-producing calcaneus osteotomy and the dorsiflexion-producing first cuneiform/first metatarsal osteotomy.

A properly corrected foot position is necessary to properly align the total ankle arthroplasty. In the revision total ankle arthroplasty setting, this is perhaps even more important because there is potentially less forgiveness as bone loss and other detriments may play a role in the final outcome. One study discussed that equal outcomes should be expected in cases where the average preoperative varus was 25° versus 5° of varus. This indicates that with proper foot alignment, a functional score and pain score are equivalent to straightforward ankle replacement.[12]

Valgus Malpositioning

Valgus in many cases is more challenging than varus. Incongruent valgus and the associated ligament insufficiency often require significant consideration in the primary total ankle arthroplasty and often a staged approach. When the progressive flatfoot deformity is either unrecognized or undertreated, this puts the totality of the total ankle and residual ligament supports at risk. In the setting of an unsatisfactory clinical outcome with valgus, an in situ total ankle arthroplasty may or may not need to be revised depending on preoperative CT.

Deltoid Incompetence

The isometric ligaments of the hindfoot are the posteromedial deltoid and the calcaneofibular ligaments. For practical considerations in the patient with flatfoot, the deep deltoid ligament (posteromedial deltoid) and the spring ligament require assessment.

If the ligaments are deemed intact and the ankle mortise is congruent on preoperative weight-bearing radiographs, then a rebalancing (without reconstruction) is often adequate. Integrity of the ligaments needs to be confirmed intraoperatively. One technique to assess is use of a larger polyethylene insert to tension the deltoid.[14,15] The clinical decision making is that if there is greater than 10° of valgus at the ankle with stress, then an extra-articular deltoid ligament reconstruction is indicated.

In a 2019 respective series of 80 patients who have undergone total ankle arthroplasty in the setting of severe valgus deformity, with a mean follow-up of 3.5 years, the study authors were able to correct the valgus from an average of 15° to a mean of 1.2°, which was maintained at final follow-up.[16]

Syndesmosis Insufficiency

Occasionally, syndesmotic widening is found in longterm flatfoot deformity. After complete reconstruction, stress radiographs should be obtained to assess its stability and potential need for repair. This is most common in previous ankle fractures with a malunion of the fibula or previous syndesmotic repair.[16]

Fixed Forefoot Varus

Ankle arthroplasty following triple arthrodesis violates the orthopaedic principle of working proximal to distal. The challenge after triple arthrodesis is that the motion segment of the total ankle is poorly tolerant of hindfoot fusion malposition. Specifically, fixed forefoot varus, from a malpositioned triple arthrodesis, will drive the ankle arthroplasty to valgus through deltoid attrition. This biomechanics effect is not always obvious when assessing the patient for total ankle arthroplasty but an intraoperative double-check of foot position before total ankle arthroplasty cuts is critical. It is recommended that the malunion be addressed with an osteotomy through the transverse tarsal joint with proper positioning of the hindfoot fusion underneath the total ankle arthroplasty. A malpositioned hindfoot can be corrected either by compensatory total ankle cuts or by a displacement calcaneal osteotomy. Takedown of a hindfoot fusion is not advised.

Flatfoot Issues (Valgus)

Pes planovalgus deformity is not an uncommon condition in the setting of revision total ankle arthroplasty. The etiology could be progressive, from conditions such as posterior tibial tendon failure after total ankle arthroplasty, or preexisting and unrecognized hindfoot deformity. In either condition, a revision surgeon should be prepared to address flatfoot deformity to preserve the best possible outcomes with revision total ankle arthroplasty.

As mentioned in previous sections, simultaneous versus staged reconstruction needs to be considered. Both are represented in a 2021 study.[17] However, in the valgus ankle revision, residual instability can be seen not only medially as expected, but also laterally. Thus, staging with the aforementioned temporary cement spacer technique gives the ankle capsule time to stabilize as the foot reconstruction heals in the setting of global ankle instability.[17]

There is anecdotal evidence regarding concerns about osteonecrosis with simultaneous retrograde talonavicular arthrodesis and total ankle arthroplasty. The

Section 8: Contemporary Surgical Techniques

combination of multisided surgery on the talus might put the blood flow to the talar body at risk.[18] These maneuvers are certainly not forbidden, but an awareness of the fragility of the blood flow to the talar body is necessary.

As with the varus deformity, the chief decision point for the foot reconstruction is whether the foot deformity is flexible (correctable) or rigid. In flexible deformities, a medial displacement calcaneal osteotomy can be performed to improve the position of the heel on weight bearing. This may have to also be augmented with a spring ligament reconstruction, or flexor digitorum longus transfer in cases of posterior tibial tendon dysfunction. In cases of rigid deformity, a subtalar joint arthrodesis is indicated.

Midfoot and forefoot stability also need to be addressed because residual forefoot varus will negate the effect of hindfoot realignment. This is often accomplished with a Cotton (plantar flexion) osteotomy, as long as the medial column joints are stable.[4] In a 2019 study on total ankle arthroplasty in patients with valgus deformity, correction was maintained at 3.5 years when following this methodology.[16]

Recurvatum

Recurvatum positioning of a primary total ankle arthroplasty results in contracture of the posterior musculature and soft tissues.[5] Awareness of the negative effect of recurvatum is paramount in planning and executing a proper revision. Adjuvant procedures of posterior capsular release and lengthening of the gastrocnemius-soleus muscle or Achilles tendon often are warranted.

The usual deformity encountered in this revision is a dorsiflexed tibial component. Most commonly the revision of the tibial component will require elevating the joint line. Joint line management is discussed later.

The other common deformity seen in this scenario is the anteriorly translated talar component. Revision of the talar component should focus on restoring the center of rotation of the ankle joint. This is done by identification of the tibial axis in the sagittal view, and lining that up with the peak of the arc of the dome of the talar component.[18,19] Accurate talar component position is an independent factor to survivorship of the ankle arthroplasty.[20]

Procurvatum

Procurvatum is an unusual presentation for revision. It occurs as a result of Achilles tendon contracture and posterior polyethylene wear. During revision, care should be taken to release the contracture and repositioning of the tibial component to neutral. The joint line will have to sit in accordance with the height of the posterior tibia available. As with recurvatum deformity, talar component position is important, and care needs to be taken

to set the talar component accurately in the anterior-posterior direction.[5]

Axial Rotation Malpositioning

Understanding axial malalignment and component malpositioning has been investigated in recent years. The popularization of patient-specific instrumentation and wider use of weight-bearing CT are the sources for this investigative boom. According to a 2020 study, it could be that axial malpositioning is far more common than previously thought.[21]

In a 2019 study of 157 total ankle arthroplasties guided by patient-specific navigation, some trends have emerged to give the revision surgeon more understanding of axial alignment. First, the external alignment jigs that rely on the tibial tubercle are subject to variability of 1.0° to 44.6°. Second, the foot position at the time of alignment tended to always be internally rotated in this series (0.7° to 38.4°). Third, when using the medial gutter versus both gutters for alignment of the talar component, there was a small amount of persistent rotation (3° to 5°). When this third trend was accounted for and corrected, medial gutter pain due to impingement was reduced more than threefold.[22] Knowing these facts about axial position can help the revision surgeon decide on full repositioning or simple additional gutter débridement.

COMPONENT FAILURE

Aseptic Loosening

Aseptic loosening is the loss of the bone-to-implant stability in the absence of infection. The major contributing factors to aseptic loosening include component migration, component undersizing (**Figure 1**), osteonecrosis, malalignment (previously discussed), and osteolysis. Osteolysis is a special consideration that is covered later. In the absence of any signs of infection, a previously well-aligned and stable implant should be evaluated for loosening if the patient begins to experience pain.[23]

Most ankle arthroplasties performed in the lower extremity ultimately depend on bone ingrowth/ongrowth to the implant. This physiologic process takes time, and therefore some component migration in the early days after implantation is expected.[22] The question of "how much is too much?" is still unknown; therefore, any measurable migration demands close observation.[24]

The components of ankle arthroplasty should have as much surface area contact as possible, and extend out to the cortical rim. This lesson was learned from experience with a first-generation implant. This implant would cover only approximately 30% of the cut talar surface,

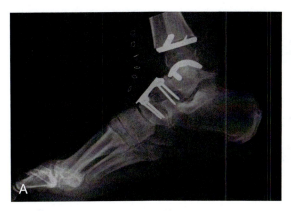 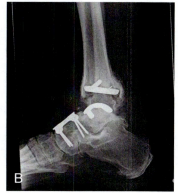 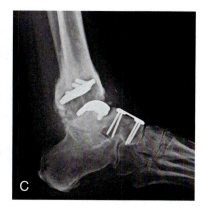

FIGURE 1 Series of lateral radiographs from immediately postoperatively to 1 year showing anterior subsidence related to inadequate coverage of the anterior tibia (CADENCE, Smith & Nephew). **A**, Immediately postoperatively with original position. **B**, Collapse of tibia into dorsiflexion at 7 months. **C**, Final position that the implant settled into at 1 year postoperatively.

and thus the incidence of subsidence was high.[25] Current fourth-generation implants are designed with the key parameters in mind: cortical contact on the tibia, full coverage of the talus, and no domed or capped design of the talus (**Figure 1**).

Modern ankle arthroplasty revision systems also accept these same tenets as key. Other unique features of modern revision systems include taking advantage of the harder bone of the talar neck by featuring extensions of the talar component that extend anteriorly.

When considering tibial placement, especially in the revision scenario, according to a 2020 study it should be noted that the tibial bone becomes significantly weaker at greater than 1 cm above the joint line.[26] Therefore, the revision surgeon needs to be aware of this fact and plan for additional methods of stability such as augments, stems, and cement.

Restoration of the joint line is something the revision surgeon should always take into account because subsidence is the most common cause of total ankle arthroplasty failure.[27] Failure to restore the joint line is likely to alter the kinematics of the ankle, appearing most noticeably as decreased range of motion.

Management of Subsidence
Tibia

As with most topics pertaining to revision ankle arthroplasty, there is scant literature support to guide the revision of the tibial component. Tibial bone loss at the time of revision can often be dramatic. The amount of bone removed for the placement of the primary implant does not correlate well with the residual defect upon removal, given the presence of cysts and any porous ingrowth often removes more of the metaphysis than the implant alone. A surgeon must assess and be prepared to reconstruct the joint line, malleoli, and metaphyseal plafond because these anatomic factors serve as the structural representation of the joint stability and ongrowth capabilities of the revised ankle.

Implant stability is paramount and can be achieved with intramedullary fixation, metaphyseal augments, cortical loading, and impaction grafting. The goal is to achieve a stable platform to transmit forces to the tibial bone.

Malleoli are attachment points for ligamentous structures needed for ankle joint stability. These may be affected by osteolysis. However, if impaction grafting is not possible, custom malleolar replacement may be used. These are obtained through preoperative three-dimensional imaging, sometimes of the opposite limb.

Prophylactic fixation of the medial malleolus is the rule rather than the exception. The prophylactic fixation should be added before removal of the primary implant to preserve the anatomic relationship if the malleoli were to fracture (**Figure 2**).

Tibial component subsidence can occur in the early postoperative period.[28,29] A surgeon must take care not to violate the anterior tibial cortex at any time of the surgery, particularly during tibial implantation. Conversion to a stemmed tibial implant is often required in this instance (**Figure 3**).

Finally, if the joint line needs further adjustment, or ankle stability is still not achieved, then additional polyethylene thickness or augmented tibial base plates can be used. A general principle is that the distal end of the polyethylene insert should match the native distal tibia. Knowledge of some standard bony landmarks such as the posterior colliculus of the medial malleolus and the distal tip of the lateral malleolus is helpful in re-creating the proper joint height.[28,29]

A comprehensive total ankle revision system will include stemmed tibial components, different thickness of tibial base plates, and a wide variety of polyethylene inserts. Adjunct equipment should include vertical

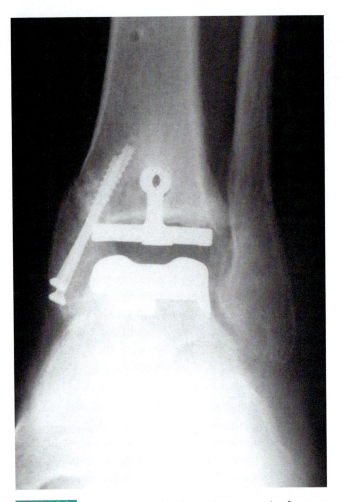

FIGURE 2 AP radiograph showing an intraoperative fracture during insertion of the Salto Talaris implant (Smith & Nephew) subsequent open reduction and internal fixation of the medial malleolus with healing.

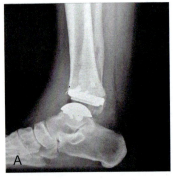 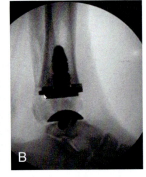

FIGURE 3 Lateral radiographs showing conversion to a stemmed tibial implant. **A**, Tibial subsidence of the INFINITY total ankle prosthesis (Stryker) at 3 months postoperatively. **B**, Revision to a stemmed implant.

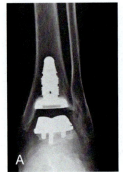 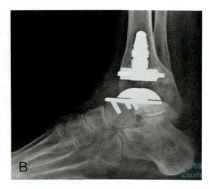

FIGURE 4 AP view of revision components featuring a stemmed tibia (INBONE II [Stryker]) (**A**) and lateral view showing broad revision talus (INVISION [Stryker]) (**B**).

cannulated screws and/or plates for prophylactic fixation of the medial malleolus (**Figure 4**).

Talus

Talus subsidence can easily escalate to a highly complex situation because of the adjacent subtalar joint. The Berlet et al talar defect classification system (**Table 2**) assists the surgeon in determining appropriate bone stock for implant stability.[27]

There are three major surgical techniques described to assist in the reconstruction of the talus damaged by subsidence. The first technique is the revision systems designed with talar neck support (Stryker Invision). By spanning over the neck of the talus, the bone is often stronger, and theoretically less vulnerable to subsidence. The second technique is a re-bar technique using large cannulated screws in the subtalar joint as reinforcement to prevent collapse and support the revision talar component.[26] The third technique has been the development of a three-dimensionally printed total talus component. The total talus has been reported to show promising outcomes when used in the primary setting. This implant uses an articulating tibiotalar and talonavicular joint with the option of a subtalar fusion to the implant.[30]

Special Failures

Joint Sepsis

Obviously a prosthetic joint infection is a devastating complication. However, at the ankle, this can become limb-threatening rather quickly. Therefore, a heightened sense of alertness should always be present because quick diagnosis and treatment can be the difference in success or failure to salvage the implant.

Acute infections, less than 3 weeks in duration, can be managed by surgical irrigation, débridement, polyethylene insert exchange, and a course of culture-specific

Chapter 29: Revision Total Ankle Arthroplasty

Table 2

Berlet et al Talar Defect Classification System

Classification	Subclassification	Description
A		Central defect (no cortical breach in any axial direction)
	A1	Small (<12 mm in greatest diameter in primary cyst or additively if polycystic disease is present)
	A2	Large (>12 mm in greatest diameter in primary cyst or additively if polycystic disease is present)
B		Peripheral defect (cortical breach in any axial direction)
	B1	1 of 4 quadrants (primary cyst or polycystic)
	B2	2 of 4 quadrants (not necessarily contiguous) (primary cyst or polycystic)
	B3	3 of 4 quadrants (primary cyst or polycystic)
	B4	4 of 4 quadrants (primary cyst or polycystic)
C	—	Subtalar breach (posterior facet)
F	—	Fractured talus (or otherwise failed bony integrity—not amenable to component revision)

Reproduced from Berlet GC, Penner MJ, Prissel MA, Butterwick DR: CT-based descriptive classification for residual talar defects associated with failed total ankle replacement: Technique tip. *Foot Ankle Int* 2018;39(5):568-572.

intravenous antibiotic therapy. This follows the established guidelines seen in total knee arthroplasty. For infections lasting longer than 3 weeks, a two-staged procedure should be considered. The first stage is a total explantation of the prothesis and implantation of an antibiotic-loaded cement spacer, followed by a period of culture-specific intravenous antibiotic therapy. A novel technique for forming the antibiotic-loaded spacer as an articulation spacer has been described in a 2020 study, and uses a surgical measuring cup.[31] These spacers have been shown to improve range of motion and to decrease length of hospital stays in the total knee arthroplasty literature.[32] The second stage is reimplantation of a total ankle arthroplasty prosthesis. However, not all patients have the physiologic capability of the final conversion. Therefore, long-term use of the articulating antibiotic-loaded spacer can be considered because it has been successful in limb salvage for more than 77% of patients in one series.[33]

Periprosthetic Fracture

Periprosthetic fracture is a complication most commonly encountered intraoperatively, but can be seen postoperatively as well. The incidence of intraoperative fracture is low (<2%).[33] This complication is best treated by identifying those patients at risk for fracture. In a retrospective study of 198 total ankle arthroplasty cases with periprosthetic fracture, preoperative CT was analyzed for osteopenia and osteoporosis.[34] Using the Hounsfield units on CT, a threshold for intraoperative or postoperative fracture was identified as less than 200 HU. In patients with a perceived risk of postoperative fracture due to osteopenia, studies from 2019 and 2021 demonstrate that consideration should be given to pretreatment with diphosphonates or prophylactic fixation of the compromised bone.[34,35]

Most periprosthetic fractures in total ankle arthroplasty occur in the medial malleolus. It is generally accepted that all periprosthetic ankle fractures be treated surgically. This is despite previous classification schemes at the ankle, and at other joints, that use implant stability as a factor in analysis. Ultimately, implant stability and nonunion risks are deemed too high to ignore as there is a correlation with the need for revision; thus, the universal recommendation is to surgically stabilize all periprosthetic ankle joint fractures.[33]

Despite the universal recommendation to treat all periprosthetic ankle fractures surgically, it is still necessary to identify the causes and risk factors that contributed to these complications. Rectifying the underlying or associated factors will ultimately lead to better patient-reported outcomes and function, such as implant malpositioning. For example, failure to reposition a varus-placed total ankle implant at the time of periprosthetic fracture fixation is associated with a decrease in American Orthopaedic Foot and Ankle Society scores, 67.3 for uncorrected position implants versus 87.6 for the corrected position implants.[36]

Other common implant position cases and risk factors to be considered as risk factors for fracture are tibial component varus, tibial component varus, talar component oversizing, hindfoot malalignment, and forefoot malalignment. Each of these positions places the ankle at risk for fracture of the medial malleolus. Osteoporosis and unrecognized intraoperative injury to the medial malleolus also are risk factors that contribute to intraoperative and postoperative medial malleolar fractures.[37]

A common practice of total ankle surgeons is prophylactic fixation of the medial malleolus. This has been derived from study of a cohort of Scandinavian Total Ankle Replacement, or STAR (Enovis) total ankle arthroplasties. In this cohort, persistent medial pain without fracture was addressed postoperatively with medial malleolar screw fixation. This resolved the pain in 60% of patients. In addition, it was found that the medial malleolus thickness in patients with pain (before the screw fixation) was 10.2 mm. A control group, not reporting medial pain, was found to have a medial malleolar thickness of greater than 12 mm.[33] Currently there is a trend toward screw prophylaxis of the medial malleolus in ankles where the thickness of the medial malleolus is at 10 mm or less.[38] Fixation options include metal screws or biocomposite screws, which can be reamed or cut if they interfere with implant positioning.

Osteolysis and Periprosthetic Cysts

Periprosthetic osteolysis and cyst formation are a poorly understood phenomena in total ankle arthroplasty. It is believed that the cause of cyst formation is not always associated with polyethylene wear, so qualifying polyethylene disease from cyst formation is important. It is suspected that some osteolysis occurs as a result of polyethylene particulate debris phagocytosis, stress shielding, and possibly fluid dynamics. Therefore, the formation of cysts may be associated with implant design and wear characteristics, or can be associated with the patient's bone quality or physiologic response.[39] Furthermore, unless preoperative CT was performed, some of the cysts may have been present preoperatively.[40]

Most arthroplasty surgeons perform annual, long-term surveillance of their joint replacements by clinical and radiographic observation. Any report of pain, or radiographic change in the implant position (including subsidence or loosening) should heighten the evaluation to advanced imaging such as single photon emission computed tomography (SPECT) or weight-bearing CT (**Figure 5**).

The osteolysis and cysts are most common immediately adjacent to the implant, in the cancellous bone. This limits visualization by direct obscurity from the implant, and indirect obscurity within the already radiolucent cancellous bone. Therefore, at the very least, CT should be considered whenever a cyst is suspected.[41] CT can provide characteristics of exact cyst location, size/volume, cortical breach, and progression (when done serially over time), all of which can help the surgeon decide whether to intervene.

Loosening can be evaluated with preoperative SPECT. As described in a 2020 study, the positive SPECT examination is closely correlated with implant loosening.[42] In this scenario with a cyst adjacent to a positive SPECT, revision should be considered.

Deciding when to intervene remains controversial. Certainly, pain directly associated with a cyst needs to be treated. Cysts that compromise the implant stability, evident by position change or subsidence, should also be treated. Serial CT should be performed every 6 months once cysts are identified larger than 1 cm at their widest dimension. Intervention for the cysts is recommended with the onset of symptoms, migration of the total ankle arthroplasty implants, or cortical erosion (**Figure 6**).

The final decision in the observation of osteolysis and cysts is whether revision arthroplasty or cyst débridement and grafting is most appropriate. In general, cysts causing implant stability compromise (ie, loosening, position

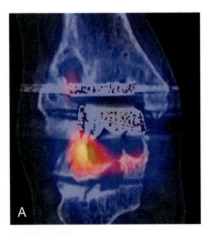
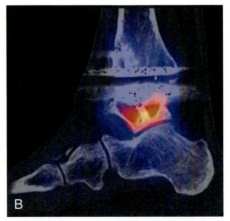
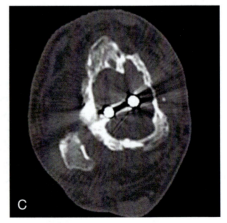

FIGURE 5 Images showing extensive osteolysis in the tibia and talus. **A** and **B**, Single-photon emission CT. **C**, CT.

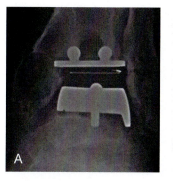 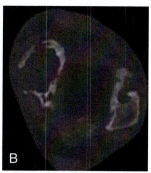 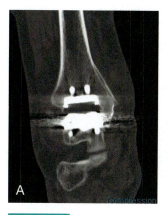 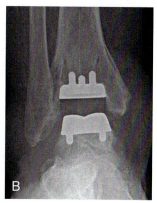

FIGURE 6 STAR ankle implant (Stryker) at 10 years with massive osteolysis of tibia with pending pathologic fracture. **A**, AP radiograph showing cysts. **B**, CT image showing pending pathologic fracture of tibia.

FIGURE 7 The talus is too large, creating impingement on malleoli. With revision, upsized polyethylene insert, and gutter débridement, the patient's symptoms were resolved. **A**, Coronal CT scan showing an oversized talus component creating impingement between talus and the ankle gutters, resulting in pain. **B**, AP radiograph showing revision of the talus component with downsizing of the talus and gutter débridement.

change, or subsidence) need to be addressed with revision arthroplasty and defect management. Cysts that are large (>1 cm) and progressive but still associated with a stable implant can be treated with polyethylene exchange and impaction grafting of cancellous allograft or autologous bone graft. Bone graft substitute such as demineralized bone matrix can be added to the mixture as well.[43]

Grafting of cysts and osteolysis is an understudied topic. But now with the abundance of total ankle arthroplasty procedures performed yearly, and many implants maturing beyond 10 years' survivorship, hopefully more research will be pursued. One study reported 27 patients who underwent grafting without revision of the implants. More than 90% had the cysts healed without recurrence at 24 months. This decreased to 60.6% at 48 months.[44]

Heterotopic Ossification

Heterotopic ossification is common in total ankle arthroplasty, with some studies estimating its asymptomatic presence at greater than 50%. In the setting of a stiff and painful total ankle, the workup should include SPECT. If there is positive signal about the heterotopic ossification, heterotopic ossification excision through either an anterior or combined anterior and posterior approach should be considered.[17,45]

Postimplant Gutter Impingement

The most common reason for repeat surgical procedures in the first 5 years of a total ankle arthroplasty is gutter pain. This pain can be generated from impingement of osteophytes, oversized talus implant, or malposition/malrotation of the talus component (**Figure 7**).

The workup includes axial CT to check on the bone-to-implant ratio and SPECT to compare patient symptoms with signal on the scan.

In the setting where the implant is appropriately sized and with neutral rotation with respect to the tibial component, a simple gutter débridement may suffice. It is preferable to take more of the bone from the talus side as opposed to the fibular or tibial sides in this procedure to avoid compromising the malleoli or the ligament attachments.

In the setting of gutter impingement with concern for malrotation or an oversized talar component, the best approach is often to revise the talus down one size if the system allows, débridement of the gutters, and removal of the heterotopic ossification.[46]

REVISION SYSTEMS

A functional revision system must have several key features:
- A mechanism for proximal tibial fixation of the revision tibial component
- A mechanism to handle bone defects left from prior implant failure on both the tibia and the talus
- A mechanism to emphasize peripheral loading of the revision implant
- A mechanism to guide alignment because the normal anatomic features are likely disrupted from the failed primary implant

SUMMARY

Total ankle arthroplasty has evolved to be the preferred option for ankle arthritis in many cases. The tipping point for the increased adoption is likely the creation of viable revision options in the event of arthroplasty failure. It is important to explore analysis of a failed total ankle arthroplasty, techniques for salvage, and revision options and techniques.

KEY STUDY POINTS

- All revisions must start with a plausible theory of why the other implant failed so that this may be addressed with technique and implant selection.
- A well-placed ankle arthroplasty situated over a malaligned foot will not enjoy long-term success. Various strategies can be employed incorporating either staged or combined foot reconstructions.
- Not all implant designs are appropriate for revisions. Peg tibial designs, although excellent for primary total ankle arthroplasty, are generally inappropriate for revision situations. Tibial fixation is paramount and this usually requires a stemmed tibial design.
- Large defects of the talus with inadequate support of the revision talus component are doomed to fail. It is generally recognized that the talus implant must be supported by three of the four talus cortices. Subtalar joint fusion is often used as an adjuvant to revision talus arthroplasty.
- Wound healing is a big challenge in revision ankle arthroplasty. Although not the subject of this chapter, preoperative vascular testing is recommended. Intraoperative careful handling of the soft tissues by avoiding the use of self-retaining retractors and limiting the use of long tourniquet time is recommended.
- Revision ankle arthroplasty will present the surgeon with many decisions to be made intraoperatively. These decisions are best made when based on solid experience with primary total ankle arthroplasty and strong grasp of the principles of total ankle arthroplasty.

ANNOTATED REFERENCES

1. SooHoo NF, Zingmond DS, Ko CY: Comparison of reoperation rates following ankle arthrodesis and total ankle arthroplasty. *J Bone Joint Surg Am* 2007;89(10):2143-2149.

2. Pedowitz DI, Kane JM, Smith GM, Saffel HL, Comer C, Raikin SM: Total ankle arthroplasty versus ankle arthrodesis: A comparative analysis of arc of movement and functional outcomes. *Bone Joint J* 2016;98-B(5):634-640.

3. Wood PLR, Prem H, Sutton C: Total ankle replacement: Medium-term results in 200 Scandinavian total ankle replacements. *J Bone Joint Surg Br* 2008;90(5):605-609.

4. Consul DW, Chu A, Langan TM, Hyer CF, Berlet GC: Total ankle arthroplasty survivorship, complication, and revision rates in patients younger than 55 years. *Foot Ankle Spec* 2022;15(3):283-290.

   This is a review of patient outcomes, complications, and implant survival in patients younger than 55 years who underwent total ankle arthroplasty at a single institution. Implant

survival was 94%, and the authors concluded that total ankle arthroplasty was safe in patients younger than 55 years. Level of evidence: III.

5. Gauvain TT, Hames MA, McGarvey WC: Malalignment correction of the lower limb before, during and after total ankle arthroplasty. *Foot Ankle Clin* 2017;22(2):311-339.

6. Tarr RR, Resnick CT, Wagner KS, Sarmiento A: Changes in tibiotalar joint contact areas following experimentally induced tibial angular deformities. *Clin Orthop Relat Res* 1985;199:72-80.

7. Deforth M, Krahenbuhl N, Zwicky L, Knupp M, Hintermann B: Supramalleolar osteotomy for tibial component malposition in total ankle replacement. *Foot Ankle Int* 2017;38(9):952-956.

8. Kim BS, Choi WJ, Kim YS, Lee JW: Total ankle replacement in moderate to severe varus deformity of the ankle. *J Bone Joint Surg Br* 2009;91(9):1183-1190.

9. Steginsky B, Haddad SL: Two-stage varus correction. *Foot Ankle Clin* 2019;24(2):281-304.

   Correction of varus malalignment may be performed at the time of total ankle arthroplasty or as a two-stage procedure. Level of evidence: V.

10. Doets HC, Van Der Plaat LW, Klein JP: Medial malleolar osteotomy for the correction of varus deformity during total ankle arthroplasty: Results in 15 ankles. *Foot Ankle Int* 2008;29(2):171-177.

11. Rushing CJ, McKenna BJ, Berlet GC: Lateral instability in total ankle arthroplasty: A comparison between Brostrom-Gould and anatomic lateral ankle stabilization (ATLAS). *Foot Ankle Spec* 2021; [Epub ahead of print].

    The purpose of this study was to compare outcomes between techniques for addressing ankle instability in the total ankle arthroplasty population. At short-term follow-up, anatomic reconstruction produced better outcomes than the traditional Broström-Gould procedure. Level of evidence: III.

12. Sung KS, Ahn J, Lee KH, Chun TH: Short-term results of total ankle arthroplasty for end-stage ankle arthritis with severe varus deformity. *Foot Ankle Int* 2014;35(3):225-231.

13. Trajkovski T, Pinsker E, Cadden A, Daniels TR: Outcomes of ankle arthroplasty with preoperative coronal-plane varus deformity of 10° or greater. *J Bone Joint Surg Am* 2013;95(15):1382-1388.

14. Gauvain TT, Hames MA, McGarvey WC: Malalignment correction of the lower limb before, during, and after total ankle arthroplasty. *Foot Ankle Clin* 2017;22(2):311-339.

15. Dodd A, Daniels TR: Total ankle replacement in the presence of talar varus or valgus deformities. *Foot Ankle Clin* 2017;22(2):277-300.

16. Demetracopoulos CA, Cody EA, Adams SB, DeOrio JK, Nunley JA, Easley ME: Outcomes of total ankle arthroplasty in moderate and severe valgus deformity. *Foot Ankle Spec* 2019;12(3):238-245.

    Patients with a valgus deformity of at least 10° who underwent total ankle arthroplasty were retrospectively reviewed.

Mean preoperative valgus deformity was 15.5° ± 5.0° and was corrected to a mean of 1.2° ± 2.6° of valgus postoperatively. Correction of coronal alignment was achieved and maintained in patients with both moderate and severe preoperative valgus malalignment. Level of evidence: IV.

17. Ebaugh MP, McGarvey WC, Penner MJ, Berlet GC: Revision total ankle arthroplasty, in Roukis T, Hyer C, Berlet GC, Bibbo C, Penner MJ, eds: *Primary and Revision Total Ankle Arthroplasty*, ed 2. Springer, 2021, pp 421-446.

   General principles of revision ankle arthroplasty were reviewed, with considerations for workup and analysis of contributing factors. Specific case discussions on workout and revision principles were conducted.

18. Younger A, Veljkovic A: Current update in total ankle arthroplasty: Salvage of the failed total ankle arthroplasty with anterior translation of the talus. *Foot Ankle Clin* 2017;22(2):301-309.

19. Veljkovic A, Norton A, Salat P, et al: Lateral talar station: A clinically reproducible measure of sagittal talar position. *Foot Ankle Int* 2013;34(12):1669-1676.

20. Escudero MI, Le V, Barahona M, et al: Total ankle arthroplasty survival and risk factors for failure. *Foot Ankle Int* 2019;40(9):997-1006.

   A predictive model was created, with four parameters identified as being statistically associated with total ankle arthroplasty metal-component revision: diabetes mellitus, poor baseline Ankle Osteoarthritis Scale score, excessively dorsiflexed talar component, and an anteriorly/posteriorly translated talus relative to the tibial axis. The presence of three parameters predicted total ankle arthroplasty survival of 0.60, whereas the presence of all four parameters predicted survival of only 0.13 in the period studied. Level of evidence: III.

21. Hintermann B, Susdorf R, Krahenbuhl N, Ruiz R: Axial rotational alignment in mobile-bearing total ankle arthroplasty. *Foot Ankle Int* 2020;41(5):521-528.

   The relative axial rotation between the talar and the tibial component was measured intraoperatively in a cohort of 58 patients who underwent mobile-bearing total ankle arthroplasty. There is a wide range of relative axial rotation between the tibial and talar component, which suggests that it is crucial to allow the talus to intraoperatively find a position that corresponds to the patient's individual anatomy. Level of evidence: III.

22. Najefi AA, Ghani Y, Goldberg A: Role of rotation in total ankle replacement. *Foot Ankle Int* 2019;40(12):1358-1367.

   There was a large variation in rotational profile of patients undergoing total ankle arthroplasty, particularly between the medial gutter line and the transmalleolar axis. Level of evidence: II.

23. Harnroongroj T, Hummel A, Ellis SJ, et al: Assessing the ankle joint line level before and after total ankle arthroplasty with the "joint line height ratio". *Foot Ankle Orthop* 2019;4(4):2473011419884359.

   The effect of joint line level on patient outcomes after total ankle arthroplasty was explored. The ratio of vertical intermalleolar distance to vertical joint line distance was defined as the joint line height ratio. The joint line height ratio was reliable and could be a clinically applicable method for assessing ankle joint line level in patients undergoing total ankle arthroplasty. Level of evidence: III.

24. Dunbar MJ, Fong JW, Wilson DA, Hennigar AW, Francis PA, Glazebrook MA: Longitudinal migration and inducible displacement of the mobility total ankle system. *Acta Orthop* 2012;83(4):394-400.

25. Hurowitz EJ, Gould JS, Fleisig GS, Fowler R: Outcome analysis of agility total ankle replacement with prior adjunctive procedures: Two to six year follow-up. *Foot Ankle Int* 2007;28(3):308-312.

26. Steginsky B, Haddad SL: *Revision Surgery of the Foot and Ankle*. Springer International Publisher, 2020, pp 335-359.

   The management of bone loss and alteration in the ankle joint center of rotation is challenging following component subsidence in total ankle arthroplasty. The authors discuss implant technology and surgical techniques in revision arthroplasty.

27. Haddad SL, Coetzee JC, Estok R, Fahrbach K, Banel D, Nalysnyk L: Intermediate and long-term outcomes of total ankle arthroplasty and ankle arthrodesis: A systemic review of the literature. *J Bone Joint Surg Am* 2007;89(9):1899-1905.

28. Cody EA, Taylor MA, Nunley JA, Parekh SG, DeOrio JK: Increased early revision rate with the INFINITY total ankle prosthesis. *Foot Ankle Int* 2019;40(1):9-17.

   A retrospective study showed a 10% revision rate of the INFINITY prosthesis at 1- to 2-year follow-up. Most common reason for revision was deep infection and tibial component loosening. Level of evidence: IV.

29. Berlet GC, Penner MJ, Prissel MA, Butterwick DR: CT-based descriptive classification for residual talar defects associated with failed total ankle replacement: Technique tip. *Foot Ankle Int* 2018;39(5):568-572.

30. Kanzaki N, Chinzei N, Yamamoto T, Yamashita T, Ibaraki K, Kuroda R: Clinical outcomes of total ankle arthroplasty with total talar prosthesis. *Foot Ankle Int* 2019;40(8):948-954.

   This study aimed to explore the short-term results and complications of total ankle arthroplasty with total talar prosthesis. The authors concluded that combined total ankle arthroplasty was a reliable procedure not only for the management of ankle osteoarthritis following avascular necrosis of talus but also of degeneration of both ankle and subtalar joints. Level of evidence: IV.

31. Short A, Penrose C, Adams S: A novel technique for creating an articulating cement spacer for ankle prosthetic joint infections. *J Foot Ankle Surg* 2020;59(1):216-219.

   The authors describe a technique for creating an articulating antibiotic cement spacer through an anterior approach in a patient with an infected total ankle arthroplasty. Level of evidence: V.

32. Nahhas CR, Chalmers PN, Parvizi J, et al: A randomized trial of static and articulating spacers for the treatment of infection following total knee arthroplasty. *J Bone Joint Surg Am* 2020;102(9):778-787.

The purpose of this multicenter, randomized clinical trial was to compare static and articulating spacers as part of the two-stage exchange arthroplasty for the management of chronic total knee periprosthetic joint infection. When the soft-tissue envelope allows and if there is adequate osseous support, an articulating spacer is associated with improved outcomes. Level of evidence: I.

33. Lazarides AL, Vovos TJ, Reddy GB, et al: Algorithm for management of periprosthetic ankle fractures. *Foot Ankle Int* 2019;40(6):615-621.

    The authors describe an algorithm for the management of postoperative periprosthetic fractures about a total ankle arthroplasty. Level of evidence: III.

34. Cody EA, Lachman JR, Gausden EB, Nunley JA, Easley ME: Lower bone density on preoperative computed tomography predicts periprosthetic fracture risk in total ankle arthroplasty. *Foot Ankle Int* 2019;40(1):1-8.

    Lower tibial Hounsfield units on preoperative CT was strongly associated with periprosthetic fracture risk with total ankle arthroplasty. In patients with tibial Hounsfield units less than 200, surgeons may consider prophylactic internal fixation of the medial malleolus. Level of evidence: III.

35. So E, Rushing CJ, Prissel MA, Berlet GC: Bone mineral density testing in patients undergoing total ankle arthroplasty: Should we pay more attention to bone quality. *J Foot Ankle Surg* 2021;60(2):224-227.

    A systematic review on bone mineral density and total ankle arthroplasty concluded that much of the focus in total ankle arthroplasty has emphasized implants and relatively little has focused on the quality of bone into which the prostheses are implanted. Level of evidence: III.

36. Tsitsilonis S, Schaser KD, Wichlas F, Haas NP, Manegold S: Functional and radiological outcome of periprosthetic fractures of the ankle. *Bone Joint J* 2015;97-B(7):950-956.

37. Manegold S, Haas NP, Tsitsilonis S, Springer A, Mardian S, Schaser KD: Periprosthetic fractures in total ankle replacement: Classification system and treatment algorithm. *J Bone Joint Surg Am* 2013;95(9):815-820, S1-S3.

38. Lundeen GA, Dunaway LJ: Etiology and treatment of delayed onset medial malleolar pain following total ankle arthroplasty. *Foot Ankle Int* 2016;37(8):822-828.

39. Schipper ON, Haddad SL, Pytel P, Zhou Y: Histological analysis of early osteolysis in total ankle arthroplasty. *Foot Ankle Int* 2017;38(4):351-359.

40. Ali-Asgar N, Ghani Y, Goldberg AJ: Bone cysts and osteolysis in ankle replacement. *Foot Ankle Int* 2021;42(1):55-61.

    Bone cysts outside of the resection margins for a total ankle arthroplasty were present in 78% of patients with ankle arthritis before undergoing surgery. In 30% of cases, cysts were greater than 5 mm in size. In 60% of cases, the cysts were not seen on plain radiographs. Level of evidence: II.

41. Yoon HS, Lee J, Choi WJ, Lee JW: Periprosthetic osteolysis after total ankle arthroplasty. *Foot Ankle Int* 2014;35(1):14-21.

42. Gurbani A, Demetracopoulos C, O'Malley M, et al: Correlation of single-photon emission computed tomography results with clinical and intraoperative findings in painful total ankle replacement. *Foot Ankle Int* 2020;41(6):639-646.

    SPECT-CT also demonstrated high consistency with intraoperative findings during revision surgery. Compared with MRI, SPECT-CT proved more useful in establishing a diagnosis of pain after total ankle arthroplasty. Level of evidence: III.

43. Jonck JH, Myerson MS: Revision total ankle replacement. *Foot Ankle Clin* 2012;17(4):687-706.

44. Gross CE, Huh J, Green C, et al: Outcomes of bone grafting of bone cysts after total ankle arthroplasty. *Foot Ankle Int* 2016;37(2):157-164.

45. Rushing CJ, Steriovski J, Hyer CF, Berlet GC: Heterotopic ossification following total ankle arthroplasty with fourth generation prostheses. *Foot Ankle Spec* 2022;15(5):448-455.

    The study reports a similarly high incidence of heterotopic ossification after total ankle arthroplasty with two different fourth-generation prostheses (INFINITY 56.5%, CADENCE 53.6%) with a trend to differences in geographic location. Level of evidence: III.

46. Gross CE, Adams SB, Easley M, Nunley JA, DeOrio JK: Surgical treatment of bony and soft tissue impingement in total ankle arthroplasty. *Foot Ankle Spec* 2017;10(1):37-42.

Index

Note: Page numbers followed by 'f' indicate figures and 't' indicate tables

A

AAFD. *See* Adult-acquired flatfoot deformity
Accessory navicular
    classification of, 37, 38f
    clinical findings, 37–38, 38f
    nonsurgical treatment, 38
    radiographic evaluation, 38, 39f
    surgical treatment, 38–39, 39f
Acetabulum pedis, 4, 5f
Achilles tendinopathy, 365–367, 367f
Achilles tendinosis, 365–366
Achilles tendon, 8, 168, 361
    contracture, 54
    diabetic foot ulcer, 71
    disorders of, 361–367
    dorsiflexion, 57
    grafting, 373
    injury, 32
    lengthening, 56–57, 75, 139, 354
    physical examination, 367
    ruptures, 367
        acute, 361–364, 362f–363f
        chronic, 364–365, 365f
        treatment, 362
    stretching programs, 239
    tendoscopy, 412–413
    Z-shaped tenotomy of, 124
ACI. *See* Autologous chondrocyte implantation (ACI)
Acral myxoinflammatory fibroblastic sarcoma, 255–256, 257f
Acute lateral ankle sprain
    classification, 387–388
    patient history, 386
    physical examination, 386
    radiographic evaluation, 386–387, 387f
    treatment, 387–388
Adult-acquired flatfoot deformity, 167
    anatomy of, 167–168
    ankle involvement, deformities with, 177–178
    classification of, 168–170, 168t–169t, 170f, 171t
    clinical presentation of, 170–171
    complications of, 178
    flexible deformities, 174
        periarticular osteotomies, 175–177, 175f–177f
        soft-tissue procedures, 175
    imaging of, 172–173, 173f
    nonsurgical treatment of, 173–174
    pathophysiology of, 167–168

physical examination of, 171–172, 172f
    posterior tibial tenosynovitis, 174
    rigid deformities, 177, 178f
    surgical treatment of, 174
AFO. *See* Ankle-foot orthosis (AFO)
Akin osteotomy, 441
Alcohol sclerosing therapy, interdigital plantar neuralgia, 87
Allograft
    arthroplasty, 120–121, 122f
    bone products, 162
    osteoarticular, 262
    prosthetic reconstruction, 262–263
    talar, 273
    transplantation, osteochondral, 419
Allograft-autograft composite, 262, 262f
AMIC. *See* Autologous matrix-induced chondrogenesis (AMIC)
Amputation
    ankle, 261–262, 351–356
    diabetic foot disease, 74–75
    disarticulation, 352
    foot, 261–262, 351–356
    hallux, 352, 353f
    hindfoot, 355, 355f
    initial wound management, 352
    lesser toe, 353, 353f
    levels of, 352–356
    metastatic carcinoma, 261
    midfoot, 354–355, 354f
    postoperative care, 356
    ray resection, 229, 353–354, 354f
    Syme ankle disarticulation, 355–356, 356f
    total ankle arthroplasty, 144
    transtibial, 356
    wound healing, 352
Aneurysmal bone cyst, 259
Ankle
    amputation, 351–356
    anatomy of, 372
    arthrodesis, 121–126, 406, 407f
    axis of rotation, 7, 7f
    biomechanics of, 3–11
        clinical, 6–10, 7f–9f
        gait and, 10–11
    bracing treatment and shoe inserts, 263
    Charcot neuroarthropathy, 75, 434–436, 435f
    children and adolescent conditions, 37–45
    chondrocytes, 111
    computed tomography, 26–27, 26f–27f
    distraction, 116
    imaging studies of, 23–34
    impingement, 405–406
    infection of, 230–231
    instability, 19

ligament injuries, 385–397
ligament repair, 406–407
magnetic resonance imaging, 29–34
muscles of, 52, 53t
nuclear medicine, 27–29, 28f
osseous grafting, 262–263, 262f
plain radiography, 23–25
posterior tibial tendon dysfunction, deformities, 177–178
prosthetic replacement, 261–262
radiographic measurements of, 24–25
sports-related injuries, 371–381
sprains, 15
stabilization, 407
structural anatomy of, 3–6, 4f–6f
surgical débridement of, 229
tenography, 25
ultrasonography, 25–26
Ankle arthritis, 109
    acute ankle arthrodesis, 126
    anatomy of, 110, 110f
    biomechanics of, 110
    clinical presentation of, 112–113
    imaging of, 112–113
    incidence and etiology, 110–112, 111f–112f
    nonsurgical treatment of, 113
        bracing, 114–115, 115f
        intra-articular injections, 114
        oral therapy, 113–114
    surgical treatment of
        arthrodesis, 121–126
        joint preservation surgery, 115–120
        joint-sacrificing surgery, 120–121
        joint-sparing procedures, 115, 116t
    total ankle arthroplasty, 133, 144–145
        arthrodesis *vs.*, 144
        clinical outcomes, 142
        complications of, 140–142, 141f
        contraindications to, 138
        design issues, 134–138
        implants, 134, 134f–137f
        indications, 138
        rationale, 134–138
        revision, 142–144, 143f
        surgical approaches, alternative, 139–140
        surgical treatment, 138–139
Ankle-foot orthosis (AFO), 17
    adult-acquired flatfoot deformity, 174
    ankle arthritis, 114–115
    Intrepid Dynamic Exoskeletal Orthosis, 19
    modifications, 18, 18t
    nonarticulated, 18
    solid-ankle, 18
    types, 18, 18t

Index

Ankle fractures
- arthroscopy, 286
- classification of, 285
- complications of, 289
- definitive management of, 286
- evaluation of, 284
- incidence of, 283–284
- initial management of, 285–286
- malleolus
  - lateral, 286, 287f
  - medial, 287, 287f
  - posterior, 287–289, 288f
- patient history of, 284
- physical examination of, 284
- postoperative management, 289
- radiographic studies of, 284–285
- syndesmosis, 289, 289f

Ankle tumors
- benign osseous, 256–260
- benign soft-tissue, 252–255
- biopsy of, 251–252
- history of, 250
- imaging of, 250–251
- incidence of, 250
- isolated limb infusion and, 263
- laboratory evaluation of, 251
- malignant osseous, 260–261
- malignant soft-tissue, 255–256
- nononcologically excised malignant, 263
- patient evaluation of, 250–252
- physical examination of, 250
- reconstructive treatments for, 261–263

Anterior ankle arthroscopy, 404
- ankle arthrodesis, 406, 407f
- ankle impingement, 405–406
- ankle ligament repair, 406–407
- fracture management, 407–408, 408f
- indications, 404, 404f
- technique, 404–405, 405f

Anterior talofibular ligament, 6, 385
- acute lateral ankle sprain, 386–387
- chronic lateral ankle ligament instability, 388–392

Anterior tibial tendon disorders, 372–373

AO/Orthopaedic Trauma Association (OTA) systems
- ankle fractures, 285
- pilon fractures, 290, 291f

Apophysitis
- Iselin disease, 43, 44f
- Sever disease, 43

ARMIS. *See* Arthroscopic reduction and minimally invasive surgery (ARMIS)

Arthritis, 111. *See also specific types*
- iatrogenic, 153
- inflammatory, 153
- posttraumatic, 138
  - calcaneal fractures, 319, 319f–320f
  - talar neck fracture, 305
- septic, 70, 226, 229

Arthrodesis
- ankle, 406, 407f, 449
- ankle arthritis, 121
  - acute, 126

arthroscopic technique, 123, 124f
- complications of, 123
- malunions, 123
- open technique, 124, 125f
- results, 124–126
- subtalar, 139
- total ankle arthroplasty, salvage of failed, 126, 127f–128f
- *vs.* arthroplasty, 144
- calcaneocuboid, 158–159, 159f
- cavovarus deformity, 60
- cuboid fractures, 330
- double, 159, 161f
- first metatarsophalangeal joint, 411–412
- hallux rigidus, 197–198, 197f
- intra-articular calcaneal fractures, 314
- minimally invasive surgery, 443
- osteonecrosis of the talus, 276
- Siffert beak triple, 60
- subtalar, 157–158, 157f, 410–411
- talonavicular, 158, 158f
- triple, 159, 160f

Arthroereisis, 42, 177

Arthrofibrosis, 411

Arthroplasty
- allograft, 120–121, 122f
- arthrodesis *vs.*, 144
- distraction, 116–118, 117f
- excisional, 215
- resection and interposition, 195

Arthroscopic reduction and minimally invasive surgery (ARMIS), 408

Arthroscopy
- ankle fractures, 286
- anterior ankle, 404–408
- first metatarsophalangeal joint, 411–412
- hallux rigidus, 195
- posterior ankle, 408–410
- subtalar, 410–411
- tendoscopy, 412413

Aseptic loosening, revision total ankle arthroplasty, 452–453, 453f

Atherosclerosis, 69

Athletic shoes, 13. *See also* Sports-related injuries
- barefoot-style running shoes, 14
- energy-storing mechanisms, 15, 15f
- maximally cushioned, 15, 15f

Autologous chondrocyte implantation (ACI), 418

Autologous matrix-induced chondrogenesis (AMIC), 420–421

Autonomic neuropathy, 68, 71

Avulsion fractures
- fifth metatarsal, 339–340, 340f
- midfoot, 327–328

B

Beam model, of medial longitudinal arch, 9, 9f

Biopsy, 229
- aneurysmal bone cyst, 259
- nerve, 55

osteochondroma, 257
- tumors, 251–252

Bipolar allograft metatarsophalangeal resurfacing, 195

Bone cysts
- aneurysmal, 258–259
- unicameral, 259, 259f

Bone grafting, osteonecrosis of the talus, 272–274, 273f–274f

Bone marrow edema, 14, 31–34

Bone marrow stimulation, 416–418

Bone transport, ring fixators and rails, 263

Boyd amputation, 355

Bracing
- ankle arthritis, 114–115, 115f
- biomechanics, 13
- treatment, 263

Brodsky classification, of Charcot neuroarthropathy, 431, 431f

Broström procedures, 5, 5f, 391

Broström repair technique, 391

Bunionette
- clinical evaluation of, 208–209, 209f
- etiology of, 208
- nonsurgical treatment of, 209
- pathoanatomy of, 208
- repair, 441–443, 443f–444f
- surgical treatment of, 209, 209f

C

CADENCE Total Ankle System, 10, 134, 136f

Calcaneal apophysitis, 43. *See also* Sever disease

Calcaneal fractures, 311, 322f
- complications of
  - calcaneal malunion, 320–321, 321f
  - posttraumatic arthritis, 319, 319f–320f
  - wound, 318–319, 318f
- epidemiology of, 311–312
- extra-articular, 317–318
- intra-articular
  - classification of, 312–313
  - displaced, 313–314, 313f
  - imaging of, 312–313, 312f–313f
  - minimally invasive techniques, for displaced, 314
  - nonsurgical treatment of, 313
  - open reduction and internal fixation, 314
  - percutaneous reduction and fixation, 314–315
  - sinus tarsi approach to, 315–316, 317f
  - tongue-type fracture, 314, 315f
  - type IV, primary arthrodesis for, 314
- pathoanatomy of, 311–312

Calcaneal gait, 11

Calcaneal malunion, 320–321, 321f

Calcaneal osteotomy, 140
- cavovarus deformity, 58–60, 59f–62f
- minimally invasive surgery, 444–445, 445f

Calcaneocuboid arthrodesis, 158–159, 159f

Calcaneocuboid joint, 4

Calcaneofibular impingement, 40-41

Calcaneofibular ligament, 4, 6, 385

462   © 2025 American Academy of Orthopaedic Surgeons   Orthopaedic Knowledge Update®: Foot and Ankle 7

acute lateral ankle sprain, 386–387
chronic lateral ankle ligament instability, 389, 391–392
Calcaneonavicular coalitions, 40, 40f
Calcaneus, 4, 153
  osteomyelitis of, 238
  stress fractures, 245, 245f
Cartilage injury, 33, 33f
Cartilage tumors, 250
Cavovarus deformity, 51
  anatomy, 52–54, 53t, 54f
  bony procedures
    calcaneal osteotomy, 58–60, 59f–62f
    claw toe correction, 62
    first metatarsal dorsiflexion osteotomy, 58
    fusion, 60–62, 62f–63f
  causes, 51, 52t
  Charcot-Marie-Tooth disease and, 51–52
  diagnosis, 54
    history of, 54–55, 55f
    imaging studies and, 55–56, 55f
    physical examination and, 54–55, 55f
  etiology, 51–52, 52t
  nonsurgical treatment, 56
  pathomechanics, 52–54, 53t, 54f
  soft-tissue procedures
    Achilles tendon lengthening, 57
    gastrocnemius recession, 56–57
    lateral ligament reconstruction, 57
    modified Jones procedure, 57
    peroneus brevis–to–peroneus longus tenodesis, 57
    plantar fascia release, 56
    posterior tibial tendon transfer, 57–58
  surgical treatment planning, 56
  trauma, lower extremity, 52
Cavus foot orthosis, 19
Cedell process, 408, 410
Cellulitis, 227–228
Charcot-Marie-Tooth (CMT) disease
  cavovarus deformity and, 51, 53, 54f
  diagnosis of, 55
  myotendinous imbalances, 56
  neuropathies, 52
Charcot neuroarthropathy, 19, 69, 76f–77f, 77, 429
  Brodsky classification of, 431, 431f
  Eichenholtz classification of, 430, 430t
  epidemiology of, 429–432
  exostectomy, 432
  infectious radiographic characteristics and, 69–70
  natural history of, 429–432
  osteomyelitis and, 70
  pathology of, 429–432
  reconstruction, 432–433
  Schön classification of, 431, 431f
  stages of, 75
  superconstructs, 433–434, 433f–434f
  surgical techniques and considerations, 432
  treatment of, 431–432
Charcot Restraint Orthotic Walker (CROW), 19, 432

Cheilectomy, hallux rigidus, 193–194, 193f, 440–441, 442f
Chondroblastoma, 257–258
Chondroma, periosteal, 257
Chondromatosis, synovial, 253
Chondromyxoid fibroma, 259
Chondrosarcoma, 260
Chopart joint, 4
Chronic lateral ankle ligament instability, 388
  patient history, 388
  physical examination, 388–389, 389f
  radiographic evaluation, 390, 390f
  treatment, 390–393, 391f–393f
Claw toe
  clinical evaluation of, 204
  correction, cavovarus deformity and, 62
  etiology of, 203–204
  nonsurgical treatment of, 205–206
  pathoanatomy of, 203–204
  surgical treatment of, 207–208, 208f
Clear cell sarcoma, 256
CMT disease. See Charcot-Marie-Tooth (CMT) disease
Coleman block test, 54, 55f, 154, 389
Compartment syndrome, midfoot, 335
Complex regional pain syndrome (CRPS), 162
  classification of, 99
  diagnosis of, 100, 100f
  epidemiology of, 99
  history and clinical examination, 100
  pathophysiology of, 99–100
  treatment of, 100–101
  type I, 99
  type II, 99
Computed tomography (CT), 26–27, 26f–27f, 322f
  acute lateral ankle sprain, 387
  adult-acquired flatfoot deformity, 173
  ankle arthritis, 113
  ankle fractures, 285
  calcaneus, stress fractures of, 245
  cavovarus deformity, 55
  chondroblastoma, 257
  cuboid fractures, 329
  deep peroneal nerve entrapment, 95
  diabetic foot disease, 69–70
  extra-articular calcaneal fractures, 317
  hallux rigidus, 192
  hallux valgus, 187
  hindfoot arthritis, 155
  intra-articular calcaneal fractures, 312
  intraosseous lipoma, 260
  lateral process fractures, 306, 306f
  metastatic carcinoma, 261
  nondiabetic foot infections, 226
  osteochondral lesion of the talus, 413–414, 414f
  osteoid osteoma, 260
  periprosthetic fracture, 455
  pilon fractures, 290
  postimplant gutter impingement, 457
  sprains, midfoot, 380
  stress fractures, 329, 378
  superficial peroneal nerve, 96

sural nerve, 98
syndesmotic sprains, 394
talar neck fractures, 300–301
tarsal coalition, 40, 40f
tarsometatarsal fractures, 331–332
total ankle arthroplasty, 138, 140, 143
tumors, 251
Controlled ankle motion boot, 19
Core decompression, osteonecrosis of the talus, 272
Corticosteroid injection
  adult-acquired flatfoot deformity, 173
  ankle arthritis, 114
  hindfoot arthritis, 156
  interdigital plantar neuralgia, 87
  lateral plantar nerve entrapment, 94
  medial plantar proper digital nerve syndrome, 98
  midfoot arthritis, 156
  plantar fasciitis, 239
Cotton osteotomy, 176, 452
Coughlin classification, hallux rigidus, 192, 193t
C-reactive protein, 70, 141, 227
CRPS. See Complex regional pain syndrome (CRPS)
CT. See Computed tomography (CT)
Cuboid fractures, 329–330, 330f
Cuneiform fractures, 330

D

Danis-Weber classification, ankle fractures, 285
Débridement
  arthroscopic, bone marrow stimulation, 417–418
  diabetic foot ulcer, 72
  posterior tibial tendon, 175
  synovectomy and, 115–116, 116f
Deep peroneal nerve entrapment, 94
  anatomy of, 94
  diagnosis of, 95
  etiology and physical examination, 94–95
  treatment of, 95
Deltoid incompetence, valgus malpositioning, 451
Deltoid ligament complex, 6, 6f
Deltoid ligament injuries, 395
  anatomy of, 396
  classification of, 396–397
  radiographic evaluation, 396
  treatment, 396–397
Deltoid-spring ligament complex, 8
Desmoid tumor, 254. See also Extra-abdominal fibromatosis
Diabetes, 352. See also Diabetic foot ulcer
  amputation, 74–75
  autonomic neuropathy, 68
  COVID-19 deaths, 67
  foot care instructions for, 77, 78t
  glycemic control, 77
  therapeutic in-depth shoes, 16
  vascular disease, 69

Index

Diabetic foot disease, 67
amputation, 73–75
Charcot neuroarthropathy and, 75–77, 76f–77f
complications of, 70–77
diabetic ulcer and, 70–73, 72f
epidemiology of, 67–68
etiology of, 68
evaluation of, 68–70
infection, 73–74, 74t
risk and preventive care, 77–79, 78t–79t
surgical complications, 77
treatment of, 70–77
Diabetic foot ulcer
classification system for, 71, 72f
management strategies of, 71–73
prevalence of, 70
risk factors for, 71
Diabetic neuropathy, 68
Digital Imaging and Communication in Medicine, 23
Digital radiography, 23
Distal interphalangeal (DIP) joint, 203
claw toe, 207
mallet toe, 206
Distal metatarsal articular angle, 185, 187
Distal tibial articular surface angle, 110, 110f
Distraction arthroplasty, 116–118, 117f
Double-crush syndrome, 86
DTML. See Deep transverse metatarsal ligament (DTML)
Dwyer closing-wedge osteotomy, 58

E

Eichenholtz classification, of Charcot neuroarthropathy, 430, 430t
Electromyography, 15, 55
Enchondroma, 257, 258f
Endoscopy
decompression, interdigital plantar neuralgia, 88
hindfoot, 408–410
peroneal tendons, 412
Energy-storing mechanisms, athletic shoes, 15, 15f
Energy-storing orthosis, 20, 20f
Epidermoid inclusion cyst, 254
Epithelioid sarcoma, 256
Erythrocyte sedimentation rate, 227
EVENup Shoe Lift, 19
Ewing sarcoma, 260–261
Exostectomy, 432
Extensor hallucis brevis tendon transfer, 191
Extensor hallucis longus tendon transfer, 191
Extra-abdominal fibromatosis, 254
Extra-articular calcaneal fractures, 317–318

F

Fat pad atrophy, 86
Felon, 227
Fibroma
ankle, 253

chondromyxoid, 259
foot, 253
nonossifying, 260
plantar, 253–254
Fibromatosis
extra-abdominal, 254
plantar, 253–254
Fibrous dysplasia, 250
Fibroxanthomas, 260. See also Nonossifying fibromas
Ficat and Arlet classification system, 271, 271t
Fine-needle aspiration biopsy, tumors, 252
First metatarsal, dorsiflexion osteotomy, 58
Fleck sign, 4, 332, 332f
Flexible pediatric flatfoot
clinical findings, 41
nonsurgical treatment, 42
radiographic evaluation, 41–42, 42f
surgical treatment, 42–43, 43f
Flexor digitorum longus tendon transfer, 175, 377
hammer toe, 206
mallet toe, 206
Flexor hallucis longus tendon transfer, 364, 377
Fluoroscopy, 24, 154
minimally invasive surgery, 440
posterior ankle arthroscopy, 409
stress, 390
syndesmotic sprain, 394, 394f
Foot
amputation, 351–356
biomechanics of, 3–11
clinical, 6–10, 7f–9f
gait and, 10–11
malalignment and alterations in, 6, 7f
bracing treatment and shoe inserts, 263
care instructions, diabetes, 77, 78t
cavovarus, 55, 55f
Charcot involvement of, 75
children and adolescent conditions, 37–45
computed tomography, 26–27, 26f–27f
deformity, 7
high-fashion footwear on, 15
imaging studies of, 23–34
magnetic resonance imaging, 29–34
muscles of, 52, 53t
nuclear medicine, 27–29, 28f
osseous grafting, 262–263, 262f
plain radiography, 23–25
prosthetic replacement, 261–262
sports-related injuries, 371–381
structural anatomy of, 3–6, 4f–6f
surgical débridement of, 229
tenography, 25
ultrasonography, 25–26
Foot-ankle offset, 9
Foot orthosis, 17. See also Ankle-foot orthosis (AFO)
ankle instability and, 19
custom, 19
Foot tumors
benign osseous, 256–260
benign soft-tissue, 252–255
biopsy of, 251–252

history of, 250
imaging of, 250–251
incidence of, 250
isolated limb infusion and, 263
laboratory evaluation of, 251
malignant osseous, 260–261
malignant soft-tissue, 255–256
nononcologically excised malignant, 263
patient evaluation of, 250–252
physical examination of, 250
reconstructive treatments for, 261–263
Forefoot, 3
fractures, 335, 336f
medial, positioning of, 17
minimally invasive surgery
arthrodesis, 443
bunion and bunionette repair, 441–443, 443f–444f
hallux cheilectomy, 440–441, 442f
metatarsalgia and lesser toe deformities, 443–444, 444f
pain, 203
supination, 172, 176
Freiberg infraction, 44–45, 209–210
surgical treatment of, 214–215, 215f
Fusion, cavovarus deformity, 60–62, 62f–63f

G

Gait
abnormality, 11
ankle arthritis, 112
calcaneal, 11
cycle, 10
steppage, 10
total ankle arthroplasty, 449
Trendelenburg, 11
waddling, 11
Ganglion, synovial, 252, 252f
Gastrocnemius recession, cavovarus deformity, 56–57
Giant cell tumor
of bone, 258–259
of tendon sheath, 253
Girdlestone-Taylor procedure, 206
Glomus tumor, 254
Glycemic control, diabetes, 77

H

Haglund deformity, 361
Hallux
amputation of, 352, 353f
osteomyelitis of, 229–230
Hallux rigidus
cheilectomy for, 440–441, 442f
classification of, 192
Coughlin classification of, 192, 193t
etiology of, 191
joint ablation procedures, 196f
arthrodesis, 197–198, 197f
bipolar allograft metatarsophalangeal resurfacing, 195
hemiarthroplasty, 195–197

interposition arthroplasty, 195
    resection arthroplasty, 195
    total joint arthroplasty, 195–197
joint-modifying procedures, 193
    arthroscopy, 195
    cheilectomy, 193–194, 193f
    osteotomy, 194–195, 194f
metatarsophalangeal joint and, 411–412
nonsurgical treatment of, 192–193
pathophysiology of, 191
physical examination of, 191–192
radiographic examination of, 192, 192f
surgical treatment of, 193
Hallux valgus
    anatomy of, 185–186, 186t
    deformity, 6, 19
    diagnostic evaluation, 186–187, 187f–188f, 187t
    nonsurgical treatment of, 187
    pathogenesis of, 185–186
    surgical treatment of, 187–189, 188f–189f
    wide toe box shoe, 13, 14f
Hallux varus, 189, 190f
    anatomy of, 190
    diagnostic evaluation of, 190, 190f
    nonsurgical treatment of, 190
    pathogenesis of, 190
    surgical treatment of, 190–191
Hammer toe
    clinical evaluation of, 204
    deformities of, 13, 14f
    etiology of, 203–204
    nonsurgical treatment of, 205–206
    pathoanatomy of, 203–204
    surgical treatment of, 206–207, 207f
Hawkins classification system, for talar neck fractures, 268, 300, 300f
Heel pad syndrome, 243–244, 244f
Heel spur, 238. See also Plantar fasciitis
Hereditary motor sensory neuropathies, 51
Heterotopic ossification, total ankle arthroplasty, 457
Hindfoot
    amputation, 352, 355, 355f
    ankle-foot orthosis, 18
    arthroscopy, 408
    axis of rotation of, 8
    Charcot neuroarthropathy of, 430, 430f, 434–436, 435f
    endoscopy, 408–410
    infection of, 230–231
    subtalar fusion, 60
    tarsal coalition, 39
    tibialis posterior tendon, 8
Hindfoot arthritis
    adjuvant treatment in, 161–162
    anatomy of, 151–152
    biomechanics of, 152–153
    calcaneocuboid arthrodesis, 158–159, 159f
    clinical presentation of, 154
    complications of, 162–163
    double arthrodesis, 159, 161f
    etiology of, 153–154
    imaging of, 154–155, 155f

nonsurgical treatment of, 155–156
pathophysiology of, 153–154
subtalar arthrodesis, 157–158, 157f
surgical treatment, 156
talonavicular arthrodesis, 158, 158f
triple arthrodesis, 159, 160f
Hintermann Series H3 Total Ankle Replacement System, 134
Hyperbaric oxygen therapy, diabetic foot ulcer, 72
Hyperesthesia, 98
Hypoesthesia, 98

I

Iatrogenic arthritis, 153
IDEO. See Intrepid Dynamic Exoskeletal Orthosis (IDEO)
Iliac crest autograft, 161
INBONE II Total Ankle System, 134, 135f
Indium-111 white blood cell scintigraphy, 70
INFINITY Total Ankle System, 134, 134f
Inflammatory arthritis, 153
Interdigital plantar neuralgia, 85
    anatomy and pathophysiology, 85–86
    diagnostic studies, 87
    history and physical examination, 86 87
    nonsurgical treatment, 87–88
    surgical treatment, 88–90, 89f–90f
Intermetatarsal ligament, 88, 152
Intra-articular calcaneal fractures
    classification of, 312–313
    displaced, 313–314, 313f
    imaging of, 312–313, 312f–313f
    minimally invasive techniques, for displaced, 314
    nonsurgical treatment of, 313
    open reduction and internal fixation, 314
    percutaneous reduction and fixation, 314–315
    sinus tarsi approach to, 315–316, 317f
    tongue-type fracture, 314, 315f
    type IV, primary arthrodesis for, 314
Intra-articular injections, ankle arthritis, 114
Intractable plantar keratosis, 210, 210f
    surgical treatment of, 215, 216f–217f
Intraosseous lipoma, 260
Intrepid Dynamic Exoskeletal Orthosis (IDEO), 19
INVISION Total Ankle Revision System, 134, 135f
Iselin disease, 43, 44f

J

Joint ablation procedures. See Hallux rigidus
Joint preservation surgery, ankle arthritis
    débridement, 115–116, 116f
    distraction arthroplasty, 116–118, 117f
    periarticular (supramalleolar) osteotomies, 118–120, 119f
    synovectomy, 115–116, 116f
Jones (metadiaphyseal) fractures, 340–341, 341f

K

Kellgren-Lawrence grades, ankle arthritis, 113
Kinos Axiom Total Ankle System, 134
Köhler disease, 44, 44f

L

Lachman test, 204
Lateral ligament reconstruction, cavovarus deformity, 57
Lateral plantar nerve
    entrapment of, 93–94
    first branch of, 243–244, 244f
Lateral process fractures, 306, 306f
Lauge-Hansen classification, ankle fractures, 285
Lesser toe
    amputation, 353, 353f
    anatomy of, 204, 205f
    deformities of
        clinical evaluation of, 204
        etiology of, 203–204
        minimally invasive surgery, 443–444, 444f
        nonsurgical treatment of, 205–206
        pathoanatomy of, 203–204
        surgical treatment of, 206–208, 207f–208f
    osteomyelitis of, 229–230
Leukocyte labeling, 28
Leukocytosis, 70
Ligament injuries, ankle, 385
    chronic lateral ankle ligament instability, 388–393, 389f–393f
    deltoid ligament, 395–397
    lateral ankle, 386–388, 387f
    syndesmosis, 393–395, 394f
Limb infusion, isolated, 263
Lipoma, 241, 241f, 255
    arborescens, 253
    intraosseous, 260
Lisfranc joint complex, 3
Lisfranc ligament, 4, 31, 152, 331–332
Lower extremity trauma, cavovarus deformity, 52
Lymphadenopathy, 228

M

MACI. See Matrix autologous chondrocyte implantation (MACI)
Magnetic resonance angiography, 251
Magnetic resonance imaging (MRI), 29–34
    Achilles tendinopathy, 365
    Achilles tendon injury, 32
    Achilles tendon ruptures, 362
    acute lateral ankle sprain, 387, 387f
    adult-acquired flatfoot deformity, 173, 173f
    aneurysmal bone cyst, 259
    ankle arthritis, 113

Index

Magnetic resonance imaging (MRI)
(Continued)
  ankle fractures, 285
  ankle impingement, 406
  arthroscopic débridement, 417–418
  autologous matrix-induced chondrogenesis, 420–421
  calcaneus, stress fractures of, 245
  cartilage injury, 33, 33*f*
  cavovarus deformity, 55
  Charcot neuroarthropathy, 431
  chondroblastoma, 257
  chronic lateral ankle ligament instability, 390
  cuboid fractures, 329
  deep peroneal nerve entrapment, 95
  deltoid ligament injuries, 396
  diabetic foot disease, 70
  extra-abdominal fibromatosis, 254
  flexible pediatric flatfoot, 42
  ganglion, 252
  giant cell tumor, of bone, 258
  hallux rigidus, 192
  higher Tesla, 30
  hindfoot arthritis, 155
  indications for, 29
  interdigital plantar neuralgia, 87
  intraosseous lipoma, 260
  ligamentous injury, 31
  lipoma, 255
  metatarsalgia, 213
  midfoot arthritis, 155
  Morton interdigital neuroma, 254
  nondiabetic foot infections, 226
  osseous injury, 30–31, 30*f*
  osteochondral lesion of the talus, 413–414, 416*f*, 416*t*
  osteoid osteoma, 260
  osteonecrosis of the talus, 270
  particulated juvenile cartilage, 420
  peroneal tendon, 412
    disorders, 374
    subluxation, 374
    tears, 377
  pigmented villonodular synovitis, 252
  plantar fascia, ruptured, 240
  plantar fasciitis, 239
  plantar heel pain, 238
  soft-tissue sarcomas, 255
  sprains, midfoot, 380
  stress fractures, 329
  superficial peroneal nerve, 96
  sural nerve, 98
  syndesmotic sprains, 394
  tarsal coalition, 40
  tarsal tunnel syndrome, 91–92
  tarsometatarsal fractures, 331, 331*f*
  tendinous injury, 31–33, 32*f*–33*f*
  tumors, 251
  unicameral bone cyst, 259
  vascular anomalies, 253
Malleolus, ankle fractures
  lateral, 286, 287*f*
  medial, 287, 287*f*

  posterior, 287–289, 288*f*
Mallet toe
  clinical evaluation of, 204
  etiology of, 203–204
  nonsurgical treatment of, 205–206
  pathoanatomy of, 203–204
  surgical treatment of, 206
Malunion
  ankle arthrodesis, 123
  ankle fractures, 289
  arthrodesis, 163
  calcaneal, 320–321, 321*f*
  talar neck fractures, 305
  total ankle arthroplasty, 144
Masquelet technique, bone formation, 262
Matles test, 362, 362*f*
Matrix autologous chondrocyte implantation (MACI), 418–419
Matrix metalloproteinases, 111
Maximally cushioned athletic shoe, 15, 15*f*
Meary angle, 25
Medial displacement calcaneal osteotomy, 175–176
Medial plantar proper digital nerve syndrome, 98–99
Melanoma, malignant, 256
Metastatic carcinoma, 261, 261*f*
Metatarsal fractures, 335
  fifth, 339, 339*f*–340*f*
    avulsion, 339–340, 340*f*
    Jones, 340–341, 341*f*
    nonsurgical treatment, 341
    surgical treatment, 341
  first, 336
    nonsurgical treatment, 337
    surgical treatment, 337
  middle, 337
    base, 339
    neck, 337
    shaft, 338–339, 338*f*
  stress, 341, 342*f*
    nonsurgical treatment, 342
    surgical treatment, 342
Metatarsalgia, 17
  clinical evaluation of, 211–212, 212*f*
  etiology of, 209–211
  Freiberg infraction, 209–210
    surgical treatment of, 214–215, 215*f*
  intractable plantar keratosis, 210, 210*f*
    surgical treatment of, 215, 216*f*–217*f*
  Morton neuroma, 210
    surgical treatment of, 215–216, 217*f*
  nonsurgical treatment of, 213–214
  pathoanatomy of, 209–211
  radiologic evaluation of, 212–213, 212*f*–213*f*
  sesamoiditis, 210–211
    surgical treatment of, 216–217
  transfer, 211
    surgical treatment of, 217–218
Metatarsal neck fractures, 337
Metatarsal shaft fractures, 338–339, 338*f*
Metatarsophalangeal (MTP) joint, 53
  bunionette deformity, 209

claw toe deformity, 204, 207–208
  first, 186, 188, 343
    arthritis, 189
    arthrodesis of, 197, 412
    arthroscopy, 411–412, 411*f*
    dislocations of, 345, 345*f*
    instability of, 186
    stabilizers of, 185, 186*t*
    turf toe injuries, 344–345, 344*t*
  hallux rigidus and, 191
  hallux valgus and, 185
  hallux varus and, 190
  hemiarthroplasty, 195
  Morton neuroma, 210
  silicone arthroplasty of, 6, 7*f*
Micronized cartilage extracellular matrix, 420, 420*f*
Midfoot, 3–4
  amputation, 74, 354–355, 354*f*
  ankle-foot orthosis, 18
  avulsion fractures, 327–328
  Charcot neuroarthropathy of, 431, 431*f*
  compartment syndrome of, 335
  cuboid fractures, 329–330, 330*f*
  cuneiform fractures, 330
  infection of, 230–231
  navicular body fractures, 328–329, 328*f*
  navicular fractures, 327
  osteotomies with fusion, 60
  sprains, 379
    patient history, 379
    physical examination, 379
    radiographic evaluation, 379–380
    treatment, 380, 380*f*
  stress fractures, 329
  tarsal coalition, 39
  tarsometatarsal fractures, 330–335
Midfoot arthritis, 17
  adjuvant treatment in, 161–162
  anatomy of, 151–152
  biomechanics of, 152–153
  clinical presentation of, 154
  complications of, 162–163
  etiology of, 153–154
  imaging of, 154–155
  nonsurgical treatment of, 155–156
  pathophysiology of, 153–154
  primary arthrodesis, for trauma, 159–161, 161*f*
  surgical treatment of, 156
    lateral column, 156–157
    medial and middle column, 156, 157*f*
Military combat injuries, 19
Minimally invasive surgery, 439
  calcaneal osteotomy, 444–445, 445*f*
  forefoot
    arthrodesis, 443
    bunion and bunionette repair, 441–443, 443*f*–444*f*
    hallux cheilectomy, 440–441, 442*f*
    metatarsalgia/lesser toe deformities, 443–444, 444*f*
  history of, 439–440

instrumentation for, 440, 440*f*
surgical technique, 440, 441*f*
Mintz classification, 414, 416*t*
Mitered joint hinge, 8, 8*f*
Moberg osteotomy, 194
Modified Broström-Evans anatomic-augmented procedure, 392
Modified Jones procedure, cavovarus deformity, 57
Modified Kidner procedure, 38
Morton interdigital neuroma, 254–255, 254*f*
Morton neuroma, 25, 85, 210, 215–216, 217*f*. *See also* Interdigital plantar neuralgia
Motor neuropathy, 71
MRI. *See* Magnetic resonance imaging (MRI)
Mulder test, 87
Multiple myeloma, 261

N

Nail disorders, 227
Naltrexone, complex regional pain syndrome, 101
Navicular, accessory, 37–39, 38*f*–39*f*. *See also* Accessory navicular
Navicular body fractures, 328–329, 328*f*
Necrotizing fasciitis, 228
Negative-pressure wound therapy, 72, 74
Nerve conduction velocity (NCV)
medial plantar proper digital nerve syndrome, 98
superficial peroneal nerve, 96
sural nerve, 98
tarsal tunnel syndrome, 91–92
Nerve syndromes, plantar heel pain
lateral plantar nerve involvement, 243–244, 244*f*
peripheral nerve involvement, 244–245
tarsal tunnel syndrome, 240–243, 241*f*–243*f*
Neurilemmoma, 255
Neurofibroma, 255
Neuromas, 88
Morton interdigital, 210, 254–255, 254*f*
recurrent, 90
Neuropathy
autonomic, 68, 71
Charcot-Marie-Tooth disease, 52
diabetic, 68
motor, 71
peripheral, 52, 68
sensory, 71
somatic sensory, 68
Nodular fasciitis, foot and ankle, 253
Nonarticulated ankle-foot orthosis, 18
Nondiabetic foot infections, 225
ankle, 230–231
deep infections, 228–229
hallux and lesser toes, osteomyelitis, 229–230
hindfoot, 230–231
history of, 225–226
imaging studies of, 226–227, 226*f*
laboratory studies of, 227

midfoot, 230–231
multidisciplinary management, 232
nail disorders, 227
physical examination of, 225–226
soft-tissue infections, 227–228
surgical débridement of, 229
surgical site infections, 231–232
Nononcologically excised malignant tumors, 263
Nonossifying fibromas, 260
Nonunion
ankle fractures, 289
arthrodesis, 162–163
talar neck fractures, 305
total ankle arthroplasty, 144
Nuclear medicine, 27–29, 28*f*, 155

O

OLT. *See* Osteochondral lesion of the talus (OLT)
Onychomycosis, 227
Open reduction and internal fixation (ORIF), 160
arthroscopy, 286
fracture management, 407–408
intra-articular calcaneal fractures, 314
pilon fractures, 290
sprains, midfoot, 380
talar neck fractures, 301–304, 302*f*–303*f*
tarsometatarsal fractures, 332–335
Orthosis
clinical applications of, 17
energy-storing, 20, 20*f*
molded thermoplastic, 18
prescription, 18
Osseous grafting, ankle and foot, 262–263, 262*f*
Osseous injury, 30–31, 30*f*
Osseous tumors
benign
aneurysmal bone cyst, 259
chondroblastoma, 257–258
chondroma, 257
chondromyxoid fibroma, 259
enchondroma, 257, 258*f*
giant cell tumor, of bone, 258–259
intraosseous lipoma, 260
nonossifying fibroma, 260
osteoblastoma, 260
osteochondroma, 256–257
osteoid osteoma, 260
periosteal chondroma, 257
subungual exostosis, 257
unicameral bone cyst, 259, 259*f*
malignant
chondrosarcoma, 260
Ewing sarcoma, 260–261
metastatic carcinoma, 261, 261*f*
multiple myeloma, 261
osteosarcoma, 260
Osteoarthritis (OA)
ankle, 110, 112
knee, 110
posttraumatic, 110–112

Osteoblastoma, 260
Osteochondral allograft transplantation, 419
Osteochondral autograft transplantation, 418
Osteochondral lesion of the talus (OLT)
arthroscopic débridement, bone marrow stimulation, 417–418
autologous chondrocyte implantation, 418
autologous matrix-induced chondrogenesis, 420–421
classification of, 413–414
clinical presentation of, 413
etiology of, 413
hyaluronic acid, 421
imaging of, 413–414, 414*f*–416*f*, 416*t*
incidence, 413
matrix autologous chondrocyte implantation, 418–419
micronized cartilage extracellular matrix, 420, 420*f*
natural history of, 413
nonsurgical treatment of, 414–415
osteochondral allograft transplantation, 419
osteochondral autograft transplantation procedure, 418
particulated juvenile cartilage, 419–420
pathoanatomy of, 413
platelet-rich plasma, 421
primary repair, 416–417, 417*f*
stem cell therapy, 420
surgical treatment of, 415–416, 417*f*
Osteochondroma, 256–257
Osteochondrosis
Freiberg infraction, 44–45
Köhler disease, 44, 44*f*
Osteoid osteoma, 260
Osteolysis, 456–457
Osteomyelitis, 74, 231*f*, 430
computed tomography, 69–70
fibula, 230
hallux, 229–230
lesser toes, 229–230
magnetic resonance imaging, 70
nondiabetic foot infections, 228–229
Osteonecrosis, 113
sesamoid, 346–347
talar neck fractures and, 304–305
Osteonecrosis of the talus
anatomy of, 267–268, 268*f*
diagnosis of, 269–271, 271*f*
etiology of, 268–269, 270*f*
Ficat and Arlet classification system for, 271, 271*t*
incidence of, 267–269
symptoms of, 269–271
total ankle arthroplasty, 138
treatments
algorithm, 276–277, 277*f*
joint-sacrificing, 274–276, 275*f*–276*f*, 275*t*
joint-sparing, 272–274, 273*f*–274*f*
nonsurgical, 271–272, 272*f*
vascular supply, 267–268, 269*f*
Osteosarcoma, 260

Index

Osteotomy
  Akin, 441
  calcaneal, 58–60, 59*f*–62*f*
  Cotton, 176, 452
  Dwyer closing-wedge, 58
  hallux rigidus, 194–195, 194*f*
  Moberg, 194
  Z-shaped, 59, 61*f*
Ottawa ankle rules, 386

P

Particulated juvenile cartilage, 419–420
Peek-a-boo heel sign, 389, 389*f*
Periarticular (supramalleolar) osteotomies,
    118–120, 119*f*
Peripheral nerve disorders, 85
  complex regional pain syndrome, 99–101,
      100*f*
  deep peroneal nerve entrapment, 94–95
  interdigital plantar neuralgia, 85–90,
      89*f*–90*f*
  lateral plantar nerve entrapment, 93–94
  medial plantar nerve entrapment, 93
  medial plantar proper digital nerve
      syndrome, 98–99
  superficial peroneal nerve, 95–97
  sural nerve, 97–98
  tarsal tunnel syndrome, 90–93, 91*f*
Peripheral neuropathy, 52, 77, 91, 123, 284
  prevalence of, 68
Periprosthetic cysts, 456–457
Peritendinitis. *See* Peroneal tenosynovitis
Peroneal tendon
  disorders, 373–374
  subluxation, 374–375, 375*f*
  tears, 375–377, 376*f*–377*f*
  tendoscopy, 412
Peroneal tenosynovitis, 375
Peroneus longus tenodesis, 57
PET. *See* Positron emission tomography (PET)
Pigmented villonodular synovitis (PVNS),
    252–253
Pilon fractures, 290
  classification of, 290, 291*f*
  clinical evaluation, 290
  initial management of, 290–291, 292*f*
  radiographic evaluation, 290
  surgical treatment of
      approaches to, 291–293, 293*f*
      external fixation, 294
      internal fixation, 293–294, 294*f*
PIP joint. *See* Proximal interphalangeal (PIP)
    joint
Pirogoff amputation, 355
Planovalgus deformity, 41
Plantar fascia, 9
  cavovarus deformity, release of, 56
  ruptured, 240
Plantar fasciitis, 239*f*
  chronic, tarsal tunnel syndrome, 242–243,
      243*f*
  nonsurgical protocol, 240
  physical examination, 239
  symptoms of, 238

treatments
    injections, 239
    nonsurgical, 239–240
Plantar fibroma, 253–254
Plantar heel pain, 237
  diagnosis of, 237–238
  disorders and treatment, 238–245
  etiologies of, 238, 238*t*
  nerve syndromes
      lateral plantar nerve involvement,
          243–244, 244*f*
      peripheral nerve involvement, 244–245
      tarsal tunnel syndrome, 240–243,
          241*f*–243*f*
  physical examination of, 238
  plantar fascia, ruptured, 240
  plantar fasciitis, 238–240, 239*f*
  rheumatologic diagnoses, 245
  stress fractures of calcaneus and, 245, 245*f*
Plantar nerve branches, 243
Platelet-rich plasma (PRP), 232, 272
  osteochondral lesion of the talus, 421
  plantar fasciitis, 239
Positron emission tomography (PET), 28
  epithelioid sarcoma, 256
  tumors, 251
Posterior ankle arthroscopy, 408
  anatomy of, 408, 409*f*
  impingement, 410
  indications, 408–409
  technique, 409
Posterior ankle impingement, 410
Posterior process fractures, 306–307
Posterior tibial tendon, 167
  attenuation of, 168
  palpation, 171
  tendoscopy, 412
Posterior tibial tendon dysfunction (PTTD),
    167, 172
  anatomy of, 167–168
  ankle involvement, deformities with,
      177–178
  clinical classification system for, 168, 169*t*
  clinical staging of, 168, 168*t*
  complications of, 178
  flexible deformities, 174–177
  imaging of, 172–173, 173*f*
  nonsurgical treatment of, 173–174
  pathophysiology of, 167–168
  posterior tibial tenosynovitis, 174
  rigid deformities, 177
  stage I, 168
  stage II, 168
  stage III, 170
  stage IV, 170
Posterior tibial tendon transfer, cavovarus
    deformity, 57–58
Posterior tibial tenosynovitis, 174
Postimplant gutter impingement, total ankle
    arthroplasty, 457
Prefabricated walking boots, 19
Pregabalin, complex regional pain syndrome,
    100
Primary arthrodesis, for type IV fractures, 314
Procurvatum, valgus malpositioning, 452

Proximal interphalangeal (PIP) joint, 204
  claw toe, 207
  hammer toe, 206–207
  mallet toe, 206
PRP. *See* Platelet-rich plasma (PRP)
Pseudomonas aeruginosa, 228
PTTD. *See* Posterior tibial tendon dysfunction
    (PTTD)
PVNS. *See* Pigmented villonodular synovitis
    (PVNS)

Q

Quigley maneuver, ankle fractures, 286

R

Radiography, 63*f*, 75, 117*f*, 212–213,
    212*f*–213*f*. *See also specific diseases
    and injuries*
  accessory navicular, 38, 39*f*
  acute lateral ankle sprain, 386–387, 387*f*
  chronic lateral ankle ligament instability,
      390, 390*f*
  deltoid ligament injuries, 396
  digital, 23
  Ficat and Arlet classification system, 271,
      271*t*
  flexible pediatric flatfoot, 41–42
  hallux rigidus, 192, 192*f*, 193*t*
  pilon fractures, 290
  plain, 23–25
      cuboid fractures, 329
      cuneiform fractures, 330
      tarsal coalition, 40
  syndesmosis injuries, 394, 394*f*
Randomized controlled trials, 19, 72, 87–88,
    114, 395
  Achilles tendinopathy, 366
  Freiberg infraction, 215
  interdigital plantar neuralgia, 88
  open reduction and internal fixation, 160
  percutaneous reduction and fixation, 315
  plantar fasciitis, 240
Range of motion (ROM), 113
  ankle arthritis, 115–116, 118
  chronic lateral ankle ligament instability,
      390
  hallux rigidus, 192
Ray resection, 229
  amputation of, 353–354, 354*f*
Recurvatum, valgus malpositioning, 452
Return to Run clinical pathway, 19
Revision total ankle arthroplasty, 142–144,
    143*f*
  component failure
      aseptic loosening, 452–453, 453*f*
      heterotopic ossification, 457
      joint sepsis, 454–455
      osteolysis and periprosthetic cysts,
          456–457, 457*f*
      periprosthetic fracture, 455–456
      postimplant gutter impingement, 457,
          457*f*
      subsidence, management of, 453–454

468   © 2025 American Academy of Orthopaedic Surgeons   Orthopaedic Knowledge Update®: Foot and Ankle 7

talus, 454, 455*t*
tibia, 453–454, 454*f*
malalignment, management of
cavus foot issues (varus), 450–451
proximal (tibial) issues, 450
valgus malpositioning, 451–452
varus malpositioning, 450, 450*t*
risk factors, 449
Rüedi-Allgöwer classification, pilon fractures, 290
Running, 10, 110, 155, 168, 334, 366, 410
shoes, 14
Running sports, 14
variability of, 15

S

Salto Talaris Total Ankle Prosthesis, 134, 136*f*
Sarcoma
acral myxoinflammatory fibroblastic, 255–256, 257*f*
clear cell, 256
epithelioid, 256
Ewing, 260–261
soft-tissue, 255, 256*f*
synovial, 255
SARS-CoV-2 (COVID-19), 67
Scandinavian Total Ankle Replacement, 134, 137*f*
Schön classification, of midfoot Charcot neuroarthropathy, 431, 431*f*
Schwannoma, 255
Semmes-Weinstein monofilament, 91
Sensory neuropathy, 71
Septic arthritis, 229
Sesamoid injuries, 345
Sesamoiditis, 210–211, 345
surgical treatment of, 216–217
Sesamoid osteonecrosis, 346*f*
fractures, 346
injuries, treatment of, 346–347
Sever disease, 43
Shoes
arch-type compatibility, 13
athletic, 13, 15*f*
components of, 15, 16*t*
design features of, 14, 14*f*
for diabetes, 16
energy-storing mechanisms, 15, 15*f*
inserts, 263
maximalist, 15, 15*f*
modifications of, 13
ambulation efficiency, 16
cavovarus deformity, 56
hallux valgus and, 187
insoles, 17, 17*f*
metatarsalgia, 214
pedorthist, 17
wedges/posts, 17
running, 14
types, 16, 16*t*
wide toe box, 13, 14*f*
zero drop, 15, 15*f*
Siffert beak triple arthrodesis, 60

Silfverskiöld test, 56, 139
adult-acquired flatfoot deformity, 171
arthrodesis, 154
Single photon emission computed tomography (SPECT), 456
heterotopic ossification, 457
postimplant gutter impingement, 457
Single photon emission computed tomography and CT (SPECT-CT), 28–29, 28*f*
Sinus tarsi approach, to intra-articular calcaneal fractures, 315–316, 317*f*
Skin ulcers, 13
Soft-tissue infections, nondiabetic foot infections
cellulitis, 227–228
necrotizing fasciitis, 228
Soft-tissue sarcomas, 255, 256*f*
Soft-tissue tumors
benign
epidermoid inclusion cyst, 254
extra-abdominal fibromatosis, 254
fibroma, 253
fibromatosis, 253–254
glomus tumor, 254
lipoma, 255
Morton interdigital neuroma, 254–255, 254*f*
neurilemmoma, 255
neurofibroma, 255
nodular fasciitis, 253
plantar fibroma, 253–254
schwannoma, 255
synovial tumors, 252–253, 252*f*
vascular anomalies, 253
malignant
acral myxoinflammatory fibroblastic sarcoma, 255–256, 257*f*
clear cell sarcoma, 256
epithelioid sarcoma, 256
melanoma, 256
soft-tissue sarcomas, 255, 256*f*
synovial sarcoma, 255
Somatic sensory neuropathy, 68
SPECT. *See* Single-photon emission computed tomography (SPECT)
Sports-related injuries, 371
anterior tibial tendon disorders, 372–373
midfoot sprains, 379–380
peroneal tendon
disorders, 373–374
subluxation, 374–375, 375*f*
tears, 375–377, 376*f*–377*f*
peroneal tenosynovitis, 375
stress fractures of, 377–379
Sprains
acute lateral ankle
classification, 387–388
patient history, 386
physical examination, 386
radiographic evaluation, 386–387, 387*f*
treatment, 387–388
midfoot, 379
patient history, 379
physical examination, 379

radiographic evaluation, 379–380
treatment, 380, 380*f*
syndesmotic, 393
classification of, 394–395
patient history, 393–394
physical examination, 393–394
radiographic evaluation, 394, 394*f*
treatment, 395
Staphylococcus aureus, 73
STAR total ankle arthroplasties, 456, 457*f*
Stem cell therapy, 420
Steppage gait, 10
Stress fractures
of calcaneus, 245, 245*f*
metatarsal, 341, 342*f*
diagnosis of, 342
nonsurgical treatment, 342
surgical treatment, 342
navicular, 329
sports-related, 377
patient history, 377–378
physical examination, 377–378
radiographic evaluation, 378, 378*f*
treatment, 378–379, 379*f*
Stride length, 10
Subluxation, peroneal tendon, 374–375, 375*f*
Subtalar arthrodesis, 157–158, 157*f*
Subtalar joint, 4
arthrodesis, 410–411
arthrofibrosis, 411
arthroscopy
indications, 410
technique, 410
motion of, 7
Subungual exostosis, 257
Superconstructs, Charcot neuroarthropathy, 433–434, 433*f*–434*f*
Superficial peroneal nerve
anatomy of, 95–96
diagnosis of, 96
entrapment of, 95
etiology of, 96
imaging/tests, 96
incidence and clinical presentation, 96
nonsurgical treatment, 96–97
surgical treatment, 97
Sural nerve
anatomy of, 97
clinical presentation of, 97–98
diagnosis studies, 98
entrapment of, 97
etiology of, 97
treatment of, 98
Syme ankle disarticulation, 355–356, 356*f*
Syndesmosis, 5, 289, 289*f*
insufficiency, 451
Syndesmotic sprains, 393
classification of, 394–395
patient history, 393–394
physical examination, 393–394
radiographic evaluation, 394, 394*f*
treatment, 395
Synovectomy, ankle arthritis, 115–116
Synovial chondromatosis, 253

Index

Synovial ganglion, 252, 252f
Synovial proliferations, 253
Synovial sarcoma, 255
Synovial tumors, 252–253, 252f

T

TAA. *See* Total ankle arthroplasty (TAA)
Tailor's bunion. *See* Bunionette
Talar fractures, 299. *See also* Talar neck
    fractures
  anatomy of, 299–300
  complications of, 304–305
  lateral process, 306, 306f
  open reduction and internal fixation,
    301–304, 302f–303f
  posterior process, 306–307
  talar body, 305–306
Talar neck fractures
  classification of, 300
  emergency treatment, 301
  Hawkins classification system for, 268, 300,
    300f
  malunion, 305
  mechanism of injury, 300
  nonunion, 305
  radiologic evaluation, 300–301, 301f
  surgical fixation, timing of, 301
Talocalcaneal coalitions, 41
Talonavicular arthrodesis, 158, 158f
Talonavicular joint, 4
Talus, 4. *See also* Osteochondral lesions of the
    talus
  anterior displacement of, 24
  articular surface of, 5–6
  body of, 5
  cone-shaped trochlear surface of, 5, 6f
  defect classification system, 454, 455t
  fractures
    lateral process, 306, 306f
    posterior process, 306–307
Tarsal coalition, 39
  clinical findings, 39–40
  nonsurgical treatment, 40
  radiographic evaluation, 39, 40f
  surgical treatment, 40–41
Tarsal tunnel syndrome, 90
  anatomy of, 90–91, 91f
  clinical outcomes, 92–93
  diagnostic studies, 91
  history and physical examination, 91
  nonsurgical treatment, 91–92
  plantar heel pain and, 240
    anatomy of, 241, 242f
    with chronic plantar fasciitis, 242–243,
      243f
    lipoma, 241, 241f
  recurrence and revision, 93
  surgical treatment, 92
Tarsometatarsal (TMT) joint, 3, 185
  anatomy of, 329–330
  first joint, stabilizers of, 185, 186t
  fractures
    classification of, 332, 333f

diagnostic studies of, 331–332, 331f–332f
  patient history of, 331
  physical examination of, 331
  surgical results and prognosis, 333–335
  treatment, 332–333
Tendinopathy, Achilles, 365–367, 367f
Tendinous injury, 31–33, 32f–33f
Tendon sheath, giant cell tumor of, 253
Tendon transfer, cavovarus deformity, 56
Tendoscopy
  Achilles tendon, 412–413
  peroneal tendons, 412
  posterior tibial tendon, 412
Tenography, 25
Tenosynovitis, 25
  peroneal, 373, 375
Terminal Syme amputation, 352
Tibialis posterior tendon, 8
  accessory navicular, 39, 39f
  dysfunction, 32
Tibial lateral surface angle, 110
Tibiofibular joint, 5
Tibiotalar joint, axis of rotation, 7
TMT joint. *See* Tarsometatarsal (TMT) joint
Toe fractures, 342–343, 343f
Tongue-type fracture, 314, 315f
Total ankle arthroplasty (TAA), 133, 144–145
  ankle arthritis, 121, 133–145
  arthrodesis *vs.* arthroplasty, 144
  clinical outcomes, 142
  complications of, 140–142, 141f
  contraindications to, 138
  design issues, 134–138
  implants, 134, 134f–137f
  indications, 138
  osteonecrosis of the talus, 275–276, 275t,
    276f
  rationale, 134–138
  revision, 142–144, 143f, 449
    component failure, 452–457
    malalignment, management of, 450–452
    risk factors, 449
  salvage of failed, 126, 127f–128f
  surgical approaches, alternative, 139–140
    concomitant procedures, 139–140
    patient-specific instrumentation, 140
  surgical treatment, 138–139
Total contact casting, diabetic foot ulcer, 71
Transfer metatarsalgia, 211
  surgical treatment of, 217–218
Transtibial amputation, 74, 356
Transverse tarsal joint, 4, 8, 152
Transverse tibiofibular ligament, 5
Trauma, 31, 94
  arthrodesis, for midfoot arthritis and,
    159–161, 161f
  cavovarus deformity, 52
  subacute, 159–161
  superficial peroneal nerve, 96
  sural nerve in, 97
Trendelenburg gait, 11
Tripod concept, 7
Truss model, of medial longitudinal arch, 9, 9f
Tumors

benign osseous, 256–260
benign soft-tissue, 252–255
biopsy of, 251–252
history of, 250
imaging of, 250–251
incidence of, 250
isolated limb infusion and, 263
laboratory evaluation of, 251
malignant osseous, 260–261
malignant soft-tissue, 255–256
nononcologically excised malignant, 263
patient evaluation of, 250–252
physical examination of, 250
reconstructive treatments for, 261–263
Turf toe injuries, 344–345, 344t

U

Ultrasonography, 25–26
  Achilles tendon ruptures, 364
  adult-acquired flatfoot deformity, 173
  chronic lateral ankle ligament instability,
    390
  diabetic foot disease, 70
  hindfoot arthritis, 155
  interdigital plantar neuralgia, 87
  metatarsalgia, 213
  midfoot arthritis, 155
  nondiabetic foot infections, 226
  peroneal tendons, 412
  tarsal tunnel syndrome, 91
  tumors, 251
  vascular anomalies, 253
Unicameral bone cyst, 259, 259f

V

Valgus deformity, 140
Valgus malpositioning, revision total ankle
    arthroplasty, 451
  axial rotation, 452
  deltoid incompetence, 451
  fixed forefoot varus, 451
  flatfoot issues, 451–452
  procurvatum, 452
  recurvatum, 452
  syndesmosis insufficiency, 451
Valgus talar tilting, 6
Vantage Total Ankle System, 134, 137f
Varus malpositioning, revision total ankle
    arthroplasty, 450, 450t
Vascular anomalies, 253
Vascular disease
  amputation and, 74
  diabetic foot disease and, 69
  posterior ankle arthroscopy, 409
Vascularized autograft, 262
Vitamin C, complex regional pain syndrome,
    101

W

Waddling gait, 11
Weber C fractures, 111